Volume 1

Organic Pharmaceutical and Medicinal Chemistry

Fundamental and Aliphatic Compounds

4th Edition

Volume 1

Organic Pharmaceutical and Medicinal Chemistry
Fundamental and Aliphatic Compounds
4th Edition

J.S. QADRY

M.Pharm. (Pb.), D.Sc. (Germany)
MSEI, FGAF (Germany), MASP (USA)

Founder Dean & Director, Sheikhawati College of Pharmacy, Dundlod, Rajasthan
Ex-Dean, Dubai Pharmacy College, Dubai, UAE
Formerly Founder Principal, Hamdard College of Pharmacy, University of Delhi
Founder Dean and Vice Chancellor, Hamdard University, New Delhi
Former President, Pharmacy Council of India
and Chairman, Board of Pharmaceutical Education and Research, A.I.C.T.E.
Special Advisor, Ministry of Public Health, Kuwait

S.S. QADRY

B.Sc. Chem. Engg. (Punjab Univ., Chandigarh)
M.Sc. Chem. Engg. (NJIT, New Jersey, USA)
Ph.D. (Univ. of Medicine and Dentistry, New Jersey, USA)

Associate Principal Scientist, Hoffmann-La Roche, N.J., USA

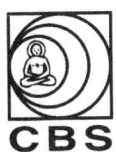

CBS

CBS Publishers & Distributors Pvt. Ltd.

New Delhi • Bengaluru • Chennai • Kochi • Kolkata • Mumbai
Hyderabad • Nagpur • Patna • Pune • Vijayawada

ISBN: 978-81-239-1918-8

Fourth Edition: 2012
Reprint: 2018, 2019

Published by **Satish Kumar Jain** and produced by **Varun Jain** for
CBS Publishers & Distributors Pvt. Ltd.,
4819/XI Prahlad Street, 24 Ansari Road, Daryaganj, New Delhi - 110002
delhi@cbspd.com, cbspubs@airtelmail.in • www.cbspd.com
Ph.: 23289259, 23266861, 23266867 • Fax: 011-23243014

Corporate Office: 204 FIE, Industrial Area, Patparganj, Delhi - 110 092
Ph: 49344934 • Fax: 011-49344935
E-mail: publishing@cbspd.com • publicity@cbspd.com

Branches:
• *Bengaluru:* 2975, 17th Cross, K.R. Road, Bansankari 2nd Stage,
  Bengaluru - 70 • Ph: +91-80-26771678/79 • Fax: +91-80-26771680
  E-mail: cbsbng@gmail.com, bangalore@cbspd.com
• *Chennai:* No. 7, Subbaraya Street, Shenoy Nagar, Chennai - 600030
  Ph: +91-44-26681266, 26680620 • Fax: +91-44-42032115
  E-mail: chennai@cbspd.com
• *Kochi:* Ashana House, 39/1904, A.M. Thomas Road, Valanjambalam,
  Ernakulum, Kochi • Ph: +91-484-4059061-65
  Fax: +91-484-4059065 • E-mail: cochin@cbspd.com
• *Kolkata:* 6-B, Ground Floor, Rameshwar Shaw Road, Kolkata - 700014
  Ph: +91-33-22891126/7/8 • E-mail: kolkata@cbspd.com
• *Mumbai:* 83-C, Dr. E. Moses Road, Worli, Mumbai - 400018
  Ph: +91-9833017933, 022-24902340/41 • E-mail: mumbai@cbspd.com

Representatives:

• Hyderabad: 0-9885175004   • Nagpur: 0-9021734563
• Patna: 0-9334159340   • Pune: 0-9623451994
• Jharkhand: 0-9811541605   • Uttarakhand: 0-9716462459

Printed at:
India Binding House, Noida, UP (India)

Preface to the Fourth Edition

Organic Pharmaceutical and Medicinal Chemistry, Vols. I, II and III have primarily been designed and written as per the courses streamlined in the Education Regulation of the Pharmacy Council of India to cater to the needs of undergraduate students of Diploma and Degree courses. The PCI has, however, now added a new dimension to the overall Pharmacy Education in India by introducing a new degree course, namely the Pharm. D. course – a course which incidentally for 15 years or so is now one and the only full-fledged degree course in all the universities in the USA. Without going into controversies raging about the rationale by calling it – Pharm. D. – a postgraduate course similar/equal to Ph.D., the fact remains that it is the first degree course, enabling the qualifiers of the same to become the regular registered pharmacist as before. My opinion with regard to the institution of Pharm. D. courses was published in The Pharma Review, December 7, Vol. 6, No. 31, under the title "Pharm. D. – A New Species in Certification of Pharmacy Degree in South Asia – At Best a Wishful Venture".

Pharma. D. course is undoubtedly a highly esteemed course which raises the status and value of pharmacists in the country of its origin. Pharm. D. graduates practice in a variety of health settings, including the community, medical institutions, healthcare facilities, hospital pharmacy and deliver pharmaceutical care services. They have in-depth clinical experiences and possess drug therapy skills as patient consultants. With the knowledge of all the aspects of drug therapy they counsel healthcare professional and patients – whom they get treated hand-in-hand with other medical personnel. We, in India, can now rightly hope to get our status elevated in the medical community after the introduction of the prestigious Pharm. D. degree in our country.

It was this changed scenario that demanded that I not only make an extensive revision of each volume, but also add new material to it in order to bring it in line with the professional requirements of the PCI after the introduction of the Pharm. D. course. This, I did, quite painstaking though it was. In doing it I had the added advantage of being personally aware of the changes introduced in the USA ever since 1991, the time when the debate for introducing Pharm. D. there was at its peak. We now hear that authorities there are thinking of increasing the Pharm. D. course to seven or eight years' duration. This is due to the fact that they want to have parity with the doctors who graduate in 10 years duration. This parity will be achieved by Pharm. D. holders by having residency course of one (general pharmacy) or two (specialty) years – one year basic residency (pharmacy practice) and two years (specialized residency in fields like infectious disease specialization, etc.). How India copes with or copies the model to achieve parity with them remains to be seen.

Irrespective of the fact what the subject is strategic consideration for introducing relevant changes in the teaching material had to be taken into account in view of the PCI's ER for Pharm. D. It was with this consideration of consistency that I decided to attempt to reform the contents of the volumes, especially those of Vols. II and III, reflecting the requirements of Pharm. D. courses as well. These changes have not been dimensionally as enormous and challenging in general pharmaceutical chemistry's branches as they are in subjects like medicinal chemistry, drug design, pharmacology-toxicology, pharmacokinetics, biochemistry, biotechnology, microbiology, pharmacy practice, patient-oriented clinical pharmacology and its application, biostatistics – statistical analysis of clinical trials, clinical intervention, pre- and post-implementation assessment, laboratory value, monitoring, literature evaluation, project, etc.

As said above, Vols. I, II and III of the book have been revised and enlarged by keeping in mind the changes that are required to be made in view of the changed circumstances, as mentioned above. Thus effort has been made by not giving more routes of synthesis, going into the depth of identification tests, emphasis on repetition of testing of usual impurities, detailed methods of analysis (assays) etc., but in diligently providing compounds' essential basic physiology, pharmacology, mechanism of action, structure activity relationship, biotransformation, substitutes, chemical nomenclature including brand names of market products.

In the new editions new chapters and a large number of new pharmaceutical and medicinal compounds have been added in Volumes II and III. I restrained myself from making any change in the rather descriptive and presentation-oriented style of the books. This I did after getting the feedback from my former students, now members of quite senior and highly placed teaching fraternity. I feel well contended to be led to the realization that the entire subject matter of Organic Pharmaceutical and Medicinal Chemistry, compressed as it is, into the three handy volumes has been welcomed and well received by all. In fact, mine is the only work on this subject which is presented (cf. preface to the first edition) in well-defined parts in three volumes. This also, in a way, makes the work unique globally. It helps in continual use of the volumes in the teaching schemes that are followed in semesters or yearly scheme classes. The readers are, however, the best judge of the usefulness or otherwise of the book.

As regards the present book, Volume I, it has been thoroughly revised in both its sections. Not only new chapters have been added, but also the old chapters have been improved and strengthened with the new additional compounds and preparations. Besides, special chapter of appendices has also been added. Each appendix carries an explanatory introductory note followed by the method of each determination.

I am sincerely thankful to Mr. S.K. Jain, the Chairman and Managing Director, and Mr. Vinod K. Jain, Production Director, of CBS Publishers & Distributors Pvt. Ltd. for their kind help and interest in the publication of this book.

I wish to express my sincere gratitude to my wife who has been encouraging me during all these years of monumental publication work of my books.

Dubai (U.A.E.)   **J.S. Qadry**
2012

Preface to the First Edition

The present book on Organic Pharmaceutical and Medicinal Chemistry is being published in three volumes. The topics dealt within volumes I to III are Fundamentals and Aliphatic Compounds, Aromatic Compounds and Natural Products, and Medicinal Chemistry respectively. The book is intended to meet the needs of the students of Diploma and Degree courses of Pharmacy in the Indian Universities.

The book contains a detailed account of chemistry of organic, pharmaceutical and medicinal compounds including the general methods of their preparation, their physical and chemical properties, and their well-established named reactions and uses. This is followed by a description of the standards and other related information on drugs and other therapeutic agents official in the Indian Pharmacopoeia.

The overall philosophy of the book is to produce a consolidated base for the study of various aspects of organic, pharmaceutical and medicinal chemistry. A considerable amount of material pertaining to the above mentioned branches of chemistry has been included in the book with a view of providing the students with a material that should last for all the years of their study in pharmacy from day one till they successfully complete the course.

It has been a long cherished desire of mine to pack in the consolidated volume all the afore-mentioned three branches of Chemistry with a solid pharmaceutical basis for the benefit of the students. But the enormity of the volume as well as the advice of many well-wishers, contributors and publishers forced me to divide the material first into two and later on into three separate volumes.

I had jointly started the work on the book soon after the publication of my earlier book on Inorganic Pharmaceutical and Medicinal Chemistry, but almost all the other members of the team originally forming the nucleus, including stalwarts like Mr. S. Sridharan, Late Dr. Ishwar Kumar and Dr. Fr. James Walker, left the Hamdard College of Pharmacy, New Delhi, which brought the project to an untimely halt. Then, as if from the blue, computer virus played havoc twice of which the worst sufferer was the publisher.

This much about the genesis and history of the book. Anyway the book is now in your hands and you are the best judge of its value and worth.

I am really thankful to the publisher for bearing with me the loss of both men and material. The good part was that he did not lose heart, nor did we.

We sincerely hope that the book will be of benefit to the students and teachers alike. Any suggestions for the improvement of the material will be appreciated.

It is a self-evident fact that no book of this size and dimension as this can be completed without the help and support of many well-wishers, friends and individuals. Hence, my sincere thanks and gratitude to all of those who helped me in various ways during the completion of this work.

I also wish to acknowledge my deepest gratitude to my contributing colleagues some of whom are not named here. However, to the following I wish to thank for their major contributions: Prof. Dr. Iqbal Ahmad, M.Sc., Ph.D. (London), Head, Department of Pharmaceutical Chemistry, Dubai Pharmacy College, Dubai; Dr. Mrs. Asha Budhiraja, Ph.D. (Bom.), Ex-Scientist, Bhabha Atomic Research Institute, Mumbai (now living in UAE); Mr. S. Zafar Qadry, M. Pharm. (Delhi), Associate Product Manager, Gulf Region, Abbotts Laboratories, Dubai; and Dr. S.S. Qadry, B.Sc. Chem. Engg. (Punjab), M.Sc. Chem. Engg. (NJIT, New Jersey, USA), Ph.D. (University of Medicine and Dentistry, New Jersey, USA), Associate Principal Scientist, Hoffmann-La Roche, USA.

I will be failing in my duty if I do not pay my special thanks to Al-Haj Saeed Bin Ahmad Al Lootah, who as the Chairman of the Governing Bodies of Dubai Pharmacy College and the Dubai Medical College has been a guiding spirit behind so many research programs and projects in this part of the world.

On a purely personal note I wish to pay my gratitude to my wife Sughra, who never grudged my long absences from her, as well as to my daughter Yasmin, who also never complained of my occasional negligencies of her during the completion of this book. Surely, they are fully aware of my deep appreciation of them for their cooperation and help.

Last but not the least I wish to record my deepest thanks to my thirty five years old friend, Mr. Sudhirbhai Shah of M/s B.S. Shah Publishers for his patience in publishing these volumes.

Dubai
2005

J.S. Qadry

Contents

Introduction

The term organic refers to plants or animal organisms, whose tissues and contents (besides of course the inorganic ones) are made up of molecules, all containing "Carbon", which like other elements of the periodic table is an element, but which has the special quality to combine and link together in chains and rings. Since the chemistry of carbon compared to other elements is very elaborate and most extensive, the organic chemistry is said to be the chemistry of carbon compounds. The organic substances are essentially the compounds of carbon with elements like hydrogen, oxygen, nitrogen and sulphur. These carbon compounds outnumber all the other existing compounds which are formed by over a hundred other existing elements. The total number of organic compounds now known is said to be over 20,00,000 and this figure is ever increasing as about 30,000 new organic compounds are added yearly. Hence, it is quite understandably impossible to include the study of such a vast subject in one chapter/book or as a part along with the inorganic chemistry. Besides, organic compounds (carbon compounds) distinguish themselves from their counterpart inorganic compounds in the following ways:

1. As stated above, organic compounds are available in large number, i.e., it is only carbon element alone, whose compounds outnumber all those compounds which are formed by rest of the elements of the periodic table.

2. Organic compounds show similar characters, i.e., they are closely related with each other as compared to the inorganic compounds which do now show similar characters and close relationship.

3. Organic compounds are complex molecules, i.e., they have very high molecular weights (e.g., the molecular weight of protein is 50,000 onwards), while the inorganic compounds have low molecular weights.

4. Organic compounds have non-ionic character, i.e., they do not ionize like the inorganic compounds and participate in ionic reactions.

5. Organic compounds exhibit isomerism, i.e., the molecular weight of an organic compound does not give any information regarding the structures. It is displayed as under:

   A. C_2H_6O has two structures to display as under:

$$C_2H_5OH \longleftarrow C_2H_6O \longrightarrow CH_3.O.CH_3$$

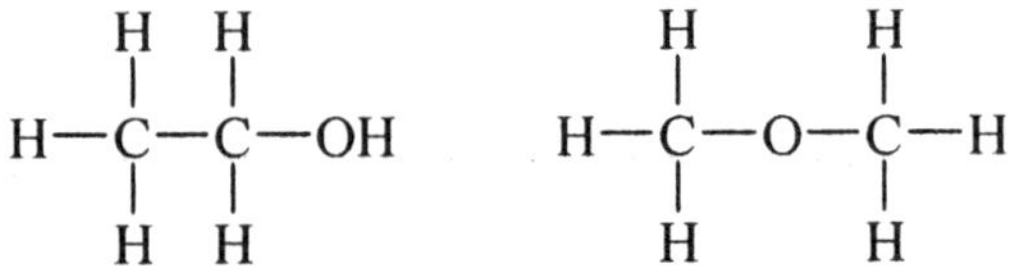

Ethyl alcohol   Dimethyl ether

B. $C_4H_{10}O$ shows seven structures, four alcohols and three ethers, as follows:

Chemical structures	*Name of compounds*
(i) $CH_3.CH_2.CH_2.CH_2OH$	*n*-Butyl alcohol

(ii)
iso-Butyl alcohol

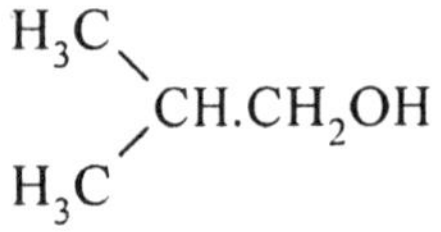

(iii)
sec-Butyl alcohol

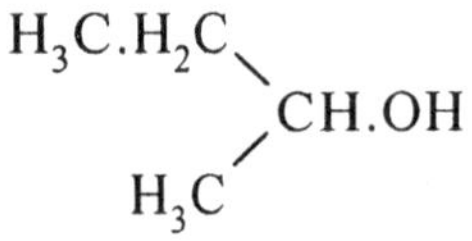

(iv)
tert-Butyl alcohol

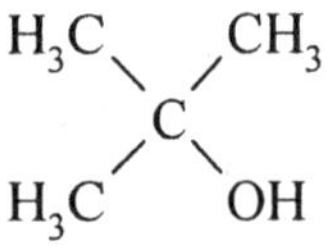

(v) $C_2H_5.O.C_2H_5$ Diethyl ether

(vi) $CH_3.O.CH_2.CH_2.CH_3$ Methyl propyl ether

(vii)
Methyl isopropyl ether

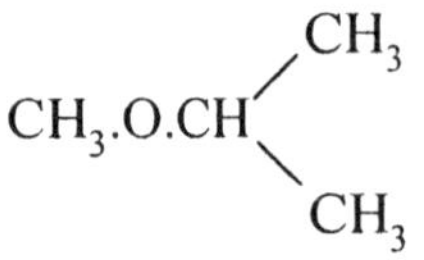

The word isomerism can be divided into two parts, namely **iso**, meaning similar and **merism** meaning structure. Isomerism thus refers to compounds which have two or more different structures but have the same molecular formula. The compounds which show isomerism are called isomers or isomerides. These different compounds, i.e., isomers have different physical and chemical properties (more details about isomerism will follow in the next chapters).

6. Most of the organic compounds are homologous and have homologous series. Due to the homologous series the study of the organic compounds becomes easier, as the members of each homologous series have similar properties. The members of homologous series can be conveniently represented by one general formula and prepared by a general method of preparation. Each member of homologous series, which may be quoted here is that of alkanes with general formula, C_2H_{2n+2} is given below.
   If $n = 1, 2, 3$ and so on, the series is as follows:

CH_4	Methane	C_2H_6	Ethane
C_3H_8	Propane	C_4H_{10}	Butane
C_5H_{12}	Pentane	C_6H_{14}	Hexane
C_7H_{16}	Heptane	C_8H_{18}	Octane

This phenomenon, like that of phenomenon of isomerism, is absent in inorganic compounds.

7. Solubility of organic compounds is peculiar and different. Important organic solvents are alcohol, ether, benzene, etc. while most of the inorganic compounds are insoluble in these organic solvents.
8. Chemical structure of organic componds is well defined and well known, while the structure of a large number of inorganic compounds is not established.

CLASSIFICATION OF ORGANIC COMPOUNDS

The existing organic compounds can be divided into two major classes as follows:

1. Acyclic or open ring (chain) compounds.
2. Cyclic or ring compounds.

To the first group of acyclic compounds belong all those organic compounds which possess an open chain of carbon atoms in their molecules. These open chain compounds or aliphatic compounds have a straight or branched chain of carbon atoms and are referred to as straight chain or branched chain aliphatic compounds, e.g.:

$$H_3C—CH_2—CH_3 \qquad \text{Propane}$$

$$H_2C=CH—CH_2I \qquad \text{Allyl iodide}$$

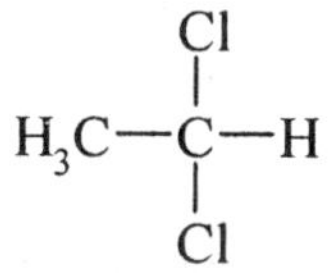

$$\underset{\underset{\displaystyle Cl}{|}}{\overset{\overset{\displaystyle Cl}{|}}{H_3C—C—H}} \qquad \text{1,1-Dichloroethane}$$

To the second group of cyclic compounds belong those compounds which have a ring of atoms. These compounds may contain one, two, three or many rings and are accordingly referred to as monocyclic, bicyclic, tricyclic and polycyclic. They are subdivided into:

(A) Homocyclic or carbocyclic and (B) Heterocyclic depending upon the ring which may have carbon atoms only, e.g., benzene, or may have other atoms, such as N, O or S, as in pyridine, furan and thiophene:

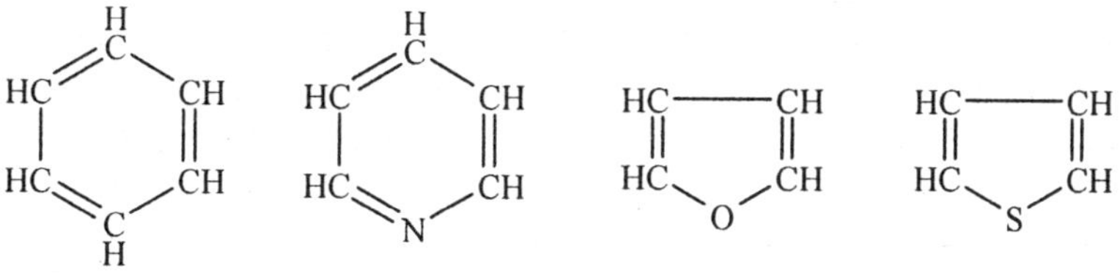

Benzene   Pyridine   Furan   Thiophene

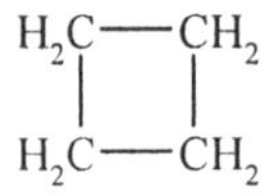

Cyclobutane 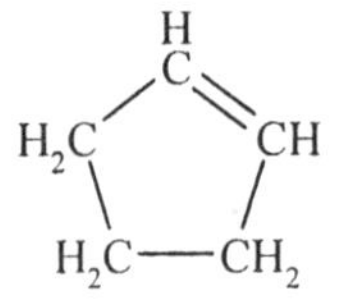   Cyclopentene 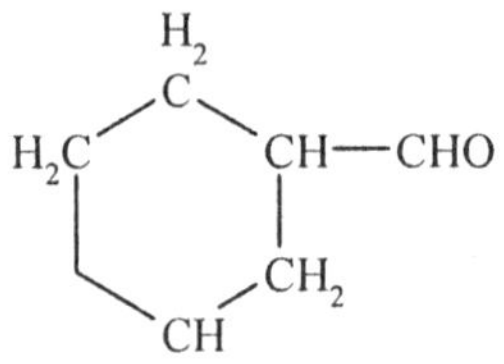   Tetrahydrobenzaldehyde

The homocyclic compounds are further subdivided into (a) Alicyclic compounds, which possess single C to C bonds in the ring. They may be saturated having different functional groups and behave more or less like aliphatic compounds; (b) Aromatic compounds, which possess alternative double and single bonds. These compounds are planar, do not show addition reactions and undergo substitution reactions despite the unsaturation in the molecule. The aromatic compounds are further subdivided into (i) benzoid aromatics which have benzene ring consisting of six carbon atoms with alternate single and double bonds, e.g., toluene, napthalene, phenol etc. and (ii) non-benzoid aromatics which contain different structural units other than benzenoid types e.g., azulene and tropolone.

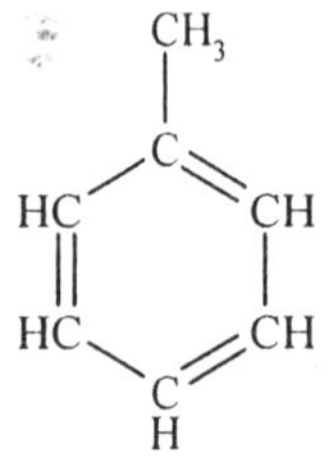

Toluene 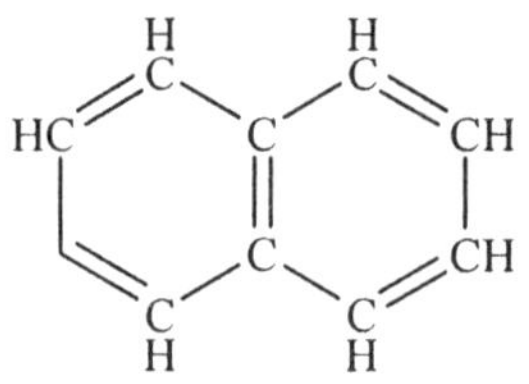   Naphthalene 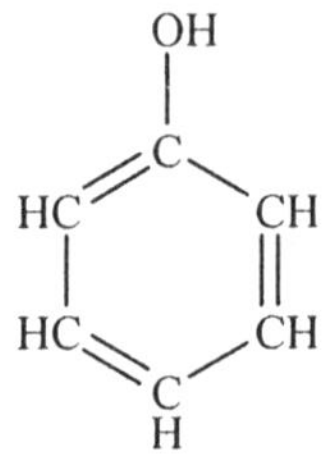   Phenol

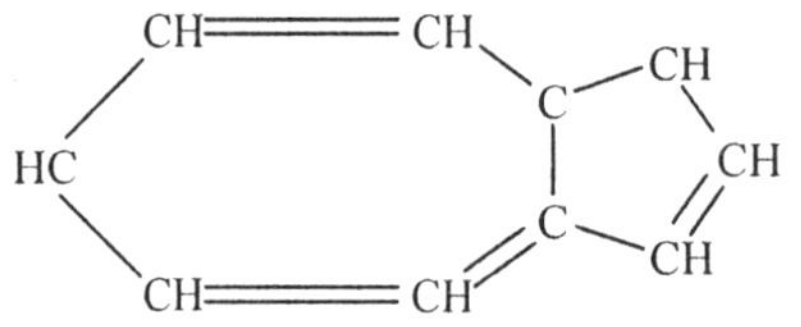

Azulene 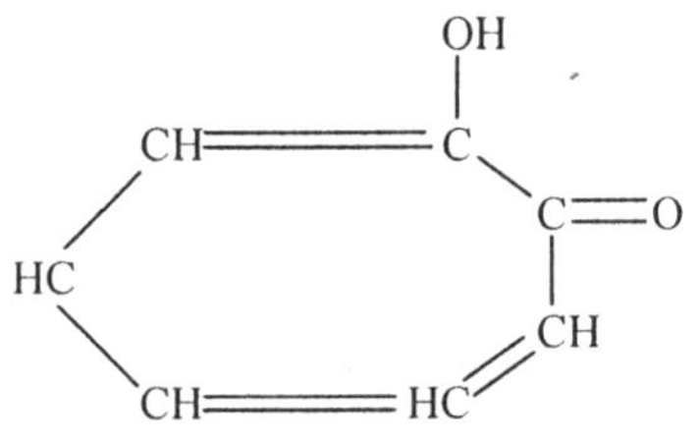   Tropolone

NOMENCLATURE AND ORGANIC FORMULA

Nomenclature

Naming of a person, place and thing is the first, foremost and most important activity of this universe. But naming of millions of chemical compounds involves special studies by chemists. This naming of chemical compounds or giving them scientific terms is referred to as nomenclature of organic compounds. In assigning an exact name to an inorganic substance, it is sufficient, as a rule, to indicate the composition of its molecule. With organic compounds, however, because of the common phenomenon of isomerism this does not hold good, as a complete and correct name of an organic compound must clearly reflect its structural formula. The nomenclature of organic compounds must make it possible to indicate clearly their structural formulae, i.e., it should enable chemists to construct the structural formulae by knowing their exact names. A structural formula can be described in words in different ways and there are different systems of organic nomenclature. An organic compound may, therefore, have several different names attached to it. The prevalent different systems of nomenclature and a number of names attributed to an organic compound makes the task of organic chemists more difficult. A detailed account of nomenclature is given separately.

Organic Formula

An organic compound, after it is isolated or synthesised, is required to be named. This is possible after its formula is known and in order to know its formula one has to first detect and know the elements followed by the determination of their proportions. Most of the organic compounds, whether synthetics or from natural sources, contain usually the elements carbon, hydrogen, oxygen and nitrogen. Besides these elements other elements that are met within the composition of organic compounds may be halogens, sulphur, phosphorus, iron, calcium, arsenic, sodium, potassium, etc. (For details see the relevant chapter.)

Purity of Organic Compounds

An organic compound whether isolated from a natural source or obtained through synthetic means is always impure, but it is required to be obtained in pure form before it is subjected to further testings. Thus molecular formula and other constituents of a compound cannot be determined, unless it is obtained in pure form. For purifying a compound all the conventional methods are used. If a substance is a solid, its melting point and mixed melting point are taken and if a substance is a liquid, its boiling point and refractive index can be determined. (For details refer to relevant chapter.) A larger proportion of organic compounds are liquids or low melting solids and they can be distilled for purification. Also many of them are not soluble in water and other highly polar solvents, but are freely soluble in non-polar organic liquids (solvents). They can thus be purified by following one of the techniques for purification, given in the next chapter.

Purification of Organic Compounds

An organic compound irrespective of its origin – whether obtained from a natural source or through synthetic reactions – is always accompanied by some substances which are referred to as impurities. These impurities may have been produced in the side reactions or may be present as such in the natural source. For chemical investigation and characterization of the organic compounds, however, it is essential that the substance must be in pure state. Though the principles and methods of purification of organic compounds are more laborious and tedious, more than one procedures are used for obtaining organic chemicals, medicines and unity compounds in pure form. Following are the methods used to purify the compounds.

Purification of Solid Organic Compounds

Extraction

(i) The extraction is the first step to purify an organic compound. If the impurities present are solid then a solvent is so chosen that it would either dissolve the compound or the impurities. The solution can be separated from solid particles by use of ordinary filtration, centrifuge or Buchner funnel using a filter pump (Fig. 2.1). The solution collected in the filtration flask is purified and evaporated to dryness if it contains organic compound.

(ii) **Use of water immiscible solvent:** If the organic compound to be extracted is soluble in water and the impurities are soluble in

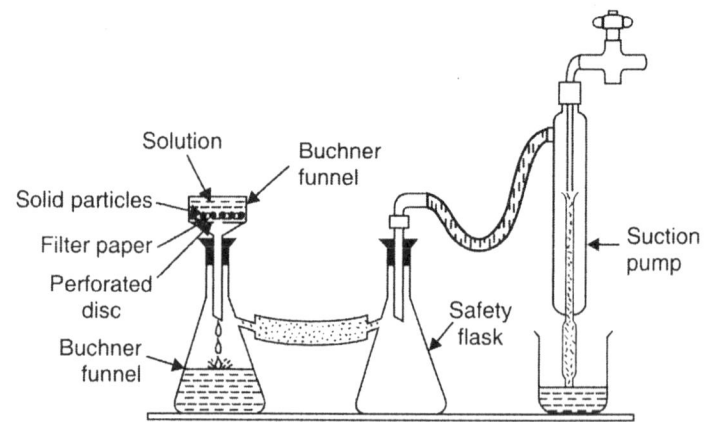

Fig. 2.1. Filter pump and Buchner funnel.

organic solvent immiscible with water, then the compound is extracted using such water immiscible solvents.

The compound dissolved in water is shaken with the solvent in a separating funnel. On standing, the mixture separates into two layers in the funnel (Fig. 2.2).

The aqueous and solvent layers are collected in two different receivers. The water layer is put again and shaken with the solvent till the colour of the solvent remains unchanged. The solvent is evaporated to get the pure organic compound. Generally diethyl ether and benzene are used as solvents for such extractions.

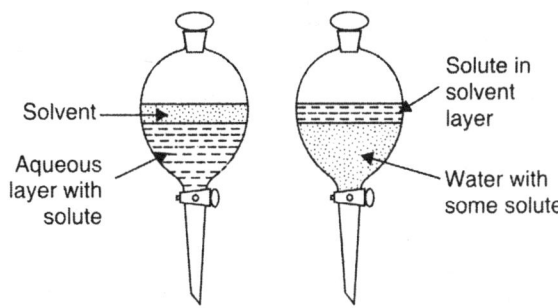

Fig. 2.2. Extraction by immiscible solvents using separating funnel.

(iii) **Soxhlet extraction:** This method is employed for the extraction of alkaloids, essential oils of flowers and leaves, vegetable colouring matter of leaves and other compounds from drugs. The crude material filled in a thimble-shaped filter paper is placed in a glass cylinder. The apparatus contains a side tube on the left, a siphon tube on the right and a water condenser on the top. The lower side of the apparatus is fitted to the flask containing a suitable solvent (Fig. 2.3).

When the flask is heated on a steam bath, the solvent vapours reach the cylinder through the side tube and condense on passing into the condenser. The condensed solvent falls on the crude drug or organic material and dissolves the desired substance/s. The solution is filtered through the filter paper and passed out back into the flask through the siphon tube. In this way, there is a continuous supply of solvent to the apparatus. The organic com-pound dissolved flows again to the flask. At the end, when the colour of the solvent is unchanged, the apparatus is disconnected, the solution of the flask is distilled off to get the solvent. The organic compound remains in the flask as a residue or a small amount.

This procedure is generally employed when the solvent is costly or a small amount of solvent is available.

Crystallization

Solid organic compounds are purified by crystallization which may be simple or fractional,

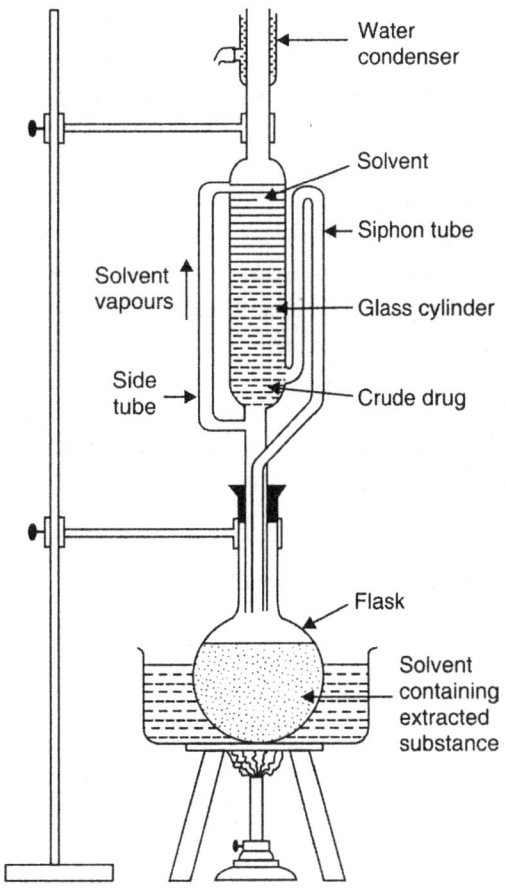

Fig. 2.3. Soxhlet apparatus.

(i) **Simple crystallization:** A solvent is used in this process which dissolves less compound at room temperature and more at higher temperature. A hot saturated solution of the organic compound is prepared and filtered with the help of a hot water funnel (Fig. 2.4). On cooling the filtrate, the compound is crystallized out. This is filtered, dried and recrystallized for further purification.

(ii) **Fractional crystallization:** If the impure compound is a mixture of two substances, both being soluble in the same solvent, the less soluble compound will be crystallized first from a saturated solution containing some quantity of other compound. This is further crystallized and recrystallized to get the pure substance.

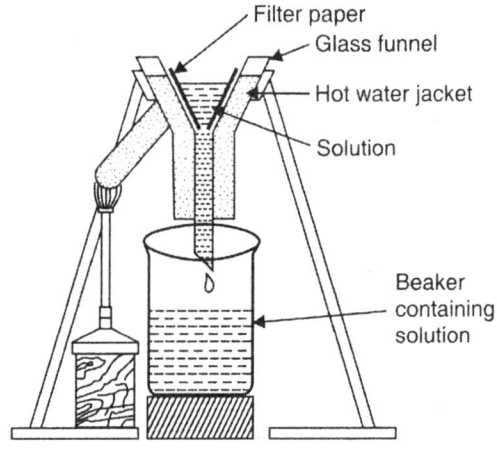

Fig. 2.4. Hot water funnel.

(iii) **Use of miscible solvents:** If a compound is very soluble in solvent A and less soluble in solvent B, A and B being immiscible, then a mixture of these two solvents is used for purification.

(iv) **Crystallization by spontaneous evaporation:** When no suitable solvent is available and the impure product is soluble in cold as well as hot solvent, then a concentrated solution is prepared and allowed to evaporate. During the course of evaporation, the solution becomes more and more concen-trated and finally results in the separation of crystals.

(v) **Sublimation:** Organic compounds such as naphthalene, anthracene, benzoic acid, camphor and indigo are heated in a dish covered by an inverted funnel containing wet cotton around the stem. The compound passes into vapour state without melting and returns to solid form on cooling. This process is called sublimation in which crystals are obtained directly from solid by heating and then cooling when other impurities do not sublime (Fig. 2.5).

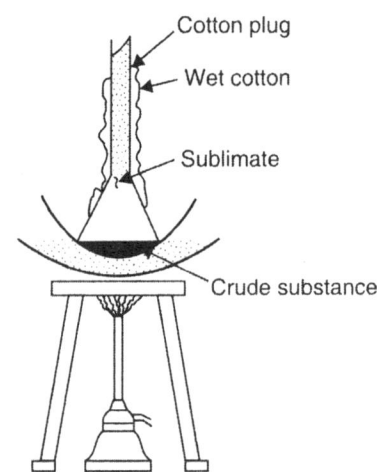

Fig. 2.5. Sublimation.

Purification of Liquids

Following methods are used for purification of liquids:

(i) The temperature at which a liquid boils is called its boiling point which is constant for every liquid under a given pressure. If the liquid has non-volatile impurities and boils without decomposition, it can be purified by distillation leaving behind the impurities. The liquid containing impurities is boiled off in flask fitted with a thermometer. The vapours when passed through a condenser are condensed and the pure liquid is collected at the given temperature in the receiver (Fig. 2.6).

(ii) **Fractional distillation:** This method is employed when the liquid to be puri-fied has another liquid as an impurity having diffe-rent b.p. The mixture of two liquids is heated in a distillation flask, the low boiling constituent distils first along with some other liquid and is collected separately. The fractions are further purified by repeating the distillation.

When the boiling points of liquids are very near to one another, a fractionating column is used to separate them. It is a long tube containing obstructions to the passage of the vapours upwards and that of liquid downwards as shown in Fig. 2.7. The column is fitted in a distillation flask. A condenser and a thermometer are fitted at the top. When the flask is heated, the liquid vapourizes and the vapours rise into the fractionating column

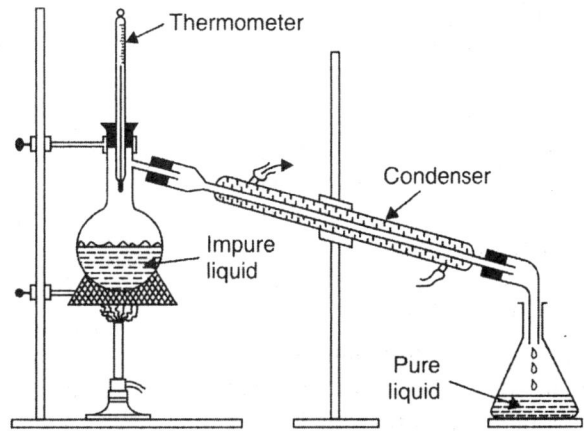

Fig. 2.6. Distillation.

when some of them condense in it and come down (Fig. 2.8).

By this process more than two liquids can be separated. In the industry specially modified fractionating columns are used.

(iii) **Distillation under reduced pressure:** Some compounds like glycerine decompose at their boiling points. Therefore, they cannot be purified by distillation under ordinary atmospheric pressure. Boiling point of a liquid is the temperature at which the vapour pressure of the liquid is equal to the atmospheric pressure. Hence, if

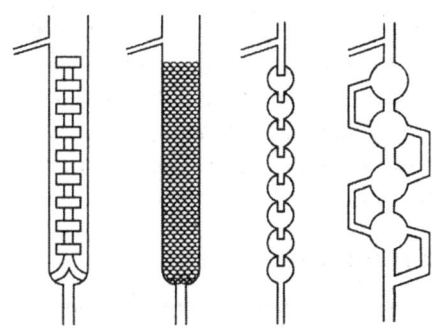

Fig. 2.7. Fractionating columns.

the pressure is reduced during boiling, the liquid will boil at lower temperature than its normal boiling point. This principle is employed in the dis-tillation under reduced pressure.

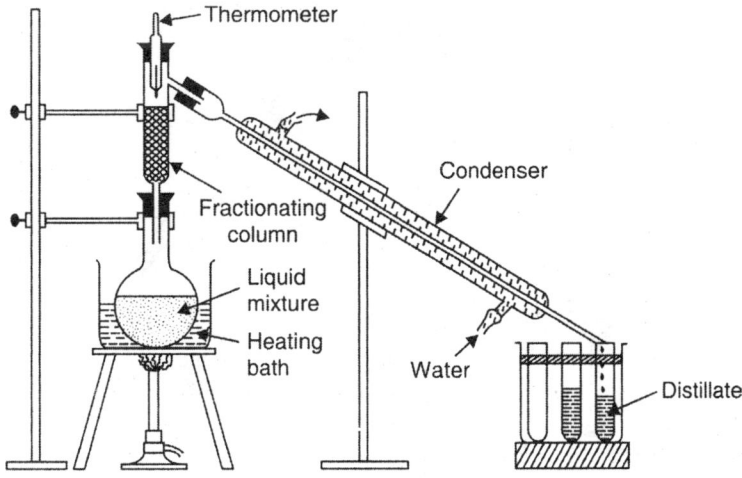

Fig. 2.8. Fractional distillation.

The organic substance, which decomposes at its boiling point, is distilled off undecomposed under reduced pressure. The vacuum is created by a pump attached to the receiver, pressure lowered is indicated by a manometer and the distillation is carried out as usual as indicated in Fig. 2.9.

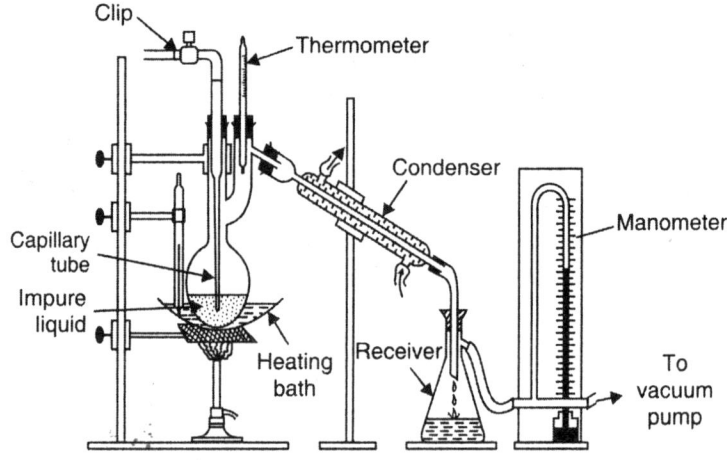

Fig. 2.9. Distillation under reduced pressure.

(iv) **Steam distillation:** This method is used in case of water insoluble mixtures which have non-volatile impurities, have a high molecular weight and possess a fairly high vapour pressure at about the boiling point of water.

Steam is passed through the impure liquid in a flask heated on a sand bath (Fig. 2.10). Vigorous boiling takes place and the vapours of the organic substance mixed with steam rise up and condense when they pass through the condenser. Thus the condensed product is a mixture of the organic substance and water. The organic compound, if immiscible with water, is separated in a separating funnel. In case the compound is partially miscible with water, it is extracted with a suitable solvent.

Salting Out Method

Many water-soluble organic compounds such as ethanol, acetone, aniline, pyridine etc. are either insoluble or sparingly soluble in solutions of salts. When solid salts like common salt, calcium chloride and sodium sulphate are added to the mixture, the organic compound is thrown out of the solution which can be separated with the help of a separating funnel or is extracted with ether.

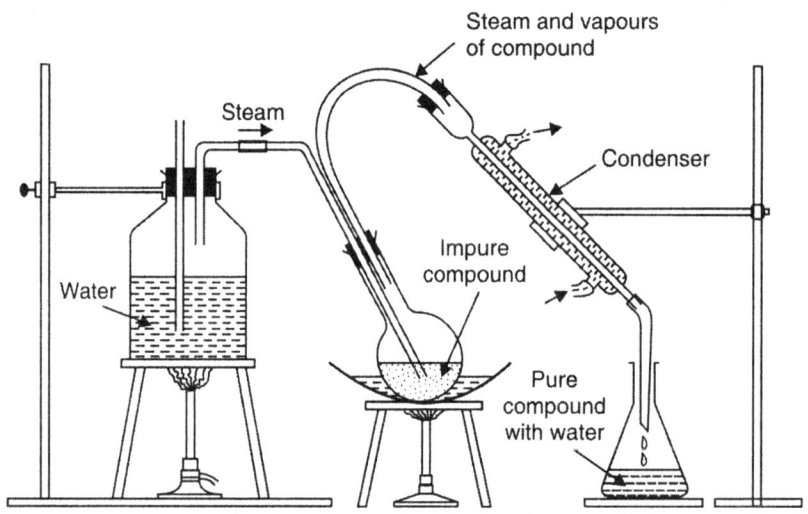

Fig. 2.10. Steam distillation.

Counter Currency Distribution

The closely related solutes are separated with the help of this automatic procedure which is based upon their slightly different partition coefficients in two immiscible liquid solvents. Experimentally a heavier solvent is placed in about 100 identical test tubes. The sample dissolved in the lighter solvent is added to test tube 1. It is shaken, allowed to settle, the upper solvent is transferred to test tube 2 and a new portion of lighter solvent is added to test tube 1. The process is repeated with test tubes 2, 3, 4 and so on. In every test tube partition of the two solutes takes place. The component soluble more in heavier solvent will pass into the lower layer and the component soluble more in lighter solvent will be retained in the upper layer.

Decolourization

Sometimes an organic compound is decolourized for purification. Animal charcoal is shaken with the liquid or the solution of the solid to be purified and boiled with it for some time. Animal charchal absorbs colour to make the compound colourless. Later charcoal is removed by filtration.

Chemical Methods of Purification

Chemical methods of purification are often used in cases where one of the two components of a mixture reacts to form a compound with a reagent added and the other remains unreacted. For example, benzoic acid and anthracene mixture when treated with sodium bicarbonate solution reacts with it to form sodium benzoate; the anthracene remaining unreacted. Sodium benzoate solution can be filtered off leaving the anthracene as a residue. Benzoic acid may be obtained by treating the filtrate with dilute hydrochloric acid when the acid precipitates. It is filtered, washed and dried. Similarly, hydrochloric acid forms hydrochlorides with aniline and amines; calcium chloride forms crystalline compounds with methanol; and sodium bisulphite gives addition products in crystalline form with carbon compounds. These compounds are separated from mixtures with the help of these reagents and after that decomposition of the salts so obtained with a suitable reagent gives organic compounds in pure form.

Drying of Organic Compounds

During the course of purification traces of moisture remain with the organic compound. If this is not removed, it may interfere with results of microanalyses and affect the fundamental properties of the compound.

Organic liquids are dried by keeping them in contact with some dehydrating agent with which they do not react. Commonly used dehydrating agents are quick lime, calcium chloride, sodium sulphate, sodium hydroxide, magnesium sulphate, metallic sodium, etc. The liquid is kept in contract with the dehydrating agent overnight or for more time and then decanted off. It is then distilled in a dry apparatus.

More solids are dried first by pressing them gently between folds of filter paper and then heated in an air oven at a suitable temperature. If the substance decomposes on heating, it may be dried in a vacuum desiccator.

Melting points and mixed melting points of solid organic compounds, and the boiling points of liquids are the usual physical constants for determining their purities.

3

Chromatography

INTRODUCTION

Chromatography in general is an analytical method in which the components to be separated are distributed between two phases, one of which is stationary (the stationary phase) while the other is mobile (mobile phase), which moves in a definite direction.

The expression chromatography (from Greek χηρομα:*chroma*, colour and γραπηειν:*graphein,* to write) is the collective term for a set of laboratory techniques for the separation of mixtures. It involves passing a mixture dissolved in a "mobile phase" through a *stationary phase*, which separates the analytes (components) to be identified/measured from other molecules (components) in the mixture based on differential partitioning between the mobile and stationary phases. Subtle differences in a compound's partition coefficient result in differential retention on the stationary phase and thus **changing/effecting the separation.**

Historical background: In the last about 60 years the chromatography, which is essentially a physical method of separation, has become the most important method for the separation of mixtures of substances. It depends upon the fact that substances with regard to their adsorption (exchange of ions) behave differently in their distribution between different solutions and simple filtration effect. In other words the components to be separated are distributed between two phases, one of which is stationary (stationary phase) while the other (the mobile phase) moves in a definite direction.

The beginning of **chromatography** goes back to Mikhail S. Tswett, a Russian botanist, who in 1906, while filtering petroleum ether extract of the leaves for separating plant pigments through calcium carbonate ($CaCO_3$), confirmed that the colouring components of the extract travel through the column at a different speed.

TYPES OF CHROMATOGRAPHIC TECHNIQUES

COLUMN CHROMATOGRAPHY (CC)

In the 1930's, R. Kuhn separated the carotenes through an aluminum oxide column, and this led H.

Brockmann to standardize the adsorbent material, the aluminum oxide. With their observations and experiments the **column chromatography** came into existence on rational basis.

PAPER CHROMATOGRAPHY (PC)

In the 1940's, A. Martin, A. Gordon, R. Synge and R. Consdan introduced the **paper chromatography**. It resembled the long-known rational form of capillary analysis, which played an important role for the analysis of homoeopathic medicines (before the introduction of paper chromatography). The paper chromatography in between was largely pushed aside or replaced by other methods. It had the disadvantage that it was difficult to have the paper manufactured with similar/constant standardized qualities.

THIN LAYER CHROMATOGRAPHY (TLC)

It was in 1960's that the chromatography was tried using adsorption-material layers on thin plates as per the experiments undertaken by the legendary German Pharmacognosist, Egon Stahl, who named this chromatographic technique as **Thin Layer Chromatography (TLC).** TLC thus became the dominant method of chromatography. It most commonly uses Silica Gel as an adsorbent. The thin layer chromatography became very popular not because of its universal applicability as a simple and quick method, which also did not require elaborate apparatuses, but it was also due to its use for identification and purity tests in the pharmacopoeias. The TLC also developed well into an important preparative chromatographic technique for preparatory chemistry and to carry out control of processes at different sites of experimentation.

GAS CHROMATOGRAPHY (GC)

Almost simultaneously in the sixties of the last century i.e. around 1960 was introduced the Gas Chromatography (GC). This branch of chromatography utilizes well designed, though complex, apparatuses, which make it possible to separate a mixture of substances which are in a position to get completely evaporated. It also requires the mixture (of substances) to be separated in very small amounts. A separating column is used, in which is introduced a granular adsorbent impregnated with heavy volatile liquids. A storming carrier gas represents the mobile phase. The ejecting gas is led through a detector, which can be constructed keeping in mind a few principles (thermal conductivity, ionization, and electron capture capacity).

The substances with lower vapour pressure get first separated after derivatization in gas chromatograph. In clinical toxicology the combination of a gas chromatograph with a mass spectrometer (GC/MS) has achieved good success. It is now possible to evaluate and identify a number of poisons through GC in combination with computer in less than an hour. With this it is also possible to identify the sample of metabolites of substances used.

HIGH PERFORMANCE (PRESSURE) LIQUID CHROMATOGRAPHY (HPLC)

A new variety of column chromatography is the High Performance (Pressure) Liquid Chromatography (HPLC). This HPLC, as compared to the old technique of separations is carried out under pressure (up to 250 atm.) and, therefore, it is extremely quick and fast (rushes in few seconds to minutes). The important filling material of 10–50 cm long column made of metal (iron) or glass is the specially developed adsorbent (mostly silica gel) with the grain size of 5 and 50 μm, which does not have much role in influencing the speed of the mobile phase passing through the size of the surface of the column. The detectors now-a-days consisting of UV-photometer and differential diffractormeter have an important role to play. The HPLC is specially suited for most of the serial chemical reactions and to compounds including isomers. Upon the optically active adsorbents it is also possible to undertake separation of racemic and isomeric substances. As far as the separation performance is concerned, the HPLC is in no way behind GC. Besides, the HPLC does not need to have only the volatile substances.

The basic methods of chromatography have experienced a number of variations. Thus the electrically loaded particles under the influence of electric field make movements; and this method, taken also in pharmacopoeias, is called **Electrophoresis** and plays important role in the analysis of proteins bodies.

SIZE EXCLUSION CHROMATOGRAPHY (SEC)

The Size Exclusion Chromatography (SEC) is used to separate the molecules in solution according to their size, and to determine the molecular weights. It is also utilised for the determination of molecular size distribution of polymers.

The technique was invented in the fifties of the last century by Grant Henry Lathe and Colin R. Ruthven, working at Queen Charlotte's Hospital, London. They later were awarded the John Scott Award for this invention. Lathe and Ruthven used starch gels as the matrix, while Jerker Porath and Per Flodin in 1959 introduced dextran gels; other gels with size fractionation properties include agarose and polyacrylamide. They developed dextran gel, which on being swollen in an aqueous medium could separate proteins on the basis of their molecular weight. This gel, named as *Sephadex* was made available commercially and has been used extensively for biopolymer separation in low pressure gel filtration chromatography (GFC) systems using aqueous mobile phase.

CHROMATOGRAPHIC PROCEDURES IN PHARMACOPOEIAS

In the Pharmacopoeias are included Paper Chromatography; Thin Layer Chromatography; Gas Chromatography; Liquid Chromatography and Size-Exclusion Chromatography.

Paper Chromatography (PC): It is of two types, Ascending PC and Descending PC. The PC is utilized to examine the radiochemical purity of some radiopharmaceuticals and for the examination and identification of isolated radiopharmaceuticals. More detailed specifications are to be found in individual monographs.

Thin Layer Chromatography (TLC): It is the most used method of chromatography in the pharmacopoeias. In this the silica gel is activated for one hour at 100–105°C. The chromatographic chamber is layered with filter paper and is fed with the required amount of mobile phase (solvent system). One waits for about one hour till the chromatographic chamber is saturated with the vapours of the mobile phase. Details of further specifications are given and to be followed in individual monographs.

Gas Chromatography (GC): The characteristics of the columns and the conditions of the chromatography are given under individual monographs. It may be required to compare the retention time and the peak's height with a standard substance. The GC may be used, for example, for the examination of fatty oils, for the presence of unknown oils and their components.

Liquid Chromatography: The pharmacopoeias utilize the HPLC for the assays (determination of contents in weight) and/or for the estimation of components in a mixture of substances.

With the above explanatory introduction on the subject of chromatography, the individual chromatographic methods are described below in student-friendly way, which will make the student understand individual method, especially the most used methods, the TLC and GC (GLC & HPLC), from the practice point of view and to motivate them to use the techniques and machines by themselves instead of watching the lab staff and teachers doing the work on their behalf.

Before switching on to the individual chromatographic procedures, one should have the very basic concept of the types of chromatography. Based on the nature of the fixed and moving phase, following are the types of chromatography: (a) Adsorption chromatography (e.g. column, thin-layer and gas-solid chromatography); (b) Partition chromatography (e.g. paper, column, thin-layer and gas-liquid chromatography); (c) Ion-Exchange chromatography.

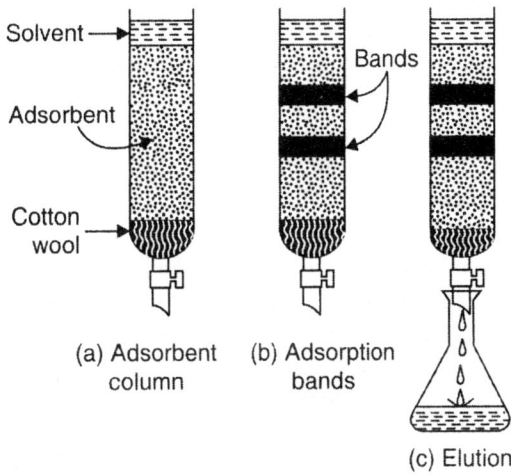

(a) **Adsorption chromatography:** This method is based on the differential adsorption of different constituents of a mixture on various adsorbents like alumina, magnesium oxide, cellulose powder, starch, silica gel, animal charcoal, etc. A column is prepared by filling any one adsorbent in a long glass tube with a stop-cork at the end. A dilute solution of the mixture is poured slowly at the top of the column. As the solution runs through the adsorbent, its different components are absorbed at different heights, called zones or bands. Different zones possess colours and travel down with different rates when a pure solvent is added to the top of the column (Fig. 3.1). The solution flowing down through the stop-cock with each band disappearing

Fig. 3.1. Adsorption chromatography.

are collected separately in different receivers. The solvent from each collected portion is removed to get the solid components which can be crystallized and subjected to desired analysis.

(b) **Partition chromatography**: Paper chromatography is a form of partition chromatography in which the stationary phase is the absorbed water always present in the filter paper, and the moving phase is a solvent previously saturated with water.

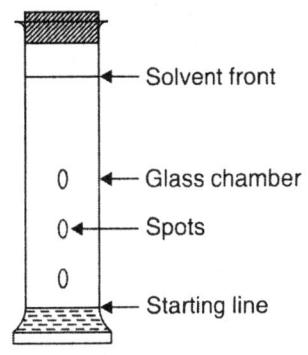

A drop of solution of mixture is applied to the paper by means of a capillary tube and the paper is dried. The paper is then placed in a suitable container called chromatographic chamber, so it can be irrigated with an organic liquid or mixture of liquids. When the solvent has travelled the required distance, the paper is removed from the container, the position of the solvent front noted and the paper is dried. Different

Fig. 3.2. Paper chromatography.

constituents of the mixture travel through different heights and correspond to the heights travelled by known substance (which can be placed similarly on the same paper as reference substances). The constituents of the mixture get separated and identified.

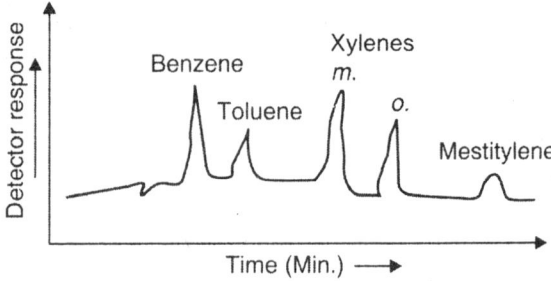

Fig. 3.3. A gas chromatogram.

The same procedure may be adopted to achieve the separation of the constituents of a mixture using thin layer plates coated with adsorbents. This is called **Thin Layer Chromatography (TLC).**

Gas chromatography: In gas chromatography the moving phase is a carrier unreactive gas such as nitrogen, helium, hydrogen, etc. The stationary phase is a liquid with a powder support and is packed in a column. The whole is placed in thermostat. The sample volatile at the column temperature is introduced in the column and the carrier gas is passed. The emerging gas with the substance's vapour is passed through a detector whose electrical response depends on the concentration of the sample in the gas stream. Since different ingredients are swept through the columns at different speeds, the emerging gas contains different consti-tuents at different times. A detector is provided with an automatic gas recorder. The record of the detector response is known as a chromatogram.

(c) Ion-exchange chromatography: It is used for the separation of ionic substances on columns of ion- exchange raisins (stationary phase) which are anionic or cationic polymers with fixed charge groups and replaceable counter ions. A sample containing organic or inorganic ions is passed through the column, the ions of the same charge as the counter ions displace the counter ions into the mobile phase and are retained on the column. The sample ions are then eluted using a suitable mobile phase, e.g. an aqueous solution containing electrolytes.

INDIVIDUAL CHROMATOGRAPHIC METHODS
COLUMN CHROMATOGRAPHY

Column chromatography is perhaps the earliest form of chromatographic technique, which can be said to be responsible for the rest of the now well established branches of chromatography. Column chromatography is a solid-liquid technique in which the two phases are a solid (stationary phase) and a liquid (moving phase). The theory of column chromatography is analogous to that of thin-layer chromatography. The most common adsorbents - silica gel and alumina - are the same ones used in TLC. The sample is dissolved in a small quantity of solvent (the eluent) and applied to the top of the column. The eluent, instead of rising by capillary action up a thin layer, flows down through the column filled with the adsorbent. Just as in TLC, there is an equilibrium established between the solute adsorbed on the silica gel or alumina and the eluting solvent flowing down through the column.

It is one of the most useful methods for the separation and purification of both solids and liquids when carrying out small-scale experiments. It is a method which is used to purify individual chemical compounds (components) from mixtures of different chemical compounds (components). Now-a-days column chromatography is mostly made use of for preparative applications on scales ranging from micrograms up to kilograms.

Apparatus: The apparatus for CC is the simplest and consists of, even for the purpose of the classical preparative chromatography, a column made of a glass tube with different diameter and length, depending upon the kind and the amount of the material to be used, ranging normally from 5 mm to 50 mm and 50 cm to 1 m respectively, with a tap at the bottom of the column (Fig. 3.4).

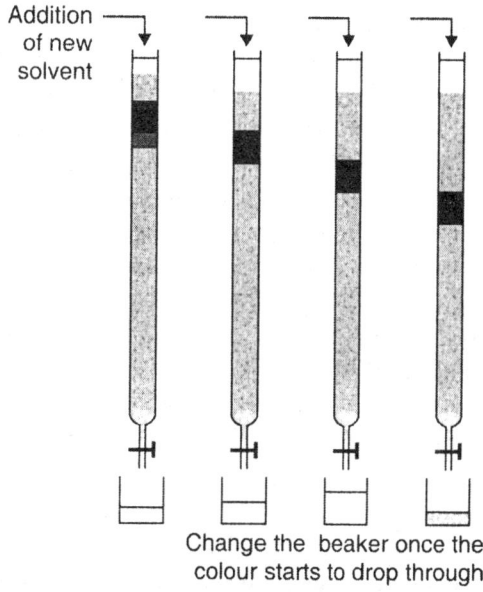

Change the beaker once the colour starts to drop through

Fig. 3.4. Four columns filled with stationary phase showing the movement of material with mobile phase at different level.

There are two methods which are generally used to prepare a column, the dry method and the wet method. In the case of dry method, the column is first filled with dry stationary phase powder, followed by the addition of mobile phase, which is put through the column in a way that the powder is completely and uniformly wet. From this point onwards the column is never allowed to run dry. In the wet method, a slurry is prepared of the eluent (mixture to be analysed) with the stationary phase powder and the slurry is then carefully poured into the column, taking care to avoid any air bubbles. A solution of the organic material is pipetted on top of the stationary phase. The upper layer is usually topped with a small layer of sand or with cotton or glass wool to protect the shape of the organic layer from the weight or stream of further addition of eluent. The eluent is periodically, but slowly, passed through the column to help travel and advance the organic material (mixture of components to be analysed). Normally a spherical eluent reservoir or a stoppered separating funnel filled with the eluent is put on top of the column to continuously feed the column with the eluent, the mobile phase.

The separation of the components takes place due to the fact that the individual components run through the column at different speed and are retained by the stationary phase from each other while they travel with the eluent/mobile phase. Thus at the end of the column they elute one by one at a time. As the chromatography process continues the eluent is collected in a series of fractions. The composition of the eluent flow can be regulated and monitored and each fraction can be analyzed for individual separated compounds/components, e.g. by using analytical chromatography, UV absorption, or fluorescence analysis. The coloured compounds (or fluorescent compounds) can be seen with the aid of a UV lamp and through the glass wall as moving bands.

Stationary phase (adsorbent): In column chromatography the *stationary phase* or *adsorbent* is always a solid material. The commonly used stationary phase is silica gel, followed by alumina. Earlier cellulose powder has also been used. The adsorbents are usually finely ground powders or gels and/or are microporous providing an increased surface area.

Mobile phase (eluent): The *mobile phase* or *eluent,* also referred as *solvent system* can be a pure solvent or a mixture of different solvents in different proportions. The solvent system is so selected that the different expected compounds get separated effectively. In laboratories usually column chromatography is run with the help of gravity force/flow. The flow rate of such a column can be increased by filling more eluent in the column above the top of the stationary phase or the flow can be decreased by regulating (lessening) the tap controls. Better flow rates can be regulated/increased by using a pump or by using compressed gas (e.g. air, nitrogen, or argon) to push the solvent through the column (flash column chromatography). The particle size of the stationary phase is generally finer in flash column chromatography than in gravity column chromatography.

Flash column chromatography: In 1978, W.C. Still introduced a modified version of column chromatography, called the flash column chromatography. This technique is very similar to the traditional column chromatography, except in this the solvent is driven through the column by applying positive pressure. This allows most separations to be performed in lesser time, with improved separations, as compared to the old method. Modern flash chromatography systems are sold as pre-packed plastic cartridges, and the solvent is pumped through the cartridge. Systems may also be linked with detectors and fraction collectors providing automation. The introduction of gradient pumps resulted in quicker separations and less solvent usage.

The diagram above shows that the blue compound/component is obviously more polar than the yellow one, as it perhaps even has the ability to hydrogen bond. It is because of this that the blue compound does not travel through the column very quickly (quickly enough compared to yellow). That means that it must get adsorbed more strongly to the silica gel or alumina than the yellow one. The less polar yellow one spends more of its time in the solvent and, therefore, it washes through the adsorbent of the column much faster to get collected as a separated component. The process of washing a compound through a column using a solvent is known as *elution*. The solvent is sometimes known as the *eluent*.

The blue compound with the rate at which it is travelling is likely to take much more time, may be it will get stuck there to the adsorbent. However, one can change the solvent during the elution by a more polar solvent once the yellow component has all been collected. The polar solvent will compete for space on the adsorbent - silica gel or alumina - with the blue compound. There will be now a greater attraction between the polar solvent molecules and the polar blue molecules. This will tend to attract any blue molecules sticking to the stationary phase back into solution. This will result in more polar solvent to spend more time with the blue compound in solution and so move faster through the adsorbent in the column for collection in eluent.

In case everything is colourless one has to collect a series of labelled tubes (collection made) and use drops for making spots through thin layer chromatography to visualize the spot/s, made from the drops of the collected eluents, and plan separation of collections made of similar spots one by one. By doing this repeatedly, one can identify which of the samples collected at the bottom of the column contain the desired and only the desired product.

Once one knows this, one can combine all of the samples which contain the desired pure product, and then remove the solvent to get the desired component/s for further chemical purposes.

PAPER CHROMATOGRAPHY

Paper Chromatography (PC) can be considered as the mother of thin layer chromatography. It is an analytical technique that involves placing of a small amount - a dot or line – of a sample mixture containing a number of compounds/components in a solution onto a strip of *chromatography paper* for separation of the components of the sample. The paper, acting as an adsorbent, is placed in a jar containing a shallow layer of solvent and sealed. As the solvent rises through the paper, regarded as a stationary phase, it meets the sample mixture which starts to travel up the paper with the solvent, the mobile phase. The paper is made of cellulose, a polar substance, and the compounds within the mixture travel farther, if they are non-polar. More polar substances bond with the cellulose paper more quickly and, therefore, do not travel as far as the other non-polar do. PC can be a **two-way paper chromatography**, also called two-dimensional chromatography, which involves using two solvents and rotating the paper 90° in between the experiment. This two-way PC is useful for separating complex mixtures of similar compounds, like amino acids. The paper chromatographic method has been largely replaced by thin layer chromatography (TLC).

Paper chromatography (PC) is of two types: **Ascending chromatography** and **Descending chromatography**.

Ascending chromatography: In this

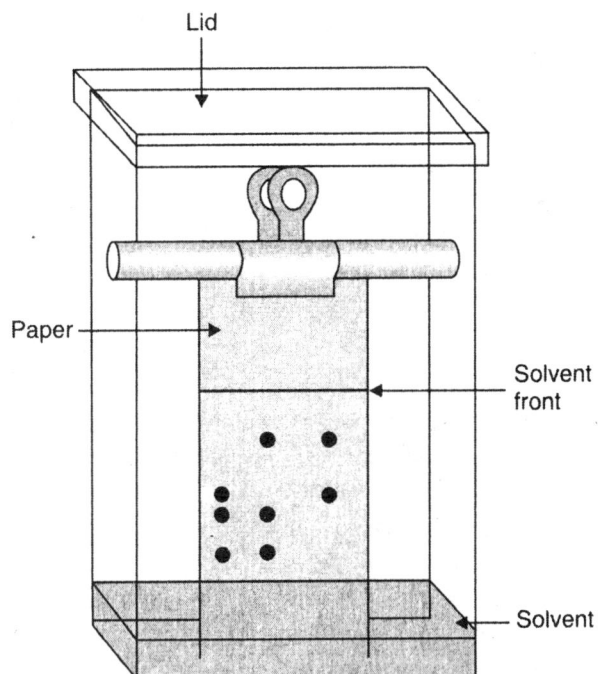

Fig. 3.5. Ascending Paper Chromatography. Chromatographic tank showing the paper chromatogram dipped in the solvent system, the mobile phase, carrying the components upwards with different speed on the stationary phase, the paper chromatogram.

kind of PC the solvent, the mobile phase, is placed as usual at the bottom of the vessel, the PC-tank containing a trough, in which the paper is supported in a way that it dips in the developing solvent (system) placed at the bottom of the tank at about a height of 25 mm. The mixture of the compounds/components dissolved in the solvent system is applied on the paper as usual before suspending the paper. The ascending chromatogram (paper) is suspended with a device which is capable of being lowered without opening the tank. This technique gives as quick a separation as that of the usual individual techniques.

Descending chromatography: In this method, the solvent is kept in a trough at the top of the chamber and is allowed to flow down the paper. The liquid moves down by capillary action as well as by the gravitational force, thus this method is also known as the gravitational method. In this case, the flow is more rapid as compared to the ascending method, and the chromatography is completed more quickly. The apparatus needed for this case is more sophisticated. The developing solvent is placed in a trough at the top which is usually made up of an inert material. The paper is then suspended in the solvent. Some substances in the mixture that cannot be separated by ascending method can sometimes be separated by the descending method. The I.P. App. 2.4.15, p. 130 gives these procedures as per the requirements of individual monographs.

R_f **values:** In the study of PC and TLC knowledge of R_f values is very important to interpret the results of the components. R_f value may be defined as the ratio of the distance travelled by the substance to the distance travelled by the solvent. R_f values are usually expressed as a fraction of two decimal places but it was suggested now that a percentage figure should be used instead. If R_f value of a solution is zero, the solute remains in the stationary phase and thus it is immobile. If R_f value = 1 then the solute has no affinity for the stationary phase and travels with the solvent front.

Procedure: The paper chromatographic technique provides an easy way to separate the components of a mixture.

(a) Place a drop of the mixture to be examined for separated components in one corner of a square of absorbent paper or in the form of small line, which should remain above the level of the solvent system.

(b) The lower edge of the paper on which drops and/or line are spotted is immersed in the solvent.

(c) The solvent is allowed to migrate up the paper sheet by capillary attraction.

(d) As the solvent rises up, the substances (components) in the drop/line are carried along at different speeds/rates.

(e) Each compound migrates at a rate that reflects (i) the size of its molecule; and (ii) tts solubility in the solvent.

(f) In a second run at right angles to the first, if done, (often using a different solvent), the various substances will be spread out at distinct spots across the sheet, forming a **chromatogram.**

(g) The identity of each spot can be determined by comparing its position with the position occupied by known substances under the **same conditions** and with the same **R_f values**.

(h) In many cases, a fragment of the paper can be cut away from the sheet and chemical analysis run on the tiny amount of substance in it.

Uses: Paper chromatography has been successfully applied as useful procedure in the study of amino acid metabolism and in the study of the transaminase system.

It is used to separate and identify all sorts of substances in forensic (police) work and forensic chemistry. Drugs from narcotics to aspirin can be identified in urine and blood samples, with the aid of chromatography.

It can also find the number of components in dyes on the foods consumed every day.

PC is used in many scientific studies to identify unknown organic and inorganic compounds. It is also used in crime scene investigation, DNA and RNA sequencing, among others.

THIN LAYER CHROMATOGRAPHY

Thin layer chromatography (TLC) is now-a-days widely employed as routine laboratory technique. TLC is very similar in many ways to paper chromatography (PC). However, in this technique in place of a stationary phase of paper, one uses a stationary phase consisting of a thin layer of adsorbent like silica gel, alumina, or cellulose spread over a glass, plastic or metal (aluminum foil) sheet or plate. In comparison to the use of paper (in PC), TLC has the advantage of being faster, affording better separations and giving better choice between different adsorbents. Besides, unlike in PC in which paper cannot be used as a stationary phase in all kinds of solvents and solvent systems, in TLC the plates can be used in all and sundry solvents and solvent systems as mobile phase.

Apparatus: The TLC Kit, which is now available globally based on Desaga German pattern having a movable applicator with an inbuilt thickness arrangement between 0 to 2 mm, has the following components:

(a) Spreader (Applicator) made of electroplated brass;

(b) Perspex Base size 114 × 23 cm to support 5 glass plates of size 20 × 20 cm and 2 plates of 20 × 5 cm;

(c) Plate Rack Aluminium for ten 20 × 20 cm plates;

(d) Spotting Termplate made of Perspex;

(e) Developing tank with lid;

(f) T.L.C. plates set of five 20 × 20 cm and two 20 × 5 cm or set of ten 20 × 10 cm and two 20 × 5 cm;

(g) Micro-pipette;

(h) Scriber for making lines made of stainless steel;

(i) Glass sprayer with rubber bellow capacity 100 ml;

(j) Instruction manual;

(k) It is same as above but the applicator is made of anodised alluminium.

Procedure: Preparation of TLC Plates: Now-a-days TLC plates are usually commercially available. This has helped the scientists and research students to save time and energy in preparing the plates through, somewhat time-consuming, the wet process of preparation (which mostly give uneven thickness of the adsorbent on the plates), drying and activation, etc. The commercially available plates in different sizes and with different kinds of adsorbents' layers are with standard particle size and this helps to improve reproducibility of results.

The plates can be prepared as and when required, and, of course, self-prepared plates are very economical. TLC plates are prepared by mixing thoroughly the adsorbent, like silica gel (say 30 g for 6 plates 20 × 20) and water (about 65 ml). This mixture, prepared carefully in a pestle and mortar, results in slurry, which is spread, in one go, over glass plates, of different sizes (30 × 30 or 30 × 10 or 30 × 5 cm) as per experimental requirement. The resultant plates are first dried on air for some minutes and then activated by heating in an oven for about 45 minutes at 110°C. The process should give plates with a thickness of the adsorbent layer of around 0.1–0.25 mm for analytical purposes and around 0.5–2.0 mm for preparative TLC.

Spotting the sample: The plate from oven is taken and the number of spots are earmarked for spotting the samples. The sample/s is/are applied on the plate, about one and a half cm from the base. The plate is then placed carefully straight down to rest it on the bottom of the TLC-tank, wherein a suitable solvent/solvent system such as petroleum ether and ethyl acetate (90:10) was put about half an hour prior to placing the TLC-plate, with a view to saturate the chamber with the vapours of the solvent, the mobile phase. The tank is then covered/sealed. The solvent travels up the plate by capillary action and meets the sample mixture. The substances/components of the mixture get dissolved in mobile phase and are carried up the plate. Different compounds/components of the sample mixture travel at different rate/speed due to the differences in their affinity and attraction to the stationary phase because of their differences in solubility in the solvent.

Also, the separation achieved with a TLC plate can be used to estimate the separation of a flash chromatography column.

Visualisation: After the solvent has travelled sufficient distance, 10 to 15 cm, the TLC plate is taken out of the tank and dried in the air in exhaust chamber. It can then be viewed in the dark room under the ultraviolet light and the position of spots and the colour of the spots noted. The composition of the solvent system may be changed using the same mixture, to get better separation of the components as seen

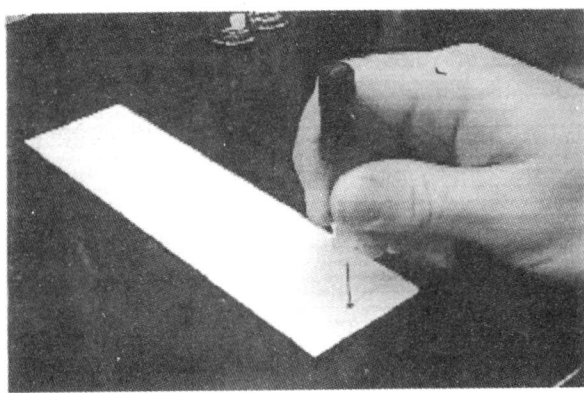

Fig. 3.6. Spotting of sample on TLC plate.

after visualising the plate as such or after spraying with reagent/s or under the UV-light. R_f values can be measured and compared with the known standard substances, if spotted along side with the mixture.

Since most of the components/chemical substances to be separated are colourless, a few methods are adopted to help visualize the spots:

- Usually a small amount of a fluorescent compound is used. Sufficient amount of manganese-activated zinc silicate is added to the adsorbent that allows the visualization of spots under ultraviolet light (UV_{254}). The adsorbent layer will thus fluoresce light green by itself, but spots of analyte quench this fluorescence.

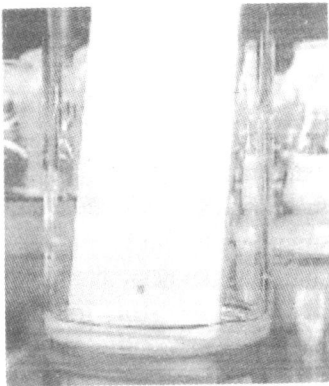

Fig. 3.7. Development of TLC plate.

- Iodine vapours are a general unspecific colour reagent.
- Specific colour reagents exist into which the TLC plate is dipped or which are sprayed onto the plate, anisaldehyde in conc. sulphuric acid, phosphomolybdic acid, 2,4-dinitrophenyl hydrazine, etc.

Like paper chromatography, two-dimensional chromatography can also be undertaken in TLC, rather more easily and for all round better results for obvious reasons. For this after the first development has taken place, the plate is put in a direction perpendicular to the first one either in the same solvent or in a different solvent system (mixture of solvents in different proportions) depending on the knowledge of the compounds/ components i.e. their polarity.

Polarity role: A good separation of compounds is based on the competition of the solute and the mobile

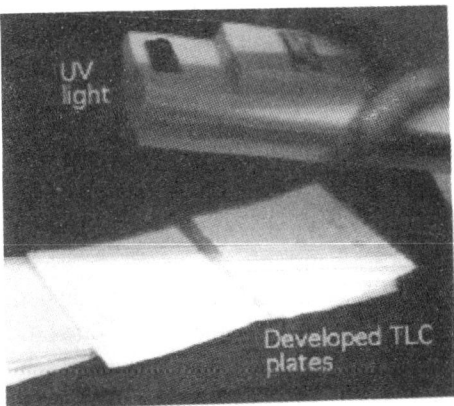

Fig. 3.8. Visualisation of TLC plate under UV light.

phase for binding places on the stationary phase. For example, if normal phase silica gel is used as the stationary phase it can be considered polar. If there are two compounds with different polarity, the more polar compound has a stronger interaction with the silica and is, therefore, more capable to dispel the mobile phase from the binding places. Consequently, the less polar compound moves higher up the plate, resulting in a higher R_f value. If the mobile phase is changed to a more polar solvent or mixture of solvents, it is more capable of dispelling solutes from the silica binding places and all compounds on the TLC plate will move higher up the plate. Practically this means that if one uses a mixture of ethyl acetate and petroleum ether as the mobile phase, adding more of ethyl acetate (up to 15%) will result in higher R_f-values for all compounds on the TLC plate.

Preparative TLC: TLC can also be used on a small semi-preparative scale to separate mixtures of up to a few hundred milligrams. The total practical method is similar to the normal TLC procedure. In preparative TLC, however, the mixture is "spotted" on the TLC plate as a thin even layer/line horizontally at the starting line, about 1.5 cm above the solvent level. When developed with solvent the compounds separate in horizontal bands rather than horizontally separated spots. Each band (or the desired component's band) is scraped off the backing material. The backing material is then extracted with a suitable solvent and filtered to give the isolated material upon the removal of the solvent. For small-scale reactions with easily separated products, preparative TLC can be far more efficient in terms of time and cost than doing column chromatography. Obviously, the whole plate cannot be chemically developed or the product will be chemically destroyed. Thus this technique is best suited to the compounds that are coloured, or visible under UV light. Alternatively, a small section of the plate can be chemically developed e.g. cutting a section out and chemically developing it, or masking most of the plate and exposing a small section to a chemical developer like iodine.

Applications of TLC: The TLC, which was developed some 50 years ago as a most important and popular technique for the phytochemists, organic chemists and scientists of other related branches of science engaged in day to day research for separation and identification of components of mixed substances, has not only survived the times as an evergreen technique, it has rather developed as a physical-analytical technique in many ways.

It has developed now as an important method for semi-quantitative determination of the individual components of somewhat complicated mixtures. Already by the last two decades the application of different TLC methods for separation and quantitative determination of a wide variety of organic, inorganic and phytochemical substances had touched sky heights. This increased interest in TLC's application has been due to the improved instrumentation and automation of various steps of TLC analysis, like gradient and forced flow methods, centrifugal development, circular rotation, planner chromatography, high pressure planner liquid chromatography, densitometry, etc. As if that was not enough further importance of TLC took place due to the coupled spectroscopic methods, such as TLC-UV-VIS, TLC-FTIR, which led to considerable enhancement of the reproducibility of TLC findings. Further TLC methods have been successfully used in many allied fields of research and development (R&D) like clinical medicine, forensic medicine, biochemistry, pharmaceutical analysis as stated above. TLC's importance in clinical pharmacology, toxicology, drugs screening, pesticides, inorganic pollutants, etc makes it the most lovable physical method of analysis.

It is now a common knowledge that the TLC and the TLC densitometry methods have been published for pharmaceutical analysis including applications such as identification, purity testing, assays, stability testing and content uniformity testing of drug products, intermediates raw materials as well as analysis of drugs and their metabolites in their biological samples. The testing is relied upon because of its simplicity, flexibility, speed of analysis and unique detection methods on both qualitative and quantitative basis. A very important advantage of TLC is that it is an open system. The samples are tested and evaluated as a whole whether they remain on the origin or travel with the solvent front (this is not always the case in HPLC). TLC has now become a crucial tool in the earlier stages of drug developments at which stage the knowledge about the impurities and degradants in drug substances and drug products is limited. It is often used as an orthogonal technique to HPLC to ensure quality of the pharmaceuticals. TLC has been taken up in almost all pharmacopoeias globally. The first analytical method was described in the European Pharmacopoeia in 1974 (Ph. Eur1) in which TLC was specified for the identification of 23 drugs.

Egon Stahl introduced the term thin layer chromatography (in German: Dunschuchtchromatography) in late 50s. From early 60s, around 1960 onwards, TLC became very popular as an analytical technique in pharmacognosy and phytochemistry and in the field of pharmacy at large. The author (J.S.Q.) was amongst one of the firsts who used TLC, GC and HPLC techniques during his research work in Germany and later during research guidance in India.

GAS CHROMATOGRAPHY

Gas Chromatography (GC), also called Gas Liquid Chromatography (GLC), is one of the chromatographic techniques used for separation of a mixture into its components in which the mobile phase is a gas, hence the name. GC is only suited to substances or their derivatives that are volatalised under the temperatures employed. GC is based on a partition equilibrium of analyte between a solid stationary phase (often a liquid silicone-based material) and a mobile gas (mostly an inert gas, e.g. helium). The stationary phase is adhered to the inside of a small-diameter glass tube (a capillary column) or a solid matrix inside a larger metal tube (a packed column).

Gas chromatography has also been referred to as **vapor-phase chromatography** (VPC), or **gas-liquid partition chromatography** (GLPC). Thus these alternative names, as well as their respective abbreviations, may be found in scientific literature. GLPC is considered by many GC practitioners as the most appropriate terminology and hence found referred by authors in their literatures.

Procedure: The apparatus or the machine used in GC is called **Gas Chromatograph.** A gas chromatograph is an instrument used in chemical analysis for separating chemical components in a complex sample. It is operated as follows:

A small amount of a mixture sample to be analyzed is drawn up into a syringe. The syringe needle is placed into a hot injector port of the gas chromatograph, and the sample is injected. The **injector** (see types of injector below) is set to a temperature higher than the components' boiling points. The components of the mixture evaporate into the gas phase inside the injector. A carrier gas, such as helium, flows through the injector and pushes the gaseous components of the sample onto the **GC column** (see types of column below). It is within the column that separation of the components takes place. The molecules get partitioned between the carrier gas (the mobile phase) and the high boiling liquid (the stationary phase) within the GC column. The components of the mixture move through the GC column and reach a **detector** (see types of detector below) at varying times due to differences in the partitioning between mobile and stationary phases. The detector sends a signal to the chart recorder which results in a peak on the chart paper. The area of the peak is proportional to the number of molecules generating the signal.

Retention time

The time taken for a particular compound to travel through the column to the detector is known as its *retention time*. This time is measured from the time at which the sample is injected to the point at which the display shows a maximum peak height for that compound.

Following instructions should be taken note of before using the gas chromatograph.

1. The syringe is washed with acetone by filling the syringe completely and ejecting the acetone onto a paper towel. The syringes are to be washed/rinsed 2–3 times.
2. Air bubbles are removed from inside the syringe by rapidly moving the plunger up and down while the needle is in the sample. Usually 1–2 µL of sample is injected into the GC.
3. The chart recorder is started on time and set to the appropriate chart speed. Set the baseline using the zero on the chart recorder. Make sure the pen is down (marking the paper) and the paper is moving.
4. The sample is injected by holding the syringe level and pushing the needle completely into the injector and quickly pushing the plunger and then pulling the syringe out of the injection port.
5. Injection time should be marked on the chart recorder. This is done by adjusting the zero just after the sample is injected. It is often convenient for one person to inject the sample while a lab partner marks the injection time at the chart recorder.
6. The syringe is to be cleaned imme-diately after injection. Syringe needles often clog quickly and must be replaced if they are not cleaned after each use.
7. The settings of the chart recorder are recorded during the run. This is needed to know the chart speed and the full-scale setting.
8. The settings of the GC are recorded during a run. A knob on the bottom centre of the GC can be turned to read column (or oven) temperature, detector temperature, and injector port temperature in °C.

Injector (or column inlet): It is used to introduce the sample to be analyzed into a continuous flow of carrier gas. The inlet is a piece of hardware attached to the head of the column.

Some common types of inlets/injectors are:

- **Split/Splitless (S/SL) injector:** It introduces the sample into a heated small chamber via a syringe through a septum. The heat facilitates volatilization of the sample and sample matrix. The carrier gas then sweeps the sample into the column.
- **On-column inlet:** The sample here is introduced in its entirety without heat.
- **Programmed Temperature Vapourising (PTV) injector:** It is a temperature-programmed sample introduction injector. It was first described by Vogt in 1979. Originally Vogt developed the technique as a method for the introduction of large sample volumes (up to 250 µL) in capillary GC. Vogt introduced the sample into the liner at a controlled injection rate. The

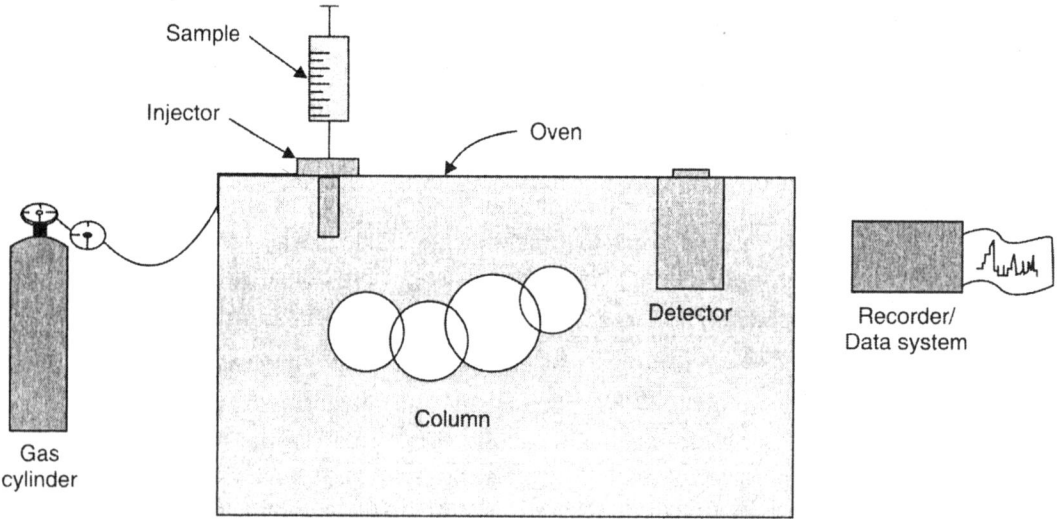

Fig. 3.9. A simplified sketch showing various parts of a gas chromatograph.

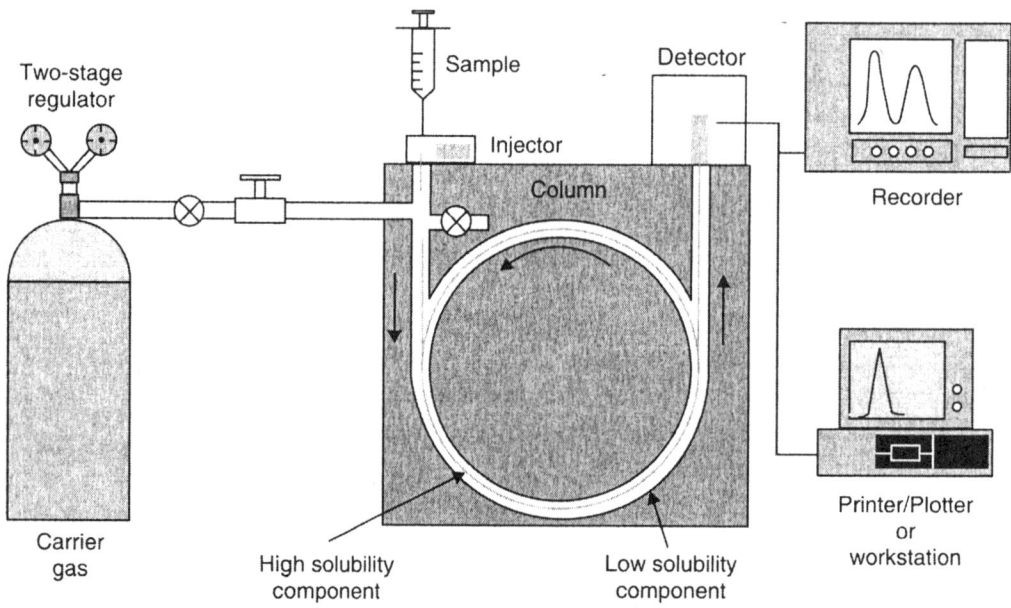

Fig. 3.10. L.S. of a simple gas chromatograph showing various parts/gadgets attached to it.

temperature of the liner was chosen slightly below the boiling point of the solvent. The low-boiling solvent was continuously evaporated and vented through the split line. This technique led to the development of the injector, PTV. By introducing the sample at a low initial liner temperature many of the disadvantages of the classic hot injection techniques were circumvented.

- **Gas source inlet or gas switching valve:** The gaseous samples in collection bottles are connected to what is most commonly a six-port *switching valve*. The carrier gas flow is not interrupted while a sample can be expanded into a previously evacuated *sample loop*. Upon switching, the contents of the sample loop are inserted into the carrier gas stream.
- **Purge-and-Trap (P&T) system:** In this system an inert gas is bubbled through an aqueous sample causing insoluble volatile chemicals to be purged from the matrix. The volatile components are 'trapped' on an absorbent column (known as a trap or concentrator) at ambient temperature. The trap is then heated and the volatile components are directed into the carrier gas stream.
- **Solid Phase Micro Extraction (SPME) system:** This system offers a convenient and low-cost alternative to P & T systems with the versatility of a syringe and simple use of the S/SL port.

Types of column used: Universally two types of column have been in use in gas chromatography. They are:

- **Packed columns:** These are 1.5–10 m in length with an internal diameter of 2–4 mm. The tubing is usually made of stainless steel or glass and contains a *packing* of finely divided, inert, solid support material (e.g. diatomaceous earth), which is coated with a liquid or solid stationary phase. The nature of the coating material determines what type of material is most strongly adsorbed. There are number of columns available which are designed to separate specific types of compounds.
- **Capillary columns:** These columns have a very small internal diameter of the order of a few tenths of millimeters, with lengths between 25–60 metres. The inner walls of the column are coated with the active materials (WCOT columns). Some columns are quasi solid filled with many parallel micropores (PLOT columns). Mostly the capillary columns are made of fused-silica with a polyimide outer coating. These columns are quite flexible and hence a very long column can be wound into a small coil.

Role of temperature (temperature programming): The temperature-dependence of molecular adsorption and of the rate of progression along the column requires a careful control of the column temperature to within a few tenths of a degree for precise work. Reducing the temperature produces the greatest level of separation, but can result in very long elution times. In some cases regulating the temperature and its ramping either continuously or in steps provides the desired separation. This is referred to as a **temperature programming**. Electronic pressure control can also be used to modify flow rate during the analysis, aiding in faster run times while keeping acceptable levels of separation.

Choice of carrier gas (mobile phase): The choice of carrier gas is important. Historically **hydrogen** being the most efficiently used and it has been providing the best separation. However, **helium** has a larger range of flow rates which are comparable to hydrogen in efficiency. Helium has the added advantage that it is non-flammable and works with a greater number of detectors. Helium, therefore, is the most common carrier gas in use globally.

Detectors: Gas chromatography makes use of a number of detectors. The most common ones are:

The flame ionization detector (FID) and the thermal conductivity detector (TCD).

Both are sensitive to a wide range of components, and both work over a wide range of concentrations. While TCDs are essentially universal and can be used to detect any component other than the carrier gas (as long as their thermal conductivities are different from that of the carrier gas, at detector temperature), FIDs are sensitive primarily to hydrocarbons and are more sensitive to them than TCD. However, an FID cannot detect water. Both detectors are also quite robust. Since TCD is non-destructive, it can be operated in-series before using an FID (destructive one), thus providing complementary detection of the same analytes.

Other detectors are sensitive only to specific types of substances, or work well only in narrower ranges of concentrations. They include:

- Discharge ionization detector (DID), which uses a high-voltage electric discharge to produce ions.
- Electron capture detector (ECD), which uses a radioactive beta particle (electron) source to measure the degree of electron capture.
- Flame photometric detector (FPD)
- Flame ionization detector (FID)
- Hall electrolytic conductivity detector (ElCD)
- Helium ionization detector (HID)
- Nitrogen phosphorus detector (NPD)
- Infrared Detector (IRD)
- Mass selective detector (MSD)
- Photo-ionization detector (PID)
- Pulsed discharge ionization detector (PDD)
- Thermal energy (conductivity) analyzer/detector (TEA/TCD)

Some gas chromatographs are connected to a mass spectrometer which acts as the detector. The combination is known as GC–MS. Some GC-MS are connected to an NMR spectrometer which acts as a back up detector. This combination is known as GC–MS–NMR. Some GC–MS–NMR are connected to an infrared spectrophotometer which acts as a back up detector. This combination is known as GC–MS–NMR–IR. It must, however, be stressed this is very rare as most analyses needed can be concluded via purely GC-MS.

ANALYSIS THROUGH GAS CHROMATOGRAPH

The retention time of each peak (in minutes) is noted and reported. Likewise the identity of each component in the mixture and the percent composition of the mixture are to be noted and reported. For determining the percent composition one has to first find the area under each curve.

$$\text{Area} = (\text{height}) \times (\text{width at } \frac{1}{2} \text{ height})$$

Note the retention time, heights, half-heights, and width at ½ heights on your GC trace. Record the calculations either in the final report or directly on the chromatograph.

Assuming that each component of the mixture causes the same response in the detector, the areas under the curves can be used to calculate percent composition of the mixture of components. (This is a reasonable assumption when the components of the mixture are very similar in structure, such as, 2-methyl-1-butene and 2-methyl-2-butene.)

% age Component 1 = [(area under peak 1)/ (total area)] × 100

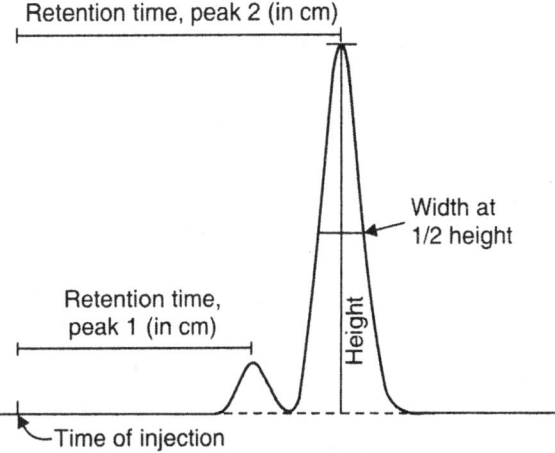

Fig. 3.11. Peaks seen in two different heights and width of a GC-printout.

Application of GC: Gas chromatography has a very wide field of application. Its first and foremost area of use is in the separation and analysis of multi component mixtures such as essential oils, hydrocarbons, solvents, etc. Many involatile substances such as amino acids, steroids and high molecular weight fatty acids can be derivatized to form volatile substances that can be separated by GC. Intrinsically, with the use of the flame ionization detector and the electron capture detector (which have very high sensitivities) gas chromatography can quantitatively determine materials present at very low concentrations. Thus the second most important application area is in pollution studies, forensic work and general trace analysis.

Gas chromatography is also widely used in applications involving food analysis. Typical applications pertain to the quantitative and/or qualitative analysis of food composition, natural products, food additives, flavour and aroma components, a variety of transformation products, and contaminants such as pesticides, fumigants, environmental pollutants, natural toxins, veterinary drugs, and packaging material.

Now-a-days gas chromatography is one of the primary analytical techniques used in every forensic laboratory. GC is widely used by forensic scientists - from analysis of body fluids for the presence of illegal substances, to testing of fibre and blood from a crime scene, and to detect residue from explosives. Scientists from Ohio University have explored another application of gas chromatography with differential mobility spectrometry as a low cost, on site detection method for ignitable liquids. Gas chromatography - mass spectrometry (GC/MS) has now become a well established method for analysis of ignitable liquids.

Gas chromatographic method is indicated to be used in quite a few monographs for identification and determination of official compounds and preparations therefrom and assay methods of some of them. Hence GC is included in its appendix 2.4.13, p. 122 in fairly good detail in relation to the monographs.

SIZE-EXCLUSION CHROMATOGRAPHY

Size exclusion chromatography (SEC) is a chromatographic technique in which the molecules in a solution are separated according to their sizes (i.e. said more correctly, as per their hydrodynamic volume). It is usually applied to large molecules or macromolecular complexes such as proteins and industrial polymers. Typically, when an aqueous solution is used to transport the sample through the column, the technique is known as **gel filtration chromatography**, versus the name **gel permeation chromatography** which is used when an organic solvent is used as a mobile phase.

The main application of gel filtration chromatography is the fractionation of proteins and other water-soluble polymers, while gel permeation chromatography is used to analyze the molecular weight distribution of organic-soluble polymers. Either technique should not be confused with gel electrophoresis, where an electric field is used to "pull" or "push" molecules through the gel depending on their electrical charges.

SEC is a widely used technique for the purification and analysis of synthetic and biological polymers, such as proteins, polysaccharides and nucleic acids. Biologists and biochemists typically use a gel medium – usually polyacrylamide, dextran or agarose – and filter under low pressure. Polymer chemists typically use either silica or cross-linked polystyrene medium under a higher pressure. These media are known as the **stationary phase**.

SEC method, as stated above, is good for the separation of larger molecules from the smaller molecules with a minimal volume of eluate. In fact various solutions can be applied without interfering with the filtration process, all while preserving the biological activity of the particles to be separated. With SEC there are short and well-defined separation times and narrow bands which lead to good sensitivity. There is also no sample loss because solutes do not interact with the stationary phase. This technique includes the disadvantages that only a limited number of bands can be accommodated because the time scale of the chromatogram is short and generally there has to be a 10% difference in molecular mass to have a good resolution. Like other forms of chromatography, increasing the column length will enhance the resolution, and increasing the column diameter increases the capacity of the column. Proper column packing is important for maximizing the resolution. SEC is utilised in a few I.P. monographs (not specifically included in this book), and it, therefore, treats this technique in appreciable detail.

Size Exclusion Chromatography (SEC) is a commonly used technique to determine the molecular size and weight of polymeric products. The retention of components is based on the size in solution so that the largest molecules are excluded from the stationary phase pores and elute earlier in the chromatogram. The smaller molecular weight components enter the stationary phase pores and, as a result, elute later in the chromatogram. SEC is utilized to qualitatively determine the molecular weight differences between two lots of polymers or quantitatively determine the number, weight, Z average molecular weights and polydispersity. Both aqueous and organic mobile phases are utilized in separate separations. Available detectors include differential refractive index (RI) and multi-angle light scattering (MALLS). With the RI detector, molecular weights are determined by standard curves generated with polymers of well-defined molecular weight. With the MALLS detector, molecular weights are determined directly based on the light scattering.

SEC is utilized to determine the molecular weight and molecular weight distribution of a number of polymers. Typically, molecular weight distribution and polydispersity are directly related to physical properties of the polymer. A routine analysis is to compare a lot of material that performs to specification to a lot that does not. The results of the analysis are often used to optimize process parameters.

LIQUID CHROMATOGRAPHY

Liquid chromatography (LC) is a separation technique in which the mobile phase is a liquid. Liquid chromatography can be carried out either in a column or a plane. Present day liquid chromatography that generally utilizes very small packing particles and a relatively high pressure is referred to as high performance liquid chromatography (HPLC).

In the **HPLC** technique, the sample is forced through a column that is packed with irregularly or spherically shaped particles or a porous monolithic layer (stationary phase) by a liquid (mobile phase) at high pressure. HPLC is historically divided into two different sub-classes based on the polarity of the mobile and stationary phases. Technique in which the stationary phase is more polar than the mobile phase (e.g. toluene as the mobile phase, silica as the stationary phase) is called normal phase liquid chromatography (NPLC) and the opposite (e.g. water-methanol mixture as the mobile phase and C18 = octadecylsilyl as the stationary phase) is called reversed phase liquid chromatography (RPLC). Ironically the "normal phase" has fewer applications and RPLC is, therefore, used considerably more.

Specific techniques which come under this broad heading are listed below. It should also be noted that the following techniques can also be considered fast liquid chromatography if no pressure is used to drive the mobile phase through the stationary phase. See also Aqueous Normal Phase Chromatography.

I.P. 2007 in its appendix gives rather a good account on Liquid Chromatography in reference to the monographs included in it. The details in relation to this technique of chromatography are not being included here.

Structure of Atom

An atom is the simplest part of an element which cannot be divided further. The atom is made up of certain fundamental particles called electrons, protons and neutrons described as the following:

1. An electron is a negatively charged particle having a magnitude of unit charge of electricity. It is a definite and universal constituent of matter. The ratio of the electronic charge, E, to the mass, m, of a single electron, E/m has been found to be 17589×10^7 emu. The mass of an electron is only 1/1837th of the mass of a hydrogen atom, the lightest atom known, i.e. 1.008/1837, which is equal to 0.000548 g.

2. A proton is a positively charged particle having a magnitude of unit charge of electricity. The mass of a proton is 1.00732 g on the chemical atomic weight scale.

3. A neutron is a chargeless particle with a mass about the same as that of a proton (or a hydrogen atom).

The nucleus of all atoms is built up of protons and neutrons. Since the positive charge on the nucleus must be balanced by the negative charge of the electrons, the number of the latter that surround the nucleus is equal to the atomic number. The total number of protons and neutrons is equal to the atomic weight of the element while the number of protons is equal to the atomic number.

According to works of Rutherford, Bohr and other workers, the positively charged nucleus is surrounded by electrons. The electrons move around the nucleus in different successive and concentric volumes in space known as **shells**. These shells are numbered as 1, 2, 3, 4, or K, L, M, N etc. and are known as Principal Quantum Numbers. Each shell has certain number of electrons and the maximum number of the electrons for each shell is fixed and denoted by $2n^2$, where n is the number of the shell. Thus the maximum number of electrons in K, L, M and N shells will be 2, 8, 18, and 32 respectively. The maximum number of electrons in the outermost shell is 8.

The shells are sub-divided into subshells indicated by 1, which have different geometric shapes and angular momentum. The subshells are known as the subsidiary of Azimuthal Quantum Number and have whole number 0 to $n - 1$. K shell has one subshell s; L shell has two subshells s and p, M shell has three s, p and d and N shell has four subshells s, p, d and f. The subshels, s, p, d and f can have maximum of 2, 6, 10 and 14 electrons, respectively.

The positions of the electrons in the various shells and subshells are represented in the following manner. Major shells in which the electrons exist are indicated by the number 1, 2, 3, ... and the subshells denoted by s, p, d, f etc. The superscript on s, p, d and f gives the number of electrons in subshells. For example, $1s^2$ indicate the presence of 2 electrons in a subshell of the first major shell (K). Similarly $4f^6$ indicates the presence of 6 electrons in the subshells of fourth major shell (N).

The subshell states s, p, d and f are further divided into a number of orbitals. An orbital may be regarded as the region around the nucleus in which there is the probability of finding the moving electrons. The total number of orbitals that a principal quantum shell can contain is given by n^2. Thus when principal quantum number is 1 (i.e., the first or K shell), then $1 = 0$; there is a single orbital in this K shell and is of s type and is known as the $1s$ orbital. When $n = 2$ (i.e. the second or L shell), then $1 = 0$ or 1. This means there are two energy subshells in the L shell. The total number of possible orbitals in L shell will be $2^2 = 4$. When $1 = 0$, this corresponds to the $2s$ orbital. When $1 = 1$, then there are three equivalent orbitals, these are the three $2p$ orbitals. When $n = 3$ (i.e., the third or M shell), then the total number of possible orbitals is 9 (3^2). This corresponds to one $3s$ orbital ($1 = 0$).

An orbital can have only two electrons having spin about their axes, some spinning in one direction and others in the opposite direction. This is indicated by the spin quantum number(s) and can have values of ½ and –½. Thus, in the s subshell having 2 electrons, there is only one orbital and it is called s orbital. Finally an electron also has a magnetic quantum number (m) and this gives the allowed orientation of the orbitals in an external magnetic field. Thus an electron is described by four quantum numbers n, l, s and m. The orbital is particular shaped space or volume within which electrons will be found. All s orbitals are spherical and are concentric about the nucleus.

The p subshells having six electrons will have three orbitals which are designated as p orbitals. The three p orbitals are directed along the coordinate axes perpendicular to each other. Each orbital consists of lobes lying along the axis, one on each side of the origin. The three p orbitals along three axes are referred as px, py, and pz respectively. These have the same energy and are distinguished from each other only in direction. Similarly d and f subshells have 5 and 7 orbitals, respectively.

The hydrogen atom is made of one proton and one electron. When the hydrogen atom is in the state of lowest energy, i.e. **ground state**, its electron will occupy the lowest energy level or the $1s$ level, when the atom is in the **excited** state, the electron will jump to higher energy level.

Helium has two electrons, hence its electron configuration in the ground is represented as $1s^2$. There are three electrons in lithium atom. Since K shell cannot occupy more than two electrons, the third electron goes to L ($n = 2$, $l = 0$, 1). Electrons occupy lowest energy levels first. Thus this third electron occupies the $2s$ orbital, and not the $2p$, because the $2p$ is a higher energy level than the $2s$. Therefore, the electronic configuration of lithium is $1s^2$, $2s^1$ where the K shell is filled first. Then the electrons enter the L shell until that is filled. In this shell the s level is filled before the p. For further study about the arrangement of electrons in orbitals Hund's rules are applied. These rules are: (i) the electrons tend to avoid being in the same orbital until all the orbitals of the subshell have at least one electron, (ii) two electrons, each singly occupying a given pair or equivalent orbitals, tend to have their spins paralelled when the atom is in the ground state. The carbon atom has six electrons which are represented as $1s^2$, $2s^2$, $2p^2$. The K shell is filled first and then electrons occupy L shell. The $2s$ orbital doubly filled before a higher level is used, then singly two of the $2p$ orbitals.

Shapes of *s* and *p* orbitals

s-subshell has only one orientation and so one *s* orbital is present in this shell. But for *p* subshell three orientations can be represented and, therefore, three *p* orbitals viz., *px*, *py* and *pz* are present in the shell. According to the wave equation the *s* and *p* orbitals have spherical and dumbbell type shapes, respectively.

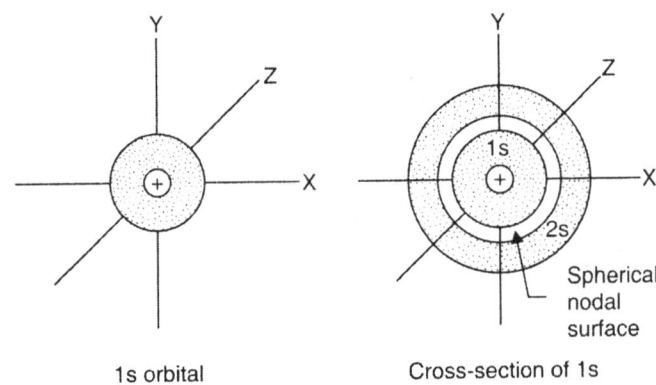

1s orbital

Cross-section of 1s and 2s orbitals

Fig. 4.1. Shapes of 1*s* and 2*s* orbitals.

Each shell contains one *s* orbital and these orbitals are represented as 1*s*, 2*s*, 3*s*, ... etc., where 1, 2, 3 are the shell numbers. The 1*s* orbital is the nearest orbital to the nucleus as it is present in the first shell. The other, *s* orbitals are far away from the nucleus as shown in Fig. 4.1.

In between two *s* orbitals there is a space where the probability of finding of electrons becomes zero. This space is called the 'spherical nodal surface'. This space is also spherical since it occurs between two spherical *s* orbitals.

As indicated above, *p* orbitals have dumbbell type shape and a plane is passed through the nucleus at right angles to the axis of the orbital where probability of finding the electrons becomes zero. This plane is called the nodal plane. In Fig. 4.2, shapes of *px*, *py* and *pz* orbitals are shown with each lobes containing the sign of wave functions as (–) and (+).

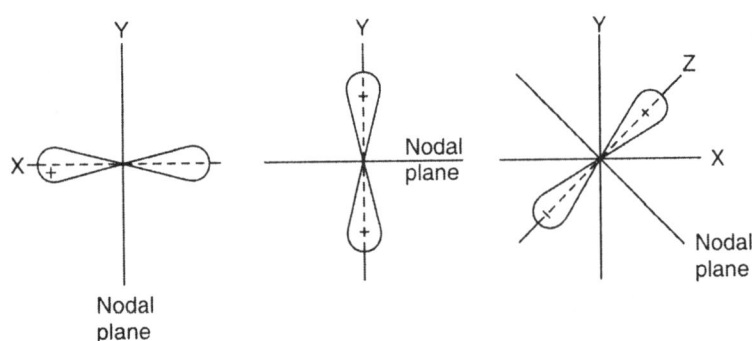

Fig. 4.2. Shapes of *px*, *py* and *pz* orbitals.

The Atomic Bonding

When a compound is formed due to reaction of molecules in a chemical change, old bonds are broken and new bonds formed. Therefore, to study the organic chemistry, we should examine the nature of different bonds formed between atoms.

The electrons of the outermost shell are the most important for the formation of chemical bonds. There are eight electrons in the outermost shell of all inert gases except helium where the outermost shell (K) cannot have more than two electrons. The inert gases usually do not undergo chemical reactions and are considered to have inert or stable electronic configuration. Thus the electronic arrangement where eight electrons are there in the outermost shell is regarded as the most stable configuration expect in cases where the outermost shell is also the first shell as in helium and the maximum number of two electrons is the stable configuration. According to Liewi and Langmuir, all other elements have a tendency to enter into chemical combination in such a manner so as to acquire inert gas type stable configuration. For obtaining stable configuration lowering of energy takes place. This tendency makes the elements undergo chemical reactions forming compounds.

Nature of Atomic Bonding

An examination of the periodic table shows that besides the inert gases, there are other three types of elements:

(i) Those having one to three electrons in the outermost shell, e.g. Na and Al.

(ii) Those having five to seven electrons in the outermost shell e.g. P, O, Cl and Br.

(iii) Those having four electrons in the outermost shell e.g., C, Si. Since the driving force for chemical combination is the tendency to acquire inert gas stable configuration, first type of elements will try to stabilize themselves by losing 1, 2 or 3 electrons because it is difficult to gain 7, 6 or 5 electrons than to lose 1, 2 or 3 electrons for obtaining stable arrangement. Similarly, the elements of the second type will try to stabilize themselves by gaining 3, 2 or 1 electrons as losing 5, 6 or 7 electrons will be more difficult. Thus the elements of the first and second type usually combine by either losing or gaining electrons.

The elements of third type, of which carbon is a representative, have to lose 4 electrons or gain 4 electrons in order to obtain inert gas configuration and if the element has balanced electropositive and electronegative characters, then either process becomes still more difficult.

In such cases, the element achieves the stable configuration by sharing of these electrons with other elements. Besides carbon, one more element is in a similar position and that is hydrogen which may attain the stable configuration by losing, gaining or sharing one electron with other elements.

ELECTRONIC THEORY OF VALENCY

The valency of an atom is determined by the electrons present in the outermost orbit of that atom. These electrons are called the valency electrons. Formation of chemical compounds from elements involves transference of valency electrons of one element to the outermost orbit of the other atoms. In this manner a chemical bond is formed and both the atoms acquire a stable configuration.

Thus valency of an atom, according to the electronic theory of valency, is the number of electrons it can lose, borrow or share with other elements. A lending atom is called electropositive while a borrowing atom is called electronegative.

Types of bonding: Formation of bonds between atoms may occur in three different ways giving three different types of bonds:

1. Electrovalent or Ionic Bond

If the outer shell of an atom is incompletely filled, it can acquire one or more electrons from another atom. This transfer of electrons leads to a stable configuration in the participating atoms. The atom which gives the electrons acquires a positive charge and the one which gets it, gains a negative charge. The charged species are known as ions and the electrostatic force between these ions of opposite charge is known as electrovalent of ionic bond.

$$A + B \longrightarrow \overset{+}{A} + \overset{-e}{B} \text{ or } \overset{+}{A} \equiv \overset{-e}{B}$$

The ions generaly have noble gas structures. These oppositely charged ions are held together by electrostatic attraction. The atoms involved are electrically neutral before combining. The element A which has lost its electron is known as electropositive whereas element B which has gained the electron is termed electronegative element. The compound formed by electron transfer is termed as electrovalent compound.

Such type of linkage is common in inorganic compounds like NaCl, K_2S and $AlCl_3$ etc. and can be explained as follows:

NaCl Na 2, 8, 1 $\xrightarrow{-1e^-}$ Na^+ 2, 8 ⎤

    Cl 2, 8, 7 $\xrightarrow{+1e^-}$ Cl^- 2, 8, 8 ⎦ NaCl

K_2S 2 (K 2, 8, 8, 1) $\xrightarrow{-2e^-}$ $2K^+$ 2, 8, 8 ⎤

   S 2, 8, 6 $\xrightarrow{+2e^-}$ S^{-2} 2, 8, 8 ⎦ K_2S

$AlCl_3$ Al 2, 8, 3 $\xrightarrow{-3e^-}$ Al^{+3} 2, 8 ⎤

   3 Cl 2, 8, 7 $\xrightarrow{+3e^-}$ $3Cl^-$ 2, 8, 8 ⎦ $AlCl_3$

Electrovalent compounds are non-volatile, high melting, soluble in polar solvents and conduct electricity in solution due to ionic nature.

2. Covalent Bond

There are many atoms in the periodic table which neither lose nor gain electrons. Such atoms combine through a process of sharing of electrons so as to acquire stable electronic configuration. Each atom contributes one electron in this process of sharing.

$$A + B \longrightarrow A : B$$

The linkage resulted by equal contribution and equal sharing of electrons is termed as covalent bond. The combination between identical atoms, e.g., atoms of hydrogen, chlorine, nitrogen, oxygen, etc. to form molecules occurs by sharing of one or more pairs of electrons. Each atom acquires the stable configuration of inert gas. Structure of compounds such as methane, ammonia, water, etc. can be satisfactorily explained by covalent bond formation.

  Hydrogen $\overset{.}{H} + \overset{.}{H} \longrightarrow H : H$

  Water $2\overset{.}{H} + : \overset{..}{O} : \longrightarrow H : O : H$

Ammonia $3\overset{\cdot}{H} + :\overset{\cdot\cdot}{\underset{\cdot}{N}}: \longrightarrow H : \overset{\cdot\cdot}{N} : H$
$ H$

Methane $4H + :\overset{\cdot\cdot}{C}: \longrightarrow H : \overset{\cdot\cdot}{C} : H$
$ H$

The electrostatic attraction between the shared pair and the nuclei of the two atoms holds the atoms together. The atoms do not contain any charge as no transfer of electrons has taken place. Therefore, covalent compounds are non-polar, low melting and generally insoluble in polar solvents.

Single, double and triple covalent bonds: The single, double and triple covalent bonds are formed by sharing one, two or three pairs of electrons, respectively, and denoted by single, double or triple lines. For example:

$:\overset{\cdot\cdot}{\underset{\cdot\cdot}{Cl}}\cdot \qquad \times\overset{\times\times}{\underset{\times\times}{Cl}}\times \qquad :\overset{\cdot\cdot}{\underset{\cdot\cdot}{O}}: \qquad \times\overset{\times\times}{\underset{\times\times}{O}}\times \qquad :\overset{\cdot}{\underset{\cdot}{N}}: \quad \overset{\times}{\underset{\times}{N}}\times$

or   or   or

$Cl—Cl \qquad O=O \qquad N\equiv N$

In such cases each of the atoms has completed its octet and acquired a noble gas configuration.

3. Coordinate of Dative Bond

This type of bond is formed when both the electrons are provided by only one of the atoms for sharing between them. The shared pair of electrons is called *lone pair*, the atom which provides the pair of *electrons* is called *donor* and the atom accepting this pair is called the *acceptor*.

Usually the donor is an atom which has already acquired stable electronic configuration and the acceptor has generally two electron deficit configuration.

$:\overset{\cdot\cdot}{A} + \overset{\cdot\cdot}{B}: \longrightarrow A:B \text{ or } A \longrightarrow B$

Sulphur dioxide is the example formed by coordinate linkage.

O S O   or   O S $\longrightarrow$ O
Sulphur dioxide molecule

This type of linkage is represented by an arrow pointing towards the acceptor atom. Coordinate compounds behave very much like covalent compounds but are usually less volatile.

EQUILIBRIUM AND REVERSIBILITY

When a chemical reaction occurs, the products are formed. The compound formed may be dissociated to give the starting reagents and the reaction can take place in both the directions. But in any direction the extent of the reverse reaction is so small that it can be neglected. Such chemical reactions may thus be regarded as proceeding to completion in one direction. For example, when a mixture of two parts of hydrogen and one part of oxygen is reacted in the presence of an electric arc at ordinary temperature, complete conversion into water is resulted. But at temperatures $1500^\circ C$ or above water vapour is decomposed into hydrogen and oxygen to some extent. The reverse reaction, thus, definitely occurs at high temperatures.

When the conditions are such that both the forward and reverse reactions can occur to a noticeable extent, the process is described as a *reversible reaction*. If the substances are reacted in a closed vessel, so that the products of the forward reaction do not escape, the reactant cannot combine completely. As soon as the products are formed, they tend to react so as to reserve the process and regenerate the reacting substance, hence the reaction is not completed in either direction. If hydrogen and oxygen were heated together in a closed space at a temperature of 2000°C, for example, some of the reacting gases would remain unchanged, no matter how long the reaction was allowed to continue. Now consider a case of a reaction which is reversible at much lower temperature, e.g., formation of hydrogen iodide. A mixture of hydrogen gas and iodine vapour will not combine completely to form hydrogen iodide if heated in a closed vessel at 450°C. In the range of this temperature hydrogen and iodine react to yield hydrogen iodide, but the latter decompose to an appreciable extent into the starting elements. The reversible nature of the reaction is indicated by writing

$$H_2 + I_2 \rightleftharpoons 2HI$$

The reversible process not only occurs in gaseous phase, but the process is reversed in liquid and solid phases also at ordinary temperature. One of the examples of reversible process is the esterification, reaction between ethanol and acetic acid leading to the formation of ethyl acetate and water as represented by the equation

$$C_2H_5OH + CH_3COOH \rightleftharpoons CH_3COOC_2H_5 + H_2O$$

Starting with equivalent of alcohol and acid, the reaction proceeds until about two-thirds of the reacting substances have been converted into ester and water. In like manner, if equivalent quantity of ethyl acetate and water are brought together, the reaction proceeds in the direction indicated by the lower arrow, until about one-third of the original substances have been converted into acid and alcohol. In other words, the reaction is reversible, a condition of equilibrium resulting when the speeds of the two reactions, indicated by the upper and lower arrows, become equal. If a fixed amount of acid is taken, and the quantity of alcohol is varied, a corresponding displacement of the equilibrium results.

It has been found that after the lapse of a sufficient interval of time, all reversible reactions reach a state of **chemical equilibrium**. This is a state in which no further change in the composition with time can be detected, provided the temperature and pressure are not altered. If the conditions are properly chosen, exactly the same state of equilibrium may be attained from either direction for a given reversible reaction. For example, at a temperature of 25°C, the equilibrium mixture consists of 12 molecular per cent of hydrogen, 12 per cent of iodine vapour and 76 per cent of hydrogen iodide, irrespective of whether the starting point is hydrogen iodide or an equivalent mixture of hydrogen and iodine.

The composition of the system at equilibrium does not change if the temperature and pressure are not altered. There are two possibilities at this stage. Either the chemical reaction has ceased entirely so that the system is stationary, or the forward and reverse reactions are taking place simultaneously at exactly the same rate. It is now universally accepted that the latter condition is actually operative and that the system is in a state of *dynamic equilibrium*.

POLARITY OF BONDS

When the atoms forming a covalent bond are identical, e.g., H–H, Cl–Cl, etc., the sharing of electrons forming the bond will be equal between the two atoms. With the two atoms having different electronegativities the sharing of electrons will be unequal and will result in the development of polarity in the molecule. Such a covalent bond will have partial ionic character. Usually most of the bonds are intermediate between ionic and covalent bonds. Carbon and hydrogen do not differ much in electronegativities and so, compounds like methane, ethane, etc. are almost non-polar or pure covalent compounds. Chlorine has a much greater electronegativity than hydrogen. When chlorine and hydrogen combine to form covalent hydrogen chloride, the electrons forming the covalent bond are displaced towards the more electronegative chlorine without any separation of the nuclei.

$$H. + .\overset{..}{\underset{..}{Cl}}: \longrightarrow H :\overset{..}{\underset{..}{Cl}}: \text{ or } HCl$$

The hydrogen atom will, therefore, be slightly positively charged and the chlorine atom slightly negatively charged. A covalent bond, such as this, in which one atom has a larger share of the electron-pair, is said to possess partial ionic character. The compounds like H_2O, NH_3, C_2H_5OH, etc., are all having partial ionic or polar character.

In a bond between two atoms having larger difference in electronegativities, the electron cloud is distorted to such an extent that one of the atoms acquires a partial negative charge (δ^-) and the other, a partial positive charge (δ^+). The polarity or charge separation in molecules results in a dipole where two equal and opposite charges are separated by a distance. The dipole moment of such a compound may be expressed as:

$$\mu = e \times d$$

where e is the charge in esu and d is the distance in Å separating the two charges. Dipole moment (μ) is expressed in Debye. The limit 10^{-18} esu cm being called as Debye (D).

The dipole moment is a vector quantity and its direction is often indicated by an arrow parallel to the line joining the points of charge and pointing towards the negative end e.g. H→Cl. The greater the value of the dipole moment, the greater is the polarity of the bond.

However, simply the presence of a polar bond in a molecule is not enough to make it polar. Thus, there may be even number of such polar bonds or dipoles in opposite directions in space making the compound, as a whole, non-polar. In fact, all molecules possessing a centre of symmetry are non-polar, the explanation of this is important. The dipole moment is really a property of every bond between two different atoms; the observed dipole moment of a molecule is the vector sum of all the individual bond moments. In carbon tetrachloride, for example, each C–Cl bond possesses a dipole moment, but since the moment is symmetrical, the four bond moments cancel each other exactly to give a resultant dipole moment of zero. The same is true for stannic chloride, *p*-dichloro-benzene and for the hydrocarbons.

The zero dipole moment of carbon dioxide indiates that the molecule is symmetrical and linear but the association of a definite moment with the water molecule and with sulphur dioxide suggests that these latter substances have angular structures as indicated above. The arrows, which point from the positive to the negative end of the dipoles, indicate the directions of the various bond

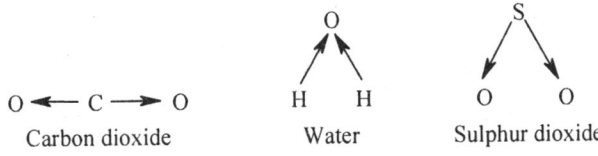

| Carbon dioxide | Water | Sulphur dioxide |

moments. In carbon dioxide, the two C–O bond moments cancel each other exactly, but the vector sums of the O–H moments in water, and S–O moments in sulphur dioxide, are not zero, since the molecules are not linear.

The dipole moments of a number of polar compounds are recorded in Table 4.1.

Table 4.1. Dipole moments (DPM) in the gaseous state in Debye unit (D)

Compound	DPM	Compound	DPM
Water	1.84	Methyl chloride	1.87
Ammonia	1.46	Acetone	2.88
Sulphur dioxide	1.63	Chlorobenzene	1.70
Hydrogen chloride	1.03	Aniline	1.53
Chloroform	1.02	Benzonitrile	4.42
Diethyl ether	1.15	Nitrobenzene	4.22
Ethanol	1.70	Toluene	0.43

In addition to these data in the table, it may be noted that hydrogen, carbon dioxide, carbon disulphide, carbon tetrachloride, stannic chloride, boron trichloride, paraffins, cyclohexane and benzene have zero moments.

Numerous applications, similar to those just described, have been made of dipole moments in the elucidation of the structures of inorganic and organic molecules. Measurements of dipole moments of benzene derivatives have confirmed that the benzene ring is a planar, regular hexagon, for only upon this basis, it is possible to explain quantitatively the observed moments

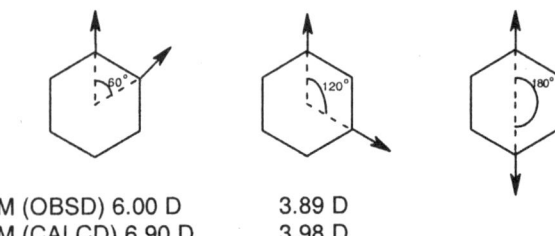

M (OBSD) 6.00 D   3.89 D
M (CALCD) 6.90 D   3.98 D

Fig. 4.3. Dipole moments of dinitrobenzene.

of ortho-, meta- and para-compounds. In ortho compounds, the bond moments of the two substituents will be co-planar and inclined at an angle of 60° and in the meta-compounds, the angle will be 120°. If the two substituents are the same, the para-component should have zero dipole moment. In the example in Fig. 4.3, the observed and calculated values of the dipole moments of the three dinitrobenzenes are given. The calculated values are based on 3.90 D for the moment of the $-NO_2$ group. In the case of o-substituted dinitrobenzene repulsion between the two groups is attributed. This makes the angle between the bond dipoles larger than 60° and the resultant dipole moment is consequently less than expected. It should be mentioned that para-compounds in which the substituents in both positions is – OR or – NR_2, do not have zero moments. The reason is that, like H_2O and NH_3 respectively, these groups have an angular structure and the group moment is not directed toward the centre of the benzene ring as it is with groups such as $-NO_2$, –CI, $-CH_3$ and –CN.

Physical and chemical properties of a molecule are concerned with bond polarities. The polarity of a bond determines the kind of reaction that can take place at that bond and even affects reactivity at nearby bonds. The polarity of bonds can lead to polarity of molecules and thus, profoundly affect melting point and solubility. (More details are beyond the scope of this book.)

5

Determination of Molecular Structure of Organic Compounds

In the determination of molecular structure of an organic compound the following steps are involved:

1. Detection of elements
2. Estimation of elements
3. Calculation of empirical formula
4. Calculation of molecular weight and molecular formula
5. Determination of molecular structure with the help of chemical reactions and spectroscopic methods

1. DETECTION OF ELEMENTS

Detection of carbon: This element is detected by heating substance strongly but carefully on a crucible lid or on a piece of platinum foil. The substance chars and gives a black carbonaceous mass, which burns away ultimately on prolonged heating. Sometimes many substances char only when heated with concentrated sulphuric acid and give dark solution showing some black particles, simultaneously some of the sulphuric acid gets reduced into sulphur dioxide, while carbon gets oxidised to oxides of carbon. There are some substances which do not get charred even when heated with concentrated sulphuric acid, e.g. acetic acid, formic acid, oxalic acid, etc.

A better and surer way for detecting carbon is by strongly heating the substance mixed with powdered copper oxide in a hard glass test tube. The carbon gets oxidised into carbon dioxide, which on being passed through lime water can be detected due to the formation of white precipitate of calcium carbonate.

Detection of hydrogen: Hydrogen element in the organic compounds is detected by the formation of drops of water in the cool part of the test tube during the above test. But in this case, care must be taken to see that both sample and the copper oxide have been dried before performing the test. (Hydrogen can also be detected together in the test as mentioned above.)

Detection of nitrogen, halogens and sulphur: All these elements are detected by **Lassaigne's test**. The organic compound is fused with metallic sodium to yield ionizable inorganic substances.

Nitrogen is converted into sodium cyanide, halogens into sodium halides and sulphur into sodium sulphide. The solution of the fused compound is boiled with freshly prepared saturated solution of ferrous sulphate and then dilute sulphuric acid is added. Development of prussian blue colour or precipitate indicates the presence of nitrogen.

Sulphur is detected in the fused mixture by adding ferric chloride. Appearance of a blood red colour confirms the presence of both of sulphur and nitrogen. If freshly prepared sodium nitroprusside is added in place of ferric chloride, a deep blue colour indicates sulphur only.

Detection of halogens is carried out by the addition of silver nitrate to the solution. A white or yellow precipitate indicates the presence of halogens. Chlorine water test is also performed for confirming bromine and iodine. If fluorine is present, the solution is acidified with glacial acetic acid, calcium chloride solution is added and allowed to stand for several hours. Formation of gelatinous calcium fluoride shows the presence of fluorine.

Besides Lassaigne's test, combustion and soda lime tests of organic compound for detection of nitrogen; oxidation of the substance with mixture of sodium carbonate and potassium nitrate to detect sulphur and Beilstein's flame test for halogen detection are also performed.

Detection of phosphorus: The compound is heated with either a fusion mixture (Na_2CO_3 + KNO_3) or concentrated nitric acid to yield phosphoric acid. The mixture so obtained is dissolved in water, boiled with nitric acid and then ammonium molybdate solution is added. If phosphorus is present, a yellow colour or precipitate is developed.

Detection of oxygen: Oxygen is detected indirectly by heating the compound alone in a dry test tube in an atmosphere of nitrogen. Drops of water are deposited in cooler part of the test tube if oxygen is present in a functional group like alcohol (–OH), aldehyde (–CHO), carboxylic (–COOH), etc., then these groups are detected by the usual conformational tests.

Detection of metals: The organic compounds containing metals are strongly heated. The organic part burns away and a residue is left if a metal is present. This residue is usually the oxide of the metal which is dissolved in an acid and is then detected by inorganic qualitative tests.

2. ESTIMATION OF ELEMENTS (QUANTITATIVE)

In determining molecular formula the next step is the quantitative analysis, i.e. estimation of elements by weight. The percentage composition of the compound is found out by weight. Different methods employed for this purpose are given below:

(I) Estimation of Carbon and Hydrogen

The principle of the estimation depends upon the method of burning of substance in oxygen as stated above. This method was derived by Liebig in 1931. An organic substance is burnt in excess of oxygen, when carbon and hydrogen present in the substance are oxidised to carbon dioxide and water. Knowing the weight of CO_2 and H_2O, the percentage composition of carbon and hydrogen is calculated.

$$2C_xHy \ + \ 5/2O_2 \ \longrightarrow \ 2xCO_2 \ + \ y/2H_2O$$
Organic substance

Apparatus: The apparatus (Fig. 5.1) employed for the purpose consists of the following units:

(i) **Oxygen supply:** The oxygen is allowed to bubble through potassium hydroxide solution

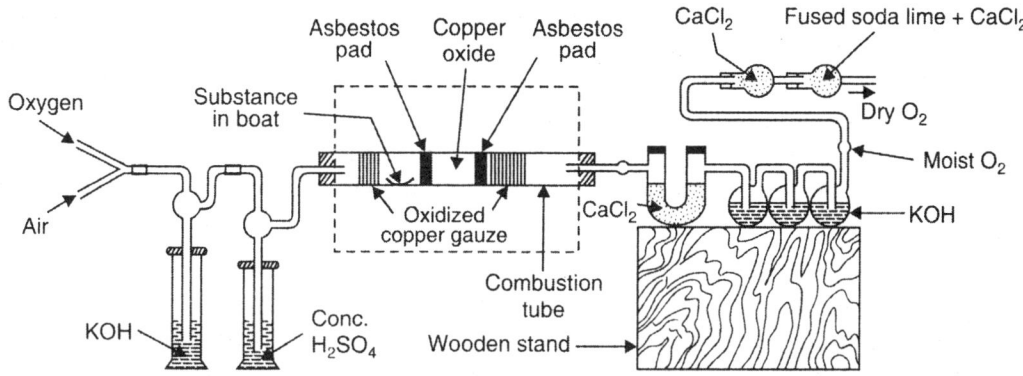

Fig. 5.1. Liebig's apparatus for estimation of carbon and hydrogen.

followed by conc. sulphuric acid and then passed through the tube charged with soda lime (CaO + NaOH). The oxygen gas thus, free from moisture and carbon dioxide, enters into the combustion tube.

(ii) **Combustion tube:** It is a hard glass tube about 90 cm in length and 1.5 cm in internal diameter and is open at both ends. It is used for the combustion of the organic substance. It has, as shown in diagram, the following zones and fittings:

(a) **An oxidised copper packing** which prevents the backward diffusion of the products of the combustion and also to heat the porcelain boat by radiation.

(b) **A porcelain boat containing a known weight** (about 0.2 g) of the organic substance.

(c) **An oxidised copper box placed towards the end** of the combustion tube to prevent any vapour of the organic substance leaving the tube unoxidised.

(d) A coarse cupric oxide is packed between two asbestos pads which oxidises organic vapour passing through it.

(e) A bright copper spiral is placed near the exit which reduces nitrogen oxides into nitrogen if formed in vapours. In this way, oxides of nitrogen are not absorbed in caustic potash solution and nitrogen gas escapes unabsorbed.

(f) If the compound contains halogens, volatile copper halides are produced and absorbed in the absorption unit. This can be prevented, if a bright silver gauze roll is placed near the exit end. This decomposes volatile copper halides forming non-volatile silver halides. Free halogens also combine with silver giving silver halides.

(g) In case the substance contains sulphur or sulphur and halogens both, a layer of lead chromate is placed near the exit. At high temperature lead chromate acts as an oxidising agent and forms non-volatile lead halides. It also reacts with sulphur dioxide formed during combustion to give non-volatile lead sulphate.

(iii) **Combustion furnace:** It is an asbestos lined semicylindrical sheet iron tray, about 80–85 cm in length. Gas burners are fitted in a row under the tray to heat the iron tube placed in the furnace. The top of the tray is covered by fire-clay tiles, which can be raised or lowered to increase or decrease the intensity of heat as required.

(iv) **Absorption apparatus:** The product of combustion containing moisture and carbon dioxide is then passed onto the absorption apparatus which consists of:

(a) A weighed U-tube packed with pumice stone soaked in concentrated sulphuric acid or anhydrous $CaCl_2$ in the tube to absorb water.

(b) A weighed U-tube containing strong solution of KOH to absorb CO_2.

(c) A guard tube filled with anhydrous $CaCl_2$ to prevent the entry of moisture from the atmosphere.

Procedure: The tube is heated strongly to dry its contents and drive out the carbon dioxide present in it by passing a current of dry and pure oxygen through it. It is then cooled and connected to the absorption apparatus. The other end of the combination tube is opened for a while and a boat containing a weighed quantity of the organic substance is introduced. The tube is heated strongly till the whole of the substance in the boat has burnt away. This takes above two hours. Finally, a strong current of oxygen is passed through the combustion tube to sweep away any traces of carbon or moisture, which may have been left in it. The two tubes are detached and the increase in weight in each of them is determined.

Calculations: Suppose the weight of the organic substance taken $= w$ g

Increase in weight of U-tube $(H_2O) = x$ g

Increase in weight of second U-tube $(CO_2) = y$ g

We know that: $\quad \dfrac{H_2O}{18} = \dfrac{2H}{2} \qquad \dfrac{CO_2}{44} = \dfrac{C}{12}$

$$
\begin{aligned}
&\text{18 g water contains hydrogen} && = 2 \text{ g} \\
&\text{1 g water contains hydrogen} && = 2/18 \times x \text{ g} \\
&x \text{ g water contains hydrogen} && = (2 \times x)/18 \\
&\text{\% of hydrogen in organic substance} && = 2/18 \times x/w \times 100
\end{aligned}
$$

Similarly,
$$
\begin{aligned}
&\text{44 g of } CO_2 \text{ contains carbon} && = 12 \text{ g} \\
&\text{1 g of } CO_2 \text{ contains carbon} && = 12/44 \text{ g} \\
&y \text{ g of } CO_2 \text{ contains carbon} && = 12/44 \times y \text{ g} \\
&\text{\% of carbon in organic substance} && = 12/44 \times y/w \times 100
\end{aligned}
$$

Example 1: 0.2613 g of an organic substance on combustion in oxygen gave 0.7310 g of carbon dioxide and 0.3527 g of water. Find out the percentage of carbon and hydrogen in the substance.

Weight of organic compound (w) = 0.2613 g

Weight of carbon dioxide (y) = 0.7310 g

Weight of water (x) = 0.3527 g

We know that: $\quad \dfrac{CO_2}{44} = \dfrac{C}{12} \qquad \dfrac{H_2O}{18} = \dfrac{2H}{2}$

Applying the formula:

$$\text{Percentage of carbon in organic substance} = \frac{12 \times y \times 100}{44 \times w} = \frac{12 \times 0.7310 \times 100}{44 \times 0.2613} = 85\%$$

Percentage of hydrogen in the given substance $= \dfrac{2 \times 100 \times x}{18 \times w} = \dfrac{2 \times 100 \times 0.3527}{18 \times 0.2613} = 15\%$

Answer: Carbon: 85%; Hydrogen = 15%.

II. Estimation of Oxygen

In a usual method, oxygen is estimated indirectly by difference calculating the total percentage of various elements and subtracting it from one hundred. The remainder will be the percentage of oxygen.

Example 2: 0.6 g of an organic substance gives 1.17 g of carbon dioxide and 0.84 g of water on combustion. Calculate its percentage composition.

$$\text{Percentage of carbon} = \dfrac{1.17 \times 12}{44} \times \dfrac{100}{0.6}$$

$$= \dfrac{117 \times 12 \times 100}{44 \times 600} \times \dfrac{585}{11} = 53.8\%$$

$$\text{Percentage of hydrogen} = \dfrac{0.84 \times 2}{18} \times \dfrac{100}{0.6}$$

$$= \dfrac{84 \times 2 \times 100}{18 \times 60} \times \dfrac{560}{18} = 31.27\%$$

Hence, percentage of oxygen $= 100 - (53.8 + 31.27) = 14.93$

However, oxygen is now estimated by any one of the following methods:

1. **Meulen's method:** In this method, a known organic compound is subjected to pyrolysis in a current of dry hydrogen. The gases produced are passed over red hot platinised asbestos. The oxygen of the substance is converted into CO, CO_2 and H_2O.

This gaseous mixture is then passed over a heated catalyst, e.g. finely divided nickel on thorium oxide in the presence of excess of hydrogen at $350^{\circ}C$. The oxides of carbon are reduced to methane and the oxygen is quantitativel converted into water vapour.

$$CO + 3H_2 \longrightarrow CH_4 + H_2O$$
$$CO_2 + 4H_2 \longrightarrow CH_4 + 2H_2O$$

The water vapour formed is absorbed in a weighed calcium chloride tube. Knowing the weight of water, the percentage of oxygen can be calculated.

$$\text{Percentage of oxygen} = \dfrac{\text{wt. of } H_2O}{\text{wt. of the substance}} \times \dfrac{16}{18} \times 100$$

2. **Aluise method:** In this method, a known weight of organic substance is decomposed by heating in a stream of nitrogen. The oxygen is converted to carbon monoxide when it is passed through on bed of granular carbon at $1100^{\circ}C$ along with other gaseous products.

$$\text{Compound} \xrightarrow{\text{Pyrolysis}} \text{Oxygen} + \text{Gaseous products}$$

$$O_2 + 2C \xrightarrow[1100^{\circ}C]{} 2CO$$

The acidic impurities obtained due to the presence of halogens, nitrogen, sulphur and phosphorus in the compound are removed by passing CO_2 gas through soda-asbestos U-tube. Pure dry CO obtained in this way is passed through a tube containing iodine pentoxide at 175°C when CO_2 is produced due to oxidation of CO.

$$5CO + I_2O_5 \xrightarrow{\text{175°C}} 5CO_2 + I_2$$

The resulting gaseous mixture of CO_2 and I_2 is passed through potassium iodide, which absorbs iodine. Carbon dioxide gas passing out is then absorbed in a weighed soda-asbestos U-tube. Knowing the weight of carbon dioxide, the weight of oxygen and hence, its percentage can be determined in the organic substance.

III. Estimation of Nitrogen

Two methods are mainly used for the estimation of nitrogen in an organic substance.

Duma's method: Nearly all the compounds containing nitrogen can be estimated by this method.

Principle:

$$C_xH_yN_z + CuO \longrightarrow xCO_2 + y/2H_2O + z/2N_2$$

This method is based on the fact that when an organic substance is burnt with cupric oxide in the atmosphere of carbon dioxide, carbon, hydrogen and sulphur are converted into their oxides and nitrogen is set free. This mixture of gases is passed through bright copper spiral. Nitrogen, if oxidised into nitrogen oxides, is reduced into nitrogen. The gaseous mixture is passed through caustic potash solution where carbon dioxide, sulphur dioxide and moisture (water) are absorbed and nitrogen is collected in a nitrometer. Knowing the volume of nitrogen gas, percentage of nitrogen can be calculated.

The apparatus (Fig. 5.2) consists of:

(i) **Carbon dioxide gas generator:** The current of oxygen is replaced in nitrogen estimation by CO_2 which is produced by heating magnesite marble and dil. HCl.

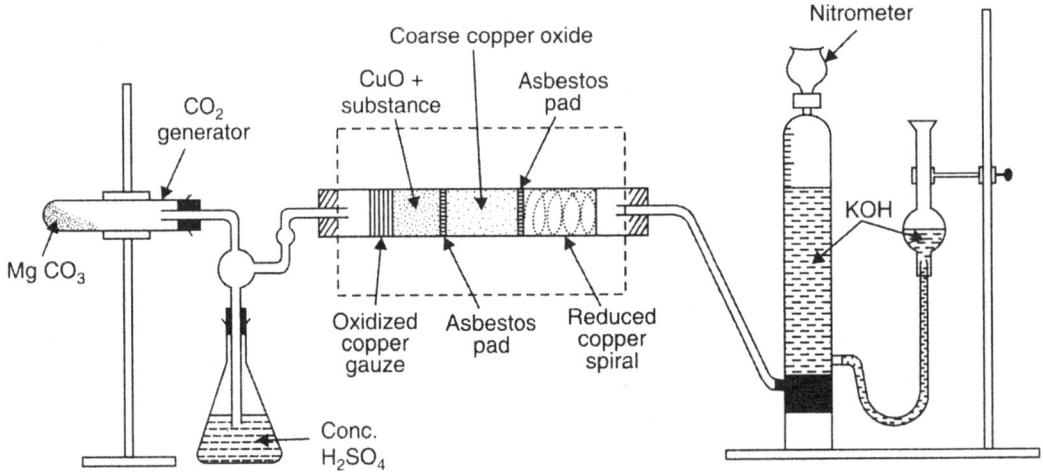

Fig. 5.2. Duma's apparatus used for estimation of nitrogen.

The generator is a hard glass tube containing the marble.

$$MgCO_3 \longrightarrow MgO + CO_2$$

$$CaCO_3 + 2HCl \longrightarrow CaCl_2 + CO_2 + H_2O$$

(ii) **Combustion tube:** The combustion tube of about 90 cm in length and 1.5 cm in diameter opens at both ends. The tube is heated in a combustion furnace as described in the case of carbon and hydrogen estimation. The other parts of the tube are:

(a) A roll of oxidised copper gauze to prevent back diffusion of the products of combustion.
(b) A weighed amount (about 200 mg) of the organic substance mixed with excess of cupric oxide.
(c) A long layer of coarse cupric oxide packed in position by asbestos plugs on either side.
(d) A bright copper spiral which reduces any oxides of nitrogen formed during combustion to nitrogen.

(iii) **Schiff's nitrometer:** It is a graduated tube filled with KOH solution, provided with a funnel, a tap at its upper end and the two side tubes near the lower end. One side tube is connected with combustion tube and the other with a 50 percent caustic potash solution reservoir with a little mercury at the bottom. Mercury allows the gas to go in the nitrometer but does not allow the back flow of the potash solution.

Procedure: The apparatus is fitted as shown in Fig. 5.2. A known weight of organic substance, mixed with CuO, is placed in the combustion tube in between oxidised copper roll and coarse copper oxide. The combustion tube is placed in the furnace. A current of CO_2 is now passed through the combustion tube. When no more air bubbles collect in the nitrometer, it shows that whole of the air has been displaced. The upper tap of the nitrometer is now opened and the reservoir is raised till the KOH solution level reaches the tap which is then closed. On heating the compound in the furnace, nitrogen is set free from the compound and is collected in the nitrometer. If any nitrogen oxide is formed, it is reduced into nitrogen by bright copper spiral, while carbon dioxide and the water are absorbed in KOH solution.

$$2NO + 2Cu \longrightarrow N_2 + Cu_2O$$

When the combustion is complete, a strong current of CO_2 is passed through the combustion tube to sweep away the traces of nitrogen. The volume of nitrogen is now carefully noted. Room temperature and pressure are also noted.

Calculation: Knowing the volume of nitrogen, temperature and pressure, the volume of nitrogen at N.T.P. is calculated. From the volume of nitrogen at N.T.P., its weight is determined from the relation that 22,400 ml weighs 28 g. Knowing the weight of nitrogen, its percentage composition is calculated.

$$\text{Percentage of } N_2 = \frac{\text{Weight of } N_2}{\text{Weight of organic compound}} \times 100$$

$$= \frac{28v}{22400} \times \frac{100}{w}$$

where v = volume of N_2 (ml)

Example 3: 0.1877 g of an organic substance when analysed by the Duma's method yielded 31.7 ml of moist nitrogen measured at 14°C and 758 mm mercury pressure. Determine the percentage of nitrogen in the substance (aqueous tension at 14°C is 12 mm).

Applying the gas equation to calculate the volume of N_2 at N.T.P.

$$\frac{P_1 V_1}{T_1} = \frac{P_2 V_2}{T_2}$$

$$P_1 V_1 T_2 = P_2 V_2 T_1$$

$P_1 = 758 \times 12.0 = 646$ mm

$P_2 = 760$ mm

$$V_2 = \frac{P_1 V_1 T_2}{P_2 T_1}$$

$T_1 = 273 + 14 = 287°$ K

$$V_2 = \frac{746 \times 31.7 \times 273}{760 \times 287}$$

$T_2 = 273°$ K

$V_1 = 31.7$ ml

$V_2 = ?$

Volume of N_2 (V_2) = 29.6 ml

Now weight of 22,400 ml of N_2 gas at N.T.P. = 28 g

1 ml of 22,400 ml of N_2 gas at N.T.P. = $\dfrac{28}{22,400}$

29.6 ml of 22,400 ml of N_2 gas at N.T.P. = $\dfrac{28 \times 29.6}{22,400}$

Weight of N_2 = 0.037 g

$$\text{Percentage of } N_2 = \frac{0.037 \times 100}{0.1877} = \frac{37,000}{1877} = 19.71\%$$

Example 4: (i) 0.15 g of a base gave on ignition 0.3882 g of CO_2 and 0.1160 g of H_2O. (ii) Its 0.31 g gave 35.5 ml of nitrogen in Duma's method at 17°C and 750 mm pressure. Calculate the percentage composition of the compound.

$$\text{Percentage of carbon} = \frac{\text{Weight of } CO_2 \times 12}{44} \times \frac{100}{w}$$

$$= \frac{0.3882 \times 12}{44} \times \frac{100}{0.15} = 70.5\%$$

$$\text{Percentage of hydrogen} = \frac{\text{Weight of } H_2 \times 2}{18} \times \frac{100}{w}$$

$$= \frac{0.1160 \times 2}{18} \times \frac{100}{0.15} = 8.6\%$$

For the second experiment:

Let V be the volume of the gas at N.T.P.

Then $\dfrac{760 \times V}{273} = \dfrac{736.6 \times 35.5 \times 273}{760 \times 290} = 33.32$ ml

$V = \dfrac{736.6 \times 35.5 \times 273}{760 \times 290} = 33.32$ ml

Weight of 33.32 ml of nitrogen at N.T.P. $= \dfrac{33.32}{22,400} \times 28$

Hence percentage of nitrogen $= \dfrac{33.32 \times 28}{22,400} \times \dfrac{100}{0.31} = 13.44\%$

Percentage of oxygen $= 100 - (70.5 + 8.6 + 13.44) = 7.46$.

Example 5: An organic compound gave the following results on analysis: (a) 0.73 g of the compound gave 1.32 g of CO_2 and 0.6 g of water. (b) 0.365 g of compound gave 56 ml of moist nitrogen at 14°C and 760 mm mercury pressure (aqueous tension is 14 mm). Calculate its percentage composition.

$$\text{Percentage of carbon} = \dfrac{1.32 \times 12}{44} \times \dfrac{100}{0.73} = 49.3\%$$

$$\text{Percentage of hydrogen} = \dfrac{0.6 \times 2}{18} \times \dfrac{100}{0.73} = 9.5\%$$

For the second experiment:

Let V_2 be the volume of the gas at N.T.P.

$$V_2 = \dfrac{P_1 V_1 T_2}{P_2 V_1} = \dfrac{746 \times 56 \times 273}{760 \times 287} = 49.99 \text{ ml}$$

Weight of 22,400 ml N_2 at N.T.P. = 28 g

1 ml of 22,400 ml N_2 at N.T.P. $= \dfrac{28}{22,400}$ g

29.99 ml of 22,400 ml N_2 at N.T.P $= \dfrac{28 \times 49.99}{22,400} = 0.062$ g

Here percentage of nitrogen $= \dfrac{0.062 \times 100}{0.365} = 17\%$

Percentage of oxygen $= 100 - (49.3 + 9.5 + 17) = 24.2\%$

Kjeldahl's method: This method is based upon the fact that when an organic substance containing nitrogen is heated strongly with conc. H_2SO_4 acid in the presence of little copper sulphate and potassium sulphate, nitrogen of organic compound is quantitatively converted into ammonium sulphate. This, on further heating with NaOH solution, evolves ammonia which is absorbed in a known volume of standard acid.

$$\text{Nitrogenous organic compound} + \text{Conc. } H_2SO_4 \xrightarrow{K_2SO_4} (NH_4)_2SO_4$$

$$(NH_4)_2SO_4 + 2NaOH \longrightarrow Na_2SO_4 + 2NH_3 + 2H_2O$$

This method is generally employed for estimation of nitrogen in food and fertilizer in which nitrogen is joined to carbon and hydrogen.

Procedure: About 0.5 g accurately weighed organic substance, 20 ml conc. H_2SO_4, 10 g potassium sulphate and one drop of mercury or few crystals of copper sulphate are taken in the Kjeldahl's flask (Fig. 5.3) and heated strongly. Potassium sulphate is used to increase the boiling point of sulphuric acid while mercury acts as a catalyst. In the beginning, the contents of the flask get darkened and then become clear, indicating that the whole nitrogen is being converted into ammonium sulphate.

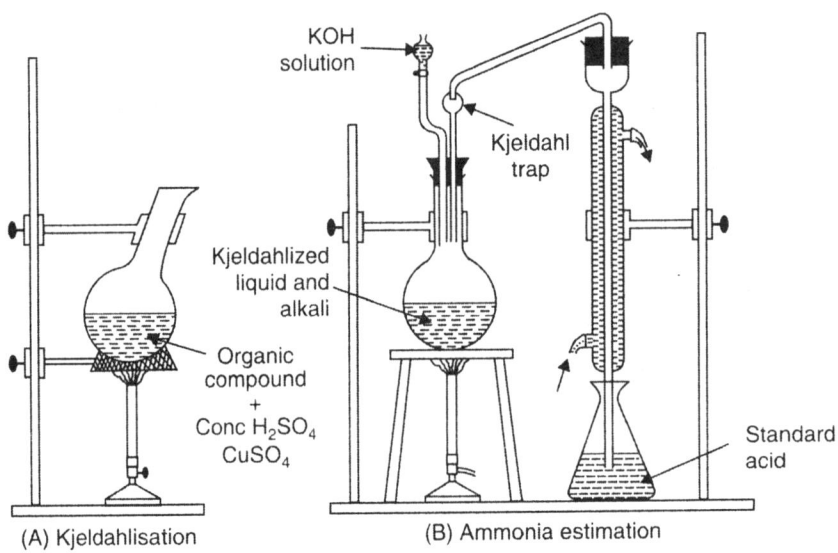

Fig. 5.3. Kjeldahl's apparatus for estimation of nitrogen.

The above contents (Kjeldahlized liquid) are taken in a flask fitted with a condenser as shown in Fig. 5.3. Sodium hydroxide solution is added from the funnel. Ammonia is evolved on heating which is bubbled in a flask containing known volume of standard acid. Some of the acid is utilized and the remaining acid is back titrated with standard alkali.

Calculation: The weight of organic substance = w g

Volume of 1 normal acid which completely neutralized ammonia = V ml

Volume of 1 N normal acid which completely neutralized ammonia = V ml

V ml of 1 normal acid = V ml of normal ammonia

1000 ml N normal ammonia $\equiv$ 17 g of $NH_3 \equiv$ 14 g of nitrogen

Amount of nitrogen present in V ml of N normal $NH_3 \equiv \dfrac{14}{1000} \times N \times V$

$$\text{Percentage of } N_2 = \frac{14}{1000} \times N \times V \times \frac{100}{w}$$

Example 6: 0.257 g of nitrogenous organic substance was Kjeldahlized and ammonia gas evolved was absorbed in 50 ml of N/10 HCl, which required 23.2 ml of NaOH for neutralization. Determine the percentage of nitrogen in the substance.

$w = 0.257$ g

$V = 50 - 23.2 = 26.8$ ml

$$\text{Amount of } N_2 \text{ present in 26.8 ml of N/10 HCl acid} = \frac{26.8}{1000} \times \frac{1}{10} \times 14$$

$$\text{Percentage of } N_2 = \frac{26.8 \times 14}{1000 \times 10} \times \frac{100}{0.257} = 15$$

Example 7: 0.24 g of an organic substance was Kjeldahlized and ammonia formed was absorbed in 50 ml of N/4 H_2SO_4 acid. The excess of acid required 77 ml of N/10 NaOH solution for complete neutralization. Calculate the percentage of nitrogen in the sample.

Wt. of the organic substance = 0.24 g, 50 ml of N/4 $H_2SO_4 \equiv 12.5$ ml of 1 N H_2SO_4

Volume of H_2SO_4 taken = 50 ml, 77 ml of N/10 NaOH $\equiv 7.7$ ml of 1 N NaOH

Volume of H_2SO_4 consumed in neutralization of ammonia = 12.5 − 7.7 = 4.8 ml

$$\text{Percentage of nitrogen} = \frac{1.4 \, NV}{w} = \frac{1.4 \times 1 \times 4.8}{0.24} = 28$$

IV. Estimation of Halogens

The following are the more common methods used for the estimation of halogens.

(a) **Carius method:** In this method, an organic compound of known weight is heated with concentrated nitric acid and silver nitrate in a sealed tube to give carbon dioxide, water and silver halide. From the amount of silver halide, the percentage of halogen is determined.

Procedure: For the estimation of halogens, a special hard glass tube known as **Carius** or **Bomb tube**, which is 20 to 50 cm long and has 2 to 2.5 cm diameter, is used. About 5 ml of conc. HNO_3 and 0.5 g of silver nitrate are kept in the tube. An accurately weighed amount (0.2 g) of organic compound is taken in a small tube and this tube is then introduced along the side of the Carius tube. Upper end of the Carius tube is sealed carefully as shown in Fig. 5.4.

Carius tube is now wrapped in asbestos paper and heated strongly in a bomb furnace for 5–6 h at 250–300°C. The furnace is put off and the tube is heated with Bunsen flame to soften when gases present inside under pressure escape. The sealed end is cut and the contents transferred into a beaker. The precipitated silver halides are washed, dried and weighed.

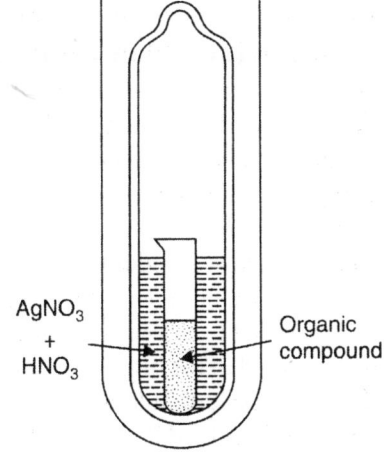

Fig. 5.4. Carius tube used for estimation of halogens.

Calculation: Molecular weight of silver chloride = 143.5 g.

One gram molecular weight of silver chloride contains 35.5 g of chloride. Hence weight of chloride present in a certain weight of silver chloride = Wt. of AgCl = $\dfrac{35.5}{143.5}$

Percentage of chlorine = Wt. of AgCl $\times \dfrac{35.5}{143.5} \times \dfrac{100}{\text{Wt. of compound}}$

Similarly, percentage of bromine = Wt. of AgBr $\times \dfrac{80}{188} \times \dfrac{100}{\text{Wt. of compound}}$

and percentage of iodine = Wt. of AgI $\times \dfrac{127}{235} \times \dfrac{100}{\text{Wt. of compound}}$

Example 8: In a Carius method 0.369 g of an organic compound when heated with conc. HNO_3 and silver nitrate gave 0.345 g of silver bromide. Calculate the percentage of bromine in the organic compound.

Wt. of organic substance taken = 0.369 g

Molecular wt. of AgBr = 108 + 80 = 188 g

Since 188 g of silver bromide contains 80 g of bromine

0.345 g of silver bromide contains $\dfrac{80}{188} \times 0.345$ g of bromine

Therefore, percentage of bromine = $\dfrac{80}{188} \times 0.345 \times \dfrac{100}{0.369} = 39.75$

Carius method is suitable for volatile compounds and the substances which are decomposed by nitric acid. With iodide compounds satisfactory results are not obtained, since silver formed is slightly soluble in concentrated nitric acid, and also iodine is liberated in the free form. With highly halogenated compounds the reaction is not complete.

(b) **Peria and Schiff's method:** This method is more suitable for those compounds which are not completely decomposed by nitric acid. In this method accurately weighed quantity (about 0.2 to 0.3 g) of the organic compound is mixed with an intimate mixture of sodium carbonate-lime mixture (1 : 4) in a platinum crucible. The crucible is filled up with more sodium carbonate-lime mixture completely and inverted on the base of bigger crucible. More sodium carbonate-lime mixture

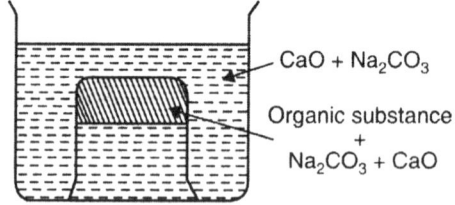

Fig. 5.5. Peria and Schiff's method for estimation of halogens.

is then filled in the bigger crucible to cover the smaller crucible completely (Fig. 5.5). The contents of the bigger crucible are heated on a blow pipe to fuse the mixture. It is then cooled and the contents dissolved in excess of dilute nitric acid when the halogen is precipitated by adding silver nitrate solution. This is separated, washed, dried and weighed. The percentage of halogen is then calculated from the weight of silver halides obtained as shown in case of Carius method.

When iodine is estimated, sodium carbonate is used in place of sodium carbonate-lime mixture, because iodine compounds react with lime to give insoluble calcium iodate.

(c) **Stepanov's method:** Accurately weighed quantity (about 0.2 g) of the organic compound is taken in a round-bottomed flask and refluxed with 98% ethanol (Fig. 5.6). Calculated amount of metallic sodium pieces are added through the condenser within half an hour and the flask is heated on a steam bath for 40 minutes to dissolve all the sodium. The halogen present in the compound is quantitatively converted into sodium halide.

$$RX + C_2H_5OH + 2Na \longrightarrow C_2H_5ONa + RH + NaX$$

After the completion of the reaction, ethanol is distilled off, residue dissolved in nitric acid and filtered. Silver nitrate solution is added to the filtrate and the silver halide precipitated is filtered, washed and dried. Knowing the weight of silver halide, the percentage of halogen can be calculated in the organic compound.

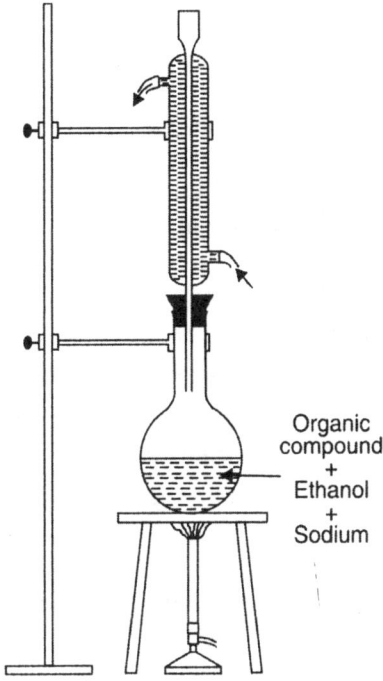

Organic compound + Ethanol + Sodium

Fig. 5.6. Stepanov's method for estimation of halogen.

(d) **Robertson's method:** This method is used for the estimation of halogen in volatile compounds. The substance is treated with a strong oxidizing agent like chromic acid and pure air is blown. The vapourized substance is passed through red hot silica tube containing finely divided platinum when the halogen is set free. This is absorbed in alkaline hydrogen peroxide and estimated by titrating against standard silver nitrate solution.

V. Estimation of Sulphur

The principle involved in the estimation of sulphur is that when an organic compound containing sulphur of calculated amount is oxidized, sulphur is converted into sulphuric acid. Barium chloride is added to it when the sulphate ions are precipitated as barium sulphate. Knowing the weight of barium sulphate, the weight of sulphur can be calculated and from this the percentage of sulphur in organic compound can be worked out. One of the two methods used is as follows:

Carius method: In this method, about 0.2 to 0.3 g of the organic compound is heated with concentrated nitric acid in a sealed Carius tube at 250–300°C for four hours. The furnace is then put off to cool to the room temperature. Carius tube is taken out and the contents are transferred to a beaker. Barium chloride solution is added to it along with a little dilute hydrochloric acid and the precipitated barium sulphate is separated and dried. From the weight of barium sulphate, the percentage of sulphur in the substance is calculated as given below:

Calculations:

Weight of organic compound = W g

Weight of barium sulphate = X g

Molecular weight of barium sulphate $(BaSO_4) = (137.4 + 32 + 64) = 233.34$

Since 233.34 g of $BaSO_4$ contains 32 g of sulphur

X g of $BaSO_4$ contains $\dfrac{32X}{233.34}$ g of sulphur

Percentage of sulphur in the compound $= \dfrac{32X}{233.34} \times \dfrac{100}{W}$

Example 9: 0.16 g of an organic compound containing sulphur was heated with concentrated nitric acid and the resultant solution on treatment with barium chloride gave 0.466 g of barium sulphate. Calculate the percentage of sulphur in the organic compound.

Wt. of the organic compound = 0.16 g

Wt. of barium sulphate = 0.466 g

Molecular weight of barium sulphate = 233.34

Since 233.34 g of $BaSO_4$ contains 32 g of sulphur

Therefore, 0.466 g of $BaSO_4$ contains $\dfrac{32 \times 0.466}{233.34}$

Percentage of sulphur $= \dfrac{32 \times 0.466 \times 100}{233.34 \times 0.16}$

$= 40.01.$

DETERMINATION OF MOLECULAR WEIGHTS AND MOLECULAR FORMULA

Molecular weight of a substance is the weight of a molecule of that substance as compared to the one-twelfth of ^{12}C isotope of carbon. The molecular weight expressed in grams is called the gram-molecular weight. In case of volatile compounds, it is expressed as the gram-molecular volume which is the volume occupied by the vapour of one gram molecular weight of a substance at N.T.P. The value at N.T.P. is 224 litres.

Molecular weight of a compound can be calculated by adding the atomic weights of all the atoms present in the molecule, e.g.

Molecular weight of C_2H_5OH = 2 (At. wt. of carbon) +

6 (At. wt. of hydrogen) +

1 (At. wt. of oxygen)

$= (2 \times 12) + (6 \times 1) + (16 \times 1)$

$= 24 + 6 + 16 = 46$

DETERMINATION OF MOLECULAR WEIGHT

Both physical and chemical methods are used for determining the molecular weight. Now-a-days, spectroscopic method (mass spectrum) is widely used for this purpose.

I. PHYSICAL METHODS

Different physical methods are used for the determination of molecular weights of volatile and non-volatile compounds.

1. Molecular Weight of Volatile Compounds

For the determination of molecular weights of volatile substances, a known weight of the compound is converted into vapour and the volume obtained is reduced to N.T.P. Knowing this volume, the weight of 22,400 ml of the vapour is calculated.

$$\text{Thus Mol. wt.} = \frac{\text{Weight of volatile compound} \times 22,400}{\text{Reduced volume at N.T.P.}}$$

By determining the vapour density (V.D.) from a convenient method, the molecular weight of a volatile compound can be calculated directly from the relationship:

$$\text{Molecular weight} = 2 \times \text{V.D.}$$

$$\text{V.D.} = \frac{\text{Weight of } V \text{ ml of vapour at N.T.P.}}{\text{Weight of } V \text{ ml of hydrogen at N.T.P.}}$$

$$= \frac{w}{V \times 0.00009}$$

$$= \frac{w}{V \times \dfrac{2}{22,400}} = \frac{w \times 22,400}{V \times 2}$$

A brief account for the various methods used is given below:

(a) **Victor Mayer's method:** In this method, a volatile compound of known weight is vapourised in Victor Mayer's tube. The vapour collected is measured at N.T.P. and the weight of 22.4 litres of vapour is determined to give the molecular weight.

(b) **Duma's method:** In this method, Duma's bulb is filled with the vapour of the volatile compound at a known temperature and pressure. The weight of the vapour in the bulb is found out to know the vapour density. From this molecular weight is calculated. This method is not generally used.

(c) **Hofmann's method:** This method is employed for those substances which decompose when boiled at atmospheric pressure. A known weight of the organic compound is introduced in a barometer tube at the top of mercury level. The tube is surrounded by a heating cover. The substance is vapourized and the volume of the vapour produced is noted at a given temperature. Molecular weight of the substance can be calculated from the weight and volume of the vapour.

2. Molecular Weight of Non-Volatile Compounds

The different methods employed for the determination of molecular weights of non-volatile compounds are given below:

   (a) Freezing point depression method.
   (b) Boiling point elevation method.

The principle involved in these methods is that every liquid freezes and boils at fixed temperature. When a solution is added to it, the lowering of freezing point or elevation of boiling point takes place which is proportional to the molecular concentration of the substance dissolved. Equimolecular quantities of different solutions dissolved in a fixed weight of the solvent will produce the same elevation in the boiling point or depression in freezing point. For example, when one gram molecular weight of any solution is dissolved in 100 g of water, the freezing point is always lowered by 18.6°C and the boiling point is raised by 52°C. These values are referred to as molecular depression constant and molecular elevation constant, respectively, for the solvent and they are denoted by K.

Let w g of a solution be dissolved in W g of the solvent causing the freezing point to be lowered by ΔT.

Hence ΔT will also be depression caused by dissolving $w/W \times 100$ g of the substance in 100 g of the solvent. If M is the molecular weight, then M g of the substance dissolved in 100 g of the solvent will cause a depression K.

Now, T is the depression by $w/W \times 100$ g

Therefore, $M = w/W \times 100 \times K/T$

$$M = \frac{w \times K \times 100}{W \times T}$$

(a) Beckmann's Freezing Point Depression Method

About 20 g of the solvent is taken in a freezing tube, surrounded by a jacket tube. This is kept in a freezing mixture along with the jacket tube. The content is stirred with a platinum stirrer and the temperature is noted when the solvent freezes.

The freezing tube is taken out and the solvent melted by warming. A known amount (w g) of the solute is added from the side tube and the temperature is pointed when the solution freezes as in the previous case. The difference of the two freezing points gives the depression ΔT. From these observations, the molecular weight is determined by the expression:

$$M = \frac{w \times K \times 100}{W \times \Delta T}$$

where w = wt. of the solute
   W = wt. of the solvent
   ΔT = F.P. depression
   K = molecular depression constant

(b) Landberger's Method of Elevation in Boiling Point

In this method, a pure solvent is boiled in a flask and the vapours are allowed to bubble in a boiling tube containing the solvent. When the solvent in the boiling tube begins to boil and the vapours pass, the temperature is noted.

A weighed amount of the solute is now added to the boiling tube, vapours are again passed and the boiling point of the solution is determined. The volume of the solution is now noted. The weight of the solution is calculated by knowing the density of the solution. Subtracting the weight of the solute from that of the solution, the weight of the pure solvent is known. The difference in the two boiling points observed is ΔT, i.e. the elevation in boiling point. The molecular weight can be calculated from the expression:

$$M = \frac{w \times K \times 100}{W \times \Delta T}$$

where w = wt. of the solute
$\quad\quad W$ = wt. of the solvent
$\quad\quad K$ = molecular elevation constant
$\quad\quad \Delta T$ = elevation in boiling point

For detail account of the above methods, a textbook of physical chemistry may be consulted.

II. CHEMICAL METHODS

Molecular weights of acids and bases are generally determined by chemical methods.

(a) Silver Salt Method for Acids

The principle involved in this method is that most of the organic acids form insoluble silver salts. When these salts are ignited, a metallic silver residue is obtained. By knowing the weights of silver salts and silver residue, the equivalent weight of the acid can be calculated.

In this method, a neutral solution is obtained by treating acid solution with ammonium hydroxide which is treated with silver nitrate solution. The precipitated silver salt is filtered, washed and dried. A known weight of this salt is ignited in a platinum crucible until a constant weight is obtained. From these observations, the equivalent weight of silver can be calculated as follows:

$\quad\quad$ Wt. of silver salt taken = W g
$\quad\quad$ Wt. of metallic silver = X g

Now, one atom of hydrogen (H) is equivalent to one atom of silver (Ag). Hence one equivalent of silver salt will contain one atom of silver in place of hydrogen in the acid molecule. Therefore, if E is the equivalent weight of the acid, then the equivalent weight of silver salt will be $(E - H + Ag)$ or $(E - 1 + 108)$ or $(E + 107)$.

Now X g of silver is obtained from W g of salt.

Therefore, 108 g are obtained from $\dfrac{W}{X} \times 108$ g of salt

Therefore, equivalent of silver salt is = $\dfrac{W}{X} \times 108$

Therefore,$\quad\quad\quad\quad\quad\quad E + 107 = \dfrac{W}{X} \times 108$

or$\quad\quad\quad\quad\quad\quad\quad E = \left(\dfrac{W}{X} \times 108\right) - 107$

Now, if n be the basicity of the acid, then

$\quad\quad$ Molecular weight of the acid $= \left[\left(\dfrac{W}{X} \times 108\right) - 107\right] \times n$

(b) Platinichloride Method for Bases

The method is based on the principle that organic bases form insoluble double salts with chloroplatinic acid, H_2PtCl_6, which when ignited leaves a residue of metallic platinum. Knowing the weights of chloroplatinate double salts and the platinum obtained, molecular weight of the base can be calculated. On multiplication of equivalent by the acidity of the base, the molecular weight is obtained.

$$\text{Wt. of platinichloride} = W \text{ g}$$

$$\text{Wt. of platinum obtained} = X \text{ g}$$

If B is the equivalent weight of the base, then the molecular formula of the platinichloride will be $B_2H_2PtCl_6$ (since the acid H_2PtCl_6 is dibasic).

Therefore, molecular weight of platinichloride $= 2B + 2 + 195 + (35.5 \times 6)$
$$= 2B + 410$$

Now one molecule of chloroplatinate on heating leaves one atom of platinum:

$$B_2H_2PtCl_6 \longrightarrow Pt$$
$$(2B + 410) \qquad 195$$

Hence, if X g of platinum is obtained from W g of salt

then, 195 g of plantinum is obtained from $\dfrac{W}{X} \times 195$ g of salt

Therefore, $B_2H_2PtC_6$ of platinum is obtained from $\dfrac{W}{X} \times 195$

or $$2B + 410 = \dfrac{W}{X} \times 195$$

or $$2B = \left[\left(\dfrac{W}{X} \times 195\right) - 410\right]$$

or $$B = 1/2\left[\left(\dfrac{W}{X} \times 195\right) - 410\right]$$

If n is the acidity of the base, then

Molecular weight of the base $= n/2 \times \left[\left(\dfrac{W}{X} \times 195\right) - 410\right]$

(c) Volumetric Method of Acids and Bases

This method is used for determination of equivalent weight of the acids and bases both. A known weight of the organic acid is dissolved in water or alcohol and the solution titrated against a standard alkali using an indicator. From the volume consumed and strength of alkali used, the weight of acid is found which would require 1000 ml of N alkali for neutralization. In this way, we obtain gram-equivalent weight of the acid. This equivalent weight multiplied by the basicity gives the molecular weight.

Let the weight of the acid used be X g and the volume of N/10 alkali used for neutralization be V ml.

Thus V ml of N/10 alkali $\equiv X$ g of acid

Therefore, 1000 ml of N alkali $\equiv \dfrac{X \times 10 \times 1000}{V}$ g of acid

Equivalent weight of the acid $= \dfrac{X \times 10 \times 1000}{V}$ g

Now, if n be the basicity of the acid, then

Molecular weight of the acid $= n \left(\dfrac{X \times 10 \times 1000}{V} \right)$

Example 10: 0.2 g of tribasic acid required for neutralization 27 ml of N/10 NaOH solution. Calculate the molecular weight of the acid.

27 ml of N/10 NaOH $\equiv$ 0.2 g of a tribasic acid.

$$\frac{1000 \text{ ml of 1 N NaOH}}{1 \text{ g eq. weight}} \equiv \frac{0.2 \times 10 \times 1000}{27}$$

Eq. wt. of the acid $\equiv 74$

Mol. wt. $\equiv$ Eq. wt. $\times$ Basicity of an acid

Mol. wt. of tribasic acid $= 74 \times 3 = 222$

Example 11: 0.177 gm of dibasic acid required 30 ml of N/10 NaOH. Calculate the mol. wt. of the acid.

30 ml of N/10 NaOH $=$ 0.177 g of dibasic acid

1000 ml of 1 N NaOH $= \dfrac{0.177 \times 10 \times 1000}{30}$

Eq. wt. of acid $= 59$

Mol wt. $=$ Eq. wt. $\times$ Basicity of acid
$$= 59 \times 2$$
$$= 118$$

III. MASS SPECTROMETER

When an organic compound is bombarded with high energy electrons in a mass spectrometer in vacuum, it is converted into positive ions by loss of an electron. This positively charged ion possessing energy immediately undergoes fragmentation into smaller ions, which in turn can undergo further fragmentation. Generally, these fragmented ions carry a unit positive charge. They are passed through negativity charged accelerating plates and then sorted out into a spectrum according to their mass to charge (m/e) ratio by the analyzing magnet. Thus, the mass spectrum is a graph of the intensity of the beams of ions plotted against the mass number and so the masses of the ions can be determined. Since most ions have unit positive charge, m/e is equivalent to m.

$$M + e \longrightarrow M^+ + 2e$$

A single molecule like methane (CH_4) may break into several positive ions corresponding to mass number of 16, 15, 14, 13, 12 and 1. Out of these, peak corresponding to 16 is the base peak and it will be most intense followed by the peaks at mass 15, 12 and 1 due to the greater stability of these ions as compared to ions corresponding to mass 14 and 13.

In mass spectrum a single molecule gives a whole spectrum of masses. The largest peak in a spectrum corresponds to the most abundant ion and is known as base peak. The base peak is used to report mass spectra in a standardised form. Its intensity is given the value of 100 and all other peaks are reported as percentages of the base peak. The base peak corresponds to the mass of parent molecule minus one electron. It provides very accurate method of determining molecular weights of organic compounds.

Mass spectrometry may be used with gases, liquids and solids and only very small amount of material is necessary. It is extremely valuable for the determination of accurate molecular weights, obtaining molecular formula, elucidation of structure, quantitative analysis of mixture, ionization potentials and bond strengths.

EMPIRICAL FORMULA

From the knowledge of percentage composition and molecular weight of a substance, we can calculate the empirical and molecular formulae. The empirical formula of a compound is the simplest formula which expresses the relative number of atoms of constituent elements present in the molecule. The steps involved in the calculation of empirical formula are given below:

   (i) The percentage of each element is divided by its molecular weight. It gives the relative number of different atoms present in the molecule.
  (ii) The relative number or different atoms obtained in the above step are divided by the lowest one amongst them to obtain the simple atomic ratio of atoms present in the molecule.
 (iii) The number expressing the atomic ratio may or may not be whole number. If it is not the whole number, then they are multiplied by suitable common factor to convert each one of them to whole numbers. Minor fractions are neglected.
  (iv) The symbols of each element present are written in a line side by side and the respective numbers giving the atomic ratio are put as subscripts at the lower right corner of each respective element. This gives the empirical formula.

Example 12: An organic compound on analysis gave the following percentage composition of the elements: Carbon 54.54%, Hydrogen 9.09% and Oxygen 36.37%. Calculate the empirical formula of the compound.

Element	At. wt.	Percentage	Relative number of atoms	Atomic ratio
Carbon	12	54.54	$\dfrac{54.54}{12} = 4.54$	$\dfrac{4.45}{2.27} = 2$
Hydrogen	1	9.09	$\dfrac{9.09}{1} = 9.09$	$\dfrac{9.09}{2.27} = 4$
Oxygen	16	36.37	$\dfrac{36.37}{16} = 2.27$	$\dfrac{2.27}{2.27} = 1$

Empirical formula of the compound is C_2H_4O.

Example 13: An organic compound containing carbon, hydrogen, nitrogen and oxygen on analysis gave the following values: Carbon 41.35%, Hydrogen 6.89%, Nitrogen 24.12% and Oxygen 27.64%. Find out the simplest formula.

Element	Percentage	At. wt.	Relative ratio	Simple ratio
C	41.35	12	3.45	2
H	6.89	1	6.89	4
N	24.12	14	1.73	1
O	27.64	16	1.72	1

Empirical formula = C_2H_4NO

DETERMINATION OF MOLECULAR FORMULA

The formula expressing the actual number of atoms of various elements present in a molecule of the compound is called the molecular formula. It may be either the same as the empirical formula or a simple multiple of it.

Therefore, molecular formula = empirical formula $\times n$, where n is a whole number. The value of n is obtained as:

$$n = \frac{\text{Molecular wt.}}{\text{Empirical formula wt.}}$$

To determine the molecular formula, the value of n is obtained and then the empirical formula is multiplied by n to get the number of atoms present in the molecular formula.

Example 14: 0.2137 g of an organic compound on combustion gave 0.4862 g CO_2 and 0.1938 g water. If 0.152 g of the same substance is dissolved in 25 g of water, a depression of 0.19°C in freezing point of water is produced (molecular depression constant is 18.5°C for 100 g of water). Find out the molecular formula of the compound.

(i) **Empirical formula:**

% of carbon $= \dfrac{12}{44} \times \dfrac{0.4862}{0.2137} \times 100 = 62.04$

% of hydrogen $= \dfrac{2}{18} \times \dfrac{0.1938}{0.2137} \times 100 = 10.08$

% of oxygen $= 100 - (62.04 + 10.08) = 27.88$

Element	At. wt.	Percentage	Relative number of atoms	Atomic ratio
Carbon	12	62.04	$\dfrac{62.04}{12} = 5.17$	$\dfrac{5.27}{1.74} = 3$
Hydrogen	1	10.08	$\dfrac{10.08}{1} = 10.08$	$\dfrac{10.08}{1.74} = 6$
Oxygen	16	27.88	$\dfrac{27.88}{16} = 1.74$	$\dfrac{1.74}{1.74} = 1$

Empirical formula is C_3H_6O.

(ii) **Molecular weight and formula:**

$$\text{Molecular weight, M} = \frac{100 \times K \times w}{W \times t}$$

where K = molecular depression constant

w = weight of the solute

W = weight of the solvent

t = depression in freezing point

$$\text{Therefore, M} = \frac{100 \times 18.5 \times 0.152}{25 \times 0.19} = 59.2$$

Empirical formula weight = $(12 \times 3) + (1 \times 6) + (16 \times 1) = 58$

Now, $\dfrac{\text{Mol. wt.}}{\text{Empirical formula wt.}} = \dfrac{59.2}{58} = 1$

Therefore, molecular formula is $(C_3H_6O)_1$ or C_3H_6O.

Example 15: (a) An organic compound which is a monobasic acid analysed for carbon, hydrogen, chlorine and oxygen was found to contain C = 18.6%, H = 1.55%, Cl = 55.84% and O = 24.8%. Calculate the empirical formula. (b) 0.2709 g of the above acid dissolved in water neutralizes 25.2 ml of N/12 NaOH solution. Calculate the molecular formula of the compound.

(a)

Element	% of element	At. wt.	Relative ratio	Simple ratio
C	18.60	12	1.55	1
H	1.55	1	1.55	1
Cl	55.84	35.5	1.55	1
O	24.8	16	1.55	1

Empirical formula is CHClO.

(b) We know that empirical formula is CHClO.

$$25.2 \text{ ml of N/12 NaOH} = \frac{0.2709 \times 1000}{25.2 \times 12}$$

Mol. wt. of acid = 129 g

Empirical formula wt. = 12 + 1 + 35.5 + 16 = 64.5 gm

$$N = \frac{\text{Mol. wt.}}{\text{Empirical formula wt.}}$$

$$N = \frac{129}{64.5} = 2$$

Mol. formula = $(CHClO)_2$ or $C_2H_2Cl_2O_2 = CHCl_2COOH$.

The compound is dichloroacetic acid.

DETERMINATION OF MOLECULAR STRUCTURE WITH THE HELP OF CHEMICAL REACTIONS AND SPECTROSCOPIC METHODS

For determining the molecular structure of an unknown compound, a detailed study of its chemical reactions is carried out. Various functional groups like $-OH$, $-COOH$, $-CHO$, $-CO$, $-NH_2$, $-CONH_2$ etc. are detected by usual tests. Specific organic qualitative methods are used for identification of natural products, such as steroids, tannins, saponins, amino acids, proteins, carbohydrates, glycosides, oils, fats etc. Compound of higher molecular weights are degraded into smaller molecules of known structures. For example, protein is hydrolyzed to yield amino acids, which are separated and identified. An organic compound having a complicated structure can also be synthesized, starting from the known molecules of low molecular weight to obtain it in its original form for verification of its structure, e.g. tridecene–2–al–(1) can be synthesized from acetylene as starting material and by converting it into phenylhydrazone derivative and its structure can be verified.

Spectroscopy is the most recent and important tool for elucidating the structures of organic compounds. The generally employed physical methods are ultraviolet (UV) (200–400 nm), visible spectroscopy (400–750 nm), infrared (IR) spectroscopy (400–650 cm^{-1}), Raman spectroscopy, nuclear magnetic resonance (NMR) spectroscopy and mass spectroscopy.

A few functional groups and unsaturations are detected with the help of UV and visible spectroscopic methods, while an IR and Raman spectra give information about the presence of various functional groups, hydrogen bonding, cis- and trans-isomers, etc. NMR is used for the correlation of hydrogens present in a molecule in different structural environments and for studying chemical exchange in active hydrogen compounds. Mass spectrometry is employed in the study of reaction mechanism and for determination of molecular weights and molecular formulae.

When sufficient evidences are obtained the structure, which best fits the facts, is accepted. Sometimes, two or more structures fit the findings almost equally well. In such cases the compound exists in both the forms which are in equilibrium. This phenomenon is known as tautomerism discussed in detail in the chapter of Isomerism.

STRUCTURAL FORMULA

Empirical and molecular formulae give the relative number and actual number of atoms, respectively, and they do not give the mode of internal linking of various atoms in the molecule. The formula showing the mode of linking of various atoms in the molecule is called the structural formula.

For determining the structural formula, a detailed study of functional groups and properties of organic compounds is done. For example, a compound having the molecular formula C_3H_7Cl can be represented as the following:

$$CH_3CH_2CH_2Cl \text{ and } CH_3 - \underset{\underset{\underset{(II)}{Cl}}{|}}{CH} - CH_3$$

$$(I)$$

Now, if the compound forms n-propanol on hydrolysis with aqueous alkali then the molecule has the structure (I) and if not it has the structure (II).

If the compound is represented by its structural formula, then it requires a lot of space and the chemical reactions cannot be represented conveniently. Therefore, short form of structural formula is used in practice and it is called **Rational formula**. It gives the complete idea about the constitution of the compound. The mode of linking between atoms usually shown by dots. For example, acetic anhydride can be represented as:

$C_4H_6O_3$

Molecular
formula

$(CH_3CO)_2O$ or

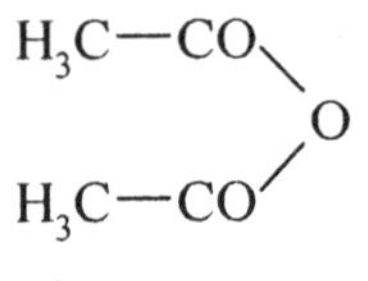

$H_3C—CO$
$\diagdown$
O
$\diagup$
$H_3C—CO$

Rational formula

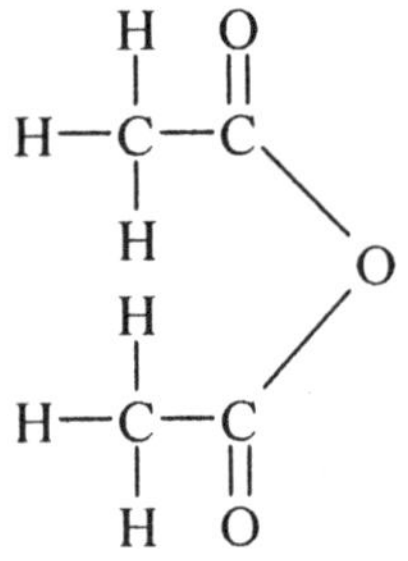

Structural formula

Nomenclature of Organic Compounds

Whenever anyone wants to get himself introduced to someone, he has to, first of all, tell his name. Thus, it is the name that matters. To study the chemistry of an organic compound, a name is first given to it. Due to the occurrence of huge number of organic compounds in this universe, there was a problem to name these compounds. The early chemists usually named the compound according to the source from which it was obtained or on the basis of its structure or properties. Thus, the names methanol (meaning spirit of wood), citric acid (from citrus plant), urea (from urine), formic acid (from formica or red ants), acetic acid (from vinegar), malic acid (from apple), etc. were based on their sources from which they were obtained. Similarly, the names of glucose (sweet), pentane (five), hexane (six), were derived from the Greek words describing their properties and structure. These names are called **trivial** or **common names**.

However, as the number of known organic compounds increased, it became very difficult to assign common names to each compound. The common names given did not have any logic and a single compound was given different names by different chemists. Keeping all these things in mind, it became apparent that it was necessary to systematize the method of nomenclature. This work began in 1892 when an International Committee of Chemists met in Geneva to give a system of naming known as the Geneva System of Nomenclature. The work was revised by the International Union of Chemists (IUC) by a committee appointed in 1922 and in 1931 and the system is known as **IUC System of Nomenclature**. Nomenclature is always undergoing revision, and the latest rules for naming the compounds are recommended by the Commission of the International Union of Pure and Applied Chemistry (IUPAC) in 1957 and 1967. The name assigned to a compound based on the IUPAC rules is known as its **systematic name**.

The names of various homologous series and their particular members are given below:

1. Saturated Hydrocarbons (Alkanes or Paraffins)

The general formula for alkanes is C_nH_{2n+2} and they are considered as the parent compounds for writing the structure of all the known organic compounds. The first four members of the family are known by their common names in all the systems. For the rest of the members, the name is simply derived from the Greek prefix for the particular number of carbons in the alkane, e.g. **pentane** for five, **hexane** for six, **heptane** for seven, **octane** for eight and so on. The hydrocarbon residues formed by the removal of one hydrogen from the alkanes are called **alkyl groups** and are named by dropping '**ane**' from the name of the corresponding alkane and then suffixing 'yl'. The examples are given in the following table:

Formula of alkane	Common name	IUPAC name	Formula of alkyl group	IUPAC name of alkyl group
C_nH_{2n+2}	Paraffins	Alkanes	R–	Alkyl
CH_4	Methane	Methane	CH_3-	Methyl
C_2H_6	Ethane	Ethane	C_2H_5-	Ethyl
C_3H_8	Propane	Propane	C_3H_7-	Propyl
C_4H_{10}	Butane	Butane	C_3H_9-	Butyl
C_5H_{12}	–	Pentane	$C_6H_{11}-$	Pentyl
C_6H_{14}	–	Hexane	$C_6H_{13}-$	Hexyl
C_7H_{16}	–	Heptane	$C_7H_{15}-$	Heptyl
C_8H_{18}	–	Octane	$C_8H_{17}-$	Octyl
C_9H_{20}	–	Nonane	$C_9H_{19}-$	Nonyl
$C_{10}H_{22}$	–	Decane	$C_{10}H_{21}-$	Decyl
$C_{11}H_{24}$	–	Undecane	$C_{11}H_{23}-$	Undecyl

The hydrocarbons having three or more carbon atoms exist in various isomeric form. For example, propyl group may be represented by two isomeric structures known as n-propyl ($CH_3CH_2CH_2-$) and isopropyl [$(CH_3)_2CH-$]; a butyl group by four isomeric structures and amyl group by five isomeric forms and so on. For example, in case of butyl radical we have:

$$CH_3CH_2CH_2CH_2- \qquad (CH_3)_2CH-CH_2- \qquad (CH_3)_3 \cdot C- \qquad CH_3-\overset{\textstyle |}{CH}-CH_2-CH_3$$

n-butyl   iso-butyl   tert-butyl   sec-butyl

2. Alkenes or Olefins

The general formula for alkenes is C_nH_{2n}. These are the unsaturated compounds containing carbon-carbon double bond. For simpler alkenes, the names used are ethylene, propylene and butylene. The butylenes are differentiated by the prefixes cis- and trans-. The other higher alkenes are referred to as pentylenes, hexylenes, heptylenes and so on. In IUPAC system, the name for a particular member of this series is derived from the name of the alkane containing the same number of carbon atoms by substituting the 'ane' suffix of alkane by 'ene'. The longest continuous chain that contains the carbon-carbon double bond is selected as the parent structure and the chain is numbered from the side of the double bond.

The hydrocarbon radicals formed by the removal of one hydrogen from the alkenes are named as alkenyl groups. Thus:

Formula of alkenes	Common name	IUPAC name	Formula of alkenyl group	IUPAC name of alkenyl group
C_nH_{2n}	Alkylenes	Alkenes	$RCH = CH-$	Alkenyl
C_2H_4	Ethylene	Ethene (Vinyl group)	$CH_2 = CH-$	Ethenyl
C_3H_6	Propylene	Propene	$CH_2 = CH \cdot CH_2-$ (Allyl group)	Propenyl
C_4H_8	Butylene	Butene	Bond at different positions	Butenyl
C_5H_{10}	Pentylene	Pentene	,,	Pentenyl
$C_{10}H_{20}$	Decylene	Decene	,,	Decenyl

3. Alkynes or Acetylenes

The general formula for alkyne family is C_nH_{2n-2} and the compounds contain carbon-carbon triple bond. The common name of the first member is acetylene. There is no relationship in the other names of alkynes. For naming the alkynes in IUPAC system, the rules are exactly the same as for the naming of alkenes, except that the ending 'ene' is replaced by 'yne'. The hydrocarbon residue obtained by removing one hydrogen from the alkyne is reported as alkynyl group. For example:

Formula of alkynes	Common name	IUPAC name	Formula of alkynyl group	IUPAC name of alkynyl group
C_nH_{2n-2}	Acetylenes	Alkenes	$RC \equiv C-$	Alkynyl
C_2H_2	Acetylene	Ethyne	$CH \equiv C-$ (Acetylide group)	Ethynyl
C_3H_4	Methyl acetylene	Propyne	$CH \equiv C- CH_2-$ (Propargyl group)	Propynyl
$C_{10}H_{18}$		Decyne		

4. Alkyl Halides

The halogen derivatives are obtained by the replacement of one or more hydrogen atoms of the hydrocarbons by halogens. Depending on the number of halogens, they are classified as mono-, di-, tri- or poly-halogen compounds.

(i) **Monohalogen derivatives:** The general formula for monohalogen derivatives or alkyl halides is R–X, where R stands for alkyl group and X for halogen. The common names are derived from the alkyl group. In IUPAC system, they are considered as halogen derivatives of alkanes. For example:

Formula	Common name	IUPAC name
R–X	Alkyl halides	Haloalkanes
CH_3Cl	Methyl chloride	Chloromethane
C_2H_5Br	Ethyl bromide	Bromoethane
C_3H_7F	Propyl fluoride	Fluoropropane
C_4H_9I	Butyl iodide	Iodobutane
$C_{10}H_{21}Cl$	Decyl chloride	Chlorodecane

(ii) **Dihalogen derivatives:** Replacement of two halogens gives dihalo derivatives. The two halogens may be attached to the same carbon atom (**gem-dihalides or alkylidene halides**) or they may be attached to adjacent carbon atoms (**vic-dihalides or alkylene halides**). In IUPAC they are considered as dihalo derivatives of alkanes. For example:

Formula	Common name	IUPAC name
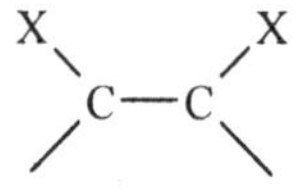 $\underset{}{\overset{X}{\underset{}{\diagdown}}}C—C\underset{}{\overset{X}{\diagup}}$	vic-dihalide or Alkylene halide	1,2-Dihaloalkane
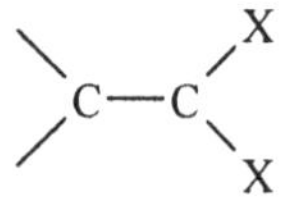 $C—C\underset{X}{\overset{X}{\diagup}}$	gem-dihalide or Alkylidene halide	1,1-Dihaloalkane
$Br–CH_2–CH_2–CH_2–Br$	Trimethylene bromide	1,3-Dibromopropane
CH_2I_2	Methylene iodide	Diiodomethane

(iii) **Tri- and polyhalogen derivatives:** These compounds, obtained by substitution of three or more hydrogens by halogens, are named similar to the dihalogen derivatives. For example:

Formula	Common name	IUPAC name
CHI_3	Iodoform	Triiodomethane
CH_3Cl_3	Chloroform	Trichloromethane
CCl_4	Carbon tetrachloride	Tetrachloromethane
$CH_2Br·CHBr·CH_2Br$	–	1,2,3-Tribromopropane
CCl_2F_2	Freon	Dichlorodifluoromethane

(iv) **Halogen derivatives of unsaturated hydrocarbons:** The common names of these compounds are derived from the names of unsaturated residues, while in IUPAC system they are regarded as the halogen derivatives of the corresponding unsaturated hydrocarbons. Thus:

Formula	Common name	IUPAC name
$CH_2 = CH–Cl$	Vinyl chloride	1-Chloroethene
$CH_2 = CH–CH_2Br$	Allyl bromide	3-Bromo-1-propene
$CH \equiv C–CH_2I$	Propargyl iodide	3-Iodo-1-propyne

5. Alcohols or Alkanols

Alcohols are the compounds having hydroxyl (–OH) functional group. The common name consists simply of the name of the alkyl group followed by the word **alcohol**. Alcohols are also named in the carbinol system in which alcohols are considered to be derived from methyl alcohol, by replacing one or more hydrogen atoms by other groups. In IUPAC system the 'e' of alkane is replaced by 'ol' to name the alcohols. The hydroxyl group may be primary, secondary or tertiary. The alcohols are classified into mono-, di-, tri- and polyhydric alcohols according to the presence of one, two, three and many hydroxyl groups in the molecule. Thus:

Formula	Common name	Carbinol name	IUPAC name
R–OH	Alkyl alcohol	Alkyl carbinol	Alkanol
CH_3OH	Methyl alcohol	Carbinol	Methanol
C_2H_5OH	Ethyl alcohol	Methyl carbinol	Ethanol
$CH_3.CH_2.CH_2–OH$	n-propyl alcohol	Ethyl carbinol	1-Propanol
$(CH_3)_3.C–OH$	t-Butyl alcohol	Trimethyl carbinol	2-Methyl-2-propanol
$(CH_3)_2.CH–CH_2OH$	Isopropyl alcohol	Isopropyl carbinol	2-Methyl-1-propanol
$C_{10}H_{21}OH$	–	Nonyl carbinol	1-Decanol

The common names of the dihydric alcohols are glycols, while their systematic names are obtained by adding suffix 'diol' after the names of parent alkanes and the positions of these groups are indicated by numbers. Thus:

Formula	Common name	IUPAC name
$CH_2OH.CH_2OH$	Ethylene glycol	Ethane-1,2-diol
$CH_3.CH_2OH.CH_2OH$	Propylene glycol	Propane-1,2-diol
$CH_2OH.CH_2.CH_2OH$	Trimethylene glycol	Propane-1,3-diol
$CH_2OH.CH_2.CH_2.CH_2OH$	Tetramethylene glycol	Butane-1,4-diol

The common name of trihydric alcohol ($CH_2OH \cdot CHOH \cdot CH_2OH$) is glycerol and that of polyhydric alcohol, $C_6H_8(OH)_6$, is sorbitol.

The IUPAC names of these important alcohols are 1,2,3-propanetriol and 1,2,3,4,5,6-hexanehexol, respectively.

6. Ethers or Alkoxyalkanes

Ethers are compounds of the general formula R–O–R′ where R and R′ may be same or different alkyl or aryl groups. To name ethers the two groups that are attached to oxygen are named and these names are followed by the word ether. The systematic name for the ethers is alkoxyalkane, e.g.:

Formula	Common name	IUPAC name
R–O–R′	Dialkyl ether	Alkoxylkane
$CH_3–O–CH_3$	Dimethyl ether	Methoxymethane
$CH_3–O–C_2H_5$	Ethyl methyl ether	Methoxyethane
$C_2H_5.O.C_2H_5$	Diethyl ether	Ethoxyethane
$C_3H_7.O.C_2H_5$	Ethyl propyl ether	Ethoxypropane

7. Aldehydes or Alkanals

The common names of aldehydes, containing –CHO functional group, have been derived from the names of the corresponding carboxylic acids by replacing **-ic acid** by **-aldehyde**. However, in

IUPAC system, the longest chain carrying –CHO group is considered the parent structure and is named by replacing the -e of the corresponding alkane by -al. Thus:

Formula	Common name	IUPAC name
R–CHO	Aldehyde	Alkanal
H.CHO	Formaldehyde	Methanal
CH_3CHO	Acetaldehyde	Ethanal
$C_2H_5.CHO$	Propionaldehyde	Propanal
C_3H_7CHO	Butyraldehyde	Butanal
$C_4H_9.CHO$	Valeraldehyde	Pentanal
$C_8H_{17}.CHO$	–	Octanal

8. Ketones or Alkanones

The common name of carbonyl compound having C = O group, where the two valencies of the carbon are satisfied with two alkyl groups, is ketone. According to the IUPAC system, the longest chain carrying the carbonyl group is considered the parent structure, and is named by replacing -e of the corresponding alkane with one. For example:

Formula	Common name	IUPAC name
R.CO.R′	Ketone	Alkanone
$CH_3CO.CH_3$	Acetone	Propanone
$CH_3CO.C_2H_5$	Ethyl methyl ketone	Butanone
$C_2H_5.CO.C_2H_5$	Diethyl ketone	3-Pentanone
$C_2H_5.CO.C_3H_7$	Ethyl propyl ketone	3-Hexanone

9. Carboxylic Acids or Alkanoic Acids

Carboxylic acids contain –COOH functional group and they are known as mono-, di-, tri-, or poly-carboxylic acids, due to the presence of one, two, three or more carboxylic groups. The common names of these compounds have been derived from the source from where they are obtained. The name in IUPAC system considers the longest chain carrying the carboxylic group as the parent structure, and is named by replacing the -e of the corresponding alkane with -oic acid. For example:

Formula	Source	Common name	IUPAC name
R.COOH	–	Monocarboxylic acid	Alkanoic acid
H.COOH	Red ant (formica)	Formic acid	Methanoic acid
$CH_3.COOH$	Vinegar (acetum)	Acetic acid	Ethanoic acid
$C_2H_5.COOH$	–	Propionic acid	Propanoic acid
$C_3H_7.COOH$	Butter (butyrum)	Butyric acid	Butanoic acid
$C_4H_9.COOH$	Root of Valerian plant	Valeric acid	Pentanoic acid
$C_9H_{19}.COOH$	Gout butter (Caper)	Capric acid	Decanoic acid
$C_{11}H_{23}.COOH$	Laurel oil	Lauric acid	Dodecanoic acid

The systematic name of dicarboxylic acid is **alkanedioic acid**. Thus:

Formula	Common name	IUPAC name
COOH.COOH	Oxalic acid	Ethanedioic acid
HOOC.CH$_2$.COOH	Malonic acid	Propanedioic acid
HOOC.CH$_2$.CH$_2$.COOH	Succinic acid	Butanedioic acid
HOOC.CH = CH.COOH	Maleic acid	Butenedioic acid
HOOC.(CH$_2$)$_3$.COOH	Glutaric acid	Pentanedioic acid
HOOC.(CH$_2$)$_4$.COOH	Adipic acid	Hexanedioic acid

The IUPAC names of tri- and poly-carboxylic acids are alkane-trioic and alkane-polyoic acids, respectively.

10. Derivatives of Carboxylic Acids

The various derivatives of carboxylic acids are given below:

(i) **Acid halides or acyl halides:** The systematic names of acid halides, obtained by replacing –OH of the –COOH group by a halogen, are derived by substituting the 'e' of alkane by 'yl halides'. Thus:

Formula	Common name	IUPAC name
R–COX	Acyl halide	Alkanoyl halides
H.COCl	Formyl chloride	Methanoyl chloride
CH$_3$.COCl	Acetyl chloride	Ethanoyl chloride
C$_2$H$_5$.COI	Propionyl iodide	Propanoyl iodide
C$_3$H$_7$.COBr	Butyl bromide	Butanoyl bromide
C$_4$H$_9$.COCl	Valeryl chloride	Pentanoyl chloride

(ii) **Acid anhydrides:** These compounds have two acyl groups attached to an oxygen atom. The common names of symmetrical anhydrides are derived from the parent acids, whereas the names of unsymmetrical anhydrides contain the names of both the parent acids. In IUPAC system they are named by replacing 'acid' by 'anhydride' from the name of the corresponding acid. For example:

Formula	Common name	IUPAC name
R.CO.O.CO.R	Acid anhydride	Alkanoic anhydride
CH$_3$.CO.O.CO.CH$_3$	Acetic anhydride	Ethanoic anhydride
C$_2$H$_5$.CO.O.CO.C$_2$H$_5$	Propionic anhydride	Propanoic anhydride
C$_3$H$_7$.CO.O.CO.C$_3$H$_7$	Butyric anhydride	Butanoic anhydride

(iii) **Esters and lactones:** The esters (R–COO·R′) are named systematically as alkyl alkanoates. The suffix 'ic acid' is replaced by 'ate' and the name of alkyl group prefixed to the word. Alkyl carboxylate is their common name.

Cyclic esters are known as **Lactones**. These are referred as α (alpha), β (beta), γ (gamma), δ (delta) lactones, depending on the size of the ring.

Formula	Common name	IUPAC name
R.COO.R′	Alkyl carboxylate	Alkyl alkanoate
HCOO.CH$_3$	Methyl formate	Methyl methanoate
CH$_3$COO.CH$_3$	Methyl acetate	Methyl ethanoate
C$_2$H$_5$COO.CH$_3$	Methyl propionate	Methyl propanoate
C$_2$H$_5$COO.C$_2$H$_5$	Ethyl propionate	Ethyl propanoate
H$_2$C——CO | | H$_2$C——O	β-Propiolactone (4-membered ring)	β-Propiolactone
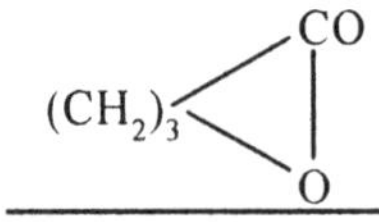 (CH$_2$)$_3$⟨CO O	γ-Butyrolactam (5-membered ring)	γ-Butyrolactone

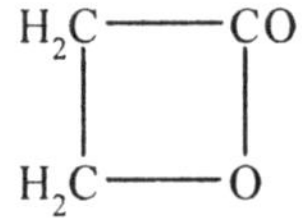

(iv) **Amides and lactams:** Acid amides are obtained by the replacement of hydroxyl group of acids (–COOH) by amino group. Their common names are derived from the names of the corresponding acids. In IUPAC system, they are named by replacing the ending 'e' of the parent hydrocarbon by 'amide'. If the nitrogen is substituted, they are named first by placing a capital 'N' before the name of the amide. Cyclic amides are called lactams and a, b, g, d etc. are written to indicate the size of the ring in the lactam. Thus:

Formula	Common name	IUPAC name
R–CO.NH$_2$	Acid amide	Alkanamide
H.CO.NH$_2$	Formamide	Methanamide
CH$_3$.CO.NH$_2$	Acetamide	Ethanamide
C$_2$H$_5$.CO.NH$_2$	Propionamide	Propanamide
C$_3$H$_5$.CO.NH$_2$	Butyramide	Butanamide
C$_2$H$_5$.CO.NH·CH$_3$	N-Methyl acetamide	N-Methyl ethanamide
C$_9$H$_{19}$.CO.NH$_2$		Decanamide
C$_3$H$_7$.CO.N(CH$_3$)$_2$	N,N-Dimethyl butyramide	N,N-Dimethylbutanamide
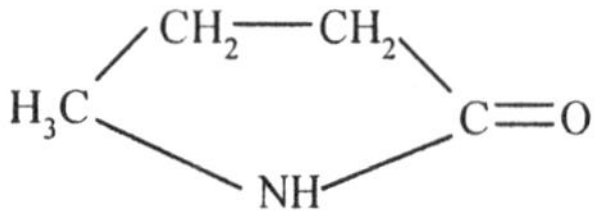 H$_3$C⟨CH$_2$—CH$_2$⟩C=O, NH	γ-Butyrolactam	γ-Butyrolactam

11. Amides or Alkyl Derivatives of Ammonia

Amines can be regarded as the alkyl derivatives of ammonia. They are classified as **primary, secondary** or **tertiary**, according to the number of groups attached to the nitrogen and followed by the word **-amine**. IUPAC names for primary, secondary and tertiary amines are aminoalkanes, alkyl aminoalkanes and dialkyl aminoalkanes, respectively.

Formula	Common name	IUPAC name
$R.NH_2$	Alkylamines	Aminoalkanes
CH_3NH_2	Methylamine	Aminomethane
$C_2H_5.NH_2$	Ethylamine	Aminoethane
$C_2H_5.NHCH_3$	Ethyl methylamine	N-Methylaminoethane
$(CH_3)_2.NH$	Dimethylamine	N-Methylaminomethane
$(CH_3)_3.N$	Trimethylamine	N,N-Dimethylaminomethane

12. Nitroalkanes

These are named as the nitro derivatives of alkanes. The common and systematic names are almost the same. The position of nitro groups is indicated in the latter system. Thus:

Formula	Common name	IUPAC name
$R.NO_2$	Nitroalkane	Nitroalkane
$CH_3.NO_2$	Nitromethane	Nitromethane
$C_2H_5.NO_2$	Nitroethane	Nitroethane
$C_3H_7.NO_2$	Nitropropane	1-Nitropropane
$C_{10}H_{21}.NO_2$	Nitrodecane	1-Nitrodecane

13. Thioalcohols or Thiols or Mercaptans

They are sulphur analogues of the alcohols. The suffix used for thioalcohols in IUPAC system is 'thiol' in place of 'ol' used in the names of alcohols. For example:

Formula	Common name	IUPAC name
R–SH	Thioalcohols or Mercaptans	Alkanethiol
CH_3–SH	Methyl thioalcohol (Methyl mercaptan)	Methanethiol
C_2H_5–SH	Ethyl thioalcohol	Ethanethiol
C_3H_7–SH	Propyl thioalcohol	Propanethiol
$C_{10}H_{21}$–SH	Decyl thioalcohol	Decanethiol

14. Thioethers

The sulphur analogues of the ethers are termed as thioethers. The common names are represented as 'thio' derivatives of the ethers, whereas in systematic nomenclature they are referred to as dialkyl sulphides. Thus:

Formula	Common name	IUPAC name
R–S–R′	Dialkyl thioethers	Dialkyl sulphides
CH_3–S–CH_3	Dimethyl thioether	Dimethyl sulphide
CH_3–S–C_2H_5	Methylethyl thioether	Ethylmethyl sulphide
C_2H_5–S–C_3H_7	Ethylpropyl thioether	Ethylpropyl sulphide

15. Alkyl Cyanides or Nitriles

The common names of alkyl cyanides, containing 'cyano' group (–CN), are written by suffixing 'cyanide' to the alkyl group, whereas systematic names are obtained by suffixing 'nitrile' to the name of the parent hydrocarbons. For example:

Formula	Common name	IUPAC name
R–CN	Alkyl cyanide	Alkanenitrile
$CH_3.CN$	Methyl cyanide or Acatonitrile	Ethanenitrile
$C_2H_5.CN$	Ethyl cyanide or Propiononitrile	Propanenitrile
$C_3H_7.CN$	Propyl cyanide	Butanenitrile
$C_9H_{19}.CN$	Nonyl cyanide	Decanenitrile

16. Cyanogen Compounds

The alkyl isocyanides ($RN \equiv C$) or carbylamines are isomeric with alkyl cyanides. Their common names are referred as alkyl isocyanides, whereas their systematic names are obtained by suffixing carbylamine to the name of alkyl group present in the molecule. For example:

Formula	Common name	IUPAC name
$(R.N \equiv C)$	Alkyl isocyanides	Alkyl carbylamines
$CH_3.NC$	Methyl isocyanide	Methyl carbylamine
$C_2H_5.NC$	Ethyl isocyanide	Ethyl carbylamine
$C_3H_7.NC$	Propyl isocyanide	Propyl carbylamine

17. Alkyl Nitrates, Nitrites, Cyanates, Isocyanates, Thiocyanates, Isothiocyanates, etc.

They are considered as alkyl derivatives of inorganic acids and names as CH_3ONO_2, methyl nitrate CH_3ONO, methyl nitrite; $C_2H_5.CNO$, ethyl cyanate; $C_2H_5.NCO$, ethyl isocyanate; R.CNS, alkyl thiocyanate; R.NCS, alkyl thioisocyanate; $R–SO_3H$, alkyl hydrogen sulphate; and $R–O.SO_2.O.R$, dialkyl sulphate are given to them.

18. Organometallic Compounds

For naming Grignard reagent, the alkyl group is written first followed by magnesium and then by the halo atom. Other organometallic compounds are likewise named giving the name of the metal. For example:

$$CH_3.MgBr \qquad C_2H_5.MgI \qquad C_2H_5.Zn.C_2H_5$$
Methyl magnesium bromide   Ethyl magnesium iodide   Diethyl zinc

$$(C_2H_5)_4PB \qquad (C_2H_5)_2Hg$$
Tetraethyl lead   Diethyl mercury

Isomerism

Compounds having the same molecular formula (composition) but showing different properties are called isomers (Greek: *iso* = equal, same; and *meros* = parts) and the phenomenon itself being known as isomerism. Isomers contain the same numbers and the same kind of atoms i.e. the same percentage composition and molecular weight, but in these molecules, the atoms are attached to one another in different ways. Thus isomers are different compounds because they have different molecular structures and so they are assigned to different chemical families. For example, ethyl alcohol and dimethyl ether have the same molecular formula C_2H_6O but both the compounds are from different chemical families. Depending on the arrangement of atoms in the molecule, the isomerism can be divided into **structural isomerism** and **stereoisomerism**.

(a) **Structural isomerism:** Structural isomerism is due to the difference in structure and results from different arrangement of atoms in the molecule, giving two or more different structural formulae.

(b) **Stereoisomerism:** When the isomers have the same formulae, but they differ from each other, only in the way the atoms are oriented in space within the molecule, the phenomenon is termed as **stereoisomerism**. The arrangement of atoms or groups in space is also referred to as **configuration** of the molecule.

The above mentioned isomerisms are exhibited in different ways which are described as follows:

STRUCTURAL ISOMERISM

In structural isomerism, there are four modes of linking of atoms due to which they differ in structural features:

1. Skeletal or chain isomerism,
2. Position isomerism,
3. Functional isomerism, and
4. Metamerism.

1. Skeletal Isomerism or Chain Isomerism

The isomers differing in the structure of carbon chain are called skeletal or chain isomers. Different arrangement of carbon atoms in the molecule show different properties. The compound butane has the molecular formula C_4H_{10}, which can be represented by two structural formulae differing only in the arrangement of atoms along the carbon chain.

$$CH_3.CH_2.CH_2.CH_3$$

n-Butane (b.p. –0.5°C)
Straight chain

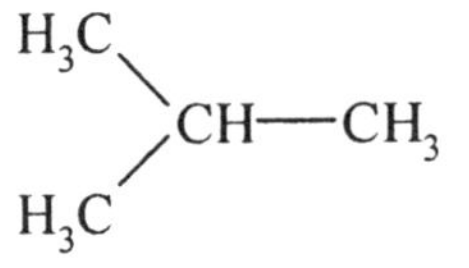

$$\begin{array}{c} H_3C \\ \diagdown \\ H_3C \end{array} CH—CH_3$$

Isobutane (b.p. –10.2°C)
Branched chain

In case of pentane (C_5H_{12}), the five carbon atoms can be represented in three different forms of chains. Similarly hexane (C_6H_{14}) has five, heptane (C_7H_{16}) has nine and octane (C_8H_{18}) has eighteen isomers. With increase in the number of carbon atoms in the molecule, the number of chain isomers increases.

The isomerism of molecular formula C_4H_8 may be represented by straight chain, branched chain or cyclic skeleton to give rise to five types of known isomers.

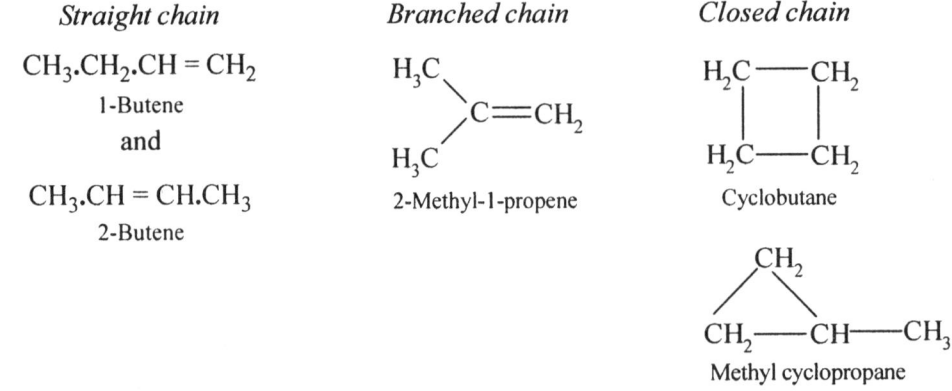

| *Straight chain* | *Branched chain* | *Closed chain* |

$$CH_3.CH_2.CH = CH_2$$

1-Butene

and

$$CH_3.CH = CH.CH_3$$

2-Butene

2-Methyl-1-propene

Cyclobutane

Methyl cyclopropane

Such isomerism is also exhibited by other classes of compounds besides the hydrocarbons. The isomerism of molecular formula $C_5H_{12}O$ (amyl alcohol) may be represented as:

(i) $CH_3.CH_2.CH_2.CH_2.CH_2.OH$

1-Pentanol

(ii) 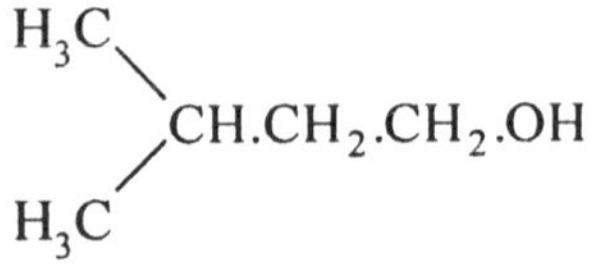 $\begin{array}{c} H_3C \\ \diagdown \\ H_3C \end{array} CH.CH_2.CH_2.OH$

3-Methyl-1-butanol

(iii) $CH_3.CH_2.CH_2.CH(OH).CH_3$

2-Pentanol

(iv) $CH_3.CH_2.CH_2.CH(OH).CH_3$

2-Pentanol

(v) 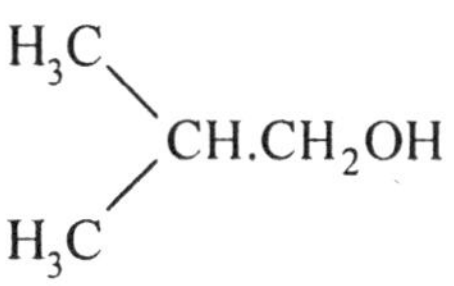
$$H_3C \diagdown$$
$$\diagup CH.CH_2OH$$
$$H_3C \diagup$$
2-Methyl-1-butanol

(vi) 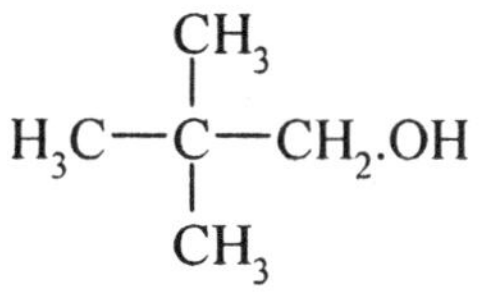
$$\overset{\displaystyle CH_3}{\underset{\displaystyle CH_3}{H_3C-\overset{|}{\underset{|}{C}}-CH_2.OH}}$$
2,3-Dimethyl-1-propanol

(vii) $(CH_3)_2 CH.CH(OH).CH_3$
3-Methyl-2-butanol

(viii) $(CH_3)_2 C(OH).CH_2.CH_3$
2-Methyl-2-butanol

2. Position Isomerism

It is shown by compounds having the same carbon skeleton but differing in the position occupied by a substituent group, e.g. the isomers of molecular formula C_3H_7Cl may be demonstrated as:

$$\overset{3}{C}H_3 . \overset{2}{C}H_2 . \overset{1}{C}H_2 . Cl$$
1-Chloropropane

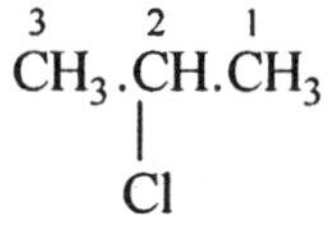

$$\overset{3}{C}H_3 . \overset{2}{\underset{|}{C}}H.\overset{1}{C}H_3$$
$$Cl$$
2-Chloropropane

In unsaturated hydrocarbons different positions of multiple bonds can be shown in a carbon chain. Thus:

Molecular formula

C_4H_8 (i) $CH_3.CH_2.CH = CH_2$ (ii) $CH_3.CH = CH.CH_3$
               1-Butene   2-Butene

C_4H_6 (i) $CH_3.CH_2.C \equiv CH$ (ii) $CH_3.C \equiv C.CH_3$
               1-Butyne   2-Butyne

The aromatic compounds show different isomeric forms which are the position isomers differing only in the position of the two substituents on the benzene ring. The isomers of three xylenes (mol. formula C_8H_{10}) may be shown as:

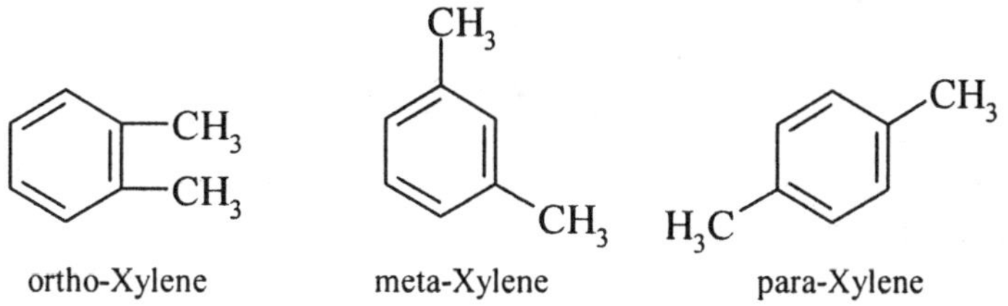

ortho-Xylene   meta-Xylene   para-Xylene

3. Functional Isomerism

This isomerism is exhibited by compounds having different functional groups, i.e., compounds with the same molecular formula but belonging to different homologous series. As the properties of a compound are due to functional group such compounds differ in their physical and chemical properties. Compounds showing this type of isomerism are termed as **functional isomers**.

(i) Ethyl alcohol and dimethyl ether are represented by the same molecular formula (C_2H_6O) but the former has alcohol linkage belonging to the class of alcohols whereas the latter having an ether linkage belongs to the class of ethers.

$$CH_3.O.CH_3 \qquad\qquad C_2H_5.OH$$

Dimethyl ether   Ethtyl alcohol

(ii) Propionaldehyde and acetone have the same molecular formula (C_3H_6O) but have aldehydic (–CHO) and ketonic (>CO) groups respectively.

$$CH_3.CH_2.CHO \qquad\qquad CH_3.CO.CH_3$$

Propionaldehyde   Acetone

4. Metamerism

This type of isomerism is shown by compounds of the same homologous series. There is an unequal distribution of carbon atoms of alkyl groups of different size on either side of the functional group in the molecule. Thus diethyl ketone and methyl propyl ketone have the same molecular formula ($C_5H_{10}O$) and the same functional group but contain different alkyl groups on either side of the carbonyl group.

$$C_2H_5.CO.C_2H_5 \qquad\qquad CH_3.CO.C_3H_7$$

Diethyl ketone   Methyl propyl ketone

Ethers and amides also show metamerism.

Molecular formula:

$C_4H_{10}O$ $C_2H_5.O.C_2H_5$ $CH_3.O.C_3H_7$

Ketone   Diethyl ether   Methyl propyl ether

$C_6H_{15}N$ $C_3H_7.NH.C_3H_7$ $C_2H_5.NH.C_4H_9$

Amine   Dipropyl amine   Butyl ethyl amine

$$CH_3.NH.C_5H_{11}$$

Methyl pentyl amine

STEREOISOMERISM

Stereoisomers are isomeric compounds of identical structure but differing in the arrangement of the atoms in three-dimensional space. This type of isomerism is divided into two classes: 1. **Optical isomerism**, and 2. **Geometrical isomerism**.

1. OPTICAL ISOMERISM

The optical isomers do not differ in their structure and so have the same physical and chemical properties except the behaviour towards plane polarized light. The property due to which the molecules rotate the plane of plane-polarized light is called as optical activity and the substances which show this property are known as **optical active compounds**.

Plane-polarized light

Among certain properties of light, one is that light is propagated by a wave motion. The vibrations occur at right angles to the direction in which the light travels. There are an indefinite number of planes passing through the line of propagation and ordinary light is vibrating in all these planes [Fig. 7.1(a)]. If we consider that we are looking into an imaginary cross-section of a beam of light, it will be observed that these vibrations occur in all directions at right angles to the line of propagation. Thus symmetry is present in ordinary light. However, if a beam of ordinary light is passed through a Nicol prism (polarizer), the beam so obtained has all the waves vibrating in one plane [Fig. 7.1(b)].

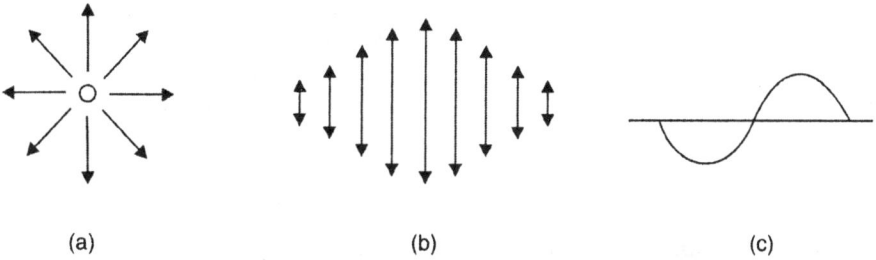

(a) (b) (c)

Fig. 7.1. Schematic representation of (a) ordinary light, (b) plane-polarized light, and (c) propagation of a light wave.

Plane-polarized light is that light whose vibrations take place in only one of these possible planes.

The rotation of the plane of polarized light is detected and measured by an instrument called the **polarimeter**, which is represented schematically in Fig. 7.2.

Polarimeter contains a light source of monochromatic beam and two Nicol or Polaroid lenses. One lens, the polarizer, is mounted in a fixed position. It transmits plane polarized light to a tube of known length, placed in between the two lenses, having glass windows on both sides. The solution to be examined for optical activity is placed in this tube. The second Nicol lens, the analyser, is mounted on a movable axis and can be rotated as desired. The angle of rotation is measured on a circular scale placed after the second lens. When the polarimeter tube is either empty or contains a solvent devoid of optical activity, it permits maximum transmission of light and indicates zero point on the scale. It indicates that the analyzer and polarizer are oriented in the same optical plane. When the analyzer is turned through an angle of 90°, a point of minimum light transmission is reached. If a solution of an optically active substance is placed in the polarimeter tube, light transmitted by the polarizer is rotated to a certain extent, either to the left or to the right. Light reaching the lens nearer to eye (analyzer) is thus diminished in intensity but by rotating the analyzer a point is obtained where the original intensity of the light is regained. In this situation, the analyzer is in alignment with the plane of light emerging from the polarimeter tube. The angle of rotation, by which the maximum intensity of light is restored in either dextro or laevo sense, is then read from the scale. If such a substance is placed in the sample tube, which does not affect the plane of polarization, then the substance is optically inactive.

These substances which rotate the plane of polarized light to right (clockwise) are referred as

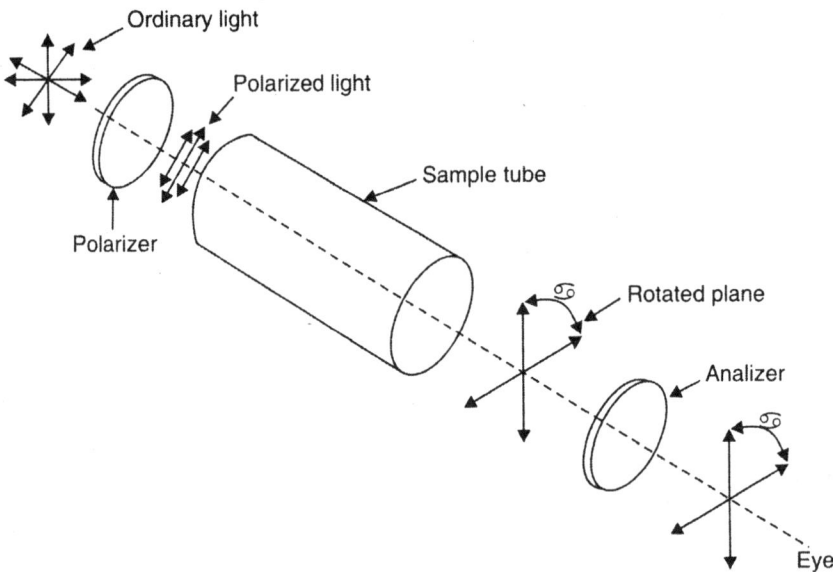

Fig. 7.2. Schematic representation of a polarimeter.

dextro-rotatory and denoted by the sign 'd' or (+) and those which rotate the light to the left (anti-clockwise) are called laevo-rotatory and indicated by sign 'l' or (–). Polarimeter is not only used for determining the rotation of plane and direction, but also the degree of rotation.

Specific Rotation

The measurement of optical activity is reported in terms of specific rotation which is the number of degrees of rotation observed if a 1-decimetre tube is used, and the compound being examined is present to the extent of 1 gm/ml. Specific rotation is a constant quantity for a given substance. This may be calculated from observations with tubes of varying lengths and at different concentrations by using the following equation:

$$[\alpha]_D^t = \frac{\alpha}{l \times C}$$

where $[\alpha]_D^t$ is the specific rotation with sodium light (D represents the D line of the sodium flame) at the temperature t, α is the observed rotation, l is the length of the tube in decimeters and C is the concentration of the solution in grams per ml.

Symmetric Molecules

The symmetry properties of a given molecule tell us whether or not the molecule is superimposable with its mirror image. A molecule is considered to be symmetric if it possesses a plane of symmetry, a centre of symmetry or an alternating axis of symmetry. A molecule has a plane of symmetry, if on passing plane or line through one half of the molecule becomes identical to the other half and both of the parts are mirror images of each other (Fig. 7.3).

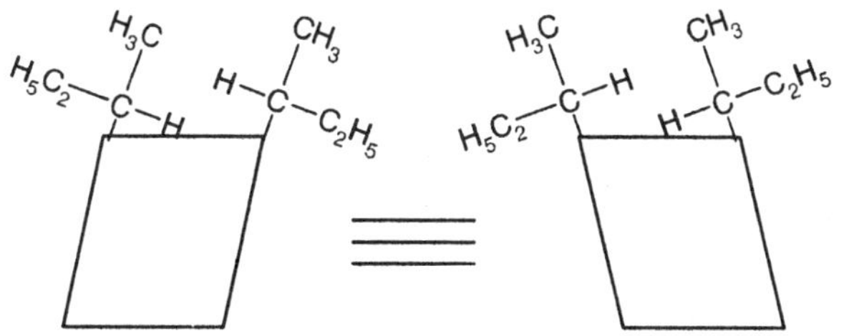

Fig. 7.3. Molecule with plane of symmetry.

Dissymmetry: Molecules that are not superimposable on their mirror images are dissymmetric. Dissymmetric molecules do not have plane of symmetry.

Enantiomers: Enantiomers are the isomers that are mirror images of each other and have the same physical properties except for the direction of rotation of the plane-polarized light. For example, two isomers of 2-methyl-1-butanol have identical physical constants like melting points, boiling points, densities, refractive indices, etc. But both of them have different directions of rotation of the light. One isomer rotates plane-polarized light to the right while the other to the left. However, the amount of rotation is exactly the same, the specific rotation of one being $+5.756°$ and of other is $-5.756°$. Thus, these molecules are so similar that they rotate the light by the same amount. The molecules are mirror images of each other and their properties are identical.

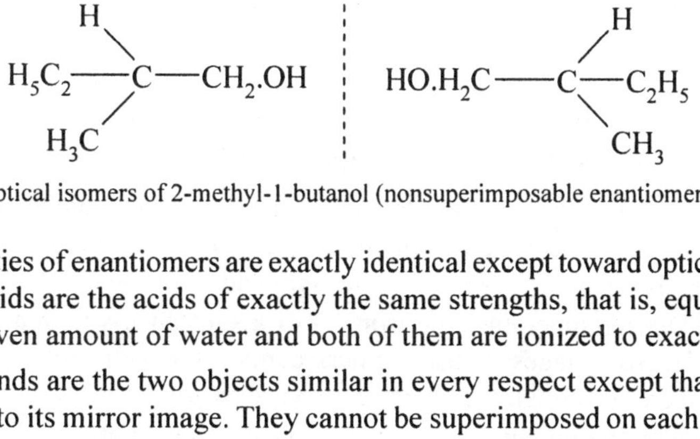

Optical isomers of 2-methyl-1-butanol (nonsuperimposable enantiomers)

Chemical properties of enantiomers are exactly identical except toward optically active reagents. The two isomeric acids are the acids of exactly the same strengths, that is, equal amounts of acids are dissolved in a given amount of water and both of them are ionized to exactly the same degree.

Right and left hands are the two objects similar in every respect except that they are related to each other as object to its mirror image. They cannot be superimposed on each other exactly. Thus, an object which cannot be superimposed on its mirror image must be asymmetric. Such pairs related to each other as an object to its mirror image are known as enantiomers.

The asymmetric carbon atom: A carbon atom to which four different groups of atoms are attached is termed as **asymmetric carbon atom**. The following molecules contain the asymmetric carbon atoms, marked as C*.

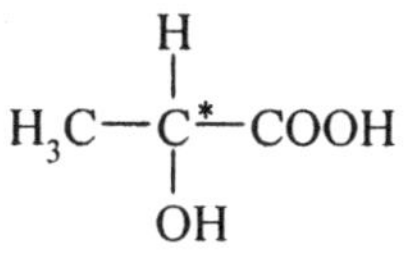

Lactic acid 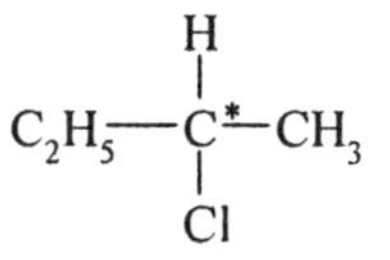   sec. Butyl chloride 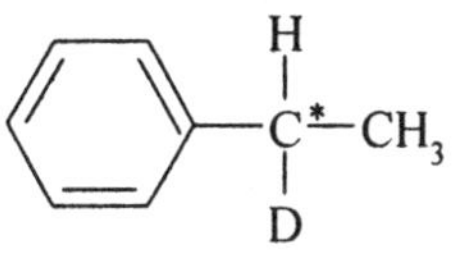   Deuterioethyl benzene

$$\underset{\text{Bromochloro-iodomethane}}{\overset{\displaystyle Cl}{\underset{\displaystyle I}{Br\!-\!\overset{*}{C}\!-\!H}}} \qquad \underset{\text{Malic acid}}{\overset{\displaystyle CH_2COOH}{\underset{\displaystyle COOH}{H\!-\!\overset{*}{C}\!-\!OH}}} \qquad \underset{\text{Tartaric acid}}{\overset{\displaystyle COOH}{\overset{\displaystyle H\!-\!\overset{*}{C}\!-\!OH}{\underset{\displaystyle COOH}{HO\!-\!\overset{*}{C}\!-\!H}}}}$$

Most of the molecules containing an asymmetric carbon are dissymetric.

Cause of Optical Activity

Le-bel and Van't Hoff gave an idea that the optical activity of molecules in solutions or in liquid state is due to the presence of the asymmetry of the substance. They suggested that carbon atom is situated at the centre of an imaginary regular tetrahedron and its four valencies are directed towards its four corners. Now, if a carbon atom is linked to four different atoms or groups the molecule becomes asymmetric. Thus, if a substance which has at least one asymmetric carbon atom, then it will be optically active. The optical activity is not due to the presence of asymmetric carbon atoms in the molecule, but whole of the compounds must be asymmetric as in case of d- and meso-tartaric acid.

If the asymmetric character of any molecule is changed, the compound becomes inactive. For example, if lactic acid is reduced, it gives propionic acid which is optically inactive.

$$\underset{\text{(Optically active)}}{\overset{\displaystyle CH_3}{\underset{\displaystyle COOH}{H\!-\!C\!-\!OH}}} \xrightarrow[\text{Reduction}]{HI} \underset{\text{(Optically inactive)}}{\overset{\displaystyle CH_3}{\underset{\displaystyle COOH}{H\!-\!C\!-\!H}}} \qquad \text{No asymmetry}$$

The number of optical isomers are calculated by 2^n where n is the number of asymmetric carbon atoms. Thus, if there is one such carbon atom, the molecule is represented by $(2^1 = 2)$, for two $(2^2 = 4)$, it will be four and for three $(2^3 = 8)$, it will be eight and so on.

Diastereomers: Diastereomers are the isomers of a substance which are not related to each other as object and mirror images. Diastereomers contain the same functional groups showing similar chemical properties, though the chemical properties are not identical.

Diastereomers have different physical constants like melting points, boiling points, solubility in a given solvent, densities, refractive indices etc. They also have different specific rotation. They may have same or opposite signs of rotation.

2,3-Dichloropentane contains two asymmetric carbon atoms, C-2 and C-3 and, therefore, the number of isomers will be $(2^2 = 4)$ four as given below:

$$\underset{\text{I}}{\overset{\displaystyle CH_3}{\overset{\displaystyle H\!-\!C\!-\!Cl}{\underset{\displaystyle C_2H_5}{Cl\!-\!C\!-\!H}}}} \qquad \underset{\text{II}}{\overset{\displaystyle CH_3}{\overset{\displaystyle Cl\!-\!C\!-\!H}{\underset{\displaystyle C_2H_5}{H\!-\!C\!-\!Cl}}}} \qquad \underset{\text{III}}{\overset{\displaystyle CH_3}{\overset{\displaystyle H\!-\!C\!-\!Cl}{\underset{\displaystyle C_2H_5}{H\!-\!C\!-\!Cl}}}} \qquad \underset{\text{IV}}{\overset{\displaystyle CH_3}{\overset{\displaystyle Cl\!-\!C\!-\!H}{\underset{\displaystyle C_2H_5}{Cl\!-\!C\!-\!H}}}}$$

Isomers I and II are the mirror images of each other but not superimpossible, and hence may be enantiomers. Similarly III and IV are enantiomers. But structures III and IV are non-superimposable, on either I or II; it is not, of course, the mirror image of either. Stereoisomers, that are not enantiomers are **diastereomers**. Compounds III and IV are diastereomers of I and II.

Isomers I and II are not interconvertible by rotation about carbon-carbon single bond, and hence, are not conformational isomers. They are configurational isomers. Structure III cannot be converted into I or II by rotation about single bonds and so here, too, they are configurational stereoisomers.

Meso Structures

2,3-Dichlorobutane has two asymmetric carbons and so exists in four stereoisomeric forms.

$$
\begin{array}{cccc}
\text{CH}_3 & \text{CH}_3 & \text{CH}_3 & \text{CH}_3 \\
| & | & | & | \\
\text{H--C--Cl} & \text{Cl--C--H} & \text{H--C--Cl} & \text{Cl--C--H} \\
| & | & | & | \\
\text{Cl--C--H} & \text{H--C--Cl} & \text{H--C--Cl} & \text{Cl--C--H} \\
| & | & | & | \\
\text{CH}_3 & \text{CH}_3 & \text{CH}_3 & \text{CH}_3 \\
\textbf{V} & \textbf{VI} & \textbf{VII} & \textbf{VIII}
\end{array}
$$

Structure V and VI are mirror images that are not superimpossible or interconvertible; they are, therefore, enantiomers, and should be capable of optical activity. Isomer VIII is a diastereomer of V and of VI. Structure VIII is the mirror image of VII and both are superimposable, i.e., VII coincides in every respect with VIII. The isomer VII contains asymmetric carbon atoms, even then it is not dissymmetric. One half of the VII or VIII is the mirror image of the other half. The isomer has a plane of symmetry and cannot be dissymmetric. Two enantiomeric forms cannot be shown for this and the isomer will not be optically active. This structure (VII) of the compounds is called a meso form.

A meso compound contains two or more asymmetric carbon atoms and its molecules are superimpossible on their mirror images. A meso compound is optically inactive because the molecule is non-dissymmetric. The rotation caused by one half of the molecule is cancelled by an equal and opposite rotation caused by the other half of molecule.

The optical inactivity in the molecules VII and VIII has also arisen due to equal and opposite activity of each half of the molecule. Thus, the optical inactivity due to the compensation of the activity of one half by the other half and this is known as the **internal compensation**. The meso molecules cannot be resolved into optically active components.

Compounds with Asymmetric Atoms Other Than Carbon

Atoms which are similar to carbon in the arrangement of valencies may behave in a similar manner when they are attached to four different groups. Thus, quaternary ammonium salts, compounds of phosphorus, arsenic, antimony, etc. have been shown to be optically active because of the asymmetric N, P, As and Sb atoms, respectively. Methylethylpropylphenyl quaternary ammonium chloride is an optically active compound containing tetravalent nitrogen.

$$\left[\begin{array}{c} CH_3 \\ | \\ N^+ \\ C_2H_5 \diagup \ | \ \diagdown C_6H_5 \\ | \\ C_3H_7 \end{array} \right]$$

Methylethylpropylphenyl quaternary ammonium chloride

Optical Isomers of Lactic Acid

Lactic acid has one asymmetric carbon atom and hence has two configurations, one of these being dextro- and other laevorotatory. These are related to each other as object and mirror image and, therefore, constitute a pair of enantiomers indicated as *d*- and *l*-forms.

$$\begin{array}{cc}
COOH & COOH \\
| & | \\
H-C-OH & HO-C-H \\
| & | \\
CH_3 & CH_3 \\
(+)\ d\text{-Lactic acid} & (-)\ l\text{-Lactic acid}
\end{array}$$

Lactic acid and other compounds containing one asymmetric carbon also occur in an optically inactive form which differ from the d- and l-acids in physical properties. This form is a mixture of equal amounts of 'd' and 'l' varieties and is known as racemic mixture of **dl** or ($\pm$) form, which can be separated into 'd' and 'l' forms. Such mixtures are optically inactive due to external compensation of the rotation.

Ordinary lactic acid is present in sour milk. It is manufactured by fermentation or by synthetic methods and is a racemic mixture and, therefore, inactive. *d*-Lactic acid may be obtained from meat extract and l-lactic acid is formed during the fermentation of sucrose by ***Bacillus acidi laevolactiti***.

Malic acid molecule contains one asymmetric carbon atom and due to this it exists in three forms – dextro, laevo and racemic forms as described above.

Isomers of Tartaric Acid

Tartaric acid is the classical example of compounds containing two similar asymmetric carbon atoms. The number of possible isomers is $2^2 = 4$ and they may be represented as:

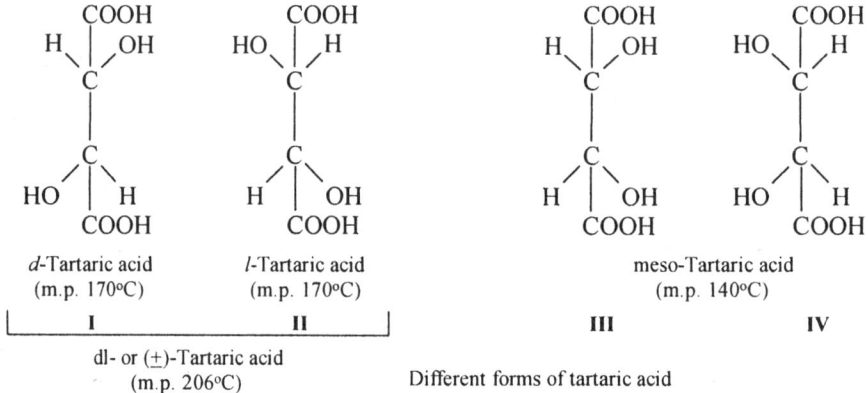

d-Tartaric acid (m.p. 170°C)	*l*-Tartaric acid (m.p. 170°C)	meso-Tartaric acid (m.p. 140°C)	
I	II	III	IV

dl- or ($\pm$)-Tartaric acid
(m.p. 206°C)

Different forms of tartaric acid

Among these formulae, I and II are related to each other as object and its mirror image and thus referred as enantiomers. Similarly, III and IV are related as mirror images but they become identical when one of the structure is rotated through 180°. Formulae I and II are not related to either III or IV as object and mirror image and so they are diastereomers. The structures III and IV have a plane of symmetry and would, therefore, be optically inactive.

Structure I rotates the plane, polarized light in clockwise direction and will be d-tartaric acid. The structure II rotates in an anti-clockwise direction and will represent l-tartaric acid. However, in case of structures III and IV, one asymmetric carbon atom rotates the light in clockwise direction whereas the other rotates equally in an anticlockwise direction. The total rotation results in zero and thus the isomer becomes optically inactive.

The optical inactivity in the molecule has arisen due to equal and opposite rotation caused by two similar asymmetric carbon atoms of the same molecules. Dextrorotation of one half of the molecule is compensated by the laevorotation of the other half. Since this compensation has arisen within the molecule itself, the molecule is said to be inactive due to **internal compensation**.

Besides these three forms, tartaric acid also exists in a racemic or *dl* or (±) form. It is obtained when symmetrical dibromosuccinic acid is heated with silver oxide and water and is inactive because of external compensation. Melting points, densities, solubilities and other physical constants of the meso- and racemic forms differ considerably from those of d- and l-forms.

Configuration: Relative and Absolute Configuration

Arrangement of atoms or groups in a molecule, that characterizes particular stereoisomer, is referred as its configuration.

Compounds containing asymmetric carbon atoms have different configurations each of which belongs to different optical isomers. For example, in case of lactic acid dextro (*d*) and laevo (*l*) enantiomers are known in which one configuration is represented as dextro lactic acid and the other as laevo lactic acid. Fisher indicated the stereochemical relationship to indicate the actual direction of rotation. Rosanoff solved this problem of assigning the configuration and selected glyceraldehyde as standard of reference and a configuration assigned to it absolutely. Accordingly, the two forms of glyceraldehyde were represented by following conventional configurations and denoted as 'D' and 'L' glyceraldehyde, respectively, not by sign of rotation.

$$
\begin{array}{cccc}
\text{CHO} & \text{CHO} & \text{CHO} & \text{CHO} \\
| & | & | & | \\
\text{H}-\text{C}-\text{OH} & \text{HO}-\text{C}-\text{H} & \text{H}-\text{C}-\text{OH} & \text{HO}-\text{C}-\text{H} \\
| & | & | & | \\
\text{CH}_2\text{OH} & \text{CH}_2\text{OH} & \text{CH}_2\text{OH} & \text{CH}_2\text{OH}
\end{array}
$$

D(+)-Glyceraldehyde   L(−)-Glyceraldehyde   D-form   L-Form

All compounds having relationship with 'D' glyceraldehyde in configuration are related to 'D' series. Similarly, those which have identity of configuration with standard glyceraldehyde must belong to 'L' series. When the configuration of an optical isomer corresponds to some compound of known configuration it is known as its relative configuration. For example, when D-glyceraldehyde is oxidized, glyceric acid is formed. The configuration of glyceric acid so obtained must be 'D' accordingly.

$$
\begin{array}{c}
\text{CHO} \\
| \\
\text{H—C—OH} \\
| \\
\text{CH}_2\text{OH}
\end{array}
\quad \xrightarrow{\text{(O)}} \quad
\begin{array}{c}
\text{COOH} \\
| \\
\text{H—C—OH} \\
| \\
\text{CH}_2\text{OH}
\end{array}
$$

D(+)-Glyceraldehyde   D(−)-Glyceric acid

It is important to note that this 'D' or 'L' prefix does not show the direction of rotation as dextro (+) or laevo (−) but only indicates the configuration at asymmetric carbon atom. The actual direction of optical rotation is usually denoted after D or L, the sign (+) corresponds to dextro and (−) to laevo, which may or may not have the same degree of rotation. Thus D-glyceric acid related to D-glyceraldehyde is laevorotatory, whereas D-glyceraldehyde itself is dextrorotatory.

R and S system: A new convention for specifying the configuration of asymmetric carbon atoms was given by Cahn, Ingold and Prelog known as **Rectus** (Latin, meaning right) and **Sinister** (Latin, meaning left) system and generally represented as R and S system. According to this system the atoms are joined to the asymmetric carbon atom directly and are arranged in a sequence as indicated below:

1. The order of priority or sequence is formed on the basis of the atomic numbers of the atoms attached directly to the asymmetric carbon. The atom having greater atomic number gets the higher priority.

In the case of CHClBr. COOH, for example, the four atoms are attached to the asymmetric carbon atom and all are different. The priority depends simply on atomic number. The atom of higher number will get higher priority. So sequence will be Br, Cl, COOH, H.

$$
\begin{array}{c}
\text{COOH} \\
| \\
\text{C} \\
\diagup \quad | \quad \diagdown \\
\text{H} \quad \text{Br} \quad \text{Cl}
\end{array}
$$

Chlorobromoacetic acid

2. When two or more same atoms are attached to asymmetric carbon atom, the atoms next to those similar atoms are taken into consideration for determination of the relative sequence. If these are also the same, then the third atoms are considered and so on. For example, for −CH$_3$ and −CH$_2$·CH$_3$, the order of priority will be −CH$_2$CH$_3$ > CH$_3$, because in methyl C− is joined to H, H, H whereas in ethyl, it is joined to C, H and H. Since carbon has a higher atomic number than hydrogen, C$_2$H$_5$ has the greater sequence.

3. For determining order of priority, multiple bonds are considered as separate single bonds.

Thus, $\overset{|}{\text{H—C}}=\text{O}$ is regarded as carbon linked to 2 oxygens and one hydrogen. The order of priority of $\overset{\text{O}}{\overset{|}{\text{—C}}}=\text{OH}$, $\overset{\text{O}}{\overset{|}{\text{C}}}\text{—H}$ and −CH$_2$−OH groups will be −COOH > −CHO > −CH$_2$OH.

According to these rules, the order of priority group and atoms in lactic acid will be OH > COOH > CH_3 > H and in glyceraldehyde OH > CHO > CH_2OH > H. The phenyl group corresponds

to $C{\overset{\diagup CH}{\underset{\diagdown C}{—}}}CH$.

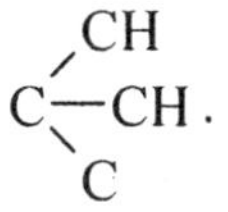

The priority order of the groups joining the asymmetric C atom is fixed and then the tetrahedral structure of the isomer is examined from the side opposite to the group having lowest priority. The arrangement of rest of the groups is viewed. If the arrangement is such that in going from top priority group to second and then to the third priority group, is in clockwise direction, the configuration is referred as 'R' or rectus configuration. On the other hand, if this arrangement is in anticlockwise direction, the configuration is decided as 'S' or sinister configuration.

Resolution

Whenever compounds possessing asymmetric carbon atom are synthesized in the laboratory, the product is always equal mixture of two enantiomers whether the starting compound is racemic mixture or an optically active compound. The products so obtained are usually optically inactive racemic mixture. However, asymmetric compounds always occur in optically active form in nature.

Propionic acid on chlorination yields *dl* or (±) chloropropionic acid which on hydrolysis gives lactic acid in racemic form. There are two identical hydrogen atoms, a and b, in the propionic acid and on chlorination replacement of one of these hydrogens gives one enantiomer and the replacement of other gives another isomer. Since there are equal chances of the substitution of the two hydrogens, the product is a racemic mixture, e.g.:

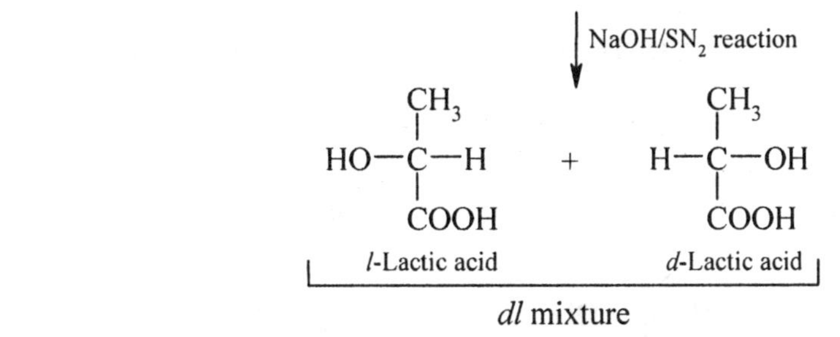

The process of separation of a racemic (*dl*) mixture into the component *d*- and *l*-enantiomers is called resolution. Most of the chemical properties of enantiomers are same. Therefore, they cannot be separated by the general procedures of separation like fractional distillation, crystallization, sublimation, chromatographic techniques, etc. The methods employed for the resolution are as follows:

(i) **Mechanical resolution (Pasteur, 1848):** When the two isomers or their salts have well-defined crystals, they can be separated by simple hand picking. Crystals of sodium ammonium tartarate, $NaNH_4 \cdot C_4H_4O_6 \cdot 2H_2O$, were separated by this manner.

(ii) **Biochemical resolution (Pasteur, 1850):** When certain microorganisms were allowed to grow in the medium of a racemic mixture of certain compounds they consumed, preferentially only one stereoisomer leaving behind the other. The other isomer left in the solution can be isolated by fractional crystallization. For example, treatment of *dl*-tartaric acid with micro-organism.

Penicillium glaucum converts it into *l*-tartaric acid because *d*-form is utilized by the organism. In this method, one half of the compound is destructed. The poisonous enantiomers cannot be separated by this method and it is not easy to find the proper organism which may consume one of the isomers.

(iii) **Chemical method of conversion to diastereomers (Pasteur, 1858):** The enantiomers have the same physical properties, while diastereomers have different physical properties. Therefore, racemic mixture may be separated conveniently by converting them to diastereomers. The diastereomers so separated may be converted then to optically active compounds. For example (±) lactic acid on treatment with *l*-brucine gives two diastereomers which may be resolved by differential solubilities. Diastereomers yield the optically active acid on hydrolysis.

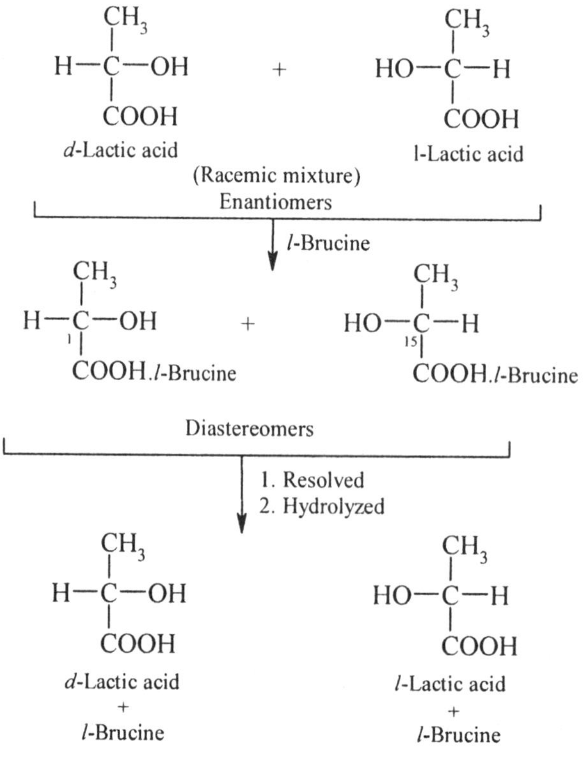

The other bases used for resolution of dl-acid mixture are (–) quinine, (+) cinchonine and (–) strychnine etc. For resolution of bases, optically active acids like (+) tartaric acid, (–) malic acid or (–) mandelic acid may be used.

This method is the best of all methods of resolution. Compounds like acids, bases, alcohols and aldehydes may be resolved by this method.

(iv) **Differential adsorption method:** When a racemic mixture is placed on a chromatographic column containing optically active substances like starch, quartz etc., the enantiomers will move down the column at different rates and this can be separated because of the adsorption selectively of the adsorbent. *dl*-Mandelic acid has been resolved by adsorption over starch in this manner.

(v) **Differential reactivity or kinetic methods:** The enantiomers react with optically active substances at different rates. Therefore, in some cases, it is possible to obtain a separation by stopping the reaction before it acquires equilibrium.

Racemization: When many optically active compounds are kept for a longer time, or heat, light etc. is applied to them, they are converted into racemic mixture. For example, when a solution of *d*-tartaric acid is heated in water, it is changed into a completely inactive mixture of the racemic tartaric acid. **The conversion of dextro or laevo compounds (optically active) to their racemic (dl) forms (optically inactive) is known as Racemization.**

Some intramolecular rearrangement is caused by light, heat or catalysts in case of racemization and optically active compound exists temporarily in equilibrium with this transformed product. The intermediate compound does not have an asymmetric carbon, so that when it again forms the asymmetric centre, both d- and l-forms are obtained in equal amounts. For example, racemization of lactic acid may be given as:

| *d*-Lactic acid | Unstable enol form | *d*-Lactic acid | *l*-Lactic acid |
| (Optically active) | | | |

dl-Lactic acid (Racemic)

Racemization generally occurs when the compounds are easily enolized. Therefore, the compounds possessing carbonyl group adjacent to asymmetric carbon atom carrying a hydrogen are easily racemized.

Walden Inversion

P. Walden, 1923: When a substituent attached to the asymmetric carbon atom is replaced by other group in a reaction, the new product formed has opposite sign in rotation to that of the starting compound. This change of **dextro form into the laevo or vice versa without recourse to resolution** is an optical inversion and a reaction in which **the inversion of configuration occurs is termed Walden inversion.** For example in the conversion of *d*-malic acid to *l*-malic acid and vice-versa, the following steps take place and the reaction shows a change in configuration.

$$\underset{\substack{\text{H}-\text{C}-\text{OH} \\ | \\ \text{COOH}}}{\overset{\text{CH}_2\text{COOH}}{|}} \xrightarrow{\text{PCl}_5} \underset{\substack{\text{Cl}-\text{C}-\text{H} \\ | \\ \text{COOH}}}{\overset{\text{CH}_2\text{OOH}}{|}} \xrightarrow{\text{AgOH}} \underset{\substack{\text{HO}-\text{C}-\text{H} \\ | \\ \text{COOH}}}{\overset{\text{CH}_2\text{COOH}}{|}}$$

d-Malic acid l-Chlorosuccinic acid l-Malic acid

I - Inversion

$$\xrightarrow{\text{PCl}_5} \underset{\substack{\text{H}-\text{C}-\text{Cl} \\ | \\ \text{COOH}}}{\overset{\text{CH}_2\text{COOH}}{|}} \xrightarrow{\text{AgOH}} \underset{\substack{\text{H}-\text{C}-\text{OH} \\ | \\ \text{COOH}}}{\overset{\text{CH}_2\text{COOH}}{|}}$$

d-Chlorosuccinic acid d-Malic acid

II - Inversion

In some cases the inversion is 100% whereas in some cases partial inversion occurs. A number of factors, like nature of compound, reagent, solvent etc., play an important role in this inversion. Perhaps, a biomolecular substitution mechanism occurs by the attack of the reagent from the opposite of the leaving group and inversion of configuration takes place.

Asymmetric Synthesis

Whenever an optically active compound is prepared in the laboratory always a racemic product is formed and to obtain the optically active compound, the racemic mixture must be resolved. However, there are enantiomers formed which are not in equal amounts and the mixture will be optically active because of unequal quantities of isomers formed. **The synthesis in which optically active compound is obtained from optically inactive compound, without recourse to resolution is called asymmetric synthesis**.

The following methods are generally used for asymmetric synthesis:

(i) **With optically active reagents, catalysts or solvent (Wald, 1904):** l-Isovaleric acid is prepared from ethyl methyl malonic acid using l-brucine. The l-form obtained is in 10% excess over the d-form.

$$\underset{\substack{\text{Ethyl methyl} \\ \text{malonic acid}}}{\underset{\substack{| \\ \text{C}_2\text{H}_5}}{\overset{\overset{\text{CH}_3}{|}}{\text{HOOC}-\text{C}-\text{COOH}}}} \xrightarrow{l\text{-Brucine}} \underset{\substack{| \\ \text{C}_2\text{H}_5}}{\overset{\overset{\text{CH}_3}{|}}{\text{HOOC}-\underset{7}{\text{C}}-\text{COOH.}}} + l\text{-Brucine.} \underset{\substack{| \\ \text{C}_2\text{H}_5}}{\overset{\overset{\text{CH}_3}{|}}{\text{HOOC}-\underset{13}{\text{C}}-\text{COOH}}}$$

l-Brucine

$$\downarrow \substack{170° \\ -\text{CO}_2}$$

$$\underset{\substack{| \\ \text{C}_2\text{H}_5}}{\overset{\overset{\text{CH}_3}{|}}{\text{H}-\text{C}-\text{COOH.}}} + l\text{-Brucine} \quad \underset{\substack{| \\ \text{C}_2\text{H}_5}}{\overset{\overset{\text{CH}_3}{|}}{\text{HOOC}-\text{C}-\text{COOH}}}$$

l-Brucine

$$\downarrow \text{HCl}$$

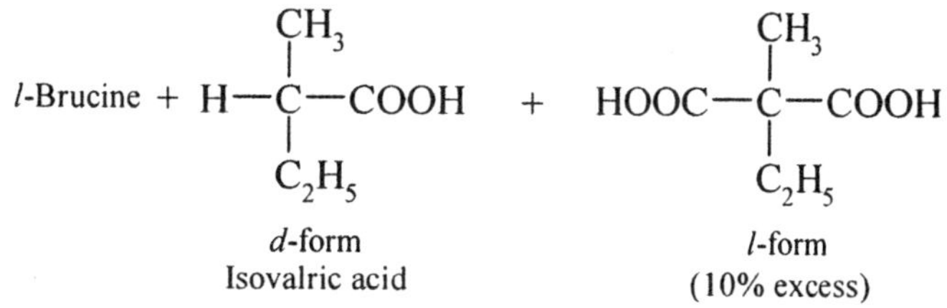

$$l\text{-Brucine} + \underset{\underset{C_2H_5}{|}}{\overset{\overset{CH_3}{|}}{H-C-COOH}} + \underset{\underset{C_2H_5}{|}}{\overset{\overset{CH_3}{|}}{HOOC-C-COOH}}$$

d-form   *l*-form

Isovalric acid   (10% excess)

A racemic mixture is obtained when pyruvic ester is reduced and then hydrolyzed. But, if pyruvic acid is esterified with an optically active alcohol like *l*-menthyl alcohol and then reduced and hydrolyzed *l*-lactic acid is produced. Thus:

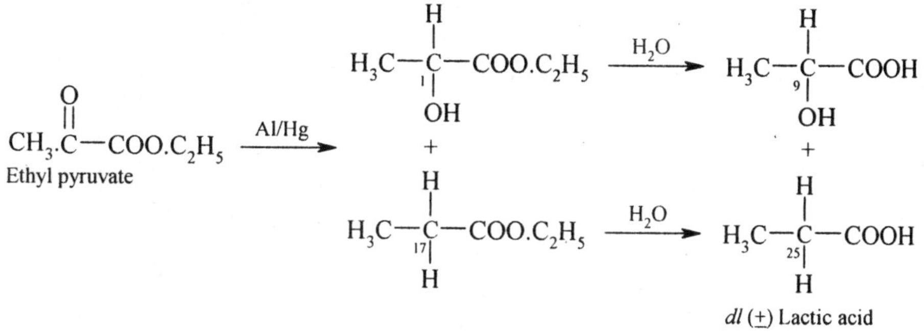

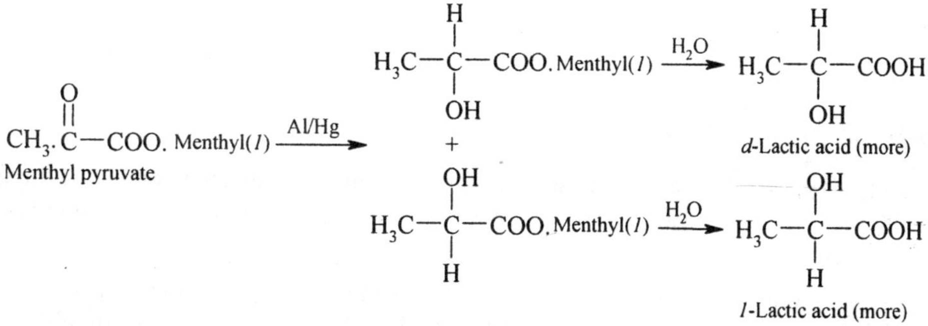

dl ($\pm$) Lactic acid

Mixed ketone on reduction with hydrogen using nickel catalyst in presence of optically active amino acids produces one enantiomer of secondary alcohols in excess.

Optically active alcohols are prepared by Grignard reagent from aldehydes when optically active ether is used as a solvent.

(ii) **With active substrate:** When optically active compound is produced from a compound which already has an asymmetric centre, then the two diastereomers are formed in unequal amount and the product is optically active. For example, 2-methylbutanal on treatment with HCN gives cyanohydrin, which is an optically active addition product.

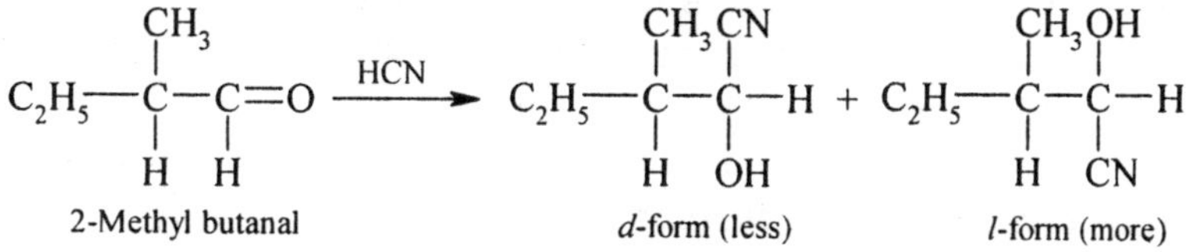

(iii) **With enzymes:** The reaction of benzaldehyde with HCN in the presence of enzyme yields optically active mandelonitrile. Hydrolysis of this compound produces 1-mandelic acid in excess.

$$C_6H_5CHO + HCN \xrightarrow{HCN} C_6H_5-\underset{\underset{OH}{|}}{\overset{\overset{H}{|}}{C}}-CN \xrightarrow{H_2O} C_6H_5-\underset{\underset{OH}{|}}{\overset{\overset{H}{|}}{C}}-COOH$$

l-Mandelonitrile   *l*-Mandelic acid

(iv) **With circularly polarised light (Kuhn and Knopf, 1930):** When optically active compounds are produced under the influence of circularly polarised light, the resulting compound is slightly optically active. If right circularly polarised light is used, the product formed is laevorotatory. This is a special synthesis of asymmetric atom known as **absolute asymmetric synthesis**.

Davis et al. (1945) reported the formation of *d*-diethyl tartaric acid ester by hydroxylation of ethyl fumarate in a beam of right circularly polarised light in a poor yield.

Ethyl fumarate $\xrightarrow[\text{Ether}]{H_2O_2}$ *d*-Diethyl tartarate

2. GEOMETRICAL ISOMERISM

The isomers which possess the same structural formula but differ in arrangement of the groups in space around the double bond are known as geometrical isomers and the phenomenon is termed as geometrical isomerism.

If two carbon atoms are attached through a double bond at the two corners then there is no free rotation and the rotation is restricted around carbon-carbon double bond. As a result of this restricted rotation, there are two types of different arrangements of the substituents in the same plane attached to these carbon atoms. The isomer which has similar groups lying on the same side of the double bond is called 'cis' (Latin, cis = same side) and the similar groups attached on the opposite side of the double bond or across the molecule is known as 'trans' (Latin, trans = across) isomer. This type of isomerism is also called as cis-trans isomerism.

The classical example of geometrical isomerism is the case of maleic and fumaric acids containing the same molecular formula $C_4H_4O_4$ but differ in most of their physical and chemical properties. They are optically inactive compounds. Maleic and fumaric acids are not the structural isomers since both are catalytically reduced to succinic acid; addition of hydrogen bromide gives bromosuccinic acid; action of water yields maleic acid and are oxidised by alkaline permanganate to tartaric acid. Thus both acids have the same structure: $HO_2C.CH = CH.COOH$, and the two possible geometrical isomers are (I) and (II)), cis and trans butenedioic acid, respectively. The spatial arrangements of the molecules are represented as follows:

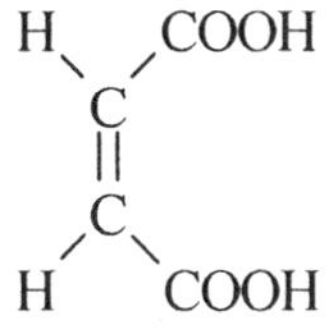

I	**II**
Maleic acid (m.p. 130°)	Fumaric acid (m.p. 287°)

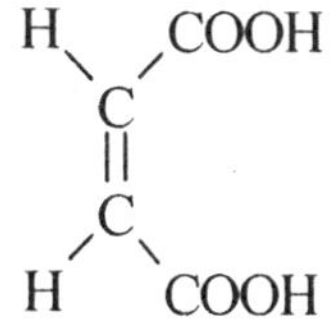

There is a hindered rotation about any carbon-carbon double linkage, but it gives rise to geometric isomerism only if there is a certain relationship among the groups attached to the double-bonded carbons. We can look for this isomerism by drawing the possible structures and then seeing, if these are indeed isomeric, or actually identical. On this bases, it is found that propylene, *1*-butene and isobutylene should not show isomerism. This conclusion agrees with the facts. Many higher alkenes may, of course, show geometrical isomerism.

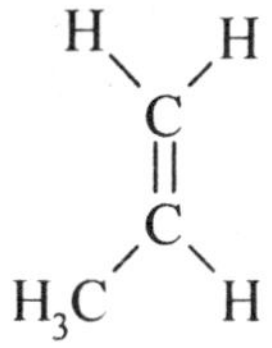

Propylene	1-Butene	Isobutylene

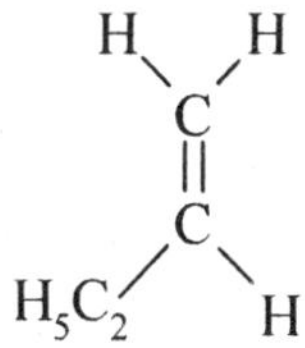

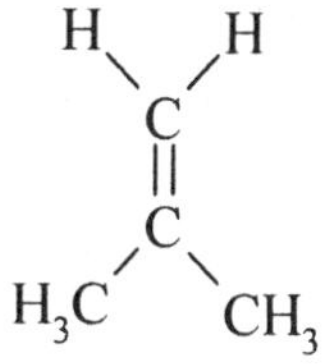

In compounds, other than hydrocarbons, it is found that 1,1-dichloro and 1,1-dibromoethenes should not show isomerism, whereas the 1,2-dichloro- and 1,2-dibromoethenes should exist in *cis* and *trans* forms.

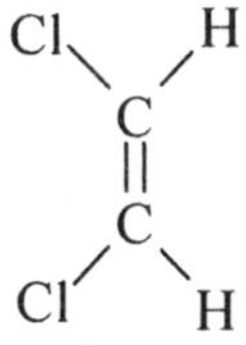

cis	*trans*	*cis*	*trans*
1,2-Dichloroethene		1,2-Dibromoethene	

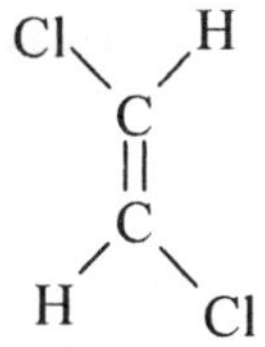

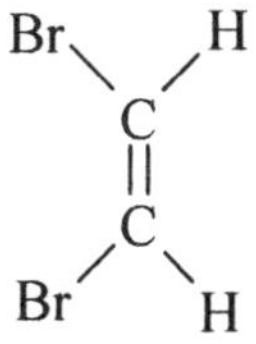

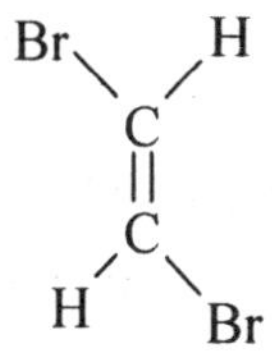

Thus if the compound has two identical groups attached to any carbon atom, then both the structures would be one and the same, and there will be no isomerism. The two groups should be attached on the different carbon atoms. It is also important to note that in cases where all the four substituents are different, then it is not possible to decide the *cis* and *trans* isomers. Other examples of geometrical isomerism are given below:

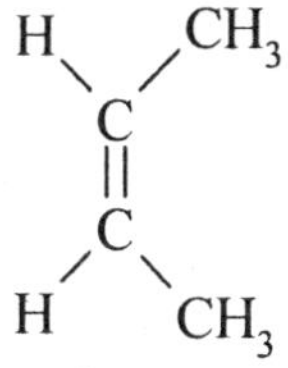

cis-2-Butene	*trans*-2-Butene	Isocrotonic acid (*cis*)	Crotonic acid (*trans*)

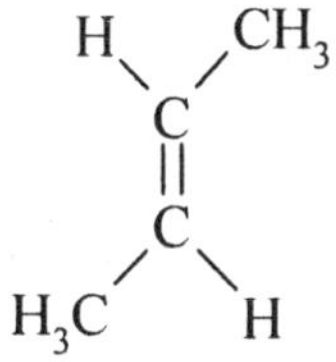

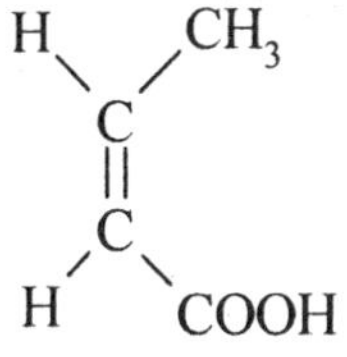

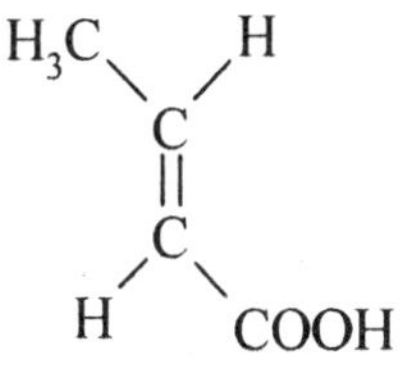

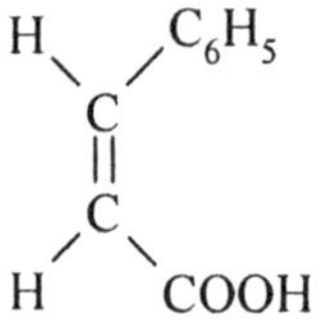

Allocinnamic acid *(cis)* 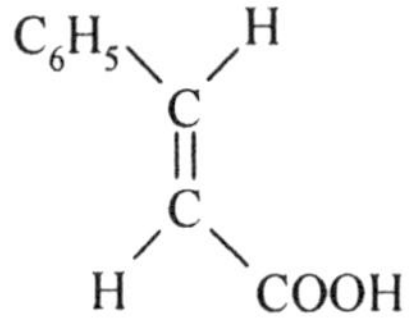 Cinnamic acid *(trans)* 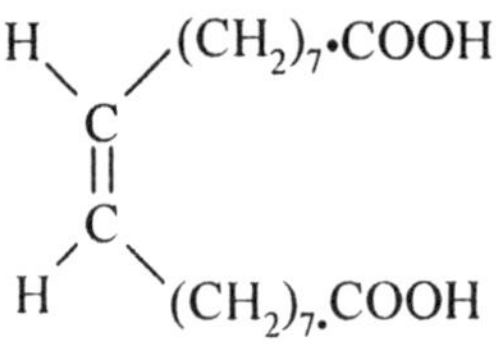 Oleic acid *(cis)* 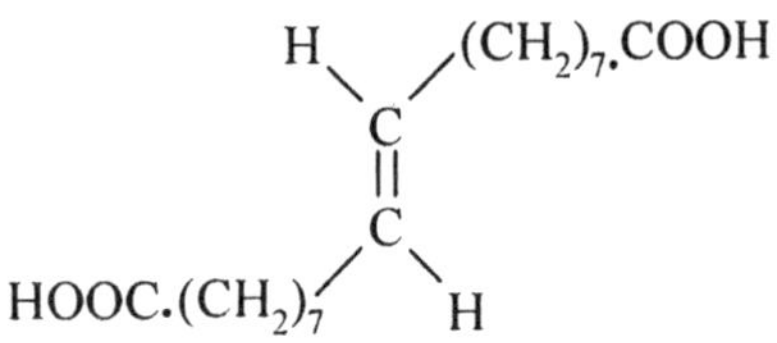 Elaidic acid *(trans)*

Properties of Geometrical Isomers

The *cis* and *trans* isomers are generally two compounds having different physical and chemical properties. The *cis* isomers usually have lower m.p. and higher density, refractive index, dipole moment etc. as compared to *trans* isomers.

In *cis* isomer, if the two groups attached are carboxylic functional groups, then it may be converted readily to anhydride on heating by losing a molecule of water; *trans* isomer may not afford the anhydride unless it is isomerized to *cis* form. For example, maleic acid readily gives an anhydride, whereas fumaric acid first isomerizes to maleic acid at much higher temperature and then forms maleic anhydride.

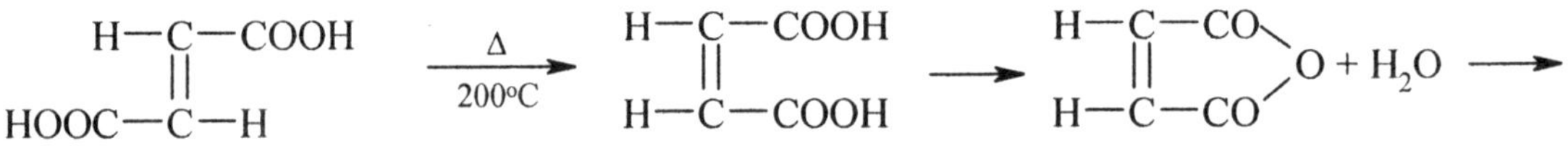

Fumaric acid *(trans)* Maleic acid *(cis)* Maleic anhydride

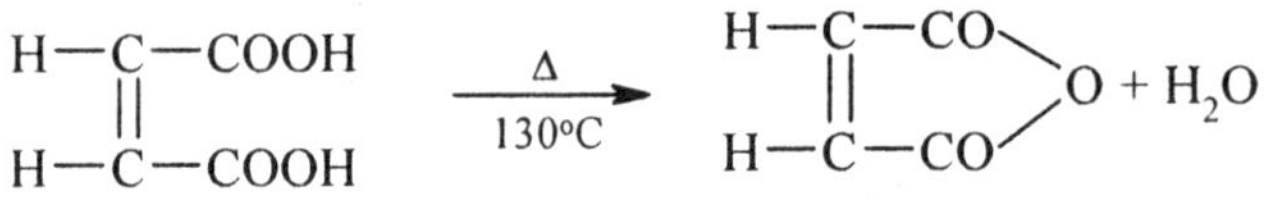

Maleic acid *(cis)* Maleic anhydride

Tautomerism (Laar, 1885)

The phenomenon of the reversible interconversion of isomers is called tautomerism.

Compounds whose structures differ markedly in arrangement of atoms, but which exist in equilibrium, are called tautomers (*tauto* = same; *meros* = parts). The most common kind of tautomerism involves structures that differ in the point of attachment of hydrogen.

A structure with –OH attached to doubly-bonded carbon is called an 'enol' ('ene' for the carbon-carbon double bond, 'ol' for alcohol). When a compound with the enol structure is prepared, a compound with the 'keto' structures is prodominated as in case of acetoacetic ester.

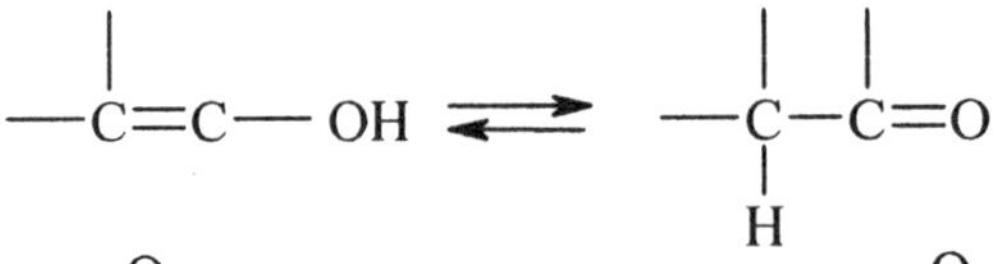

Keto-enol tautomerism

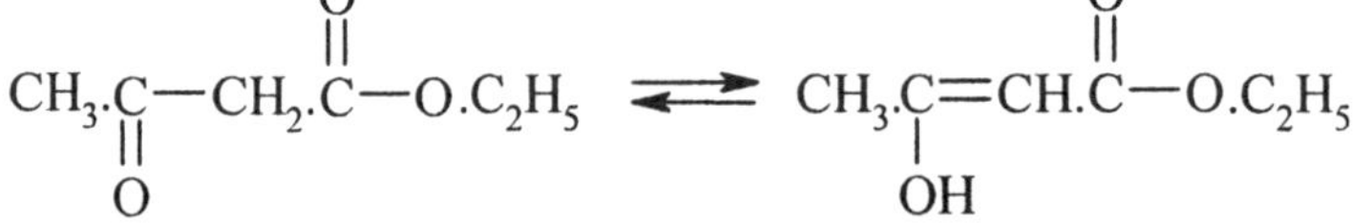

Keto form (93%) Enol form (7%)

There is an equilibrium between the two structures, but it generally lies very much in favour of the keto form. When acetylene is hydrated, vinyl alcohol is formed, but it is rapidly converted into an equilibrium mixture that is almost all acetaldehyde.

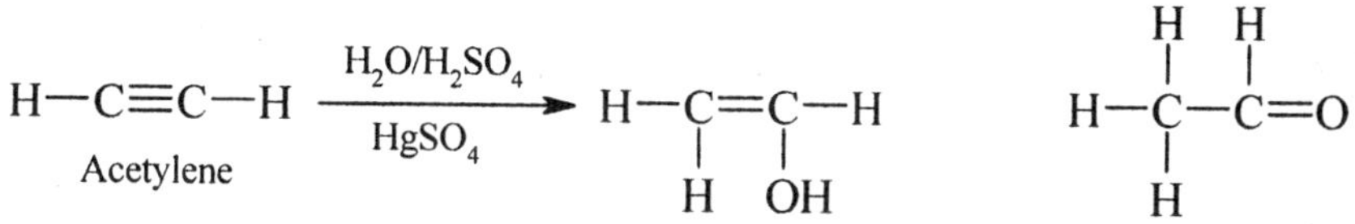

$$H-C\equiv C-H \xrightarrow[\text{HgSO}_4]{\text{H}_2\text{O/H}_2\text{SO}_4} H-\overset{|}{\underset{|}{C}}=\overset{|}{\underset{|}{C}}-H$$

Acetylene   H OH
Vinyl alcohol   Acetaldehyde

Rearrangements of this keto-enol kind take place very easily because of the polarity of the O–H bond. A hydrogen ion separates readily from oxygen, but when a hydrogen ion returns, it may attach itself either to oxygen or to carbon. When it returns, it may readily come off again, but when it attaches itself to carbon, it tends to stay there.

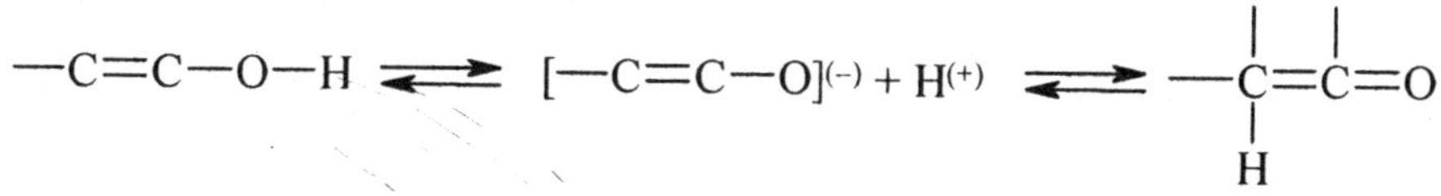

$$-C=C-O-H \rightleftharpoons [-C=C-O]^{(-)} + H^{(+)} \rightleftharpoons -\overset{|}{\underset{|}{C}}=\overset{|}{C}=O$$

Keto-enol tautomerism

The other examples of tautomerism involving different types of compounds are given below:

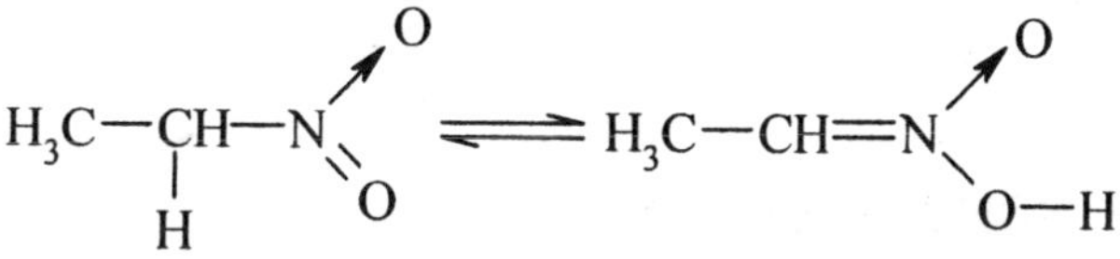

$$H_3C-\overset{|}{\underset{H}{CH}}-N\overset{\nearrow O}{\searrow_O} \rightleftharpoons H_3C-CH=N\overset{\nearrow O}{\searrow_{O-H}}$$

Nitro form   Acinitro form

(b) Nitroso-isonitroso system

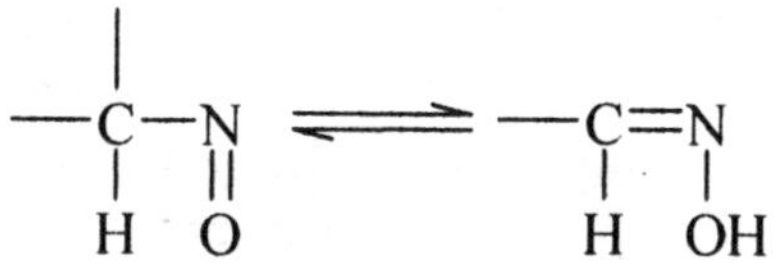

$$-\overset{|}{\underset{H}{C}}-\overset{}{\underset{O}{N}} \rightleftharpoons -\overset{}{\underset{H}{C}}=\overset{}{\underset{OH}{N}}$$

Nitroso form   Isonitroso form
or
oxime form

(c) Lactam-lactim system

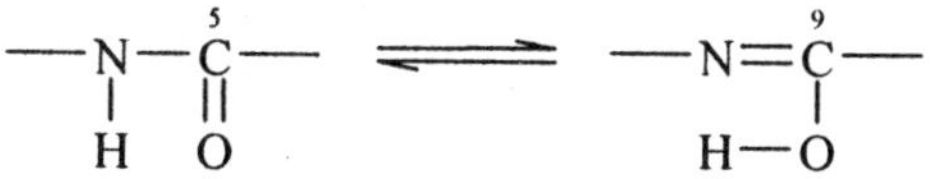

$$-N-\overset{5}{\underset{O}{C}}- \rightleftharpoons -N=\overset{9}{C}-$$

Lactam form   Lactim form

Alkanes or Paraffins
(Saturated Hydrocarbons)

INTRODUCTION

Hydrocarbons are the saturated simplest organic compounds containing only carbon and hydrogen. These are represented by a general formula C_nH_{2n+2} (where $n = 1, 2, 3, 4, ...,$ and so on). They are stable compounds and do not react with reagents like potassium permanganate, potassium dichromate, chromic acid, nitric acid, sulphuric acid and sodium hydroxide. Due to this inertness, they are known as paraffins (Latin, *parum* = little, *affinis* = affinity).

HYBRIDIZATION OF BOND ORBITALS

The atomic weight of carbon is six and its electronic configuration is represented as:

$$C^6 \quad 1s^2 \quad 2s^2 \quad 2px^1 \quad 2py^1 \quad 2pz$$

The carbon atom has one electron in each $2px$ and $2py$ orbital. So the hydrogen atom should combine with these two impaired electrons to form a divalent compound like CH_2. But carbon atom binds with four hydrogen atoms and it exhibits tetravalency in all organic compounds. For achieving a tetrahedral carbon atom, one electron of $2s$ orbital gets promoted to empty $2pz$ orbital and in this way four unpaired electrons are present for combining to four hydrogen atoms.

$$C^6 \quad 1s^2 \quad 2s^1 \quad 2px^1 \quad 2py^1 \quad 2pz^1 \quad \text{promotion of one electron}$$

From this electronic configuration, it is clear that carbon should form three bonds of one kind by combination with three p orbitals and one bond of another kind by linking the s orbital. Among four bonds, the three σ bonds will be similar in all respects and one bond formed by using s orbital will be different. But in methane, all the four bonds are equivalent in every respect.

To account for the equivalent bonds, it is suggested that $2s$ and $2p$ orbitals of carbon in excited state are mixed up to form four equivalent orbitals. This method, in which the greatest degree of directional character of orbitals is found, is called as hybridization. The resulting new orbitals are known as hybdirized orbitals. Depending on the number of orbitals in mixing up the hybridization may be of three types:

(i) **Tetrahedral hybridization:** If one electron of $2s$ and three electrons of $2p$ orbitals are hybridized resulting the four equivalent orbitals, then the hybridization is called tetrahedral or sp^3 hybridization. The characteristics of such orbitals are: (a) the hybridized orbitals are much more strongly directed than either $2s$ or $2p$ orbitals; (b) they are exactly equivalent to each other and (c) the orbitals are greatly concentrated along the four directions of a regular tetrahedron having an angle of $109.5°$, i.e., they are as far away from each other as possible in such arrangements. The hybrid orbital has three-fourths p character and one-fourth s character. Such shape of the orbital gives more space for overlapping and so the bonds formed by hybrid orbitals are stronger (Fig. 8.1). This hybridization takes place in saturated organic compounds.

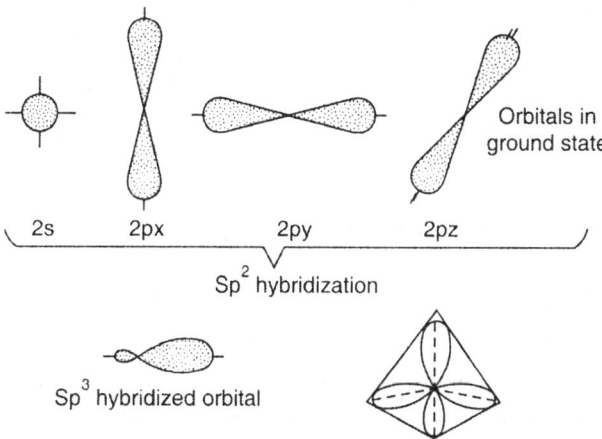

Fig. 8.1. Hybridization of $2s$ and $2p$ orbitals in alkanes.

(ii) **Trigonal hybridization:** In this hybridization, one electron of $2s$ orbital and two electrons of $2p$ orbitals take part in hybridization. These three orbitals are mixed up resulting in three equivalent coplanar orbitals pointing at angles of $120°$. The $2pz$ orbital remains undisturbed. Thus, there will be three equivalent valencies in one plane and a fourth valency pointing at right angle to this plane. The hybrid orbitals have two-thirds p character and one-third s character. The shape of trigonal hybrid orbital (sp^2) is the same as that of tetrahedral hybrid orbital (sp^3). The three equivalent orbitals are directed towards the corner of a trigon, and therefore, this is called trigonal hybridization. The three orbitals form 6 bonds. There is still an unhybridized half-filled p-orbital which combines by side-wise overlapping to unhybridized p-orbital of another carbon, resulting in π bond. The electrons involved in the formation of π bonds are mobile electrons and give rise to unsaturation, as in case of ethylene (Fig. 8.2).

(iii) **Diagonal hybridization:** Only one $2s$ and $2p$ orbitals are mixed up resulting in two equivalent hybrid orbitals. The process is called sp hybridization. In this method the $2py$ and $2pz$ orbitals remain undisturbed. The hybridized orbitals have 50% s and 50% p character. It has the same shape as that of sp^2 hybrid orbital. From these two s and p orbitals, two σ bonds are formed by co-axial overlapping, pointing in opposite directions along a straight line in the same plane having a bond angle of $180°$. There are still two unhybridized $2py$ and $2pz$

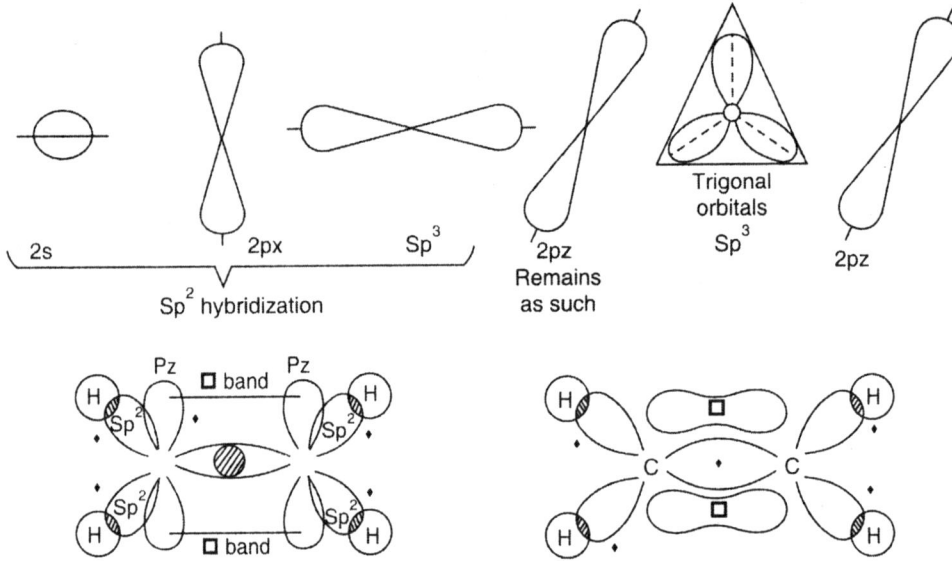

Fig. 8.2. Trigonal hybridization and molecular orbitals in ethylene molecule.

orbitals. These orbitals overlap sidewise to two unhybridized orbitals of another carbon, forming two π bonds as in case of acetylene (Fig. 8.3).

Occurrence: Petroleum and natural gas are the main sources of alkanes. Petroleum usually contains alkanes having upto forty carbon atoms in their molecules. Natural gas obtained from

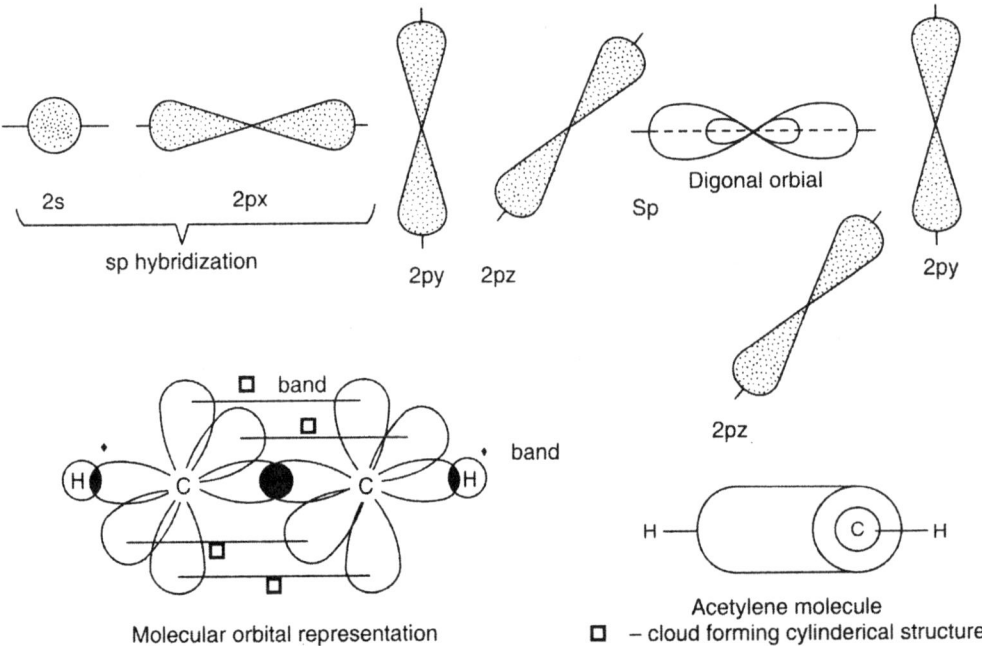

Fig. 8.3. Diagonal hybridization and molecular orbitals of acetylene.

petroleum wells contains only lower gaseous hydrocarbons like methane, ethane, propane and butane. Wax, obtained from petroleum wells and from bees, is a mixture of higher solid alkanes. Decaying process of animals and plants gives lower members like methane.

Nomenclature: The following three systems are generally adopted for naming the paraffins:

(i) **The common system:** In this system, first four alkanes of the homologous series are called as methane, ethane, propane and butane. The higher members are named by prefixing Greek numeral to the suffix 'ane'. Thus the members containing molecular formula C_6H_{14}, C_7H_{16} and C_8H_{18} are termed as hexane, heptane and octane respectively.

Alkanes may have primary (1^0), secondary (2^0), tertiary (3^0) and quaternary (4^0) carbon atoms when their valencies are satisfied with one, two, three and four other carbon atoms, respectively.

When one hydrogen is removed from alkanes, alkyl radicals result e.g. methyl group CH_3^-, propyl group $CH_3CH_2CH_2^-$, isobutyl group $(CH_3)_2CH–CH_2^-$, etc.

(ii) **As derivatives of methane:** Alkanes are named as derivatives of methane obtained by the replacement of its hydrogen atom(s) by various alkyl groups. For example, ethane is named as methyl methane, propane as dimethyl methane, isobutane as trimethyl methane and so on. This system of naming is not very much in use.

(iii) **IUPAC system:** Alkane is the name of paraffins in IUPAC system. In this system, the common names of the paraffins have been retained for the straight chain alkanes.

$$CH_3.CH_2.CH_2.CH_3$$
n-Butane

$$\overset{\displaystyle CH_3}{\underset{2}{|}} \\ \underset{3}{CH_3} — \underset{2}{CH} — \underset{1}{CH_3}$$
2-Methylpropane

$$\overset{\displaystyle CH_3}{\underset{2}{|}} \\ \underset{1}{CH_3} — \underset{2}{CH} — \underset{3}{CH_2} — \underset{4}{CH_2} — \underset{5}{CH_3}$$
2-Methylpentane

More details about the IUPAC nomenclature have been discussed in chapter dealing with nomenclature.

Isomerism: Only chain isomerism occurs in alkanes. In the first three alkanes, methane, ethane and propane, there is no other possible arrangement of carbon and hydrogen atoms for writing the structural formula. However, butane can be represented by two structural formulae, pentane by three, hexane by five, heptane by nine and octane by eighteen isomers. Details of structural isomerism are given in chapter on isomerism.

General Methods of Preparation of Alkanes

The members of a homologous series can be prepared by similar general methods. The alkanes are not obtained in pure form from their natural sources, i.e., petroleum and gas. Therefore, synthetic methods are preferred to get them in pure form.

1. **Hydrogenation of unsaturated hydrocarbon:**

$$R.CH = CH.R + H_2 \xrightarrow{\text{Ni } 300^0 C} R.CH_2.CH_2.R$$
Alkane   Alkane

$$CH_2 = CH_2 + H_2 \xrightarrow[\text{room temp.}]{\text{Pd}} CH_3.CH_3$$
Ethylene   Ethane

$$CH \equiv CH + H_2 \xrightarrow[\text{room temp.}]{Pd} CH_3.CH_3$$
Acetylene

This reaction is generally referred as Sabatier and Sendern's reaction. Methane cannot be prepared by this method.

2. **From alkyl halides:**

   (i) By reduction of alkyl halides with zinc and hydrochloric acid, hydriodic acid, zinc copper couple and alcohol, aluminium and alcohol, sodium amalgam or lithium aluminium hydride.

$$R{-}X + 2H \xrightarrow{Zn-HCl} RH + HX$$
Alkyl   Alkane
halide

$$C_2H_5I + 2H \xrightarrow{Na-Hg}_{C_2H_5OH} C_2H_6 + HI$$
Ethyl   Ethane
iodide

   Pure hydrocarbons are obtained in good yield by this method.

   (ii) **Wurtz reaction:** Higher alkanes are obtained by heating alkyl halides with sodium metal in ether.

$$RX + 2Na + XR \xrightarrow{\Delta} R{-}R + 2NaX$$
Alkyl   Alkane
halide

$$CH_3I + 2Na + ICH_3 \xrightarrow{\Delta} CH_3{-}CH_3 + 2NaI$$
Methyl   Ethane
iodide

Mechanism

$$C_2H_5I + Na \longrightarrow C_2H_5 + 2NaI$$
Ethyl   Sodium   Ethyl (free) Sodium
iodide   atom   radical   iodide

$$2C_2H_5 \longrightarrow C_2H_5C_2H_5$$

   (iii) **Frankland method:** Higher alkane are also obtained when alkyl halides are heated with zinc in an inert solvent.

$$RX + Zn + XR \xrightarrow{Ether} R-R + ZnX_2$$

$$C_2H_5I + Zn + IC_2H_5 \qquad C_2H_5C_2H_5 + ZnI_2$$
Butane

3. **From metal salts of carboxylic acids:**

   (i) By decarboxylation of sodium salts of fatty acids with soda lime (NaOH + CaO).

$$R.COONa + NaOH \xrightarrow[\Delta]{CaO} R.H + Na_2CO_3$$
Sod. salt
of acid

$$C_2H_5COONa + NaOH \xrightarrow[\Delta]{CaO} C_2H_6 + Na_2CO_3$$
Sod. propionate   Ethane

The yields are generally poor, but this method can be used for reducing the number of carbon atoms in a carbon chain.

(ii) By the electrolysis of salts of monocarboxylic acids in aqueous solution (Kolbe's electrolytic reaction – 1848).

$$2R.COONa + 2H_2O \longrightarrow R.R + 2CO_2 + 2NaOH + H_2$$

Mechanism:

$$\underset{\text{Sod. acetate}}{CH_3.COONa} \longrightarrow \underset{\text{At anode}}{CH_3COO^-} + \underset{\text{At cathode}}{Na^+}$$

$$CH_3.COO^- \xrightarrow{-2e^-} 2CH_3.COO \longrightarrow 2CH_3 + 2CO_2$$

$$CH_3 + CH_3 \longrightarrow CH_3.CH_3$$

$$Na^+ + 2e^- \longrightarrow 2Na \xrightarrow{2H_2O} 2NaOH + H_2$$

The other products are also formed due to disproportionation of free radicals.

4. **Reduction of alcohols, ketones and fatty acids:**

(i) $\underset{\text{Ethanol}}{C_2H_5OH} + 2HI \xrightarrow[150^{\circ}C]{Red\ P} \underset{\text{Ethane}}{C_2H_6} + H_2O + I_2$

(ii) $\underset{\text{Acetone}}{CH_3.CO.CH_3} + 4HI \xrightarrow[150^{\circ}C]{Red\ P} \underset{\text{Propane}}{CH_3.CH_2.CH_3} + H_2O + 2I_2$

(iii) $\underset{\text{Acetic acid}}{CH_3.COOH} + 6HI \xrightarrow[150^{\circ}C]{Red\ P} \underset{\text{Ethane}}{CH_3.CH_3} + 2H_2O + 3I_2$

Higher alkanes are prepared from fatty acids which are easily obtained by the hydrolysis of fats and oils.

5. **From Grignard reagent:** By treating Grignard reagents with compounds containing active hydrogen like water, alcohol, amines, acids etc.

$$\underset{\substack{\text{Ethyl mag.}\\ \text{bromide}}}{C_2H_5MgBr} + \underset{\text{Water}}{HOH} \longrightarrow \underset{\text{Ethane}}{C_2H_6} + MgBrOH$$

$$C_2H_5MgI + \underset{\text{Ethanol}}{HO.C_2H_5} \longrightarrow C_2H_6 + MgIOC_2H_5$$

$$CH_3MgBr + \underset{\text{Amine}}{H_2NR} \longrightarrow \underset{\text{Methane}}{CH_4} + Mg(Br)HNR$$

The yields of hydrocarbons are quantitative.

6. **From elements (total synthesis):** Lower alkanes like CH_4 and C_2H_6 can be prepared from carbon and hydrogen elements by passing electric arc (temperature about 1200°C) in hydrogen gas between carbon electrodes.

$$C + 2H_2 \longrightarrow \underset{\text{Methane}}{CH_4}$$

$$2C + 3H_2 \longrightarrow \underset{\text{Ethane}}{C_2H_6}$$

General physical properties of alkanes:

1. The hydrocarbons from C_1 to C_4 are colourless, odourless gases, while pentane to heptadecane (C_5 to C_{17}) are colourless liquids. Higher alkanes are colourless and odourless solids.
2. The alkanes are nonpolar solvents and are insoluble in polar solvents like water, but are soluble in organic nonpolar solvents, like benzene, ether, carbon tetrachloride, etc.
3. Their b.p., m.p., density, etc. increase with increase in number of carbon atoms, whereas solubility decreases with increase in their molecular weight.

Table 8.1. Physical Constants of Some Alkanes

Name	Formula	M.P. (°C)	B.P. (°C)	Density (at 20°C)
Methane	CH_4	−183	−162	–
Ethane	$CH_3.CH_3$	−172	−88.5	–
Propane	$CH_3.CH_2.CH_3$	−187	−42	–
n-Butane	$CH_3.(CH_2)_2.CH_3$	−138	0	–
n-Pentane	$CH_3.(CH_2)_3.CH_3$	−130	36	0.626
n-Hexane	$CH_3(CH_2)_4.CH_3$	−95	69	0.659
n-Heptane	$CH_3.(CH_2)_5.CH_3$	−90.5	98	0.684
n-Octane	$CH_3.(CH_2)_6.CH_3$	−57	126	0.703
n-Nonane	$CH_3(CH_2)_7.CH_3$	−54	151	0.718
n-Decane	$CH_3(CH_2)_8.CH_3$	−30	174	0.730
n-Undecane	$CH_3(CH_2)_9.CH_3$	−26	196	0.740
n-Dodecane	$CH_3(CH_2)_{10}.CH_3$	−10	216	0.749
n-Tridecane	$CH_3(CH_2)_{11}.CH_3$	−6	234	0.747
n-Tetradecane	$CH_3.(CH_2)_{12}.CH_3$	5.5	252	0.764
n-Pentadecane	$CH_3.(CH_2)_{13}.CH_3$	10	166	0.769
n-Hexadecane	$CH_3.(CH_2)_{14}.CH_3$	18	280	0.775
Isobutane	$(CH_3)_2.CH.CH_3$	−159	−12	–
Isopentane	$(CH_3)_2.CH.CH_2.CH_3$	−160	28	0.620
Neopentane	$(CH_3)_4.C$	17	9.5	–
Isohexane	$(CH_3)_2.CH(CH_2)_2.CH_3$	−154	60	0.654

4. The boiling point of a branched alkane is lower than its isomeric straight chain structure.
5. Hydrocarbons with even number of carbon atoms have higher m.p. than the next higher and next lower alkanes having odd number of carbon atoms.

General Chemical Properties of Alkanes

Alkanes are saturated compounds, therefore, they are quite inert towards common reagents, like acids, alkalis and oxidising agents. These compounds are in sp^3 hybdirized state and the four hybrid orbitals are directed towards the corners of a regular tetrahedron and are at an angle of 109.5° to each other. The 6 bonds are formed by overlapping of orbitals and due to remarkable stability of the 6 bonds these compounds are chemically inert towards even strong acids and alkalis.

In saturated hydrocarbons, there are no centres of high or low electron density and so there is no question of attacking electrophilic or nucleophilic reagents. Generally, free radical substitution reactions take place in alkanes. The important chemical reactions are as follows:

1. **Halogenation:** Alkanes react with halogens in the presence of heat, sunlight or U.V. light resulting in the successive replacement of hydrogen atoms with halogens. The extent to which halogenation occurs depends on the amount of halogen used. Thus chlorination of methane takes place as shown below:

$$CH_4 + Cl_2 \xrightarrow{\text{Sunlight}} HCl + CH_3Cl \text{ (Methyl chloride)}$$

$$CH_3Cl + Cl_2 \xrightarrow{\text{Sunlight}} HCl + CH_2Cl_2 \text{ (Methylene chloride)}$$

$$CH_2Cl_2 + Cl_2 \xrightarrow{\text{Sunlight}} HCl + CHCl_3 \text{ (Chloroform)}$$

$$CHCl_3 + Cl_2 \xrightarrow{\text{Sunlight}} HCl + CCl_4 \text{ (Carbon tetrachloride)}$$

In higher alkane mixtures all possible products are obtained from a single molecule. This type of replacement is known as substitution reaction in which an atom or a group of the compounds is replaced by another atom without undergoing any change in structure of the molecule. Ethane can yield only haloethane; propane, *n*-butane; and isobutane can form two isomers each, n-pentane can give three isomers, and isopentane, four isomers.

Mechanism: Halogenation takes place by free radical mechanism, for example, in case of chlorination of methane:

(i) $Cl_2 \longrightarrow 2Cl$. Chain-initiating step

(ii) $Cl. + CH_4 \longrightarrow HCl + CH_3$ ⎫
(iii) $CH_3 + Cl_2 \longrightarrow HCl + Cl$. ⎬ Chain-propagating step

$CH_3 + Cl. \longrightarrow CH_3.Cl$ ⎫
$CH_3 + CH_3 \longrightarrow C_2H_6$ ⎬ Chain terminating step

Similarly bromination takes place, but the reaction is not so vigorous as chlorination. In case of iodine the reaction is reversible.

$$CH_4 + I_2 \rightleftharpoons CHI_3 + HI$$

2. **Nitration:** When a hydrogen atom is replaced by nitro group ($-NO_2$) the reaction is called nitration. Nitration of alkanes is carried out in vapour phase between 150–475°C to give nitroalkanes.

$$\underset{\text{Alkane}}{RH} + HO.NO_2 \xrightarrow{\Delta} \underset{\text{Nitroalkane}}{R\!-\!NO_2} + H_2O$$

$$\underset{\text{n-Hexane}}{C_6H_{13}H} + HO.NO_2 \xrightarrow{400°C} \underset{\text{Nitrohexane}}{C_6H_{13}\!-\!NO_2} + H_2O$$

Nitration also proceeds by a free radical mechanism as in chlorination of methane.

3. **Sulphonation:** When a hydrogen atom is replaced by a sulphonic group ($-SO_3H$), then the reaction is termed as sulphonation. For sulphonation of alkanes concentrated sulphuric acid containing sulphur trioxide, known as oleum, is used. Hexane and higher hydrocarbons are sulphonated with fuming sulphuric acid at higher temperature to give alkane sulphonic acids.

$$C_6H_{13}H + HO.SO_3H \xrightarrow[400^\circ C]{SO_3} C_6H_5.SO_3H + H_2O$$
$\quad$ Hexane* $\qquad\qquad\qquad\qquad\qquad$ Hexane
$\qquad\qquad\qquad\qquad\qquad\qquad\quad$ sulphonic acid

Sulphonation also proceeds through a free radical mechanism.

4. **Chlorosulphonation:** Treatment of alkane with chlorosulphuric acid in the presence of light and pyridine catalyst yields alkane sulphonyl chloride by a free radical mechanism.

$$RH + HO.SO_2Cl \xrightarrow[C_5H_5N]{Light} RSO_2Cl + HCl$$

5. **Isomerization:** The process in which a compound is converted into its isomeric form is termed as isomerization. n-Alkanes, when heated with anhydrous aluminium chloride and hydrochloric acid at about $200^\circ C$ under pressure, isomerize to the branched chain isomers, e.g.:

$$\underset{\text{n-Hexane}}{C_6H_{14}} \xrightarrow[200^\circ C/35\ atm.]{AlCl_3/HCl} \underset{\text{2-Methyl pentane}}{CH_3.\overset{\overset{\displaystyle CH_3}{|}}{C}HCH_2.CH_2.CH_3} + \underset{\text{3-Methyl pentane}}{CH_3.CH_2.\overset{\overset{\displaystyle CH_3}{|}}{C}H.CH_2.CH_3}$$

6. **Pyrolysis (Thermal decomposition or cracking):** Decomposition of a compound by the action of heat alone is known as pyrolysis (Greek *pyr* = fire, *lysis* = losing, i.e. cleavage by heat).

Alkanes, when subjected to high temperature and pressure break up into smaller molecules. This process can occur either by the rupture of carbon hydrogen bonds when alkenes are formed or by cleavage of carbon-carbon bonds to give mixture of lower hydrocarbons. For example, pyrolysis of n-hexane may yield the following possible products:

$$\underset{\text{n-Hexane}}{C_6H_{14}}
\begin{cases}
\longrightarrow \underset{\text{Pentane}}{C_5H_{12}} + \underset{\text{Methane}}{CH_4} \\
\longrightarrow \underset{\text{Butene}}{C_4H_8} + \underset{\text{Ethane}}{CH_3.CH_3} \\
\longrightarrow \underset{\text{Butane}}{C_4H_{10}} + \underset{\text{Ethene}}{CH_2.CH_2} \\
\longrightarrow \underset{\text{Propane}}{C_3H_8} + \underset{\text{Propene}}{C_3H_6} \quad \text{etc.}
\end{cases}$$

Pyrolysis of alkanes, particularly when petroleum is concerned, is known as cracking. Large alkanes are converted into smaller alkanes, alkenes and hydrogen. Pyrolysis of alkanes to give alkenes is catalysed by the oxides of chromium, molybdenum, vanadium etc. When catalysts like silica, alumina, zinc oxide etc. are employed, then the lower alkanes are produced.

The reaction is also carried out by a free radical mechanism.

7. **Reaction with ketones:** Tertiary alkanes react with ketones in the presence of conc. sulphuric acid to yield tertiary alcohol.

$$(CH_3)_3.CH \ + \ CH_3.\overset{\overset{O}{\|}}{C}.CH_3 \longrightarrow (CH_3)_3.C - \underset{\underset{OH}{|}}{C}.(CH_3)_2$$

$$\underset{\text{Isobutane}}{} \qquad \underset{\text{Acetone}}{}$$

2,3,3-Trimethyl-2-butanol

8. **Alkylation:** Alkylation is the process in which an alkyl group is introduced in place of hydrogen of a molecule. Tertiary alkanes react with unsaturated hydrocarbons in the presence of catalysts, like concentrated sulphuric acid, boron trifluoride etc., thus:

$$(CH_3)_3CH \ + \ CH_2 = \underset{\underset{CH_3}{|}}{C} - CH_3 \longrightarrow (CH_3)_3.\overset{\overset{CH_3}{|}}{C}.CH.CH_2.CH_3$$

$$\underset{\text{Isobutane}}{} \qquad \qquad \underset{\text{2,2,4-Trimethylpentane}}{}$$

2-Methylpropene

9. **Oxidation:** On oxidation alkanes give different products under different conditions:

   (i) **Combustion:** The reaction of alkanes with oxygen to form carbon dioxide, water and heat is called combustion in which alkanes are completely oxidized.

$$2C_2H_6 + 7O_2 \longrightarrow 4CO_2 + 6H_2O + 736 \text{ KCal.}$$

   Such reactions occur in the internal combustion engine. The mechanism of this reaction is extremely complicated and is not yet fully understood. The reaction is exothermic and yet requires a very high temperature.

   (ii) **Incomplete oxidation:** Partial combustion of alkanes takes place in a limited supply of air when carbon known as lamp black is formed.

   (iii) **Catalytic oxidation:** Lower alkanes are oxidized to aldehydes, ketones and acids in the presence of metallic catalysts at high temperature and pressure.

$$\underset{\text{Methane}}{CH_4} + O \xrightarrow[400°C/200 \text{ atm.}]{Cu} \underset{\text{Methanol}}{CH_3OH} \xrightarrow{[O]} \underset{\text{Formaldehyde}}{H.CHO} \xrightarrow{[O]} \underset{\text{Formic acid}}{H.COOH}$$

   Higher alkanes produce long chain fatty acids on oxidation, e.g.

$$R.CH_3 + 3O_2 \xrightarrow[\substack{\text{acetate} \\ \text{Air } 100°C \ [O]}]{\text{Manganese}} \underset{\text{Higher fatty acids}}{2R.COOH} + 2H_2O$$

   (iv) **Chemical oxidation:** Tertiary alkanes are oxidized with reagents like $KMnO_4$ or $K_2Cr_2O_7$ to alcohols. The other alkanes are inert to these oxidising agents.

$$\underset{\text{Isobutane}}{(CH_3)_3} \longrightarrow \underset{\text{tert-Butyl alcohol}}{(CH_3)C - OH}$$

10. **Aromatization:** Alkanes containing six or more carbon atoms give aromatic compounds when they are heated under pressure in the presence of chromic oxide or aluminium oxide catalyst.

n-Hexane   Benzene

The volatile alkanes show toxicity. Propane and butane have a light narcotic action, which is more pronounced with higher alkanes. More dangerous is the contamination of technical products with carbon dioxide. Benzene has narcotic action like that of ether, but the excitation is very prominent and it results in respiratory failure. Since it is quickly destroyed, death cases from benzene drinking are very few. However, small quantities of benzene if inhaled produce euphoria which may result in addiction for benzene. It irritates mucous and skin. Similarly the high boiling petroleum has a more prominent local action than benzene.

CYCLOALKANES

The cycloalkanes contain a closed chain or ring of carbon atoms bearing certain resemblance in properties with aliphatic compounds. Inspection of molecular formulae shows that the two ends of a saturated hydrocarbon chain do not end in CH_3 group but these ends are joined together with the formation of rings. Simple saturated alicyclic hydrocarbons, known also as homocyclic or carbocyclic, have the general formula C_nH_{2n}, which is isomeric with those of alkenes. The difference being that they do not contain any double bond but possess a ring structure. They may be simple saturated or unsaturated hydrocarbons or compounds containing different functional groups like –OH, –CHO, –COOH, etc. All these compounds differ from aliphatic compounds in possessing a cyclic structure.

Cycloalkanes from a homologous series contains in its molecule two hydrogen atoms less (in saturated cycloalkanes) than the corresponding open chain alkane.

Nomenclature: Since these compounds are made up of methylene groups joined together to form a ring, they in common system are known as the polymethylenes. The number of carbon atoms in the ring is indicated by a Greek or Latin prefix. The simplest cycloalkane has at least three methylene groups with the formula C_3H_6. Thus C_3H_6 is known as trimethylene, C_4H_8 as tetramethylene, C_5H_{10} as pentamethylene and so on.

According to IUPAC system, they are named as cycloalkanes. The names of cycloalkanes are taken from the names of the corresponding open-chain saturated hydrocarbons, preceded by the prefix cyclo to the corresponding alkane. The common names and IUPAC names are given below under each cycloalkane structure:

Common name	Trimethylene	Tetramethylene	Pentamethylene	Hexamethylene
IUPAC name	Cyclopropane	Cyclobutane	Cyclopentane	Cyclohexane

Unsaturated cyclic hydrocarbons containing one, two and three double bonds are known as cycloalkenes, cycloalkadienes and cycloalkatrienes respectively. The position of double bonds is mentioned by Arabic numerals. For example:

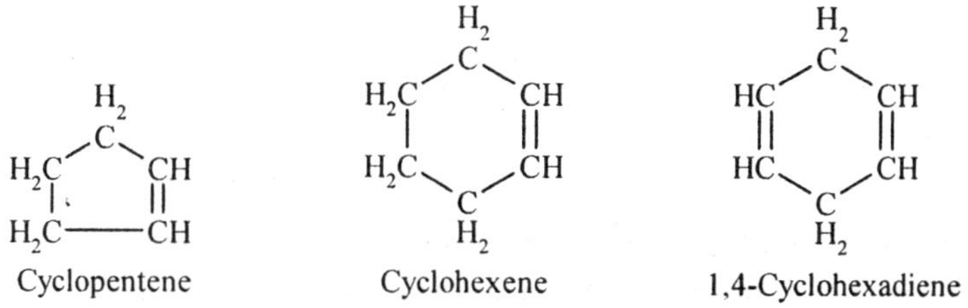

Cyclopentene   Cyclohexene   1,4-Cyclohexadiene

For convenience, cycloalkane rings are often represented by simple geometric figures: a triangle for cyclopropane, a square for cyclobutane, a pentagon for cyclopentane, a hexagon for cyclohexane and so on. It is understood that two hydrogens are attached at each corner of the figure unless some other group or double bonds is indicated. For example:

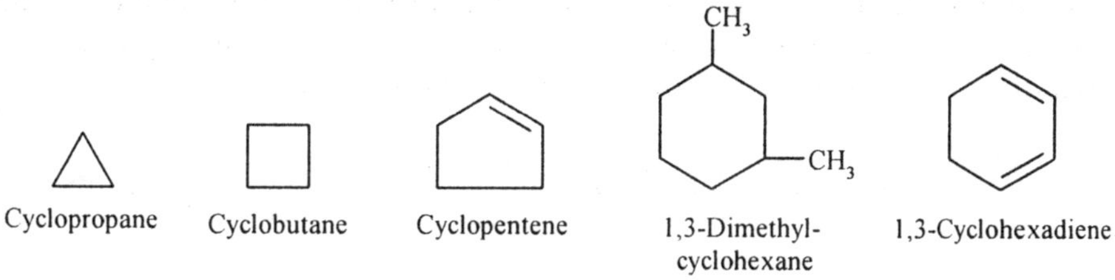

Cyclopropane   Cyclobutane   Cyclopentene   1,3-Dimethyl-   1,3-Cyclohexadiene
cyclohexane

Cycloalkanes are found widely in nature. Five- and six-membered cycloalkanes are met with in petroleum. Naphthenes contain mainly these compounds with small amount of naphthenic acids, which are cyclopentane monocarboxylic acids. Three-, four- and five-membered rings occur in terpenes. Some cyclopentene derivatives of fatty acids occur naturally and are important in medicine.

General Methods of Preparation of Cycloalkanes

Cycloalkanes may be prepared from open chain compounds by cyclization. The following general methods are normally used for their synthesis:

1. **Freud's method (1882):** α,γ-Dihalogen derivatives having terminal halogens on treatment with sodium or zinc in the presence of catalysts, like NaI and Na_2CO_3 give the corresponding cycloalkanes.

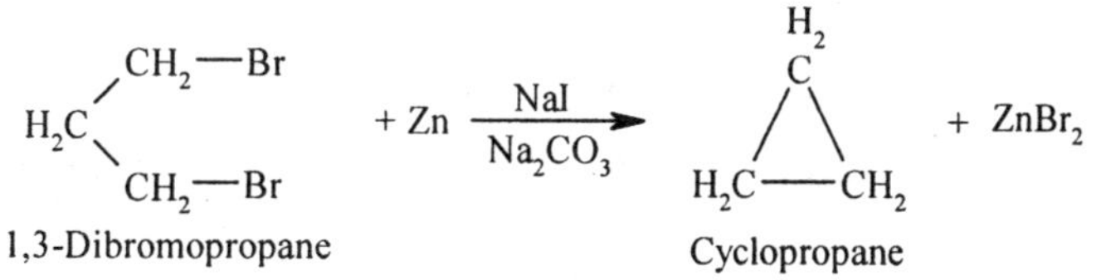

1,3-Dibromopropane   Cyclopropane

However, by this method compounds containing more than six carbon atoms are produced in poor yields. Such compounds undergo Wurtz reaction under these conditions.

2. **Wislicenus method (1893):** Dry distillation of barium or calcium salts of carboxylic acids yields cyclic ketones, which on reduction with Zn–Hg and HCl (Clemmensen's reduction) form cycloalkanes, e.g.

$$\begin{array}{c} CH_2.CH_2.COO \\ | \quad\quad\quad\quad\; {\Large\rangle} Ba \\ CH_2.CH_2.COO \end{array} \xrightarrow{\text{Heat}} \begin{array}{c} CH_2 —CH_2 \\ | \quad\quad\quad\;\; {\Large\rangle} CO + BaCO_3 \\ CH_2 —CH_2 \end{array}$$

Barium adipate   Cyclopentanone

$$\begin{array}{c} CH_2 —CH_2 \\ | \quad\quad\quad\;\; {\Large\rangle} CO + 4(H) \\ CH_2 —CH_2 \end{array} \xrightarrow[\text{HCl}]{\text{Zn—Hg}} \begin{array}{c} CH_2 —CH_2 \\ | \quad\quad\quad\;\; {\Large\rangle} CH_2 + H_2O \\ CH_2 —CH_2 \end{array}$$

Cyclopentane

This method is useful for the preparation of only five, six and seven carbon ring cycloalkanes. According to Ruzicka thorium and yttrium salts give better yields of cyclic ketones. The governing feature is that the two anionic groups in the same molecule are kept on close proximity to one another by the metallic action during the pyrolysis.

3. **Perkin's method (1883):** Many cyclic compounds may be prepared by condensing certain dihalogen of alkanes with sodium malonic ester or sodium acetoacetic ester.

(i) α,β-Dibromides condense with one molecule of malonic ester in the presence of two molecules of sodium ethoxide to form cycloalkane-1,1-dicarboxylic ester, which on hydrolysis and decarboxylation yields cycloalkane.

$$\begin{array}{c} CH_2—Br \\ | \\ CH_2—Br \end{array} \xrightarrow[-NaBr]{Na^+\bar{C}H(CO_2.C_2H_5)_2} \begin{array}{c} CH_2.CH(CO_2.C_2H_5)_2 \\ | \\ CH_2.Br \end{array} \xrightarrow{C_2H_5ONa/-H^+}$$

$$\begin{array}{c} CH_2—\bar{C}.(CO_2.C_2H_5)_2 \\ | \\ CH_2—Br \end{array} \xrightarrow{-Br^-} \begin{array}{c} CH_2 \\ | \quad\quad {\Large\rangle} C.(CO_2.C_2H_5)_2 \\ CH_2 \end{array} \xrightarrow[2.\ HCl]{1.\ KOH}$$

$$\begin{array}{c} CH_2 \\ | \quad\quad {\Large\rangle} C.(CO_2H)_2 \\ CH_2 \end{array} \xrightarrow[-CO_2]{\Delta} \begin{array}{c} CH_2 \\ | \quad\quad {\Large\rangle} CH—COOH \\ CH_2 \end{array} \xrightarrow[-CO_2]{\Delta} \begin{array}{c} \overset{H_2}{\underset{}{C}} \\ {\Large\triangle} \\ H_2C—CH_2 \end{array}$$

(ii) The above α,β-dibromides also condense with two molecules of sodium malonic ester to yield cyclobutane as follows:

$$\begin{array}{c} CH_2.Br \\ | \\ CH_2.Br \end{array} \overset{+\ 2CHNa.(CO_2C_2H_5)_2}{\underset{\text{Monosodium ester}}{\xrightarrow{\quad\quad\quad}}} \xrightarrow{-2NaBr} \begin{array}{c} CH_2—CH.(CO_2C_2H_5)_2 \\ | \\ CH_2—CH.(CO_2C_2H_5)_2 \end{array}$$

$$\xrightarrow{2C_2H_5.ONa} \begin{array}{c} CH_2—C.Na.(COOC_2H_5)_2 \\ | \\ CH_2—C.Na.(COOC_2H_5)_2 \end{array} \xrightarrow[-2NaI]{I_2} \begin{array}{c} CH_2—C.(COOC_2H_5)_2 \\ | \\ CH_2—C.(COOC_2H_5)_2 \end{array}$$

$$\xrightarrow[\text{2. Decarboxylation}]{\text{1. Hydrolysis}} \begin{array}{c} CH_2—CH_2 \\ | \quad\quad | \\ CH_2—CH_2 \end{array}$$

Cyclobutane

The cycloalkanes containing three to seven carbon atoms may be prepared by using the appropriate dihalogen derivatives of alkanes under suitable reaction conditions.

(iii) Acetoacetic ester may be used to prepare ring compounds like:

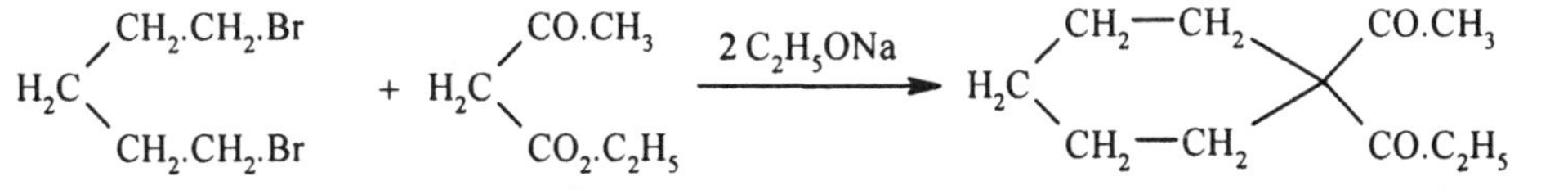

1,5-Dibromopentane Acetoacetic ester 1-Acetylcyclohexane-1-carboxylic ester

Cyclohexylmethyl ketone

Except for the four carbon atom rings, it is possible to prepare ring containing three, five, six and seven carbon atoms by using acetoacetic ester. When acetoacetic ester is reacted with 1,3-dibromopropane, formation of dihydropyran takes place.

4. **Dieckmann's method (1901):** The esters of dicarboxylic acids like adipic, pimelic or suberic acid undergo intramolecular condensation like Claisen condensation in the presence of sodium or better with sodium ethoxide to give five-, six- or seven-membered cyclic ketones.

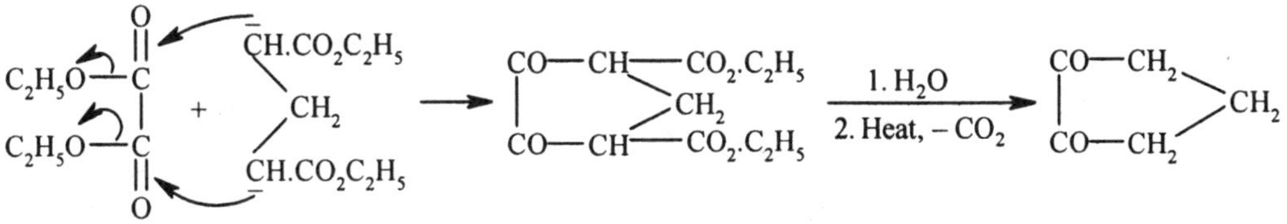

5. **Internal Grignard condensation:** The aliphatic ketones containing terminal halogen atoms form Grignard reagents with magnesium in ether which yield spontaneously cyclic tertiary alcohols, e.g.

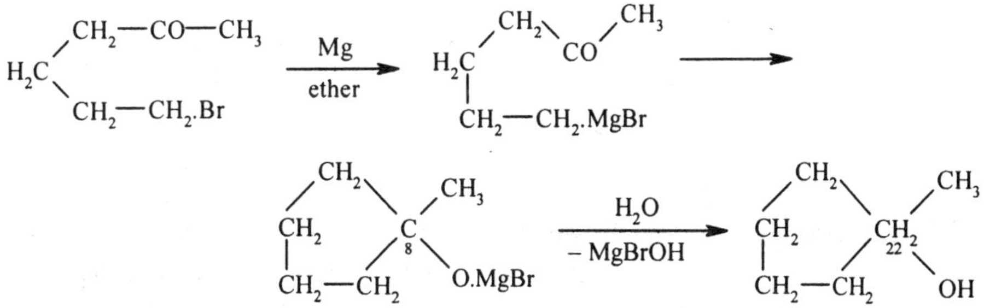

6. **Thorpe-Ziegler's method:** Intermolecular cyclization of β-dinitriles takes place giving cyclic compounds when they are treated with bases, like tertiary metallic alkyl amines, e.g.

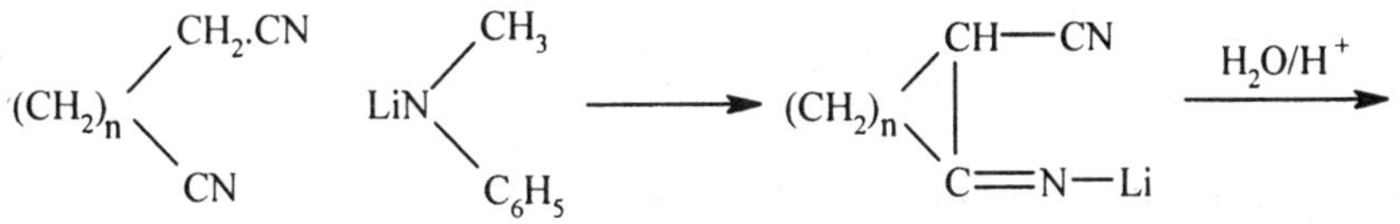

β-Dinitrile N-Lithium-N-methyl aniline

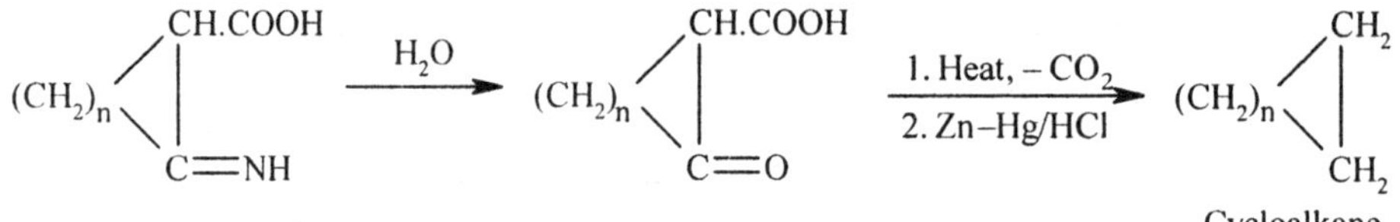

$$(CH_2)_n \overset{CH.COOH}{\underset{C=NH}{\diagdown}} \xrightarrow{H_2O} (CH_2)_n \overset{CH.COOH}{\underset{C=O}{\diagdown}} \xrightarrow[2.\ Zn-Hg/HCl]{1.\ Heat,\ -CO_2} (CH_2)_n \overset{CH_2}{\underset{CH_2}{\diagdown}}$$

Cycloalkane

Five- and six-membered ring compounds are prepared in good yields by this method. If in this reaction an ordinary base is used as a catalyst, then it would undergo intramolecular addition at the –C–N group. N–Lithium–N–methyl aniline used as a base catalyst is sterically hindered, so the reaction with CN group is minimized.

7. **Diels-Alder reaction:** When an unsaturated compound is added to a conjugated diene, a cyclic compound is formed readily without elimination of any compound. The unsaturated compound must have an electron withdrawing group like carbonyl or carboxyl groups and is termed as dienophile, e.g. acrylic aldehyde, maleic anhydride etc. The other components may be dienes of various types: alicyclic, semicyclic compounds containing two double bonds in conjugation. In this reaction no catalyst is required. The two compounds are heated together or heated in a solvent like benzene e.g.

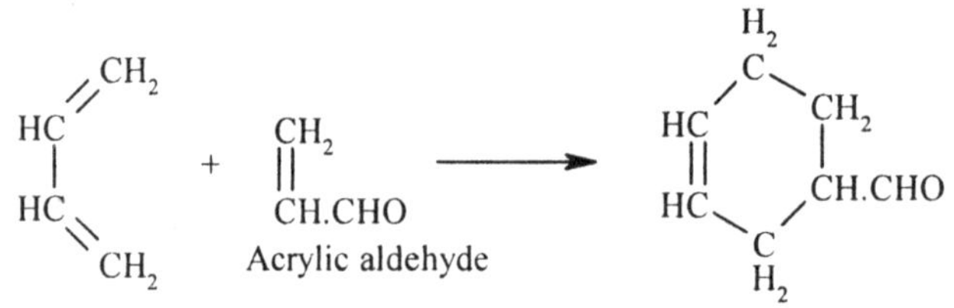

Butadiene + Acrylic aldehyde → Tetrahydrobenzaldehyde

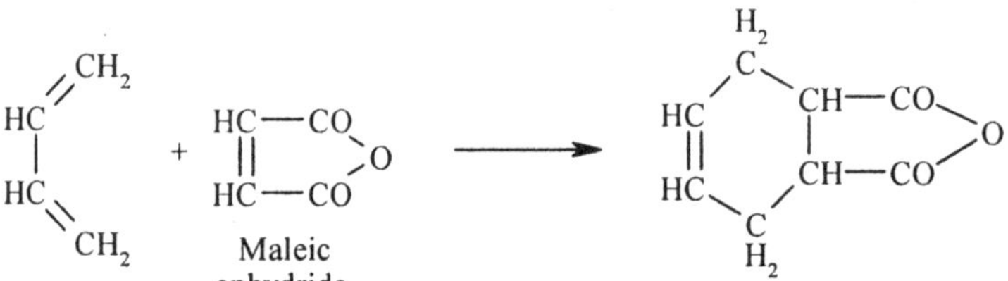

Butadiene + Maleic anhydride → Tetrahydrophthalic anhydride

8. **Internal pinacol formation:** Various types of bifunctional compounds undergo intermolecular reactions under suitable conditions to form cyclic compounds. For example cyclic 1,2-ditertiary alcohols have been made by reduction of diketones.

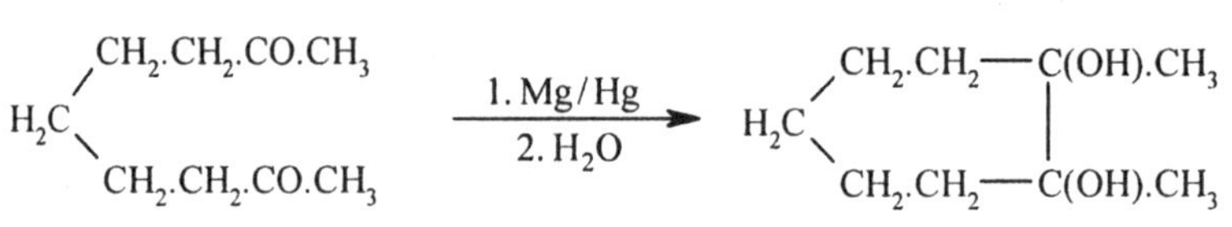

$$H_2C \overset{CH_2.CH_2.CO.CH_3}{\underset{CH_2.CH_2.CO.CH_3}{\diagdown}} \xrightarrow[2.\ H_2O]{1.\ Mg/Hg} H_2C \overset{CH_2.CH_2-C(OH).CH_3}{\underset{CH_2.CH_2-C(OH).CH_3}{\diagdown}}$$

9. **Addition of carbenes to alkenes:** Dihalocarbenes obtained by the reaction of potassium tertiary butoxide and chloroform or bromoform added to alkenes by cis-addition to yield alicyclics.

$$CHCl_3 + (CH_3)_3C—OK \xrightarrow[-(CH_3)_3.C.OH]{} :CCl_3^- \xrightarrow[-Cl]{} :CCl_2$$

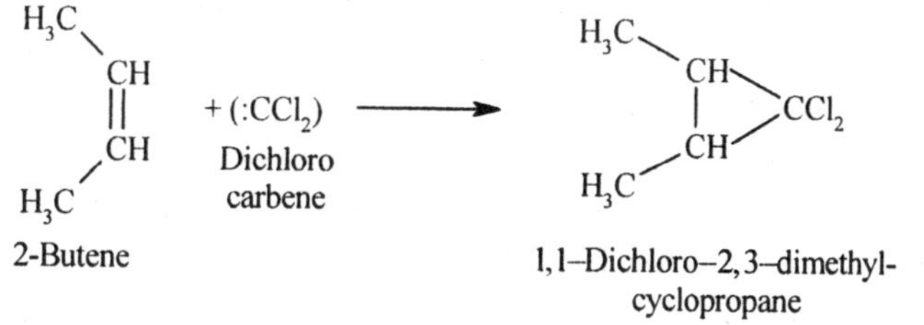

2-Butene + (:CCl₂) Dichloro carbene ⟶ 1,1–Dichloro–2,3–dimethyl-cyclopropane

10. **Condensation of unsaturated compounds:** Polymerization of unsaturated compounds like cinnamic acid takes place to give truxillic and truxinic acids in the presence of light, as under.

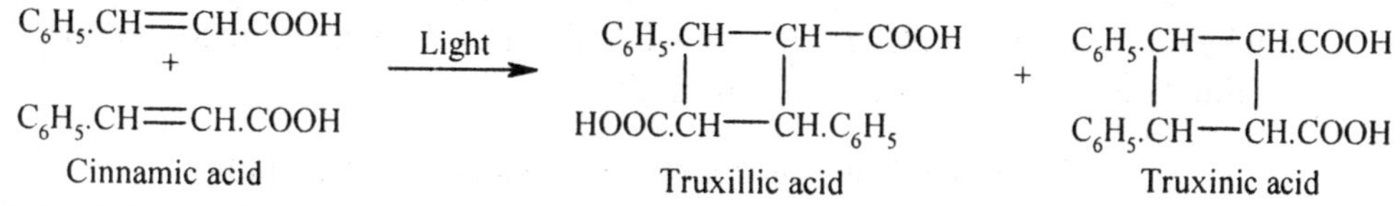

$$C_6H_5.CH{=}CH.COOH$$
$$+$$
$$C_6H_5.CH{=}CH.COOH$$
Cinnamic acid

$\xrightarrow{Light}$

$$\begin{array}{l} C_6H_5.CH—CH—COOH \\ \qquad | \qquad | \\ HOOC.CH—CH.C_6H_5 \end{array}$$
Truxillic acid

$+$

$$\begin{array}{l} C_6H_5.CH—CH.COOH \\ \qquad | \qquad | \\ C_6H_5.CH—CH.COOH \end{array}$$
Truxinic acid

11. **Reduction of aromatic compounds:** Hydrogenation of benzene derivatives in the presence of a nickel or platinum catalyst gives cyclic compounds. In this way, benzene itself yields cyclohexane, aniline yields cyclohexylamine, and phenol yields cyclohexanol:

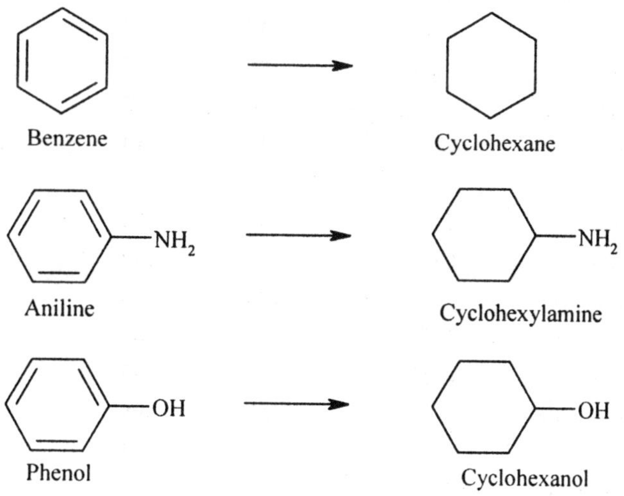

Benzene ⟶ Cyclohexane

Aniline ⟶ Cyclohexylamine

Phenol ⟶ Cyclohexanol

12. **Addition of methylenes:** Addition of alkenes with diazomethane leads to the formation of cyclopropanes in one step operations, e.g.

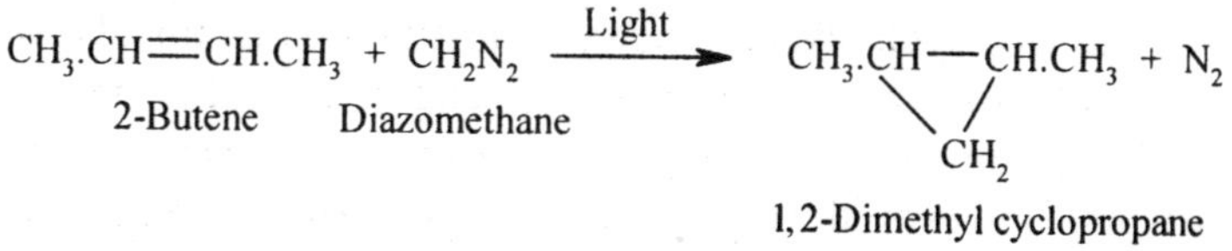

$$CH_3.CH{=}CH.CH_3 + CH_2N_2 \xrightarrow{Light} \begin{array}{c} CH_3.CH—CH.CH_3 \\ \diagdown \quad \diagup \\ CH_2 \end{array} + N_2$$
2-Butene   Diazomethane

1,2-Dimethyl cyclopropane

GENERAL PHYSICAL PROPERTIES OF CYCLOALKANES

1. The physical properties of cyclic aliphatic hydrocarbons are similar to those of the corresponding open-chain hydrocarbons. However, the boiling points and densities of cyclic compounds are somewhat higher.
2. The first two members, i.e. cyclopropane and cyclobutane are gases at room temperature, while higher cycloalkanes are colourless liquids having pleasant odour.
3. Their physical constants like b.p., m.p. and sp. gr. increase with increase in molecular weights as shown in Table 8.2.
4. They are nonpolar or weakly polar compounds and therefore, they are soluble in non-polar or weakly polar solvents like carbon tetrachloride, ligroin and ether. They are not dissolved in highly polar solvents and in water.
5. Their heat of combustion follows an irregular pattern revealing that cyclopentane and cyclohexane molecules are most stable while other cycloalkanes are less stable. This can be explained on the basis of Baeyer's strain theory.

Table 8.2. Physical constants of alicyclic compounds

Compound	Formula	B.P. ^{o}C	M.P. ^{o}C	Sp. gr. at $20^{o}C$	Heat of combustion
Cyclopropane	C_3H_5	−33	−127	−	499.8
Cyclobutane	C_4H_8	13	−80	0.704	655.6
Cyclopentane	C_5H_{10}	49	−94	0.746	793.5
Cyclohexane	C_6H_{12}	81	7	0.778	944.4
Cycloheptane	C_7H_{14}	118	−12	0.810	1108.1
Cyclooctane	C_8H_{16}	149	14	0.830	1268.8
Cyclononane	C_9H_{18}	172	11	0.845	1429.2
Cyclodecane	$C_{10}H_{20}$	201	9.6	−	1586.0
Methyl cyclopentane	$CH_3.C_5H_9$	72	−142	0.749	−
Methyl cyclohexane	$CH_3.C_6H_{11}$	100	−126	0.769	−
1,3-cyclopentadiene	C_5H_6	42	−85	0.798	−
Cyclopentene	C_5H_8	46	−93	0.774	−
1,3-Cyclohexadiene	C_6H_8	80.5	−98	0.840	−
Cyclohexene	C_6H_{10}	83	−104	0.810	−
1,4-Cyclohexadiene	C_6H_8	87	−49	0.847	−

GENERAL CHEMICAL PROPERTIES OF CYCLOALKANES

Similar to alkanes, the saturated cycloalkanes undergo substitution reaction. However, cycloalkanes having rings of 3- or 4-carbon atoms are unstable and tend to break the ring forming open chain aliphatic compounds by addition reaction. They show the chemical reactions of both saturated and unsaturated hydrocarbons. However, the type of reaction is dependent on the size of the ring.

1. **Reaction with halogen:** Cyclopropane and cyclobutane react with chlorine and bromine to form addition products by breaking the ring. However, cycloalokanes react with these halogens in sunlight to yield substitution products.

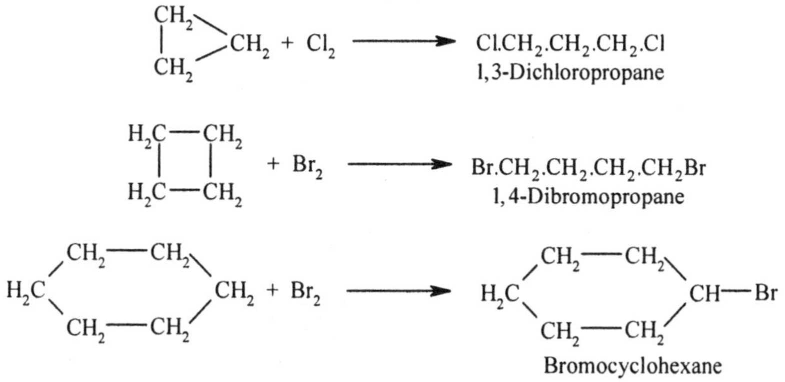

$$\begin{array}{c} CH_2 \\ | \quad \diagdown CH_2 \\ CH_2 \end{array} + Cl_2 \longrightarrow \begin{array}{c} Cl.CH_2.CH_2.CH_2.Cl \\ 1,3\text{-Dichloropropane} \end{array}$$

$$\begin{array}{c} H_2C-CH_2 \\ |\qquad| \\ H_2C-CH_2 \end{array} + Br_2 \longrightarrow \begin{array}{c} Br.CH_2.CH_2.CH_2.CH_2Br \\ 1,4\text{-Dibromopropane} \end{array}$$

$$\begin{array}{c} CH_2-CH_2 \\ H_2C \diagup \qquad\quad \diagdown CH_2 \\ CH_2-CH_2 \end{array} + Br_2 \longrightarrow \begin{array}{c} CH_2-CH_2 \\ H_2C \diagup \qquad\quad \diagdown CH-Br \\ CH_2-CH_2 \end{array}$$
Bromocyclohexane

2. **Reaction with halogen acids:** Cyclopropane and cyclobutane react with hydrochloric and hydrobromic acids to form addition products. Higher cycloalkanes do not react with these acids.

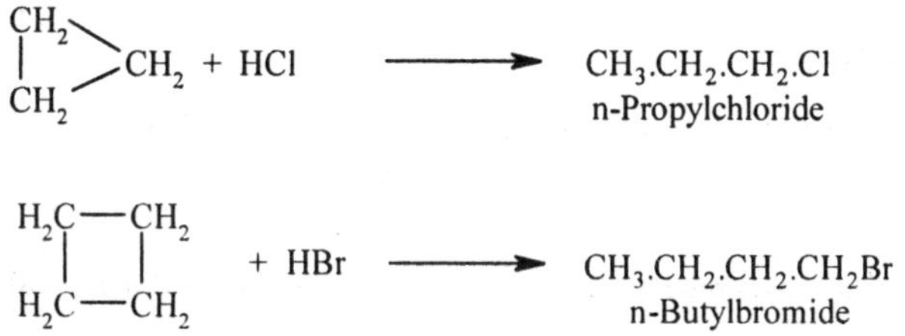

$$\begin{array}{c} CH_2 \\ | \quad \diagdown CH_2 \\ CH_2 \end{array} + HCl \longrightarrow \begin{array}{c} CH_3.CH_2.CH_2.Cl \\ n\text{-Propylchloride} \end{array}$$

$$\begin{array}{c} H_2C-CH_2 \\ |\qquad| \\ H_2C-CH_2 \end{array} + HBr \longrightarrow \begin{array}{c} CH_3.CH_2.CH_2.CH_2Br \\ n\text{-Butylbromide} \end{array}$$

3. **Reduction:** However, cycloalkanes upto five carbon atoms when hydrogenated in the presence of Ni or Pt as catalysts produce the corresponding straight chain aliphatic hydrocarbons higher ones are not easily reduced.

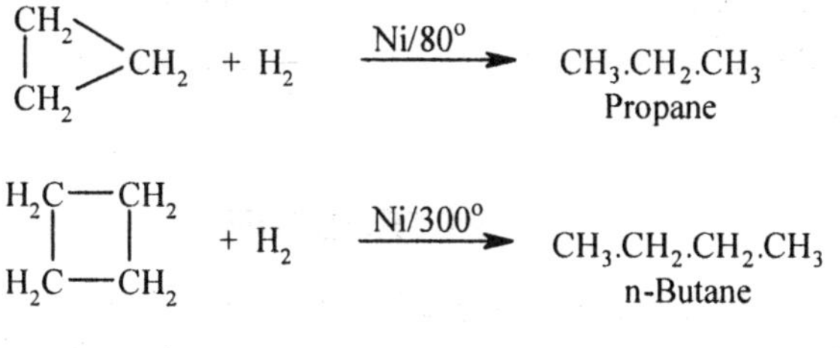

$$\begin{array}{c} CH_2 \\ | \quad \diagdown CH_2 \\ CH_2 \end{array} + H_2 \xrightarrow{Ni/80^\circ} \begin{array}{c} CH_3.CH_2.CH_3 \\ Propane \end{array}$$

$$\begin{array}{c} H_2C-CH_2 \\ |\qquad| \\ H_2C-CH_2 \end{array} + H_2 \xrightarrow{Ni/300^\circ} \begin{array}{c} CH_3.CH_2.CH_2.CH_3 \\ n\text{-Butane} \end{array}$$

4. **Oxidation:** Cycloalkanes are not oxidized by cold aqueous $KMnO_4$ or ozone. Oxidation with alkaline $KMnO_4$ gives dicarboxylic acids, as shown hereunder.

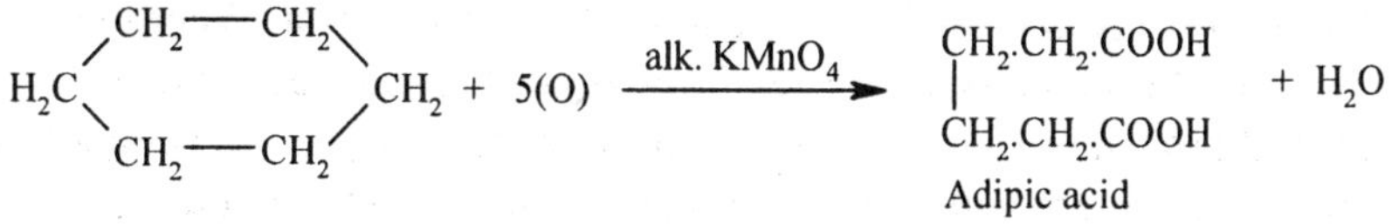

$$\begin{array}{c} CH_2-CH_2 \\ H_2C \diagup \qquad\quad \diagdown CH_2 \\ CH_2-CH_2 \end{array} + 5(O) \xrightarrow{alk.\ KMnO_4} \begin{array}{c} CH_2.CH_2.COOH \\ | \\ CH_2.CH_2.COOH \end{array} + H_2O$$
Adipic acid

5. **Ring expansion:** Diazomethane reacts with cycloalkanes to form their higher homologues by the insertion of methylene group in the ring, e.g.

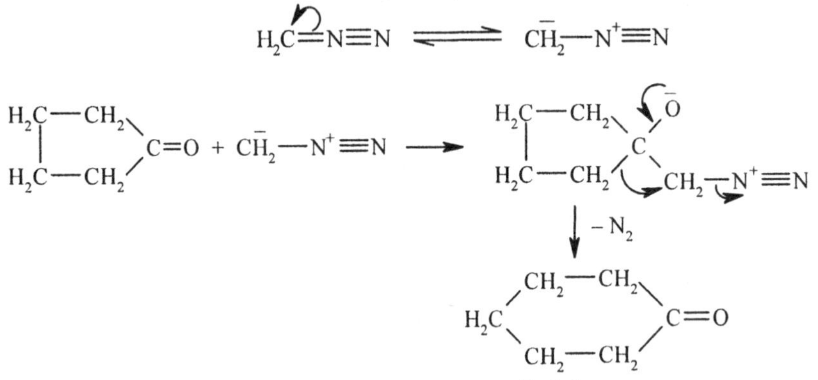

$$H_2C=N\equiv N \rightleftharpoons CH_2-N^+\equiv N$$

$$\underset{\text{Cyclohexanone}}{}$$

Cyclohexanone

6. **Rearrangement:** Cycloalkyl amines undergo ring expansion or ring contraction on treatment with nitrous acid. If the amino group is attached to the ring then the ring is contracted. On the other hand, if the amino group is separated from the ring by a carbon atom ring expansion takes place.

Ring contraction:

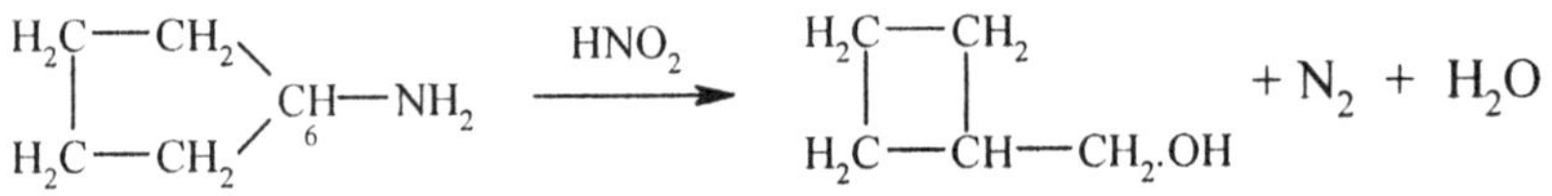

Cyclopentylamine $\xrightarrow{HNO_2}$ Cyclobutyl methyl alcohol $+ N_2 + H_2O$

Ring expansion:

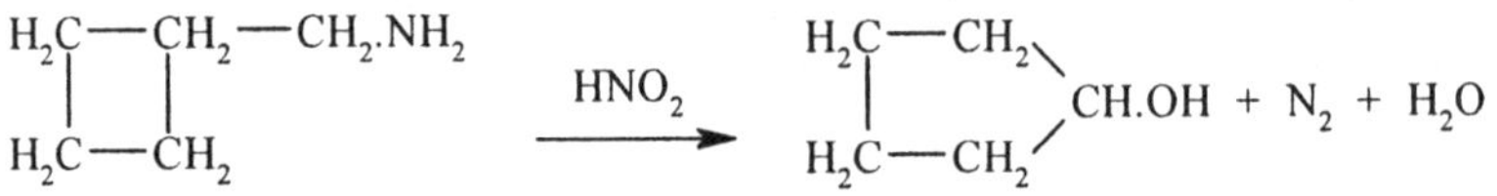

Cyclobutyl methyl amine $\xrightarrow{HNO_2}$ Cyclopentanol $+ N_2 + H_2O$

PETROLEUM

Petroleum (Latin *petra* = rock, *oleum* = oil) is a hard coloured oil found in beds beneath the surface of earth from where it is obtained by the mining process and is, therefore, called as **mineral oil** or **crude oil**. The gases obtained with this liquid are known as natural gases.

It is found under the rocky belt of the earth's crust, often floating over salt water (Fig. 8.4). Most of the world's supply of petroleum is at present obtained from Russia, Venezuela, Mexico, Romania, Iraq and some other Middle East countries. United States produces about 30% of the total world's output which is about ten million barrels of petroleum daily. India on the other hand has very poor production of petroleum amounting to about 0.4% of the world's output.

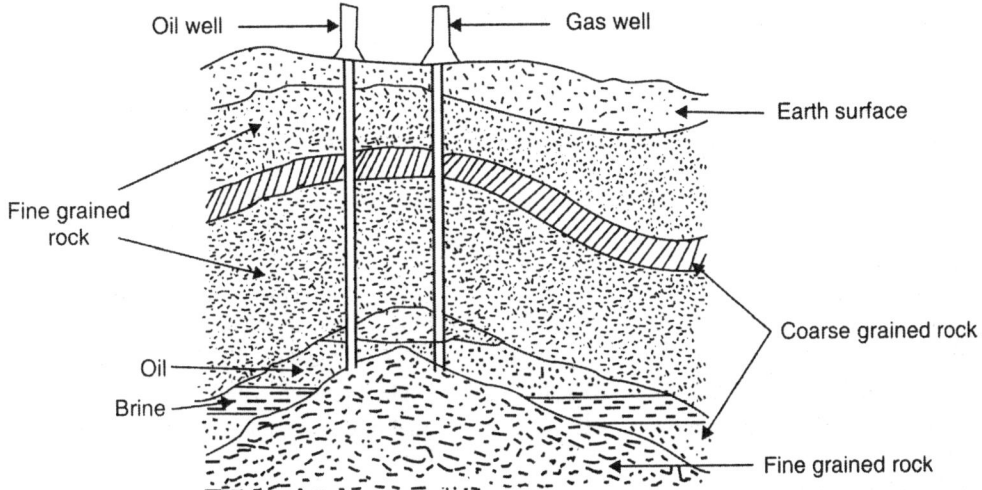

Fig. 8.4. Occurrence and drilling of crude petroleum.

Composition of petroleum: Petroleum is a highly complex mixture of hydrocarbons having varying proportions of oxygen, sulphur and nitrogen containing products. Its composition varies with the place of origin. It is a mixture of hydrocarbon gases, liquids and solid. The natural gases mainly present are methane (84%), propane (4%) and butane (2%) and other hydrocarbons (2%). Other main substances found in the petroleum are:

1. **Hydrocarbons:** Paraffins (alkanes, containing upto 40 carbon atoms), olefins or unsaturated hydrocarbons, cycloalkanes, aromatic compounds like benzene, toluene, etc.).
2. Impurities derived from organic compounds of nitrogen (e.g. quinoline) and sulphur compounds (like mercaptans).
3. Impurities derived from animals and plants (like chlorophyll, haemin, green and red colouring matters).
4. Optically active organic compounds.

Petroleum obtained from Pennsylvania (USA), Romania and Middle East is rich in alkanes and is known as **paraffinic oil**, whereas the oil obtained from Russia, Venezuela etc. is rich in cycloalkanes and is known as **asphaltic oil**.

Discussion on mining of petroleum and refining of crude oil is outside the scope of this book. However, it may be added.

The crude petroleum obtained by mining process is a high boiling viscous and dark-coloured mixture of dissolved gases and liquids. It has an unpleasant smell due to the presence of sulphur-containing impurities of sand and sea water. Separation of this crude oil by fractional distillation is done to get more useful and more consumable products.

In the following two tables (Tables 8.3 and 8.4) are given the different fractions obtained from the crude petroleum with their boiling ranges, composition and uses. The various compounds which are obtained from different hydrocarbons of petroleum give some idea about the composition and importance of petroleum.

Table 8.3

Fraction	Boiling range ^oC	Approximate composition	Uses
1. Uncondensed gases	Upto 30°	C_1 to C_5	Fuel gases, synthesis of organic compounds, production of carbon black, refrigerant, manufacture of gasoline, rubber, etc.
2. Crude Naphtha (16%) Further fraction gives:	20–150°	C_5 to C_{10}	
(i) Petroleum ether	30–70°	C_5 to C_6	Solvent for fat oil, varnish, rubber and dry cleaning
(ii) Petrol or gasoline	70–120°	C_6 to C_8	Engine fuel, dry-cleaning and for petrol air gas
(iii) Benzene	120–150°	C_8 to C_{10}	Dry cleaning and solvent for oil, fat and varnish
3. Kerosene (25–30%)	150–250°	C_{10} to C_{15}	Fuel, illuminant, oil gas
4. Gas oil or heavy oil (25–30%) Refractionation gases: (i) Gas oil (ii) Fuel oil (iii) Diesel oil	250–400°	C_{12} to C_{18}	Fuel in diesel engine, cracked to yield more gasoline
5. Residue oil (30%) above 400° Further fractionation gives:		C_{17} to C_{40}	Lubrication
(i) Lubricating oil		C_{17} to C_{20}	Candles, boot polish, wax paper etc.
(ii) Paraffin wax		C_{20} to C_{30}	Candles, boot polish, wax paper
(iii) Vaseline		C_{20} to C_{30}	Toilet goods, ointments, lubrication
(iv) Pitch or residue		C_{30} to C_{40}	Road surfacing, paints etc.
6. Petroleum cake			As fuel

Table 8.4. Petrochemicals

Hydrocarbons	Compounds obtained
1. Methane	Chloromethanes, methanol, acetylene, formaldehyde, formic acid, methyl ether, dimethyl sulphate, ethylene glycol, methyl amine, hexamethylenetetramine, hydrogen cyanide, acrylonitrile, chlorofluoromethane derivatives, freon, etc.
2. Ethane	Ethyl chloride, acetic acid, ethyl bromide, nitroethane, ethlene, acetaldehye, acetic anhydride, ethyl acetate, diethyl ether, etc.
3. Ethylene	Ethanol, ethylene glycol, ethylene oxide, ethylene chloride, ethylene chlorohydrine, vinyl chloride, butadiene, acetaldehyde, acetic acid, ethyl acetate, ethyl ether, crotonaldehyde, butyraldehyde, butanol-1, butyric acid, crotonic acid, ethyl chloride, tetraethyl lead, ethylene bromide, thiodiglycol, glyoxal, acrylonitrile, acrylic acid, etc.
4. Propane	Propanol, propionic acid, nitromethane, nitroethane, nitropropane, ethylene propyl ether, amines, acetone, cyanohydrine, etc.
5. Propene	Alkyl alcohol, alkyl chloride, glycerol, isopropyl alcohol, isopropyl amine, acetone, cyanohydrine, propylene oxide, propylene glycol, propionaldehyde, propionic acid, n-propyl alcohol, acrolein, acrylic acid, etc.

(Contd.)

	Hydrocarbons	Compounds obtained
6.	Butanes	Butanol, butadiene, methyl ethyl ketone, ethyl butyl ketone, tert-butyl alcohol, butyl rubber, iso-octane, etc.
7.	Pentanes	Amyl alcohols, amyl chlorides, amyl amines, amyl mercaptans, pentylenes, amyl phenols, etc.
8.	Butenes	Butanols, butadiene, thiophene, etc.
9.	n-Hexane	Benzene, DDT, gammexane ($C_6H_6Cl_6$)
10.	n-Heptane	Toluene, benzoic acid, saccharin, etc.
11.	Acetylene	Carbon black, vinylacetylene, chloroprene, acetaldehyde, acetic acid, peracetic acid, vinyl chloride, chloroethenes, vinyl acetate, methyl vinyl ether, butadiene, acrylonitrile, etc.
12.	Diolefins	Hexamethylenediamine, 4-vinyl cyclohexane, isoprene, etc.
13.	Cycloalkanes	Benzene, toluene, xylenes, adipic acid, hexamethylenediamine, etc.
14.	Toluenes	Benzyl chloride, benzal chloride, benzotrichloride, benzyl alcohol, benzaldehyde, benzoic acid, T.N.T., toluenesulphonic acids, p-toluenesulphonamide, phthalic anhydride, phthalamide, phthalamic acid, phthalimide, tert-phthalic acid, etc.

OFFICIAL COMPOUNDS AND PREPARATIONS

Paraffin Hard (Hard Paraffin)

It is a purified mixture of solid hydrocarbons (paraffins) obtained from petroleum or from schale oil.

Description: Hard paraffin is a colourless or white, translucent mass, which mostly shows crystalline structure. It is colourless, tasteless, slightly greasy in touch and burns with a luminous flame. It is insoluble in water and alcohol but is soluble in chloroform and solvent ether. Its melting range is 50 to 75°C (Appendix I).

Reaction (pH): A solution prepared by boiling 5 g in 10 ml of alcohol, previously neutralised to solution of litmus, is neutral to litmus.

Tests for purity: It is tested for readily carbonisable substances and sulphated ash, which should not be more than 0.1% (Appendix II).

Readily carbonisable substances: I.P. procedure for readily carbonisable substance is as follows:

Place 5 ml of the melted hard paraffin in a glass-stoppered test tube which has been rinsed with chromic acid, then rinsed with water and dried. Add 5 ml of sulphuric acid (having between 94.5% to 95.5% of H_2SO_4) and heat in a boiling water-bath for ten minutes. After the test tube has been in the bath for thirty seconds, remove it quickly and while holding the stopper in place, give three vigorous vertical shakes over an amplitude of about 12 cm. After shaking, replace the test tube in the bath. Repeat the process every thirty seconds. Do not keep the test-tube out of the bath more than three seconds for each shaking period. At the end of ten minutes, from the time when first placed in the water bath, remove the test tube. The hard paraffin remains unchanged in colour and the acid does not become darker than the standard colour by mixing in a similar test tube 3 ml of ferric chloride C.S., 1.5 ml of cobaltous chloride C.S., 0.5 ml of cupric sulphate C.S., the mixture being over laid by 5 ml of melted Hard Paraffin.

Uses: It is used as a pharmaceutical aid, as an ingredient of paraffin ointment, simple ointment and wool alcohol ointment.

LIGHT LIQUID PARAFFIN

It is a purified mixture of liquid saturated hydrocarbons obtained from petroleum and consists of mainly C_{15} to C_{20} hydrocarbons.

Description: It is a transparent, colourless, non-fluorescent, odourless and tasteless oily liquid, which is practically insoluble in water and in alcohol but is soluble in chloroform and solvent ether. It is miscible with almost all the fixed and volatile oils. Its sp. gr. (wt/ml) at 20°C is 0.820–0.880 g (Appendix III) and dynamic viscosity at 37.8°C is not greater than 30 (Appendix V).

Test for purity: It is tested for weight per ml, dynamic viscosity tests for acidity and alkalinity, readily carbonisable substances (see under Hard Paraffin) and sulphur compounds.

Sulphur compounds are tested by mixing 4 ml with 2 ml of ethyl alcohol and 2 drops of a clean saturated solution of lead monoxide in solution of sodium hydroxide and heating the mixture at 70°C for ten minutes with frequent shaking. The mixture should remain colourless.

Storage: It is used as a pharmaceutical aid, in ointments and cosmetic products, such as sunscreen oils, baby and cleansing creams.

LIQUID PARAFFIN

Synonyms: White mineral oil, liquid petrolatum.

Liquid paraffin is a purified mixture of liquid hydrocarbons obtained from petroleum. The hydrocarbons usually present range from C_{18} to C_{24}. Tocopherol in not more than 10 ppm may be added as a stabilizer (it acts as an antioxidant to avoid peroxide formation).

Description: It is transparent colourless, oily liquid and is almost free from fluorescence by day light. It is odourless and tasteless when cold but develops a faint odour of petroleum, when heated. It is practically insoluble in water and alcohol, but is soluble in chloroform, solvent ether and volatile oils. Its sp. gr. at 25°C is 0.860 to 0.904 and kinematic viscosity at 37.6°C is not less than 64 cp (Appendix II and Appendix V).

Test for purity: It is tested for acidity, alkalinity, readily carbonisable substances, sulphur compounds (see under light liquid) and solid paraffins.

Solid paraffins: If present in more than required proportions will separate and cause cloudiness when the dried oil is kept in a mixture of ice and water for four hours.

I.P. test is as follows:

Place a suitable quantity, previously dried by heating at 1000°C for two hours and cool in a desiccator over sulphuric acid in a cylindrical glass vessel. The vessel has a capacity of about 120 ml and an internal diameter of about 25 mm. Close the vessel and immerse in a mixture of ice and water, the liquid is sufficiently clear after four hours and a black line, 0.5 mm in width, held vertically behind the vessel, can be easily seen.

Storage: It is preserved in a well-closed container away from light.

Uses: It has been used as a laxative and intestinal lubricant for a long time. It can be given very successfully for softening the content of lower intestine, especially during the treatment of haemorr-hoides. It should not be given for longer period and is administered only at bed time. It is not advisable to give it to infants.

Dose: 8–30 ml.

Preparations: It is used in the following I.P. preparations:

(a) Liquid paraffin emulsion (I.P. p. 1518)

(b) Emulsifying ointment (I.P. 85)

(c) Wool alcohol ointment (I.P. 85)

WHITE SOFT PARAFFIN

Synonym: White Petroleum Jelly.

It is a purified mixture of semisolid hydrocarbons obtained from petroleum and the mixture is bleached or decolourised as much as possible.

Description: It is white, transparent, soft mass, unctuous to touch, odourless and tasteless. It is only slightly fluorescent by day light even when melted. It is practically insoluble in water and alcohol, but is soluble in chloroform, solvent ether and light petroleum. Its weight per ml at 69°C is 0.815 to 0.880 g and melting range is 38–56°C (Appendix I).

Tests for purity: It is tested for weight per ml, melting range, reaction, fixed oils, fats and resin, foreign organic matter and sulphated ash (Appendix II).

Foreign organic matter is tested by heating. It volatilises, without emitting an acrid odour. Fixed oils, fats and resin are tested as per the following I.P. method:

Digest 10 g with 50 ml solution of sodium hydroxide at 100°C for thirty minutes and allow the aqueous layer to separate. On acidifying the aqueous layer with dilute sulphuric acid, no precipitate or oily matter is produced.

Uses: Like liquid paraffin, it is used as a pharmaceutical aid. It is preferred as a household topical dressing. It is considered as a simple and effective application for burns.

Preparations: It is an ingredient of emulsifying ointment.
Paraffin ointment, simple ointment (I.P., p. 1520)
Wool alcohol ointment (I.P. 85).

YELLOW SOFT PARAFFIN

Synonym: Yellow Petroleum Jelly.

It is a purified mixture of semi-solid hydrocarbons obtained from petroleum.

Description: It is a pale, yellow translucent, soft mass, unctuous to touch, odourless and tasteless. It is not more than slightly fluorescent by day light. It is practically insoluble in water and alcohol, but is soluble in chloroform, solvent ether and light petroleum (40–60°C). Its melting range is 38–60°C (Appendix I).

Tests for purity: It is tested for melting point, reaction, fixed oils, fats and resin (I.P. 1519), foreign organic matter (see in white soft paraffin above), yellow colouring matter and sulphated ash (Appendix II).

Yellow colouring matter is tested by boiling yellow soft paraffin (5 g) with alcohol (10 ml) and noting the colour of alcohol, which is not coloured yellow.

Uses: It is an important pharmaceutical aid and is an ingredient of many ointments, like dithramol (I.P. 1049), paraffin ointment, simple ointment, wool alcohol ointments etc.

VASELINE: Vaseline is another preparation consisting of soft paraffin and is prepared and marketed by the Chesebrough Manufacturing Company (discovered by Chesebrough in 1871). It is official in some official books including DAB-2 Addendum, and is used as an ointment base. It is a very homogenous base as compared to other varieties of soft paraffins. It has the advantage of being an ointment base of better chemical stability. The distribution of vaseline ointment on the skin is said to be uniform and its film is highly stable and firm.

ICHTHAMMOL[1]

Synonym: Ammonium Ichthosulphonates, Ichthyol.

Ichthammol consists mainly of a mixture of ammonium salts of sulphuric acids derived from the hydrocarbons (oily substance) produced by destructive distillation of a bituminous schist or shale or from other sources and has ammonium sulphate and water in its composition. It contains not less than 10.5% w/w of organically combined sulphur, calculated with reference to the substance dried to constant weight at 105°C and not more than 25 of the total sulphur in the form of sulphates.

Description: It is almost black viscid liquid with strong characteristic odour, soluble in water, partly soluble in alcohol and in solvent ether, miscible with glycerin and fixed oils.

Tests for identity: (i) On being warmed with equal volume of solution of sodium hydroxide, ammonia is evolved. (ii) The dark resinous precipitate produced on the addition of hydrochloric acid to a clear solution of ichthammol is insoluble in solvent ether.

Tests for purity: It is tested for solubility in glycerol, loss on drying (not more than 5% at 105°C) and sulphated ash (Appendix II).

Assay: Ichthammol is assayed for (i) organically combined sulphur and (ii) sulphur in the form of sulphates. The organic sulphur is determined indirectly by subtracting the percentage of sulphur present as inorganic sulphurs from the total sulphur. The assay procedures as given in I.P. are given below:

For organically combined sulphur: Weigh accurately about 0.5 g and mix with 4 g of anhydrous sodium carbonate and 3 ml of chloroform in a porcelain crucible of about 50 ml capacity. Warm and stir until all the chloroform is evaporated. Add 10 g coarsely powdered copper nitrate, mix thoroughly and heat the mixture very gently with a low flame. After the initial reaction has subsided, increase the temperature slightly until most of the material has blackened. Cool and place the crucible in a large beaker, add slowly 20 ml of hydrochloric acid, and when the reaction ceases, add 100 ml of water and boil until all the copper oxide is dissolved. Filter the solution. Dilute the filtrate with 400 ml of water, heat to boiling and add 20 ml of solution of barium chloride. Set aside for two hours, filter off the precipitate, wash with water, dry and ignite. Each g of residue is equivalent to 0.1374 g of sulphur. From the percentage of total sulphur thus obtained, subtract the percentage of sulphur in the form of sulphates.

---

1. Ichthamol is not included in I.P. 2007. However, it continues to be official in other pharmacopoeias and compendia, etc.

For sulphur in the form of sulphates: Dissolve 2 g in 100 ml of water, add 2 g of cupric chloride, dissolve in 80 ml of water and add sufficient water to make 200 ml, shake well and filter. Heat 100 ml of the filterate, equivalent to 1 g of ichthammol being tested, near to boiling. Add 1 ml of HCl and 5 ml of solution of barium chloride drop by drop, and heat on a water-bath. Filter and wash the precipitate with water, dry and ignite. Each gram of residue is equivalent to 0.1374 g of sulphur present in the form of sulphates.

Uses: It is an antiparasitic and irritant. As an antiseptic, it is used in some diseases.

CYCLOPROPANE

Mol. Form.: C_3H_6 Mol. Wt. 42.08

Cyclopropane (C_3H_6) contains not less than 99.0 percent v/v of C_3H_6. It was first isolated in 1882, but it came to be known as an important inhaling anaesthetic in 1929, when it was first used in 1934. It was considered to be the most potent gaseous anaesthetic in those days. It is used in combination with oxygen in ratio of 15 : 85 volumes of cyclopropane and oxygen respectively. Its administration is normally done after the patient has been given premedication with depressant drugs, like barbiturates. In 2 or 3 minutes the anaesthesia is induced. Since it is a potent anaesthetic agent, the high percentage of oxygen in its mixture provides enough oxygen to the tissues.

Preparation: Cyclopropane can be prepared from open chain compounds through reactions which lead to cyclizations, e.g. by the action of sodium or zinc on 1,3-dibromopropane.

(See also cycloalkanes preparation and properties on pages 107 and 112).

Description: It is a colourless gas which has characteristic odour (like light petroleum) and pungent taste. It is inflammable and its mixtures with oxygen or air are explosives. It is freely soluble in water (1 vol. in 2.85) and very soluble in alcohol in solvent ether and in chloroform.

It is also compressed in metal cylinders which are maintained at 25°C for at least six hours prior to withdrawing sample for tests and assay.

Tests for purity: It is tested for acidity or alkalinity, carbon dioxide, halogens, propylene, allene and other unsaturated hydrocarbons.

In the purest form, as it is inhaled to produce general anaesthesia, it should fully comply with the tests for purity (I.P., p. 982).

Acidity and alkalinity: Add 0.3 ml of solution of methyl red and 0.3 ml of solution of bromothymol blue to 400 ml of boiling water and boil the solution for five minutes. Pour 100 ml of the boiling solution into each of three colour comparison tubes of clear glass of approximately the same size and marked 'A', 'B' and 'C' respectively. To tube B add 0.2 ml of 0.01 N hydrochloric acid and to tube C add 0.4 ml of 0.01 N hydrochloric acid. Stopper each of the tubes and cool them to room temperature. Pass a volume of gas equivalent to 2000 ml measured at normal temperature and pressure through the solution in tube B at a rate requiring about thirty minutes for the passage of the gas. The colour of the solution in cylinder B is not deeper than the orange-red colour produced in tube C and the yellow green produced in cylinder A.

Assay: It is assayed by treating the gas with sulphuric acid in a mercury charged micrometer. Cyclopropane gets absorbed by ring fission resulting in the formation of propyl hydrogen sulphate as shown below:

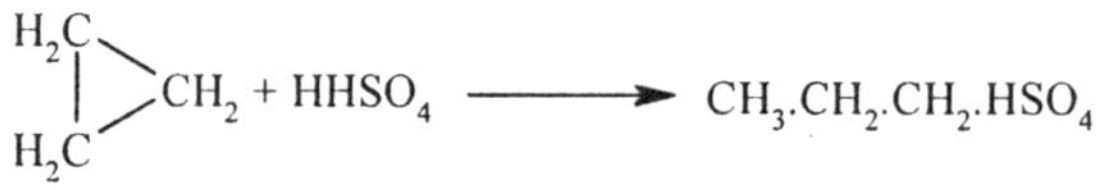

$$\underset{H_2C}{\overset{H_2C}{\big|}}\!\!\!>\!\!CH_2 + HHSO_4 \longrightarrow CH_3.CH_2.CH_2.HSO_4$$

Not less than 99% v/v cyclopropane should be absorbed.

Uses: It is used as a general anaesthetic. It has stronger narcotic action than ethylene and hence it is required in lesser concentrations. For full anaesthetic action 12–25% of cyclopropane in oxygen is used. However, the danger of explosion is less with ethylene. Cyclopropane is as lethal as ether (also see above).

Labelling: The metal cylinder containing cyclopropane is painted orange and carries a label stating the name of the gas. The label also states that cyclopropane is inflammable and its mixture with oxygen or air may explode if brought in contact with a flame or other cause of ignition. In addition the name of the gas or the symbol C_3H_6 is stencilled in paint on the shoulder of the cylinder.

Caution: Cyclopropane is highly inflammable. Do not use where it may be ignited.

Alkenes or Olefins
(Unsaturated Hydrocarbons)

INTRODUCTION

The compounds of this class have one double bond and they are represented by the general formula C_nH_{2n}. The lower members of the series react with chlorine to form oily products and, therefore, are referred to as **olefins** (Olefiant = oil forming). Since alkenes contain less than the maximum quantity of hydrogens, they are known as **unsaturated hydrocarbons**. The simplest and the first member of the series is ethylene, having the formula C_2H_4. The unsaturation or the double bond can be satisfied by reagents other than hydrogen and gives rise to the characteristic chemical properties of alkenes.

According to quantum mechanics, in alkenes the carbon atoms are in sp^2 hybridized state, and are formed by the mixing of one 's' and two 'p' orbitals. The sp^2 orbitals lie in one plane and are directed towards the corners of an equilateral triangle. The angle between any pair of orbitals is thus $120°$. The trigonal arrangement permits the hybrid orbitals to be as far apart as possible.

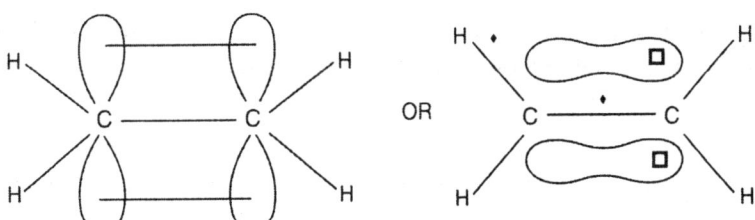

Fig. 9.1. Formation of a double bond in ethylene molecule.

In ethylene two carbon atoms are joined by axial overlapping of p-orbitals forming a σ-bond. Each carbon atom forms two C–H bonds by overlapping of $1s$ orbital of hydrogen and sp^2 orbital of carbon and forms four σ-bonds. The remaining unpaired electron at each carbon atom is in a p-orbital which is perpendicular to the plane of three σ-bonds of the carbon. These p-orbitals overlap in a parallel way giving pi (π) bond formation. This type of overlapping in bond is relatively poor and so pi (π) bond is less stable than σ bond.

Occurrence

Alkenes seldom occur free in nature due to their reactivity. Lower alkenes occur in coal gas in very small amount. Ethylene is present in natural gas in about 20% amount.

NOMENCLATURE

The following three systems are used for naming alkenes:

1. **The common system:** The common names of the first few alkenes are given by replacing 'ane' of alkanes with 'ylene' e.g., ethylene ($CH_2 = CH_2$), propylene ($CH_3.CH = CH_2$), butylene ($CH_3.CH_2.CH = CH_2$), amylene ($C_3H_7.CH = CH_2$) for ethane, propane, butane and pentane, respectively.

   The radicals derived from alkenes by removal of a hydrogen are referred as:

   $CH_2 = CH$ Vinyl $CH_2 = CH.CH_2$ Allyl
   $CH_3.CH = CH$ Propyl $CH_3CH = CH.CH_2$ Crotyl

2. **As derivatives of ethylene:** Alkenes are regarded as the derivatives of ethylene in this system. The alkenes are named by adding the name of alkyl groups in place of hydrogen atoms in ethylene. For example methylethylene ($CH_3.CH = CH_2$), ethylethylene ($CH_3.CH_2.CH = CH_2$), trimethylethylene ($(CH_3)_2.C = CH.CH_3$) and so on.

3. **IUPAC system:** In this system the ending 'ane' of the corresponding alkane is replaced by 'ene'. The longest chain of carbon atoms containing the double bond is considered the parent alkene. The carbon chain is then numbered from the end nearer to the double bond. Rules of nomenclature are discussed in detail in the chapter on nomenclature.

ISOMERISM

The first two members of the series, ethene and propene, are represented only by one structural formula. Other alkenes show the following types of isomerism.

1. **Chain isomerism:** Alkenes show chain isomerism due to different arrangement of carbon atoms along a carbon skeleton. For example 1-butene and 2-methylpropene may be represented as:

   $CH_3.CH_2.CH = CH_2$ $\begin{array}{c} H_3C \\ \\ H_3C \end{array}\!\!\!> CH = CH_2$

   1-Butene   2-Methylpropene

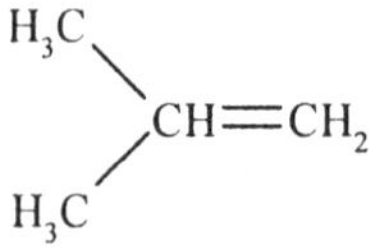

2. **Position isomerism:** The difference in the position of the double bond in the same structure gives rise to position isomerism, e.g.

   $CH_3.CH_2.CH = CH_2$ $CH_3.CH = CH.CH_3$
   1-Butene   2-Butene

3. **Ring chain isomerism:** Alkenes and cycloalkanes have the same general formula C_nH_{2n} where alkenes are open chain compounds with a double bond and cycloalkanes are cyclic saturated

compounds. For example, propene and cyclopropane are the isomeric forms. Similarly, butene is isomeric with cyclobutane.

$$CH_3.CH=CH_2 \qquad H_2C-\!\!-\!\!CH_2 \qquad CH_3.CH_2.CH=CH_2 \qquad \begin{array}{c} H_2C-\!\!-\!\!CH_2 \\ | \qquad | \\ H_2C-\!\!-\!\!CH_2 \end{array}$$

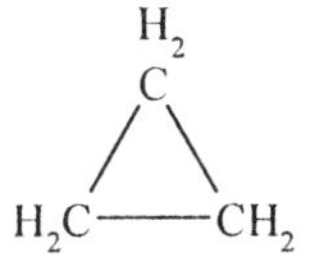

Propene   Cyclopropene   1-Butene   Cyclobutane

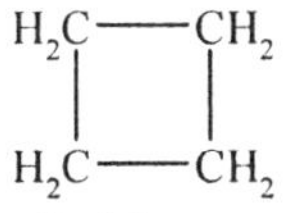

4. **Geometrical isomerism:** Except ethene and propene all other alkenes exhibit geometrical isomerism, i.e., they are represented as **cis** and **trans** forms in the unsaturated compounds where rotation around the double bond is restricted. For example, two forms of 2-butene are represented as:

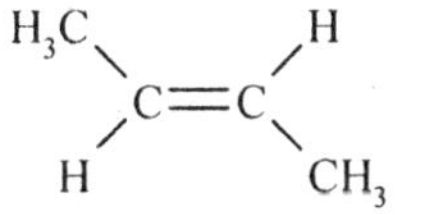

cis-2-Butene 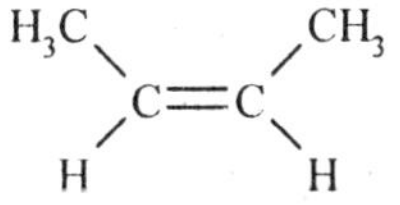   *trans*-2-Butene

(See also chapter on Isomerism).

GENERAL METHODS OF PREPARATION

Alkenes are prepared by the following general methods:

1. **Dehydration of alcohols:** Alkenes can be prepared from an alcohol by dehydration, i.e., elimination of a molecule of water in the presence of an acid at high temperature.

$$CH_3.CH_2.CH_2.CH_2.OH \xrightarrow[140-170°C]{75\%\,H_2SO_4} CH_3.CH_2.CH = CH_2 + H_2O$$

       n-Butyl alcohol   1-Butene

The other dehydrating agents are P_2O_5, H_3PO_4, Al_2O_3. The ease of dehydration in case of alcohol is in the order:

Tertiary > Secondary > Primary

The dehydration of secondary and tertiary alcohol is carried out using dilute sulphuric acid, e.g.

$$CH_3.CH_2.CH.OH.CH_3 \xrightarrow[100°C]{60\%\,H_2SO_4} CH_3.CH = CH.CH_3$$

       sec-Butyl alcohol   2-Butene

$$(CH_3)_2.C.OH.CH_3 \xrightarrow[85-90°C]{20\%\,H_2SO_4} (CH_3)_2.C = CH_2$$

       tert-Butyl alcohol   Isobutylene

2. **Dehydrohalogenation of alkyl halides:** On heating alkyl halides with alcoholic potassium hydroxide hydrogen halide is eliminated and the alkene is obtained. For example:

$$CH_3.CH_2.CH_2.Cl \xrightarrow[-HCl]{alc.\,KOH} CH_3.CH = CH_2 \xleftarrow[HCl]{alc.\,KOH} \begin{array}{c} Cl \\ | \\ CH_3.CH.CH_3 \end{array}$$

    n-Propyl chloride   Propylene   Isopropyl chloride

$$CH_3.CH_2.CH_2.CH_2.Cl \xrightarrow[-HCl]{\text{alc. KOH}} CH_3.CH_2CH = CH_2$$

n-Butyl chloride   1-Butene

In this case dehydrohalogenation takes place in the following order:
tert-alkyl halide > *sec*-alkyl halide > *pri*-alkyl halide, e.g.:

$$CH_3.CH_2.\underset{\underset{Cl}{|}}{CH}.CH_3 \xrightarrow{\text{alc. KOH}} CH_3.CH = CH.CH_3 + CH_3.CH_2.CH = CH_2$$

2-Butene (80%)   1-Butene (20%)

sec-Butyl chloride

For different halogens the ease of dehydrohalogenation is in the order, Iodine > Bromine > Chlorine.

3. **Dehalogenation of vicinal dihalides:** Vicinal dihalides have two halogens on the adjacent carbon atoms. When these compounds are heated with zinc dust in alcohol the halogen molecule is eliminated forming alkenes.

$$R.\underset{\underset{X}{|}}{CH} - \underset{\underset{X}{|}}{CH_2} + Zn \xrightarrow[\Delta]{CH_3OH} R.CH = CH_2 + ZnX_2$$

Alkene

$$CH_3.\underset{\underset{Br}{|}}{CH}.\underset{\underset{Br}{|}}{CH}.CH_3 + Zn \xrightarrow[\Delta]{CH_3OH} CH_3.CH = CH.CH_3 + ZnBr_2$$

2-Butene

Metallic sodium may also be used in place of zinc. Higher alkene is formed when a gem-dihalide containing two halogens on the same carbon atom is heated with a catalyst.

$$2CH_3CH \underset{Br}{\overset{Br}{<}} + 4Na \xrightarrow{\text{Ether}} CH_3.CH = CH.CH_3 + 4NaBr$$

1,1-Dibromoethane   2-Butene

4. **Partial reduction of alkynes:** Alkynes when hydrogenated partially with hydrogen in the presence of a catalyst like platinum, palladium or nickel produce alkenes.

$$R.C \equiv C.R \xrightarrow[H_2]{Pt.} R.CH = CH.R$$

Alkyne   Alkene

$$CH_3.C \equiv C.CH_3 \xrightarrow[H_2]{Pd.} CH_3.CH = CH.CH_3$$

Propylene   Propene

5. **Electrolysis of salts of dicarboxylic acids:** The sodium or potassium salts of dicarboxylic acids like disodium succinate on electrolysis in aqueous solution yield alkenes.

$$\begin{array}{l} CH_2\!\!-\!\!COO.Na \\ | \\ CH_2\!\!-\!\!COO.Na \end{array} \xrightarrow{\text{Electrolysis}} \begin{array}{l} CH_2\!\!-\!\!COO^- \\ | \\ CH_2\!\!-\!\!COO^- \end{array} + 2Na$$

Disodium   Succinate
succinate   dianion

At anode:

$$CH_2\text{—}COO^- \atop CH_2\text{—}COO^- \quad \xrightarrow{-2\bar{e}} \quad CH_2\text{—}COO^\bullet \atop CH_2\text{—}COO^\bullet \quad \xrightarrow{-CO_2} \quad CH_2 \atop CH_2$$

Ethene

At cathode: $\quad 2Na^+ \xrightarrow{+2\bar{e}} 2Na \xrightarrow{2H_2O} 2NaOH + H_2$

6. **Pyrolysis or cracking:** Higher alkanes when subjected to high temperature and pressure decompose to give a mixture of lower paraffins and alkenes.

$$CH_3.(CH_2)_4.CH_3 \xrightarrow[200\,atm.]{500^\circ C} CH_3.CH = CH_2 + CH_3.CH_2.CH_3$$

n-Hexene $\hspace{5cm}$ Propene $\hspace{2cm}$ Propane

Alkenes are also produced when esters and amines oxides are heated e.g.

$$R.CH_2.CH_2.O.COCH_3 \xrightarrow{500^\circ C} R.CH = CH_2 + CH_3.COOH$$

Ester $\hspace{5cm}$ Alkene

$$R.CH_2.CH_2.\overset{+}{N}.(CH_3)_3 \xrightarrow{150^\circ C} R.CH = CH_2 + (CH_3)_2.NOH$$

Amine oxide $\hspace{4cm}$ Alkene $\hspace{2cm}$ Dimethyl
$\hspace{11cm}$ hydroxylamine

7. **Decomposition of quaternary ammonium hydroxide:** Quaternary ammonium salts, the compounds of nitrogen in which it is linked by four covalent and one electrovalent bond, are converted into alkenes on heating alone.

$$(C_2H_5)_4N^+.OH^- \longrightarrow CH_2 = CH_2 + (C_2H_5)_3N + H_2O$$

Tetraethyl ammonium $\hspace{2cm}$ Ethene $\hspace{1.5cm}$ Triethylamine
hydroxide

GENERAL PHYSICAL PROPERTIES

1. The first three members of alkene series are gases, the alkenes containing five to fifteen carbon atoms are liquids and the higher members are solids.
2. Alkenes are insoluble in water but they are soluble in certain organic solvents, like alcohols, ether, esters etc. They are lighter than water.
3. They have characteristic odour and burn with luminous smoky flame.
4. They are less volatile than alkanes and are weak polar compounds. Their boiling and melting points and specific gravities are higher than the corresponding alkanes and show a regular increase with increase in molecular weight (see Table 9.1).

GENERAL CHEMICAL PROPERTIES

The alkenes are more reactive than alkanes due to the presence of double bond in the molecule. The double bond is made of a strong σ bond and a weak pi (π) bond. The reaction would involve the breaking of this weaker bond to form the two new σ (sigma) bonds in its place yielding saturated compounds.

A reaction in which two molecules combine to form a single molecule product is called an addition product. The reagent is simply added to the organic molecule which contains multiple

Table 9.1. Physical constants of alkenes

Compound	Formula	B.P. °C	M.P. °C	Sp. gr. at 20°C
Ethene	$CH_2 = CH_2$	−102	−169	−
Propene	$CH_3CH = CH_2$	−48	−185	0.514
1-Butene	$CH_3.CH_2.CH = CH_2$	−6.5	−185	0.595
cis-2-Butene	$CH_3.CH = CH.CH_3$	4	−139	0.621
trans-2-Butene	$CH_3.CH = CH.CH_3$	1	−106	0.604
1-Pentene	$CH_3.CH_2CH_2.CH = CH_2$	30	−165	0.641
cis-2-Pentene	$CH_3.CH_2.CH = CH.CH_3$	38	−151	0.656
trans-2-Pentene	$CH_3.CH_2.CH = CH.CH_3$	36	−140	0.648
3-Methyl-2-butene	$(CH_3)_2.CH.CH = CH_2$	25	−138	0.640
2-Methyl-2-butene	$(CH_3)_2.C = CH.CH_3$	39	−140	0.660
1-Hexene	$CH_3(CH)_3.CH = CH_2$	63.5	−140	0.674
1-Heptene	$CH_3(CH_2)_4.CH = CH_2$	95	−120	0.697
1-Octene	$CH_3(CH_2)_5.CH = CH_2$	122	−102	0.715
1-Nonene	$CH_3(CH_2)_6.CH = CH_2$	150	−95	0.732
1-Decene	$CH_3(CH_2)_7.CH = CH_2$	171	−87	0.743

bonded atoms. There is a cloud of pi (π) electrons above and below the place of these atoms. These pi (π) electrons are less involved than the σ (sigma) electrons in holding together the carbon nucleus and are bonded less tightly. These loosely held pi (π) electrons are particularly available to the reagents which are deficient in electrons. In many reactions the carbon-carbon double bond serves as a source of electrons, i.e., it acts as a base. The compounds with which it reacts are acids, which are deficients in electrons. These acidic reagents (seeking a pair of electrons) are called electrophilic (Greek: electron-loving) reagents.

Besides the addition reactions, alkenes undergo the free-radical reactions (substitution reactions of alkenes) due to the presence of alkyl groups. The important addition and substitution reactions of alkenes are summarized below:

A. Addition Reactions

1. **Hydrogenation:** Alkanes are formed when alkenes are reacted with hydrogen gas in the presence of catalysts, like Ni, Pt, Pd, etc.

$$CH_3.CH = CH_2 + H_2 \xrightarrow[200°C]{Ni} CH_3.CH_2.CH_3$$

Propene → Propane

The addition of hydrogen to an unsaturated compound is known as hydrogenation. Hydrogenation involves breaking of a pi (π) bond in alkene and of H–H bond of hydrogen with the formation of two C–H bonds.

2. **Addition of halogens:** Alkenes are reacted readily with chlorine or bromine to give saturated compounds that contain two halogen atoms attached to adjacent carbons. Iodine generally does not react with alkenes, e.g.

$$CH_2 = CH_2 + Br_2 \longrightarrow \underset{\underset{\displaystyle Br}{|}}{CH_2} - \underset{\underset{\displaystyle Br}{|}}{CH_2}$$

Ethene

1,2-Dibromoethane

$$CH_3.CH = CH_2 + Cl_2 \xrightarrow{\;CCl_4\;} \underset{\underset{\displaystyle Cl}{|}}{CH_3.CH} - \underset{\underset{\displaystyle Cl}{|}}{CH_2}$$

Propene

1,2-Dichloropropane

The reaction is carried out simply by mixing together the two reactants at room temperature usually in an inert solvent like carbon tetrachloride.

3. **Addition of hydrogen halides:** An alkene is converted by aqueous solution of halogen acids into the corresponding alkyl halide. The order of reactivity of the halogen acids is HI > HBr > HCl.

$$CH_2 = CH_2 + HCl \longrightarrow CH_3.CH_2Cl$$

Ethene   Ethyl chloride

$$CH_3.CH = CH_2 + HBr \longrightarrow \underset{\underset{\displaystyle Br}{|}}{CH_3.CH}.CH_3$$

Propane

2-Bromopropane

Propane on addition with the halogen acid could yield either n-propyl halide or the isopropyl halide depending upon the orientation of addition. Actually, it is found that the isopropyl halide is formed in higher yield.

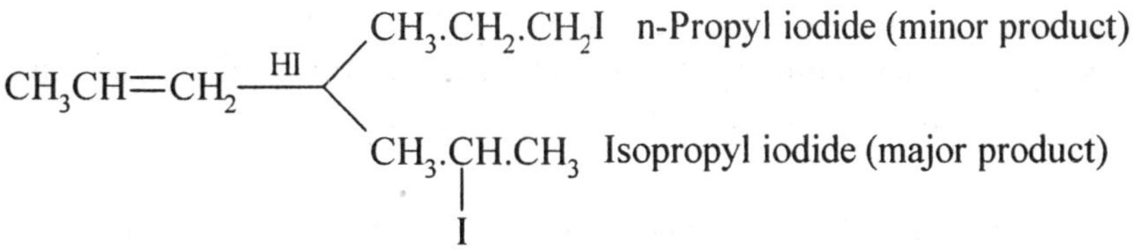

$$CH_3CH{=}CH_2 \xrightarrow{\;HI\;} \begin{cases} CH_3.CH_2.CH_2I \quad \text{n-Propyl iodide (minor product)} \\[2ex] \underset{\underset{\displaystyle I}{|}}{CH_3.CH}.CH_3 \quad \text{Isopropyl iodide (major product)} \end{cases}$$

Markovnikoff, a Russian chemist, observed a large number of such additions and showed that where two isomeric products are possible one is in major quantity. He stated, "In the ionic addition of an acid to the carbon-carbon double bond (C = C) of an alkene, the hydrogen of the acid attaches itself to the carbon atom that already holds the great number of hydrogens." This statement is generally known as Markovnikoff's rule.

Kharasch and Mayo (1930) found that in the presence of peroxides the addition occurs according to anti-Markovnikoff's rule, especially in the addition of hydrogen bromide to alkenes. The presence or absence of peroxides has no effect on the orientation of addition of hydrogen chloride, hydrogen iodide, sulphuric acid, water, etc.

The mechanism of the peroxide effect is a free-radical chain reaction, the peroxide generating the free radical as follows:

$$RO.OR \longrightarrow 2RO^{\bullet}$$

Peroxide

$$HBr + RO^{\bullet} \longrightarrow ROH + Br^{\bullet}$$

$$R.CH = CH_2 + \overset{\bullet}{Br} \longrightarrow R\overset{\bullet}{C}HCH_2Br$$

$$R\overset{\bullet}{C}HCH_2Br + HBr \longrightarrow RCH_2CH_2Br^{\bullet} + Br^{\bullet} \text{ and so on.}$$

4. **Addition of hypohalous acids:** Alkenes react with hypohalous acids to form halohydrins, the compounds containing halogen and hydroxyl groups on adjacent carbon atoms. Usually the reaction is carried out by treating the alkene with chlorine or bromine water.

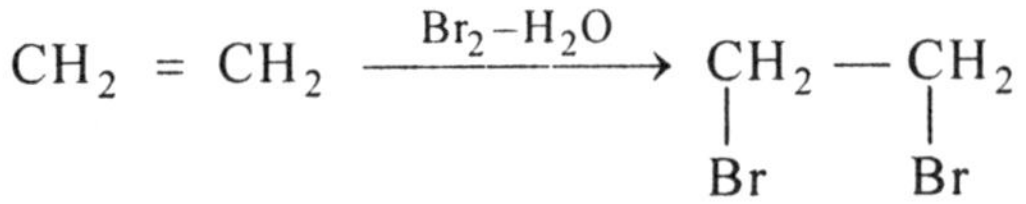

$$CH_2 = CH_2 \xrightarrow{\ Br_2-H_2O\ } \underset{\underset{Br}{|}}{CH_2} - \underset{\underset{Br}{|}}{CH_2}$$

Ethylene bromohydrin
(2-bromoethanol)

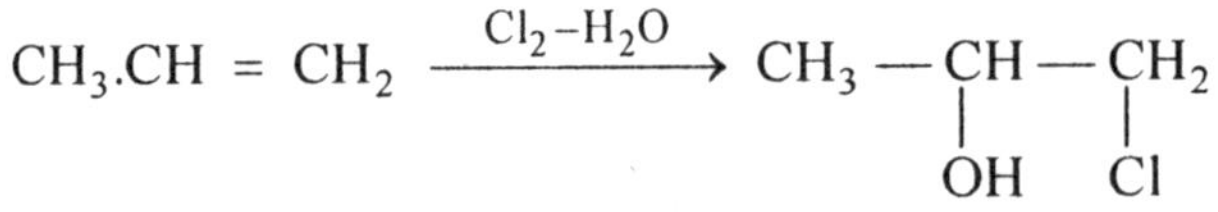

$$CH_3.CH = CH_2 \xrightarrow{\ Cl_2-H_2O\ } CH_3 - \underset{\underset{OH}{|}}{CH} - \underset{\underset{Cl}{|}}{CH_2}$$

Propylene chlorohydrin
(1-chloro-2-propanol)

The mechanism of such addition is probably via the formation of the chloronium ion (Cl^+):

$$ClOH + H^+ \rightleftharpoons ClOH_2^+ \rightleftharpoons Cl^+ + H_2O$$

$$CH_2 = CH_2 + Cl^+ \longrightarrow Cl.CH_2.CH_2^+ \xrightarrow{H_2O} ClCH_2.CH_2.OH_2^+ \xrightarrow{-H^+} Cl.CH_2.CH_2.OH$$

Halohydrins regenerate the alkenes on being treated with zinc dust in acetic acid.

5. **Addition of sulphuric acid:** Alkenes react with cold concentrated sulphuric acid to form alkyl hydrogen sulphates. These compounds are formed by addition of hydrogen ion of one side of the double bond and bisulphate ion to the other.

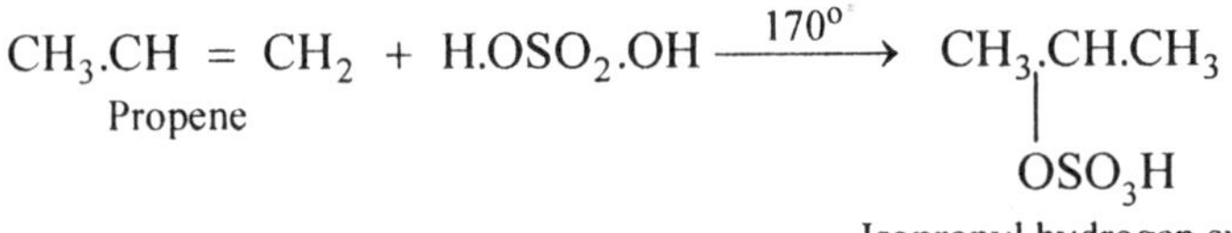

$$\underset{\text{Propene}}{CH_3.CH = CH_2} + H.OSO_2.OH \xrightarrow{170^\circ} CH_3.\underset{\underset{OSO_3H}{|}}{CH}.CH_3$$

Isopropyl hydrogen sulphate

In the product the carbon is attached to oxygen and not to sulphur. The addition of sulphuric acid to unsymmetrical alkenes takes place in accordance with Markovnikoff's rule. These products are decomposed on boiling with water to give the corresponding alcohol.

$$\underset{\text{Ethyl hydrogen sulphate}}{CH_3.CH_2.OSO_3H} \xrightarrow{H_2O \text{ heat}} \underset{\text{Ethyl alcohol}}{CH_3.CH_2.OH} + H_2SO_4$$

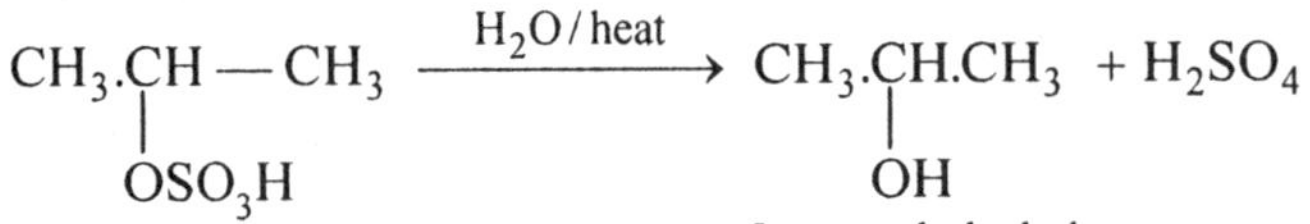

$$\underset{\underset{OSO_3H}{|}}{CH_3.CH} - CH_3 \xrightarrow{H_2O/\text{heat}} CH_3.\underset{\underset{OH}{|}}{CH}.CH_3 + H_2SO_4$$

Isopropyl hydrogen
sulphate

Isopropyl alcohol

6. **Addition to water (hydration):** Addition of water to the alkenes in the presence of acid yields alcohols. The addition follows the Markovnikov's rule e.g.

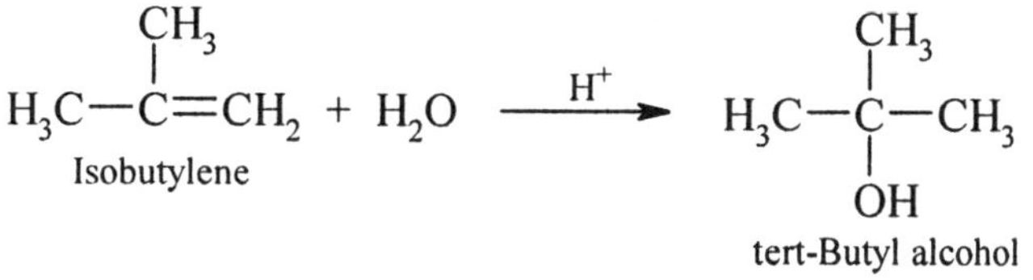

$$H_3C-\underset{\underset{Isobutylene}{}}{\overset{\overset{CH_3}{|}}{C}}=CH_2 + H_2O \xrightarrow{H^+} H_3C-\underset{\underset{OH}{|}}{\overset{\overset{CH_3}{|}}{C}}-CH_3$$

Isobutylene

tert-Butyl alcohol

7. **Addition of alkanes (alkylation):** Alkanes are added to alkenes in presence of acid catalysts like HF, H_2SO_4 or $AlCl_3$ to give branched alkanes. For example, isobutane is added to isobutylene to form iso-octane in the presence of hydrogen fluoride.

$$(CH_3)_2 = CH_2 + HCH_2.CH(CH_3)_2 \xrightarrow{HF} (CH_3)_3C.CH_2CH(CH_3)_2$$

Isobutylene   Isobutane   Iso-octane

8. **Addition of oxygen:** Addition of oxygen or air to lower alkenes takes place at high temperature and pressure in the presence of silver catalyst to form epoxides.

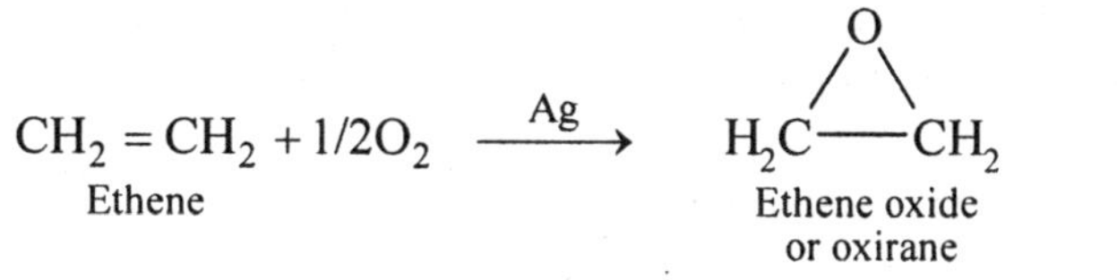

$$CH_2 = CH_2 + 1/2O_2 \xrightarrow{Ag} \overset{\overset{O}{\diagup\diagdown}}{H_2C-\!\!-\!\!-CH_2}$$

Ethene

Ethene oxide
or oxirane

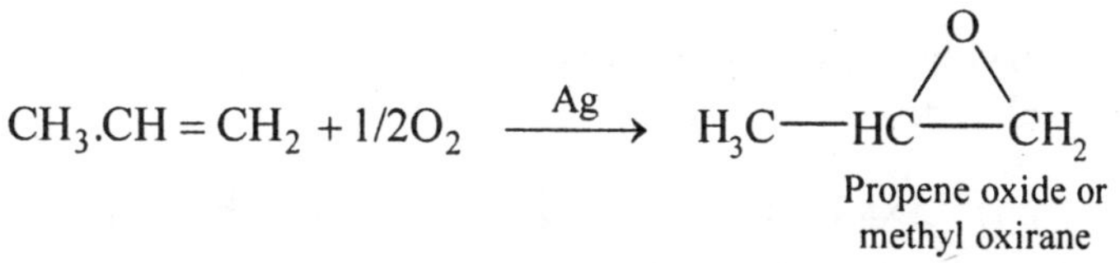

$$CH_3.CH = CH_2 + 1/2O_2 \xrightarrow{Ag} \overset{\overset{O}{\diagup\diagdown}}{H_3C-HC-\!\!-\!\!-CH_2}$$

Propene oxide or
methyl oxirane

Epoxides are also formed when alkenes are mixed with per acids like perbenzoic acid.

9. **Addition of ozone (ozonolysis):** Ozone is added to alkene in an inert solvent like solvent ether or carbon tetrachloride to form ozonide. On hydrolysis or reduction of the products carbonyl compounds are obtained.

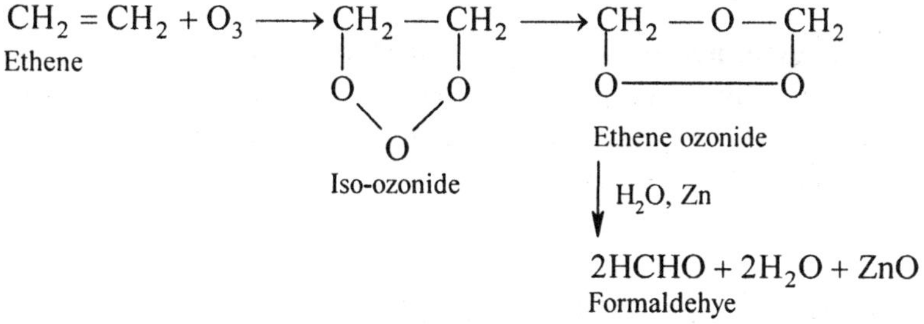

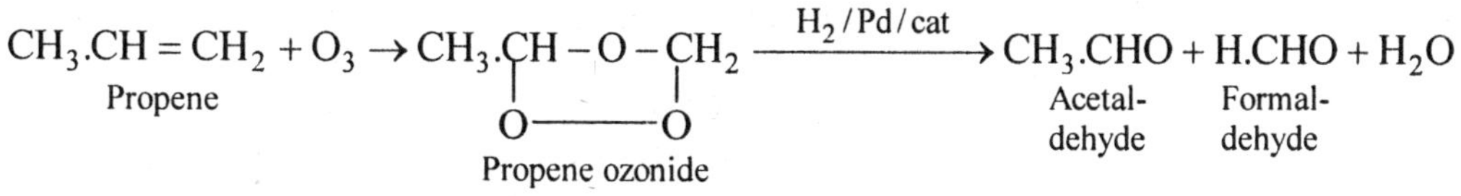

$$CH_2 = CH_2 + O_3 \longrightarrow \underset{\underset{Iso\text{-}ozonide}{}}{\overset{}{CH_2 - CH_2}} \longrightarrow \underset{\underset{Ethene\ ozonide}{}}{\overset{}{CH_2 - O - CH_2}}$$

Ethene

Iso-ozonide

Ethene ozonide

$$\downarrow H_2O, Zn$$

$2HCHO + 2H_2O + ZnO$
Formaldehye

$$CH_3.CH = CH_2 + O_3 \rightarrow \underset{\underset{Propene\ ozonide}{}}{\overset{}{CH_3.CH - O - CH_2}} \xrightarrow{H_2/Pd/cat} CH_3.CHO + H.CHO + H_2O$$

Propene

Propene ozonide

Acetal-   Formal-
dehyde   dehyde

The complete process of preparing the ozonide and decomposition is known as **ozonolysis** and is useful for determining the position of double bond in an alkene and to prepare carbonyl compounds. The tri-substituted alkenes give the mixture of the aldehyde and ketone while tetra-substituted alkenes give only ketones on ozonolysis.

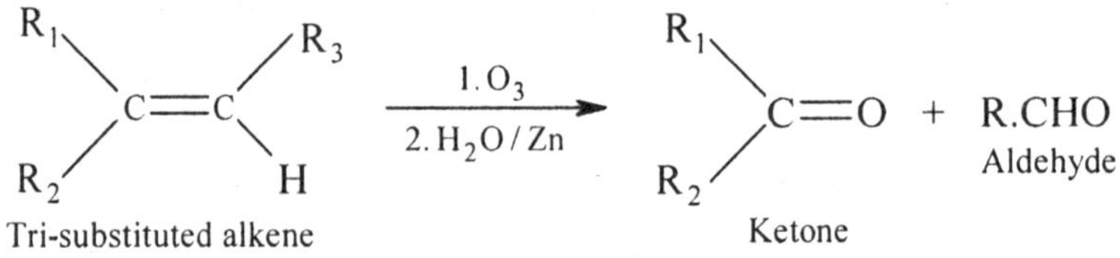

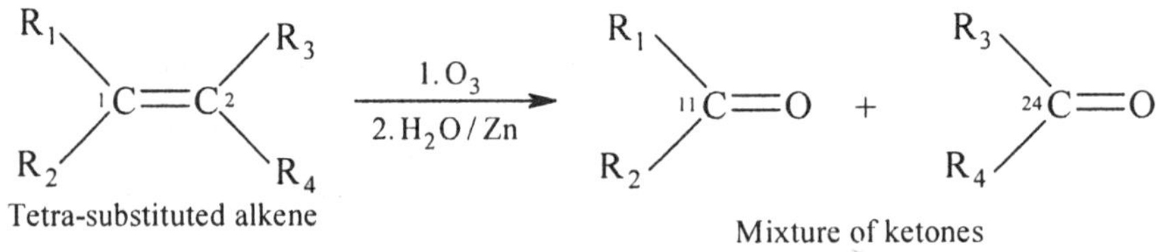

$$\underset{\text{Tri-substituted alkene}}{\overset{R_1}{\underset{R_2}{>}}C=C\overset{R_3}{\underset{H}{<}}} \xrightarrow[\text{2. H}_2\text{O / Zn}]{\text{1. O}_3} \underset{\text{Ketone}}{\overset{R_1}{\underset{R_2}{>}}C=O} + \underset{\text{Aldehyde}}{\text{R.CHO}}$$

$$\underset{\text{Tetra-substituted alkene}}{\overset{R_1}{\underset{R_2}{>}}{}^1C=C^2\overset{R_3}{\underset{R_4}{<}}} \xrightarrow[\text{2. H}_2\text{O / Zn}]{\text{1. O}_3} \underset{\text{Mixture of ketones}}{\overset{R_1}{\underset{R_2}{>}}{}_{11}C=O + \overset{R_3}{\underset{R_4}{>}}{}_{24}C=O}$$

10. **Addition of hydrogen peroxide:** A mixture of hydroperoxide and peroxides is obtained when alkenes are added to hydrogen peroxide in acid catalyst.

$$\underset{\text{Isobutylene}}{(CH_3)_2C=CH_2} + H_2O_2 \xrightarrow{H^+} \underset{\text{tert-Butylhydroperoxide}}{(CH_3)_3C-O-O-H} \xrightarrow{(CH_3)_2=CH} \underset{\text{tert-Butylperoxide}}{(CH_3)_3C-O-O-(CH_3)_3}$$

11. **Addition of nitrosyl halides:** Addition of alkenes to nitrosochloride and nitrosobromide gives crystalline nitrosohalides.

$$\underset{\text{Ethene}}{CH_2=CH_2} + \underset{\substack{\text{Nitroso-}\\\text{bromide}}}{NO-Br} \longrightarrow \underset{\text{Intermediate carbonium ion}}{(\overset{+}{C}H_2-CH_2NO)} \xrightarrow{Br^-} \underset{\substack{\text{Ethene nitrosobromide}}}{\underset{Br}{\overset{|}{CH_2-CH_2.NO}}}$$

$$\underset{\text{Propene}}{CH_3.CH=CH_2} + \underset{\text{Nitrosochloride}}{NO-Cl} \longrightarrow (CH_3\overset{+}{C}H.CH_2NO) \xrightarrow{Cl^-} \underset{\text{Propene nitrosochloride}}{CH_3.CHCl.CH_2NO}$$

12. **Addition of alkene (dimerization):** Two molecules of isobutylene are condensed by sulphuric or phosphoric acid to give a mixture of two alkenes of molecular formula C_8H_{16}. Hydrogenation of these products yields an alkane containing the same number of carbon atoms, i.e. 2,2,4-trimethyl pentane, as shown below:

$$2CH_3-\overset{\overset{\displaystyle CH_3}{|}}{C}=CH_2 \xrightarrow[80°C]{H_2SO_4} \left[\underset{\text{2,4,4-trimethyl-1-pentene}}{CH_2=\overset{\overset{\displaystyle CH_3}{|}}{C}.CH_2.C.(CH_3)_3} \right] \xrightarrow[Ni]{H_2} \underset{\text{2,2,4-Trimethylpentane}}{(CH_3)_2CH.CH_2.C(CH_3)_3}$$

$$\underset{\text{2,4,4-Trimethyl-2-pentene}}{(CH_3)_2C=CH.C(CH_3)_3}$$

Since the alkenes produced contain exactly twice the number of carbon and hydrogen atoms as that of original compound they are known as dimers of isobutylene and the process is termed as dimerization. Trimerization and polymerization also take place when three or more alkene molecules are added respectively.

$$CH_2 = CH_2 + CH_2 = CH_2 \xrightarrow[\substack{1.\,\text{High temp.}\\2.\,\text{Catalyst}\\3.\,\text{Pressure}}]{} CH_2 = CH.CH_2.CH_3 \xrightarrow{nCH_2 = CH_2} CH_2 = CH(CH_2)_n.CH_3$$
$$\text{Butene} \qquad\qquad\qquad\qquad\qquad \text{Polymer}$$

Polythene and polybutene plastics are manufactured by this process.

13. **Isomerization:** When alkenes are heated at high temperature or at low temperature in the presence of catalysis like aluminium trichloride or aluminium trisulphate they undergo isomerization. The double bond is shifted towards the centre of the molecule, e.g.

$$CH_3.CH_2.CH_2.CH = CH_2 \xrightarrow[AlCl_3]{200-300^\circ C} CH_3.CH_2.CH = CH.CH_3$$
$$\text{1-Pentene} \qquad\qquad\qquad\qquad \text{2-Pentene}$$

Sometimes migration of an alkyl groups takes place alongwith the double bonds as:

$$\overset{\displaystyle CH_3}{\underset{}{\overset{|}{CH_2}}}.CH = CH_2 \xrightarrow[AlCl_3]{200-300^\circ C} CH_2 = CH.(CH_3)_2$$
$$\text{1-Butene} \qquad\qquad\qquad\qquad \text{Isobutylene}$$

14. **Hydroboration:** Alkenes react readily with diborane in a solvent like ether at room temperature to form trialkylborane. The oxidation of these products gives alcohols.

$$CH_2 = CH_2 + (BH_3)_2 \longrightarrow CH_3CH_2.BH_2 \xrightarrow{CH_2 = CH_2} CH_3.CH_2)_2 BH \xrightarrow{CH_2 = CH_2}$$
$$\text{Ethene} \qquad \text{Diborane}$$

$$(CH_3.CH_2)_3B \xrightarrow[NaOH]{3H_2O} 3CH_3.CH_2.OH + B(OH)_3$$
$$\text{Triethyl borane} \qquad\qquad \text{Ethanol} \qquad \text{Boric acid}$$

15. **Addition of acid anhydrides, acid chlorides etc.:** Condensation of alkene takes place with acid anhydrides in the presence of a catalyst like zinc chloride, to give unsaturated ketones.

$$CH_2 = CH_2 + (CH_3.CO)_2O \xrightarrow{ZnCl_2} CH_2 = CH.CO.CH_3 + CH_3.COOH$$
$$\text{Ethene} \qquad \text{Acetic anhydride} \qquad\qquad \text{Methyl vinyl ketone}$$

Acid chloride, alkyl chloride and α halogenated ether also condense with alkenes in the presence of $AlCl_3$.

$$CH_2 = CH_2 \xrightarrow{CH_3COCl} CH_3.CO.CH_2.CH_2Cl$$

$$CH_2 = CH_2 \xrightarrow{(CH_3)_3CCl} (CH_3)_3.C.CH_2.CH_2.Cl$$

$$CH_2 = CH_2 \xrightarrow{CH_3.O.CH_2.Cl} CH_3.O.CH_2.CH_2CH_2Cl$$

16. **Addition of methylene:** Reaction of alkene with methylene in light gives cycloalkanes as:

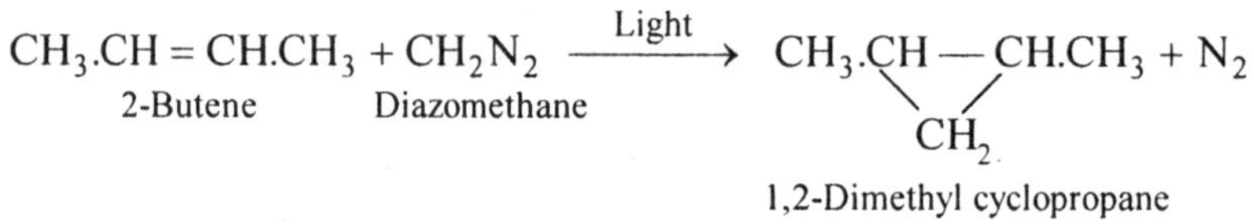

$$CH_3.CH = CH.CH_3 + CH_2N_2 \xrightarrow{\text{Light}} CH_3.CH \overset{\displaystyle}{\underset{\underset{\displaystyle CH_2}{\diagdown \diagup}}{-}} CH.CH_3 + N_2$$

2-Butene   Diazomethane

1,2-Dimethyl cyclopropane

Chloroform reacts with 2-butene in the presence of potassium tert-butoxide to produce the cyclic compound.

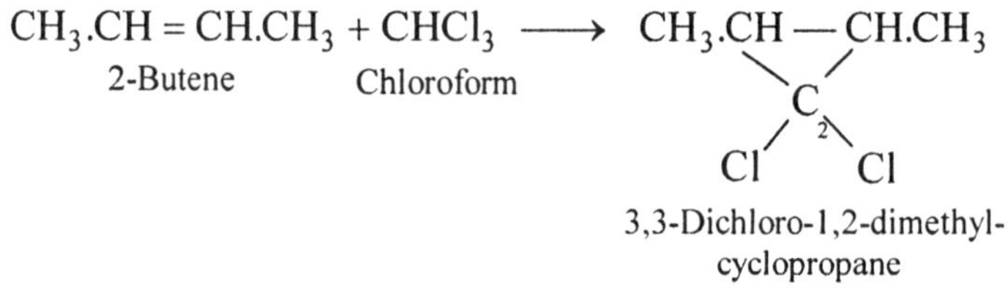

$$CH_3.CH = CH.CH_3 + CHCl_3 \longrightarrow CH_3.CH - CH.CH_3$$

2-Butene   Chloroform

$$\underset{\displaystyle Cl \quad Cl}{\overset{\displaystyle C_2}{}}$$

3,3-Dichloro-1,2-dimethyl-
cyclopropane

17. **Oxidation reactions:** Different products are obtained on oxidation of alkenes under different experimental conditions.

(i) **Oxidation with mild oxidizing agents:** Dihydroxy compounds known as vicinal glycols are obtained when alkenes are oxidized with dil. alkaline $KMnO_4$ at low temperature.

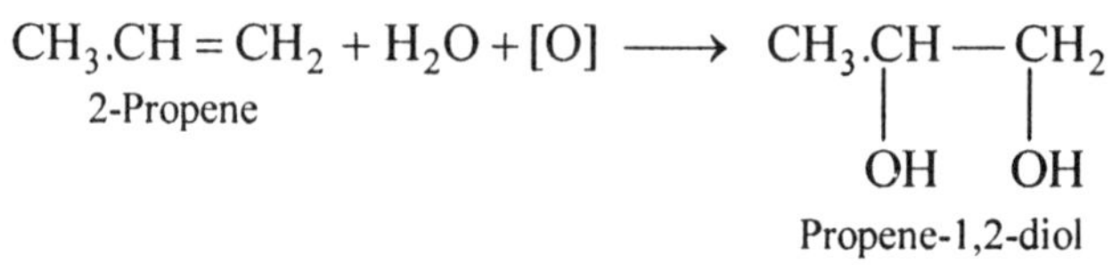

$$CH_3.CH = CH_2 + H_2O + [O] \longrightarrow CH_3.\underset{\displaystyle OH}{CH} - \underset{\displaystyle OH}{CH_2}$$

2-Propene

Propene-1,2-diol

Treatment of alkenes with osmium tetraoxide also gives glycols as follows:

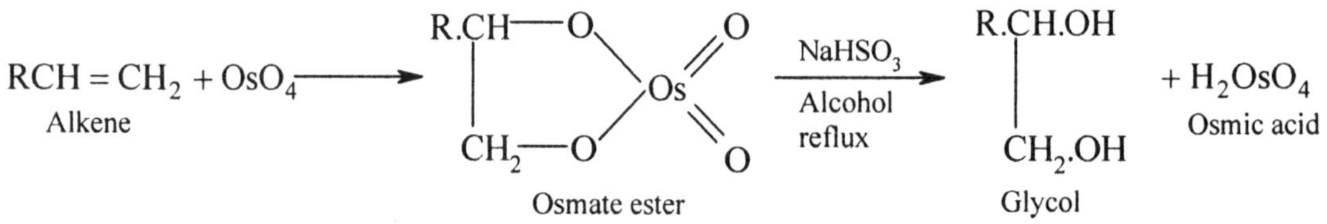

$$RCH = CH_2 + OsO_4 \longrightarrow \underset{\text{Osmate ester}}{\overset{\displaystyle R.CH-O}{\underset{\displaystyle CH_2-O}{\diagup\diagdown}Os\overset{\displaystyle O}{\underset{\displaystyle O}{\diagup\diagdown}}}} \xrightarrow[\substack{\text{Alcohol}\\ \text{reflux}}]{NaHSO_3} \underset{\text{Glycol}}{\overset{\displaystyle R.CH.OH}{\underset{\displaystyle CH_2.OH}{|}}} + \underset{\text{Osmic acid}}{H_2OsO_4}$$

Alkene

(ii) **Oxidation with periodic acid or lead tetraacetate:** Oxidation of alkenes with moderately oxidizing agents results in the formation of glycols which are then oxidized to aldehydes or ketones.

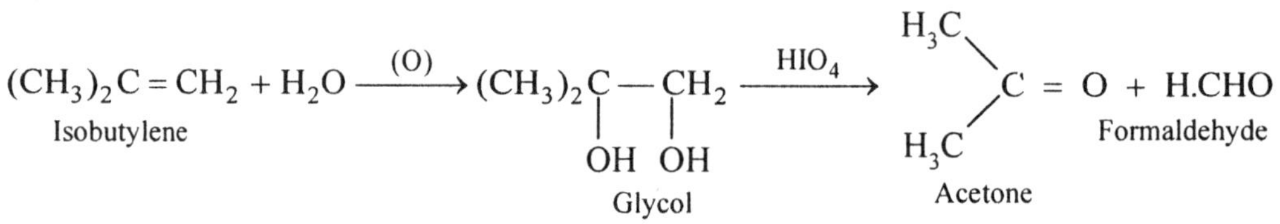

$$(CH_3)_2C = CH_2 + H_2O \xrightarrow{(O)} (CH_3)_2\underset{\displaystyle OH}{C} - \underset{\displaystyle OH}{CH_2} \xrightarrow{HIO_4} \underset{\displaystyle H_3C}{\overset{\displaystyle H_3C}{\diagup\diagdown}}C = O + H.CHO$$

Isobutylene   Glycol   Acetone   Formaldehyde

(iii) **Oxidation with acidic potassium permanganate or potassium dichromate:** With such reagents alkenes are oxidized to glycol, to carbonyl compounds and then to acids.

$$CH_3.CH = CH_2 + H_2O \xrightarrow[\text{acid}]{KMnO_4} CH_3.CH - CH_2 \xrightarrow[\text{acid}]{KMnO_4} CH_3CHO + H.CHO$$

$$\underset{\text{Propane}}{} \qquad \underset{\begin{array}{cc}| & | \\ OH & OH \\ \text{Glycol}\end{array}}{} \qquad \underset{\text{Acetaldehyde}}{} \quad \underset{\text{Formaldehyde}}{}$$

$$\downarrow [O] \qquad \downarrow [O]$$

$$CH_3.COOH \quad H.COOH$$
$$\text{Acetic acid} \qquad \text{Formic acid}$$

$$(CH_3)_2 C = CH_2 + H_2O + [O] \xrightarrow[\text{acid}]{K_2Cr_2O_7} (CH_3)_2.\underset{\underset{CH_2.OH}{|}}{C} - OH \rightarrow CH_3.CO.CH_3 + H.CHO$$

$$\underset{\text{Acetone}}{} \qquad \downarrow [O]$$

$$H.COOH$$
$$\text{Formic acid}$$

(iv) **Combustion:** Alkenes are burnt in air and form carbon dioxide and water on complete oxidation.

$$C_2H_4 + 3O_2 \longrightarrow 2CO_2 + 2H_2O$$

B. Reactions of Alkyl Group

Substitution reactions: The alkyl group of alkene undergoes substitution reaction with chlorine at a temperature of 500–600°C. The double bond of alkene is not cleaved but hydrogen of alkyl group is replaced by chlorine.

$$CH_3.CH = CH_2 + Cl_2 \xrightarrow{500°C} \underset{\text{Allyl chloride}}{CH_2 = CH.CH_2Cl} + HCl$$

If there are more than one alkyl groups then the substitution occurs at the carbon α to the double bond or at allylic carbon atom, e.g.

$$\underset{\text{1-Butene}}{CH_3.CH_2.CH = CH_2} + Cl_2 \xrightarrow{500°C} \underset{\text{3-Chloro-1-butene}}{CH_3.CHCl.CH = CH_2} + HCl$$

Ethylene (Ethene) $CH_2 = CH_2$: Ethylene, a colourless gas, with sweet odour and taste is compressed in steel cylinders. 1000 ml under normal conditions weigh 1.26 g. It is soluble in conc. H_2SO_4, water and alcohol. It decolourises bromine water, with the help of which it can be estimated. Though it was first isolated in 1669, its use as an anaesthetic was made in 1923. It is used as general anaesthetic by inhalation. It is quickly absorbed, is free of excitation, remains unchanged and is quickly excreted. It should be pure and free from acetylene carbon monoxide, phosphine, etc. Only if oxygen supply is impaired or decreased, it can possibly act as lethal. Unfortunately, its use as an anaesthetic cannot be common because of its being highly inflammable. Its mixture with oxygen and air are very dangerous and are extremely explosive, especially in presence of fire and sparks. Hence, to avoid this danger, it has to be very carefully used and prepared highly technically. Ethene is also used as an agent for ripening fruits and vegetables like potatoes, oranges and bananas. The gas is not official in I.P. It can be prepared by dehydration of alcohol (see also general methods for alkenes).

$$CH_3.CH_2.OH \xrightarrow[\text{or } H_2SO_4/170°C]{Al_2O_3/360°C} CH_2 = CH_2$$

It is mentioned here not because of its any medical use, but because of its historic importance.

Alkynes
(Unsaturated Hydrocarbons)

INTRODUCTION

The unsaturated hydrocarbons containing one triple bond are called **alkynes** or **acetylenes**. They have four hydrogen atoms less than the corresponding alkanes and are represented by the general formula C_nH_{2n-2}. The simplest member of the alkyne family is acetylene C_2H_2. The carbon-carbon triple bond is the distinguishing feature of the alkyne structure.

$$H : C ::: C : H \qquad H - C \equiv C - H$$

Acetylene   Acetylene

The nature of a carbon-carbon triple bond is almost the same as that of a double bond. The difference is that *sp* hybridization takes place in alkynes, i.e., formed by mixing of one *s* and one *p*-orbital. These *sp* orbitals lie along a straight line that passes through the carbon nucleus, the angle between the two orbitals is thus $180°$. This linear arrangement permits the hybrid orbitals to be as far apart as possible. Thus acetylene is a linear molecule in which all four atoms are lying along a single straight line.

In forming the *sp* orbitals each carbon atom has used only one of its three *p* orbitals, and two *p* orbitals have remained as such. Each of these are made up of two equal lobes, whose axis lies at right angles both to the axis of the other *p* orbital and to the line of the *sp* orbitals. Each orbital contains only one electron. The *p* orbital of one carbon atom can overlap with a *p* orbital of the other carbon atom. The electrons are paired in this way and consequently, two *p* bonds are formed.

The carbon-carbon triple bond is thus made up of one strong σ-bond and two weaker π-bonds. The total bond strength of a triple bond is 123 kcal. The C–C distance is 1.20 Å in alkynes, as compared to 1.34 Å in alkene and 1.54 Å in alkane. The free rotation of carbon atoms around triple bond is highly restricted as in case of alkenes.

Occurrence of alkynes: Like alkenes, alkynes do not occur free in nature due to their reactivity. However, they are produced by combustion of coal and decomposition of organic substances. The main sources of alkynes are coal gas and petroleum.

Nomenclature: The following systems are used for naming alkynes:
1. **Common or trivial system:** Acetylene (C_2H_2) is the first member of alkyne series. The common names of other alkynes do not bear any relationship and are based on the names of related compounds, e.g., acetylene ($CH \equiv CH$), crotonylene ($CH_3.C = C.CH_3$), etc.
2. **Acetylene derivative system:** Acetylene is considered to be the parent member of alkyne series. The other alkynes are named as alkyl derivatives of acetylene, like acetylene ($CH \equiv CH$), methyl acetylene ($CH_3.C \equiv CH$), ethyl methyl acetylene ($CH_3C \equiv C.C_2H_5$), etc.
3. **IUPAC system:** In this system 'ane' of the alkanes is replaced by 'yne'.

This suffix also indicates the presence of a triple bond. In long carbon skeleton the carbon atoms are numbered from the lower alkyl group around the triple bond, e.g., ethyne ($CH \equiv CH$), propyne ($CH_3.C \equiv CH$), 2-butyne ($CH_3.C \equiv C.CH_3$), 1-butyne ($CH_3.CH_2.C \equiv CH$), 2-pentyne ($CH_3.CH_2.C \equiv C.CH_3$), 3-methyl-1-butyne ($(CH_3)_2CH.C. \equiv CH$), etc. The nomenclature of alkynes is given in the chapter on nomenclature.

Isomerism: The first two members, ethyne and propyne, do not exhibit any type of isomerism. The other alkynes exhibit the following types of isomerism:
1. **Chain isomerism:** It is due to different arrangement of atoms in a carbon chain as represented by two formulae as in case of C_5H_8.

$$CH_3.CH_2.CH_2.C \equiv CH \qquad \overset{\overset{\textstyle CH_3}{|}}{CH_3.CH}.C \equiv CH$$
1-Pentyne   3-Methyl-1-butyne

2. **Position isomerism:** This isomerism is exhibited by various structures which may be represented by changing the position of the triple bond in a chain e.g.:

$$CH_3.CH_2.C \equiv CH \qquad\qquad CH_3.C \equiv C.CH_3$$
1-Butyne   2-Butyne

3. **Functional isomerism:** Alkynes are the isomeric forms of dienes. Thus, butyne and butadiene have the same formulae C_4H_6.

$$CH_3.CH_2.C = CH \qquad\qquad CH_2 = CH.CH = CH_2$$
1-Butyne   1,3-Butadiene

General Methods of Preparation

General methods of preparation of alkynes are similar to that of alkenes which are as follows:

1. Dehydrohalogenation of alkyl dihalides: Treatment of dihaloalkanes with excess of alcoholic potassium hydroxide or sodamide eliminates two molecules of halogen acid and formation of alkyne takes place. Both types of dihalides, gem- and vic-dihalides, yield alkyne in this process. The reaction occurs in two stages, first an olefinic halide is formed which on further elimination of a molecule of haloacid gives the desired product.

$$\underset{\substack{\text{Ethylene dibromide} \\ \text{(vic-dibromide)}}}{\overset{\displaystyle CH_2\!-\!CH_2}{\underset{\displaystyle Br \quad\; Br}{|\qquad |}}} \xrightarrow[-HBr]{\text{Alc. KOH}} \underset{\text{Vinyl bromide}}{H_2C{=}CH.Br} \xrightarrow[-HBr]{\text{Alc. KOH}} \underset{\text{Ethyne}}{HC{\equiv}CH}$$

$$CH_3.CH.Br_2.CH_3 \xrightarrow[-HBr]{\text{Alc. KOH}} CH_3.CBr{=}CH_2 \xrightarrow[-HBr]{\text{Alc. KOH}} CH_3.C{\equiv}CH$$

2,2-Dibromopropane   2-Bromopropene   Propyne
(gem-dibromide)

vic-Dihalides are prepared by treating alkene with halogen, while the reaction of aldehydes or ketones with phosphorus pentachloride gives gem-dichlorides.

2. **Dehalogenation of tetrahalides:** Treatment of tetrahalo alkanes in which active metals like zinc or magnesium yield alkynes.

$$CH_3.CBr_2.CHBr_2 + 2Zn \longrightarrow CH_3.C \equiv CH + 2ZnBr_2$$

1,1,2,2-Tetrabromopropane

This method is severely limited by the fact that these halides are themselves prepared from the alkynes.

3. **Electrolysis of salts of unsaturated dicarboxylic acids:** The method is the extension of Kolbe's electrolytic method in which a suitable unsaturated dicarboxylic acid is employed in this reaction. For example, potassium fumarate on electrolysis gives ethyne.

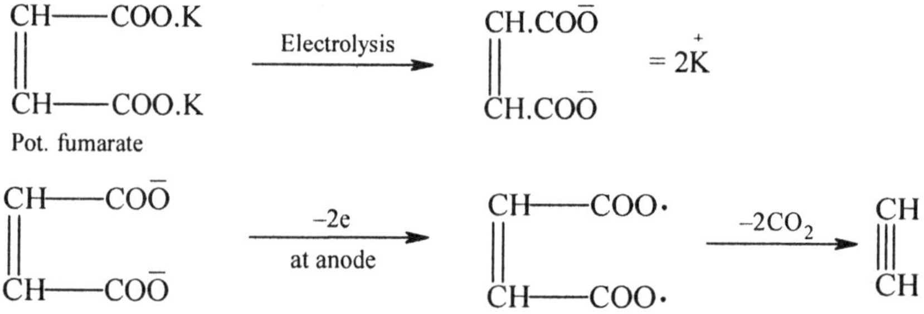

4. **Hydrolysis of alkynides:** Alkynides are the metal derivatives of alkynes which on treatment with water or dilute acids produce alkynides.

$$CH \equiv C.Ag + H_2O \xrightarrow{H^+} CH \equiv CH + AgOH$$

Silver ethynide

$$CH_3C \equiv C.Na + H_2O \xrightarrow{H^+} CH_3.C \equiv CH + NaOH$$

Sodium propynide

If the alkynides are tested with alkyl halides then higher alkynes are produced.

$$CH \equiv C.Na \xrightarrow[-NaBr]{CH_3Br} CH_3.C \equiv CH$$

Sodium acetylide   Propyne

$$Na.C \equiv C.Na \xrightarrow[-2NaBr]{2CH_3Br} CH_3.C \equiv C.CH_3$$

Disodium acetylene   Butylene

$$CH_3.C \equiv CNa \xrightarrow[-NaI]{C_2H_5I} CH_3.C \equiv C.C_2H_3$$

Sodium propynide   2-Pentyne

5. **Decarboxylation of acetylenic acids:** Sodium or potassium salts of unsaturated acids containing a triple bond on decarboxylation at higher temperature with soda lime give alkynes. For example:

$$CH_3.C \equiv C.COOH \xrightarrow{\text{NaOH}} CH_3.C \equiv C.COONa \xrightarrow[\Delta]{\text{NaOH, CuO}} CH_3C \equiv CH + Na_2CO_3$$

$$\underset{\text{Tetrolic acid}}{} \qquad\qquad \underset{\text{Sodium tetrolate}}{} \qquad\qquad\qquad \underset{\text{Propyne}}{}$$

General Physical Properties

The physical properties of alkynes are similar to alkenes and alkanes. However, they are less volatile than the corresponding alkenes or alkanes.

The first three members of alkyne series are gases, next members from C_5 to C_{13} are liquids and higher ones are solids. Ethyne has garlic odour while all other members are odourless and colourless compounds. The physical constants like b.p., m.p., heats of combustion, sp. gr. etc. show a regular increase with increase in molecular weights as shown in Table 10.1.

Table 10.1. Physical constants of alkynes

Compound	Formula	B.P. °C	M.P. °C	Sp. gr. at 20°C	Heat of combustion
Ethyne	$CH \equiv CH$	–84	–81	–	310.6
Propyne	$CH_3.C \equiv CH$	–23.2	–103	–	463.1
1-Butyne	$CH_3.CH_2.C \equiv CH$	8.1	–126	0.650	420.6
2-Butyne	$CH_3.C \equiv C.CH_3$	27.0	–32	0.691	–
1-Pentyne	$CH_3.(CH_2)_2.C \equiv CH$	40.2	–106	0.690	778.0
2-Pentyne	$CH_3.CH_2.C \equiv C.CH_3$	56.0	–109	0.711	774.3
3-Methyl-1-butyne	$(CH_3)_2.CH.C \equiv CH$	29.0	–	0.665	–
1-Hexyne	$CH_3.(CH_2)_3.C \equiv CH$	71.5	–132	0.716	935.5
2-Hexyne	$CH_3.(CH_2)_2.C \equiv C.CH_3$	84.0	–88	0.732	935.5
3-Hexyne	$CH_3.CH_2.C \equiv C.CH_2CH_3$	81.7	–105	0.724	935.5
1-Heptyne	$CH_3.(CH_2)_4.C \equiv CH$	99.7	–81	0.733	1092.9
1-Octyne	$CH_3.(CH_2)_5.C \equiv CH$	126.2	–79	0.746	1250.3
1-Nonyne	$CH_3.(CH_2)_6.C \equiv CH$	150.8	–50	0.757	1407.8
1-Decyne	$CH_3.(CH_2)_7C \equiv CH$	174.0	–44	0.766	1565.2

General Chemical Properties

Alkyne chemistry is the chemistry of the carbon-carbon triple bond. They behave in a manner similar to typical alkenes. Like alkenes, they undergo electrophilic addition reactions due to the availability of the loosely held electrons. The alkyl group attached to a carbon atom involved in triple bond formation is generally unreactive or inert.

A. **Addition reactions:** Alkynes react with two molecules of the reagent of addendum instead of one as in case of alkenes. The addition of reagents to the triple bond takes place in a manner similar to the double bond.

1. **Addition of hydrogen:** Alkynes react with hydrogen gas in the presence of a catalyst like Ni, Pt or Pd to give alkene and then alkane as:

$$\underset{\text{Ethyne}}{CH \equiv CH} + H_2 \xrightarrow{Ni} \underset{\text{Ethene}}{CH_2 = CH_2} \xrightarrow{H_2/Ni} \underset{\text{Ethane}}{CH_3.CH_3}$$

If the palladium catalyst, inactivated with traces of heavy metal salts or quinoline (Lindlar's catalyst), is used, then the reduction does not proceed beyond the alkene stage. Such partial catalytic hydrogenation of alkynes has important application in synthetic chemistry as in case of sex harmone series.

$$\underset{\text{Propyne}}{CH_3C \equiv CH} \xrightarrow{H_2\,/\,\text{Lindlar's cat.}} \underset{\text{Propene}}{CH_3.CH = CH_2}$$

trans-Alkene is obtained by reduction of alkynes with sodium or lithium in liquid ammonia. But the alkyne is almost entirely converted into cis-form when it is hydrogenated with Lindlar's catalyst.

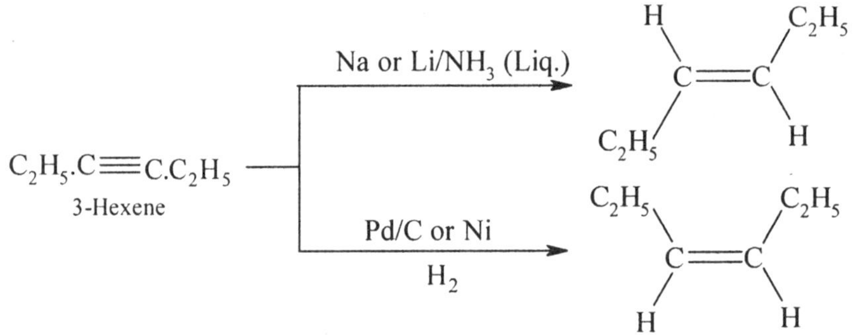

trans-3-hexene

cis-3-hexene (98–99%)

2. **Addition of halogens:** One or two molecules of halogens can be added to alkynes giving dihalides or tetrahalides respectively. Addition takes place readily with chlorine and bromine while iodine reacts slowly.

$$CH_3 \equiv H_2 \xrightarrow{Br_2} \underset{\text{1,2-Dibromopropene}}{CH_3\underset{\mid \atop Br}{C} \equiv \underset{\mid \atop Br}{CH}} \xrightarrow{Br_2} \underset{\text{1,1,2,2-Tetrabromopropane}}{CH_3.C.Br_2CHBr_2}$$

3. **Addition of halogen acids:** Addition of one molecule of halogen acid with alkyne gives an unsymmetrical halide. When another molecule of hydrogen halide is combined, dihaloalkane is formed. The order of reactivity is HI > HBr > HCl > HF. Hydrofluoric acid reacts only under pressure. The addition can take place in the dark, but is catalysed by light or metallic halides. The addition is according to the Markownikoff's rule, as previously noted. The reaction of hydrogen chloride with acetylene takes place sluggishly.

$$CH \equiv CH + HCl \longrightarrow \underset{\text{1-Chloroethene}}{CH_2 = CH.Cl} \xrightarrow{\text{HCl}} \underset{\text{1,1-Dichloroethene}}{CH_3CHCl_2}$$

$$\underset{\text{Propyne}}{CH_3.C \equiv CH} + HBr \longrightarrow \underset{\text{2-Bromopropene}}{CH_3.CBr = CH_2} \xrightarrow{\text{HBr}} \underset{\text{2,2-Dibromopropane}}{CH_3.CBr_2.CH_3}$$

Peroxides have the same effect on the addition of hydrogen bromide in alkynes as for the alkenes. Anti-Markownikoff's product is obtained in the presence of a peroxide as:

$$\underset{\text{Propyne}}{CH_3.C \equiv CH} + HBr \xrightarrow{\text{Peroxide}} \underset{\text{1-Bromopropene}}{CH_3.CH = CH.Br} \xrightarrow{\text{HBr}} \underset{\substack{| \\ Br \\ \text{1,2-Dibromopropane}}}{CH_3.CH.CH_2Br}$$

4. **Addition of hypohalous acids:** Alkynes when reacted with hypochlorous or hypobromous acids yield di-haloaldehyde or di-haloketones.

$$CH \equiv CH + HOCl \longrightarrow HO.CH = CHCl \longrightarrow (HO)_2CH.Cl_2 \downarrow -H_2O$$

$$\underset{\text{Dichloroacetaldehyde}}{CHCl_2.CHO}$$

$$CH_3.C \equiv CH + HOBr \longrightarrow CH_3.C(OH) = CHBr \longrightarrow CH_3C(OH)_2.CHBr_2 \downarrow -H_2O$$

$$\underset{\text{1,1-Dibromoacetone}}{CH_3.CO.CHBr_2}$$

The addition takes place according to Markownikoff's rule as explained earlier.

5. **Addition of water (hydration):** Alkynes are added to one molecule of water in the presence of proper catalysts like sulphuric acid and mercurous sulphate to form aldehydes and ketones. Enolic compound is formed initially by the addition of water to alkyne which is readily rearranged to form a more stable carbonyl or keto form by migration of hydrogen from oxygen to carbon with simultaneous shift of the double bond.

$$\underset{\text{Ethyne}}{CH \equiv CH} + H_2O \xrightarrow[\text{H}_2\text{SO}_4]{\text{Hg/HgSO}_4} \underset{\substack{| \\ \text{Enol (unstable)}}}{\overset{OH}{CH = CH_2}} \longrightarrow \underset{\text{Acetaldehyde}}{CH_3.CHO}$$

$$\underset{\text{Propyne}}{CH_3.C \equiv CH} + H_2O \xrightarrow[\text{H}_2\text{SO}_4]{\text{Hg/HgSO}_4} \underset{\substack{| \\ \text{Unstable}}}{CH_3 - \overset{OH}{C} = CH_2} \longrightarrow \underset{\text{Acetone}}{CH_3 - \overset{O}{\overset{\|}{C}} - CH_3}$$

6. **Addition of ammonia and hydrogen cyanide:** Addition of ammonia to alkynes in the presence of alumina and/or hydrogen cyanide in a mixture of cupric chloride and ammonium chloride at high temperature takes place to yield nitriles.

$$CH \equiv CH + NH_3 \xrightarrow[300-350^\circ]{Al_2O_3} CH_3.C \equiv N + H_2$$

$$CH \equiv CH + HCN \xrightarrow[H^+]{Cu_2Cl_2/NH_4Cl} CH_2 = CH.C \equiv N$$
$$\underset{\text{Acrylonitrile}}{}$$

7. **Addition of carboxylic acids and their derivatives:** Alkynes react with carboxylic acids and their derivatives in the presence of catalysts like mercuric oxide, boron trifluoride etc. to yield vinyl esters.

$$\underset{\text{Ethyne}}{CH \equiv CH} + CH_3.COOH \xrightarrow[\substack{(CH_3.COO)_2 Zn \\ 200^\circ C}]{\text{HgO or}} \underset{\text{Vinyl acetate}}{CH_2 = CH.OOC.CH_3} \xrightarrow[\substack{HgO \\ 200^\circ C}]{CH_3.COOH} \underset{\text{Ethyl diacetate}}{CH_3.CH(O.OCCH_3)_2}$$

$$\underset{\text{Propyne}}{CH_3.C \equiv CH} + CH_3.COOH \xrightarrow[200^\circ C]{BF_3} \underset{\alpha\text{-Methyl vinyl acetate}}{CH_2 = C(CH_3).O.OC.CH_3}$$

$$CH \equiv CH + \underset{\text{Acetyl chloride}}{CH_3.COCl} \xrightarrow{BF_3} \underset{\beta\text{-Chlorovinyl methyl ketone}}{CHCl = CH.CO.CH_3}$$

8. **Addition of alcohols:** Vinyl ethers are formed when a molecule of alcohol is added to alkynes in alkaline medium.

$$CH \equiv CH + C_2H_5OH \xrightarrow{NaOH} \underset{\text{Ethyl vinyl ether}}{CH_2 = CH.O.C_2H_5}$$

9. **Reaction with formaldehyde:** Ethyne and formaldehyde interact in the presence of sodium alkoxide as catalyst to form diaddition product, butyne diol as well as mono-addition product propargyl alcohol in small quantity.

$$CH \equiv CH + HCHO \xrightarrow{C_2H_5.ONa} \underset{\text{Propargyl alcohol}}{HOCH_2 - C \equiv CH} \xrightarrow[C_2H_5ONa]{CH \equiv CH} \underset{\text{2-Butynediol}}{HO.CH_2C \equiv C.CH_2.OH}$$

10. **Addition of ozone and ozonalysis:** Alkynes form ozonide with ozone and these compounds are decomposed by water to form dicarbonyl compounds. The products so obtained are then oxidized to acids by hydrogen peroxide formed in the reaction.

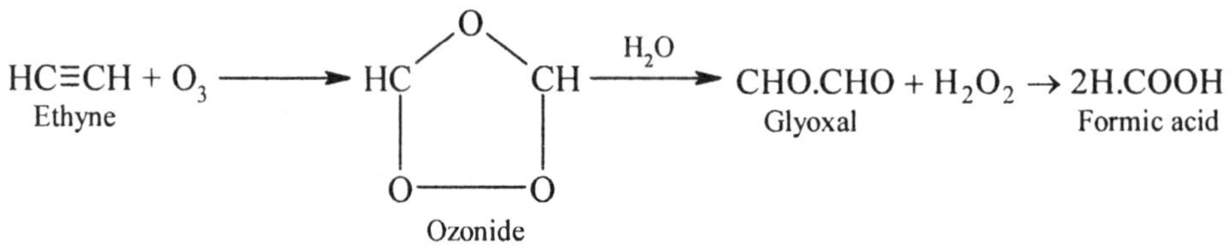

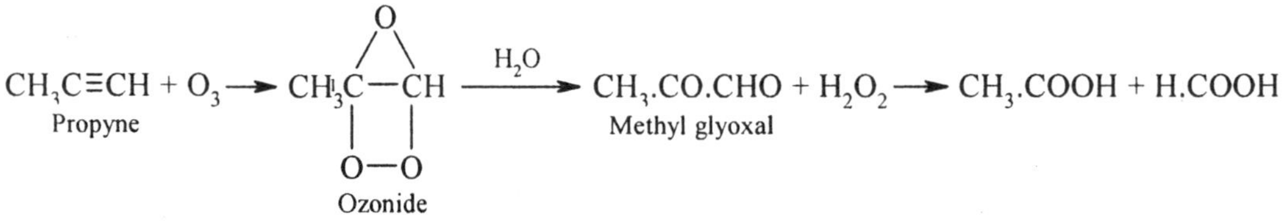

$$\underset{\text{Ethyne}}{HC \equiv CH} + O_3 \longrightarrow \underset{\text{Ozonide}}{\overset{\displaystyle O}{HC \diagup \diagdown CH}} \xrightarrow{H_2O} \underset{\text{Glyoxal}}{CHO.CHO} + H_2O_2 \rightarrow \underset{\text{Formic acid}}{2H.COOH}$$

$$\underset{\text{Propyne}}{CH_3C \equiv CH} + O_3 \longrightarrow \underset{\text{Ozonide}}{CH_3C - CH} \xrightarrow{H_2O} \underset{\text{Methyl glyoxal}}{CH_3.CO.CHO} + H_2O_2 \longrightarrow CH_3.COOH + H.COOH$$

11. **Polymerization:** Alkynes are polymerized to yield linear or cyclic compounds depending on the reaction conditions.

$$\underset{\text{Ethyne}}{2CH \equiv CH} \xrightarrow{Cu_2Cl_2/NH_4Cl} \underset{\text{Vinyl acetylene}}{CH_2 = CH.C \equiv CH} \xrightarrow{C_2H_2} \underset{\text{Divinyl acetylene}}{CH_2 = CH.C \equiv C.CH.CH_2}$$

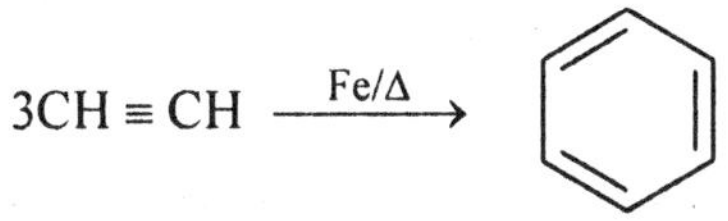
3CH ≡ CH
Fe/Δ

Benzene

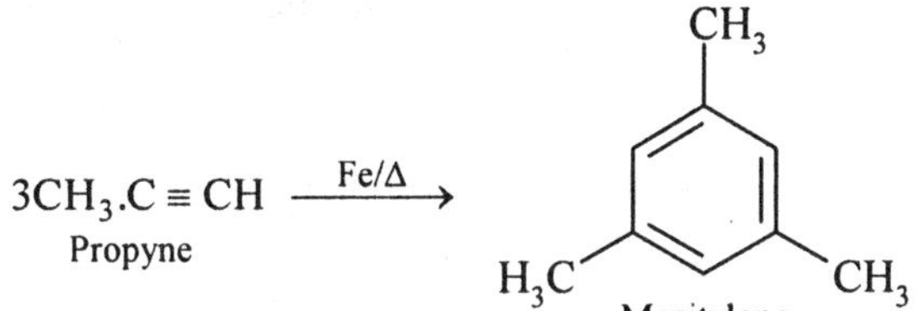
3CH3.C ≡ CH
Propyne
Fe/Δ
CH3
H3C
CH3

Mesitylene

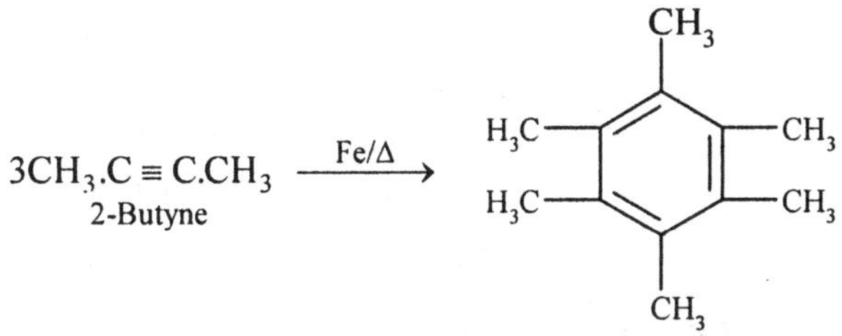
3CH3.C ≡ C.CH3
2-Butyne
Fe/Δ
CH3
H3C
CH3
H3C
CH3
CH3

Hexamethyl benzene

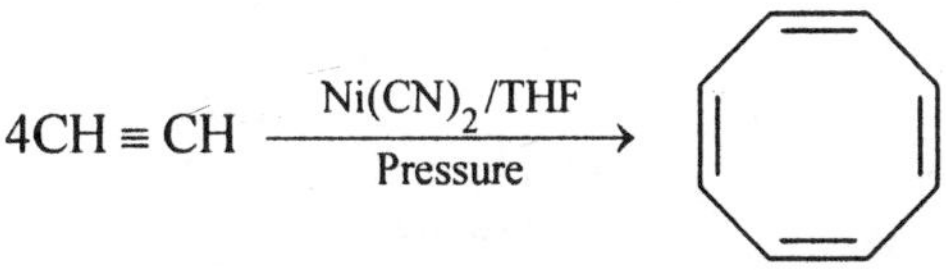
4CH ≡ CH
Ni(CN)2/THF
Pressure

Cyclo-octatrene

B. **Oxidation reactions:** Various oxidation products are obtained under different oxidizing conditions.

1. **Oxidation with strong alkaline potassium permanganate:** Carboxylic acids containing generally lesser number of carbon atoms are formed with strong alkaline $KMnO_4$.

$$CH_3.C \equiv CH + 2H_2O + 2[O] \xrightarrow[-2H_2O]{KMnO_4} \underset{\text{Methyl glyoxal}}{CH_3.CO.CHO} \xrightarrow{H_2O + O} \underset{\text{Acetic acid}}{CH_3.COOH} + H.COOH$$

$$CH \equiv CH + 2H_2O + 2[O] \xrightarrow[-2H_2O]{KMnO_4} \underset{\text{Glyoxal}}{CHO.CHO} \xrightarrow[-2H_2O]{KMnO_4} \underset{\text{Oxalic acid}}{HOOC.COOH}$$

2. **Oxidation with acidic potassium dichromate:** Carboxylic acids are formed on oxidation of alkynes with acidic $K_2Cr_2O_7$.

$$CH \equiv CH + H_2O + O \xrightarrow[H^+]{K_2Cr_2O_7} CH_3.COOH$$

3. **Oxidation with selenium dioxide:** Selenium dioxide oxidation of alkyne affords dicarbonyl compounds.

$$CH \equiv CH \xrightarrow[SeO_2]{2(O)} CHO.CHO$$

$$\underset{\text{2-Butyne}}{CH_3.C \equiv C.CH_3} \xrightarrow[SeO_2]{2(O)} \underset{\text{Butadinone}}{CH_3.CO.CO.CH_3}$$

4. **Combustion:** Alkynes on burning in air produce heat and carbon dioxide.

$$2CH \equiv CH + 5O_2 \longrightarrow 4CO_2 + 2H_2O + 312 \text{ kcal.}$$

C. **Isomerization:** Isomerization takes place when alkynes are treated with alkali. The reaction is reversible when the product is treated with sodamide.

$$\underset{\text{1-Butyne}}{CH_3CH_2C \equiv CH} \underset{NaNH_2}{\overset{\text{Alc. KOH}}{\rightleftharpoons}} \underset{\text{2-Butyne}}{CH_3C \equiv C.CH_3}$$

D. **Formation of metal derivatives (alkynides):** Alkynes are acidic in nature and the hydrogen atom attached to a triple bond can be replaced by metals forming alkynides. Acetylene forms metallic derivatives by replacement of one or both hydrogen atoms by passing over heated sodium or on treatment with sodium in ammonia.

$$\underset{\text{Ethylene}}{CH \equiv CH + Na} \xrightarrow[-H]{110^o} \underset{\substack{\text{Monosodium}\\\text{acetylide}}}{CH \equiv C.Na} \xrightarrow[-H]{110^o/Na} \underset{\substack{\text{Disodium}\\\text{acetylide}}}{NaC \equiv CNa}$$

$$CH \equiv CH + K.NH_2 \xrightarrow[-NH_2]{\text{Xylene}} \underset{\substack{\text{Potassium}\\\text{acetylide}}}{CH \equiv C.K} \xrightarrow[-NH_3]{KNH_2/\text{Xylene}} \underset{\substack{\text{Dipotassium}\\\text{acetylide}}}{K.C \equiv C.K}$$

$$CH \equiv CH + \underset{\substack{\text{Grignard}\\\text{reagent}}}{RMgX} \longrightarrow \underset{\substack{\text{Acetylene}\\\text{Grignard reagent}}}{CH \equiv C.MgX} + R.H$$

$$CH_3C \equiv CH + NaNH_2 \longrightarrow \underset{\text{Sodium propynide}}{CH_3.C \equiv C.Na} + NH_3$$

Heavy metal ions like Cu^+, Ag^+, etc. give insoluble metal acetylides. When acetylene gas is passed into cuprous ammonium hydroxide solution, a reddish-brown precipitate of cuprous acetylides is produced.

$$CH \equiv CH \xrightarrow{Cu(NH_3)_2OH} \underset{\substack{\text{Copper}\\\text{acetylide}}}{CH \equiv C.Cu} \xrightarrow{Cu(NH_3)_2OH} \underset{\substack{\text{Dicopper}\\\text{acetylide}}}{CuC \equiv C.Cu}$$

Similarly:

$$CH \equiv CH \xrightarrow{\text{Ag(NH}_3)_2.\text{NO}_2} \underset{\text{Silver acetylide}}{CH \equiv C.Ag} \xrightarrow{\text{Ag(NH}_3)_2.\text{NO}_2} \underset{\substack{\text{Disilver acetylide} \\ \text{(white)}}}{Ag.C \equiv C.Ag}$$

Uses: Alkynides are used for the preparation, purification, separation and identification of alkynes.

DIENES

Dienes or diolefines are simply alkenes that contain two carbon-carbon double bonds in the molecule. They are bifunctional compounds and have essentially alkene like properties. The general formula of these hydrocarbons is C_nH_{2n-2} which is the same as that of alkynes.

Dienes are named by the IUPAC system in the same way as alkenes, except that the ending **-diene** is used with two numbers to indicate the positions of the two double bonds. This system is used to name the compounds containing any number of double bonds, e.g.:

$$\underset{\text{1,3-Butadiene}}{CH_2 = CH.CH = CH_2} \quad \underset{\text{1,4-Pentadiene}}{CH_2 = CH.CH_2.CH = CH_2} \quad \underset{\text{1,3,5-Hexatriene}}{CH_2 = CH.CH = CH.CH = CH_2}$$

The properties of compounds containing two double bonds may be similar or different from alkenes depending upon the positions of the double bonds in the molecule. Thus dienes are divided into three main classes according to the arrangement of double bonds.

1. **Dienes with conjugated double bonds:** When the double and single bonds are present alternately in the molecule, the compound is said to have conjugated double bonds. Thus:

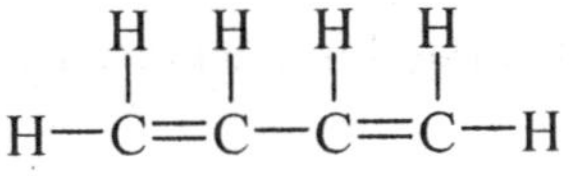

1,3-Butadiene   1,3-Pentadiene

2. **Diene with isolated double bonds:** In these dienes the double bonds are separated from each other by at least two single bonds, e.g.:

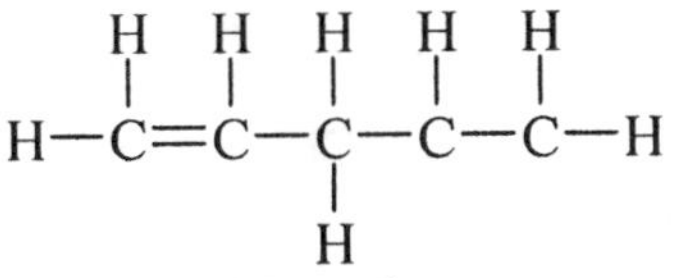

1,4-Pentadiene   1,4-Pentadiene

The double bonds in these dienes behave like independent double bonds. In such dienes the reactions of alkenes or double bonds are shown twice due to the presence of two double bonds.

3. **Dienes with cumulated double bonds or allenes:** In such dienes the double bonds are also known as allenes.

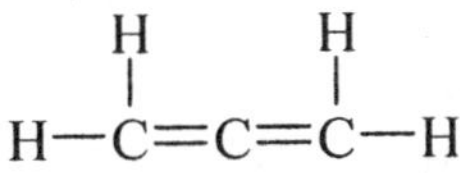

Allenes   or   Allenes

Among these dienes the conjugated dienes are the most important which have different properties from isolated or cumulated dienes.

The compounds containing three, four or many double bonds are known as trienes, tetraenes, polyenes respectively and all of them are classified according to the above classification. In IUPAC system they are named by replacing the 'ane' of the corresponding alkane by 'diene', triene and polyene. The positions of double bonds are indicated by numbering the carbon atoms.

Dienes have the same chemistry as that of alkenes. They are usually prepared by adopting the same methods used to prepare alkenes.

Preparation of Conjugated Dienes

The simplest and most important conjugated dienes are 1,3-butadiene and isoprene or 2-methyl butadiene. They may be prepared by the following methods:

1. **Dehydration of alkanes or alkenes:** n-Butane or butene are dehydrogenated when passed over heated chromic oxide to give butadiene.

$$CH_3.CH_2.CH_2.CH_3 \xrightarrow[-H_2]{Cr_2O_3/\Delta} \begin{bmatrix} CH_3CH_2.CH = CH_2 \\ \text{1-Butene} \\ CH_3.CH = CH.CH_3 \\ \text{2-Butene} \end{bmatrix} \xrightarrow[-H_2]{Cr_2O_3/\Delta} CH_2 = CH.CH_2 = CH_2 \\ \text{1,3-Butadiene}$$

Similarly, isoprene is synthesized from 2-methyl butane.

$$(CH_3)CH.CH_2.CH_3 \xrightarrow[-H_2]{Cr_2O_3/\Delta} CH_2 = \overset{\overset{\displaystyle CH_3}{|}}{C} - CH = CH_2$$
$$\text{2-Methyl butane} \qquad\qquad \text{Isoprene}$$

2. **Dehydration of diols:** 1,4-butanediols when dehydrated in the presence of phosphoric acid eliminate two molecules of water to give butadiene.

$$CH_2OH.CH_2.CH_2.CH_2OH \xrightarrow[-2H_2O]{H_3PO_4/270°C} CH_2 = CH.CH = CH_2$$
$$\text{Butane-1,4-diol} \qquad\qquad\qquad \text{1,3-Butadiene}$$

3. **By decomposition of cyclohexene:** Cyclohexene, when passed over heated nickel chromium catalyst, is decomposed to yield butadiene.

$$C_6H_{10} \xrightarrow[\Delta]{Ni/Cr} CH_2 = CH - CH = CH_2 + CH_2 = CH_2$$
$$\text{Cyclohexene} \qquad\qquad \text{Butadiene}$$

4. **By passing ethyl alcohol and acetaldehyde over heated catalyst:** Silica gel and tantalum oxide are used as catalysts in this reaction:

$$C_6H_5.OH + CH_3.CHO \longrightarrow CH_2 = CH - CH = CH_2$$
$$\text{Ethanol} \quad \text{Acetaldehyde} \qquad \text{Butadiene}$$

Properties

Butadiene is a gas at room temperature (b.p. $-2.6°C$) whereas isoprene is a liquid having b.p. $30°C$. The heats of combustion and hydrogenation of butadiene and isoprene are lower than the expected values. The bond distances of carbon atoms in butadiene have intermediate values due to resonance.

As far as the chemical properties are concerned conjugated dienes exhibit the usual reactions of alkenes such as addition reactions, though such additions undergo more readily.

Conjugated dienes when reacted with one molecule of addendum give usually a mixture of 1,4- and 1,2-addition products in which 1,4-addition product predominates.

$$CH_2Cl.CHCl.CH = CH_2 \xleftarrow{\ Cl_2\ } CH_2 = CH.CH = CH_2 \xrightarrow{\ Cl_2\ } CH_2Cl.CH = CH.CH_2.Cl$$

3,4-Dichloro-1-butene   Butadiene   1,4-Dichloro-2-butene
(1,2-addition product)   (1,4-addition product)

To account for such anomalous behaviour Thiele (1899) gave **Theory of Partial Valency.** According to this the valencies of carbon atoms involved in double bond formation are not fully satisfied and each carbon is left with some residual or partial valency. The addition to double bond occurs through these residual valencies. He also suggested that in case of conjugated dienes the partial valencies of carbon atoms 1 to 4 are free, while those of carbon 2 and 3 get mutually satisfied and hence the addition to 1,3-butadiene is not as dominant as that of 1,4-addition.

Each carbon atom of butadiene is considered to be in sp^2 hybdirized state so that each carbon has an unhybridized p-orbital.

The mobile bonds are formed by sideways overlapping of these p-orbitals. Thus the p-orbital at C-2 can overlap with either p-orbital of C-1 or that of C-3. The orbital at C-3 can also overlap with that of C-2 or C-4 to form bonds in the same way. Delocalized bond orbitals are formed over all the four carbon atoms and delocalized electron imparts greater stability (Fig. 10.1).

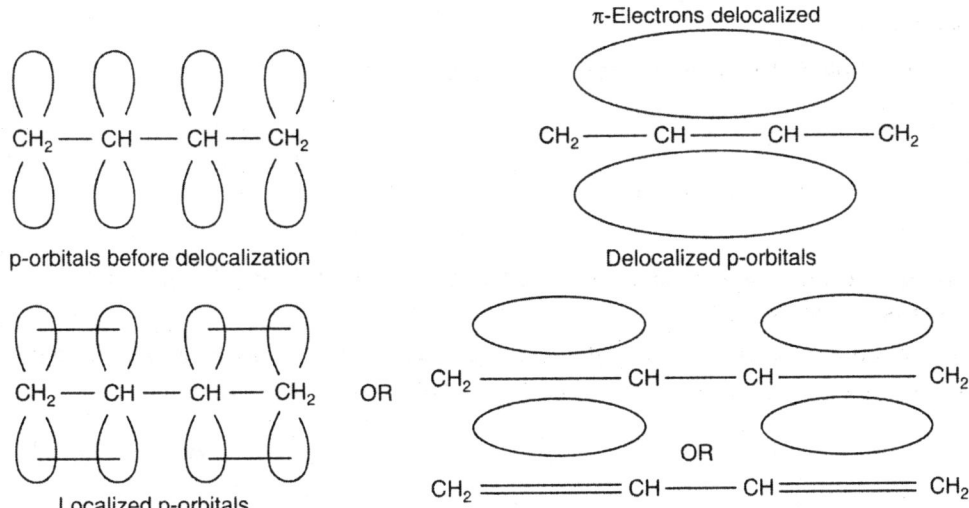

Fig. 10.1. Hybridization in butadiene molecule.

Some important reactions of conjugated dienes are mentioned below:

1. **Diels-Alder reactions:** Conjugated dienes add to alkenes by 1,4-addition to yield cyclic compounds. This is the most important type of the class of reactions spoken as Diels-Alder reaction (1928). The alkene is usually reformed as dienophile and is generally having electron attracting groups like –COOH, –CN, –COR etc. The compound formed by the condensation of dienes and

dienophile is known as the **adduct**. The adduct is usually a six-membered ring, the addition taking place in the 1,4-position, e.g.:

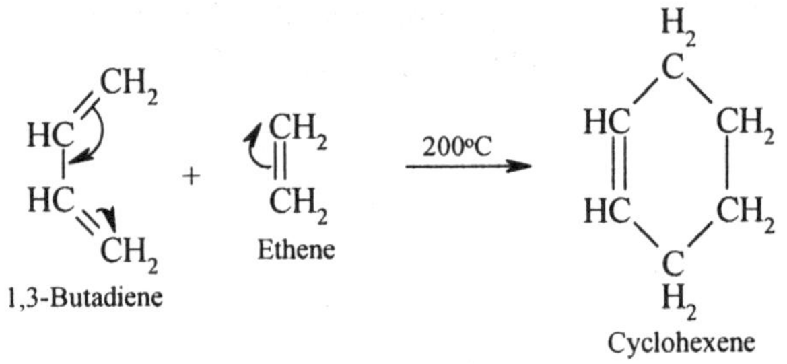
200ºC
1,3-Butadiene
Ethene
Cyclohexene

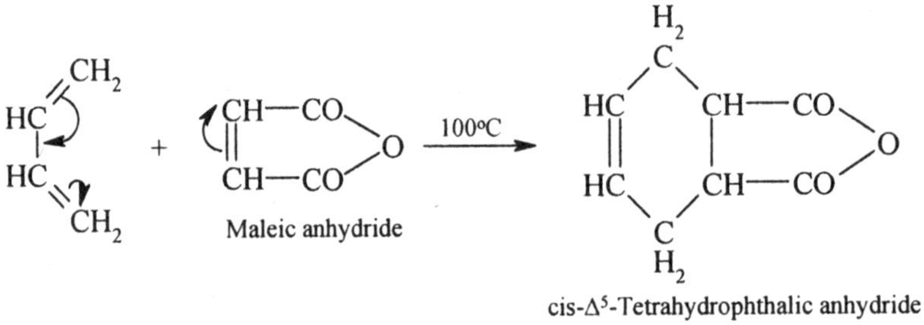
100ºC
Maleic anhydride
cis-Δ5-Tetrahydrophthalic anhydride

The Diels-Alder reaction requires no catalyst, the two compounds are heated together or heated in some solvent like benzene. The mechanism of the reaction is still uncertain but the most favoured one is mentioned above.

2. **Combination with sulphur dioxide:** Conjugated dienes react with SO_2 to form cyclic sulphones. Thus:

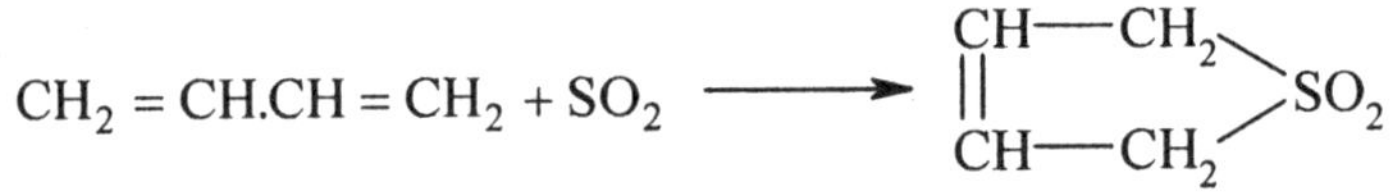

3. **Polymerization:** Conjugated dienes polymerize either by 1,4- or 1,2-addition in the presence of an acid or peroxide as a catalyst.

When 1,4-addition occurs to give polymers in acidic medium it may be either cis or trans. The natural rubber is cis-1,4-polyisoprene and *gutta percha* is trans-1,4-polyisoprene as shown below:

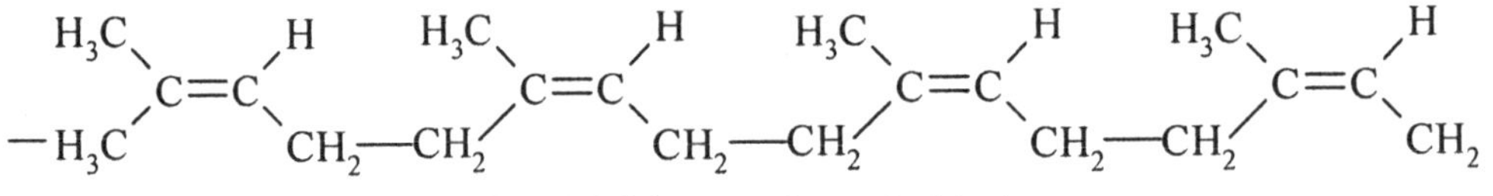

cis-1,4-Polyisoprene (natural rubber)

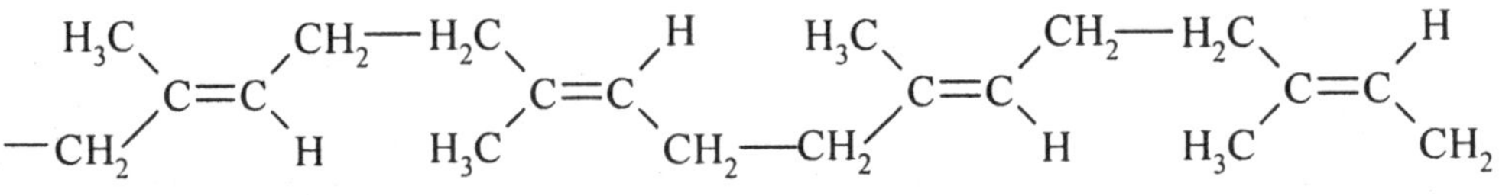

trans-1,4-Polyisoprene (gutta percha)

4. **Addition of halo acids:** Addition of halo acids to 1,3-butadiene yields both 1,2- and 1,5-products, the proportions in which they are obtained are markedly affected by the temperature at which the reaction is carried out. Reaction at $-80^{\circ}C$ yields a mixture containing 20% of 1,4-product and 80% of the 1,2-product. Reaction at higher temperature $40^{\circ}C$ yields a mixture of quite different composition, 80% 1,4- and 20% 1,2-products.

$$CH_2 = CH.CH = CH_2 + HBr \longrightarrow \underset{\substack{| \\ Br \\ \text{1,2-product}}}{CH_3.CH - CH = CH_2} + \underset{\substack{| \\ Br \\ \text{1,4-product}}}{CH_3.CH = CH.CH_2}$$

5. **Ozonolysis:** Carbonyl compounds are formed on ozonolysis of dienes.

$$\underset{\text{2-Methyl butadiene}}{\overset{\overset{\displaystyle CH_3}{\displaystyle |}}{CH_2 = C - CH = CH_2}} \xrightarrow[\text{2. }H_2O/Zn]{1.O_3} \underset{\text{Methyl glyoxal}}{HCHO + CH_3.CO.CHO + HCHO}$$

Uses: Butadiene and isoprene are used to produce natural rubber, leather substitutes and emulsion paints.

Preparation of Allenes

Allene or propadiene is the first compound of the series and hence these are known as **allenes**. They may be prepared by the following methods.

1. **From trihalopropane:** Formation of allene takes place when trihalopropanes are treated with alcoholic potassium hydroxide.

$$\underset{\substack{\text{1,2,3-Tribromo-} \\ \text{propane}}}{\overset{\displaystyle CH_2.Br}{\underset{\displaystyle CH_2.Br}{\overset{\displaystyle |}{\underset{\displaystyle |}{CH.Br}}}}} \xrightarrow[-HBr]{\text{Alc. KOH}} \underset{\substack{\text{2,3-Dibromo-} \\ \text{propene}}}{\overset{\displaystyle CH_2}{\underset{\displaystyle CH_2.Br}{\overset{\displaystyle ||}{\underset{\displaystyle |}{C.Br}}}}} \xrightarrow[-ZnBr_2]{Zn/C_2H_5OH} \underset{\text{Allene}}{\overset{\displaystyle CH_2}{\underset{\displaystyle CH_2}{\overset{\displaystyle ||}{\underset{\displaystyle ||}{C}}}}}$$

2. **From olefins:** Alkenes when treated with bromoform in the presence of potassium t-butoxide and then with magnesium in ether yield allenes.

$$CHBr_3 + \underset{\text{Pot. tert butoxide}}{(CH_3)_3C.OK} \longrightarrow \underset{\substack{\text{Dibromo} \\ \text{carbene}}}{CBr_2} + (CH_3)_3C.OH + KBr$$

$$R.CH = CH.R + CBr_2 \longrightarrow \underset{\substack{\diagdown \diagup \\ C \\ \diagup \diagdown \\ Br \quad Br}}{R.CH \quad\quad CH.R} \xrightarrow[\text{ether}-Br]{Mg} \underset{\text{Substituted allene}}{R.CH = C = CH.R}$$

Allenes are highly reactive and rearrange readily to form acetylene derivatives. For example, formation of sodium derivative of acetylene takes place when allene is treated with sodium.

$$\underset{\text{Allene}}{CH_2 = C = CH_2} \xrightarrow[\text{ether}]{Na} \underset{\substack{\text{Sodium methyl} \\ \text{acetylide}}}{CH_3.C \equiv C.Na}$$

In allenes the central carbon atom is in *sp* hybridized state and so the allene molecule is a linear molecule like acetylene. The other carbon atoms which are involved in the formation of double bonds are in sp^2 hybridized state. The molecular orbital formula of allene is shown in Fig. 10.2:

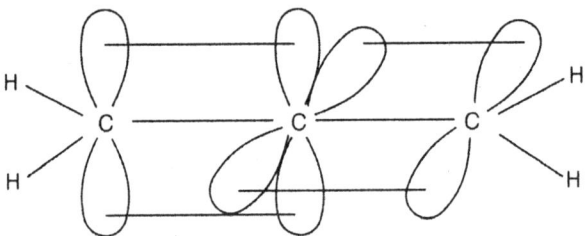

Fig. 10.2. Molecular orbital formula of allene.

If different groups are attached on the terminal carbon atoms like a.b.C=C=C.a.b., then the two enantiomorphic forms will exhibit and it will show the optical activity.

Halo Hydrocarbons

Organic compounds obtained by the replacement of one or more hydrogen atoms of hydrocarbons (alkanes, alkenes or alkynes) by halogen atoms (fluorine, chlorine, bromine or iodine) are known as halo hydrocarbons. They do not occur in nature and are entirely prepared synthetically. One or all hydrogen atoms may be highly reactive and are used for the preparation of many organic compounds. They also find uses as solvents, medicines, fungicides, insecticides, refrigerants, etc.

Halogen derivatives of alkanes, alkenes and alkynes are termed as alkyl halides (haloalkanes), alkenyl halides (haloalkenes) and alkynyl halides (haloalkynes) respectively. They are represented by the general formula RX, where R may be an alkyl, alkenyl or alkynyl group and X may be any halogen. Halogen derivatives of the alkanes are divided into mono-, di-, tri-, etc. substitution products according to the presence of one, two, three halogen atoms in the molecules.

Nomenclature

The common names of monohalogen derivatives are derived from those of the corresponding hydrocarbons and they are named as the halide of the corresponding alkyl group. Both the names are called separately. The alkyl group is written first followed by halogen atom, e.g.:

$CH_3.Cl$	Methyl chloride	$CH_3.CH_2.CH_2.CH_2.Br$	n-Butyl bromide
$CH_3.CH_2.Br$	Ethyl bromide	$(CH_3)_2CH.CH_2.Cl$	Isobutyl chloride
$CH_3.CH_2.CH_2.I$	n-Propyl iodide	$(CH_3)_3C.I.$	tert-Butyl iodide
$CH_3.CH-CH_3$ $\quad\quad\vert$ $\quad\quad I$	Isopropyl iodide	$CH_3.CH_2.CH.CH_3$ $\quad\quad\quad\quad\vert$ $\quad\quad\quad\quad F$	sec-Butyl fluoride

In IUPAC system alkyl halides are called as halogen derivatives of hydrocarbons. The number of halogen is called first followed by the name of the alkane and both the words are combined to get one word. In long chain compounds the position of halogen atom is indicated by numbering the carbon atoms, e.g.:

$CH_3.F$	Fluoromethane	$CH_3.CH_2.CH_2.CH_2.Br$	1-Bromobutane
$CH_3.Br$	Bromomethane	$(CH_3)_2CH.CH_2.Br$	1-Bromo-2-methylpropane

$CH_3.Cl$　　　　Chloromethane　　$CH_3.CH_2.\underset{|}{C}H.CH_3$　　　2-Bromobutane

Br

$CH_3.CH_2.CH_2.Cl$　1-Chloropropane　$(CH_3)_3C.Br$　　　　2-Bromo-2-methylpropane

$CH_3.\underset{|}{C}H.CH_3$　　　2-Chloropropane

Cl

Details on nomenclature of halogen derivatives are given in a separate chapter.

Isomerism

Two types of isomerism occur in higher halogen derivatives.

1. **Chain isomerism:** This isomerism is exhibited due to different arrangement of carbon alignment in carbon chain. Thus, two isomeric forms occur in case of butyl chloride.

$$CH_3.CH_2.CH_2.CH_2.Cl \qquad\qquad (CH_3)_2.CH.CH_2.Cl$$

n-Butyl chloride$$Isobutyl chloride

2. **Position isomerism:** In higher homologues the difference in the position of halogen atom in the chain shows the following type of isomerism, e.g.:

$$CH_3.CH_2.CH_2.CH_2.Br \qquad CH_3.\underset{|}{C}H.CH_2.CH_3$$

1-Bromobutane$$Br

2-Bromobutane

General Methods of Preparation of Alkyl Halides

The following methods are used for the preparation of alkyl halides.

1. **Halogenation of hydrocarbons:** Under the influence of ultraviolet light or temperature, direct halogenation of alkanes gives alkyl halides. Formation of isomeric products depends upon the replacement of hydrogen; n-butane and isobutane can afford two isomers each, n-pentane can form three isomers and isopentane four isomers.

$$CH_3.CH_3 \xrightarrow[\text{light } 25^\circ C]{Cl_2} CH_3.CH_2.Cl$$

Ethane$$Ethyl chloride

$$CH_3.CH_2.CH_3 \xrightarrow[\text{light } 25^\circ C]{Cl_2} CH_3.CH_2.CH_2.Cl + CH_3.\underset{|}{C}H.CH_3$$

Propane$$n-Propyl chloride$$Cl

(45%)$$Isopropyl chloride

(55%)

The reaction with chloride takes place readily. Bromine reacts slowly to give the corresponding bromides but in different proportions:

$$CH_3.CH_3 \xrightarrow[\text{light } 127^\circ C]{Br_2} CH_3.CH_2.Br$$

$$CH_3.CH_2.CH_3 \xrightarrow[\text{light } 127^\circ C]{Br_2} CH_3.CH_2.CH_2.Br + CH_3.\underset{|}{C}H - CH_3$$

3%$$Br

97%

Thus chlorination gives mixture in which no isomer predominates. But in case of bromination, one isomer may be formed in excess yielding 97–99% of the total product.

The reaction with iodine is reversible. In this case an oxidizing agent like HNO_3 or iodic acid is used.

$$CH_4 + I_2 \longrightarrow CH_3I + HI$$

$$5HI + HIO_3 \longrightarrow 3I_2 + 3H_2O$$

Halogenation may take place until all the hydrogen atoms are replaced by halogen atoms. For example, chlorination of methane gives carbon tetrachloride as the final compound.

$$\underset{\text{Methane}}{CH_4} \xrightarrow[-HCl]{Cl_2/Sunlight} \underset{\substack{\text{Methyl} \\ \text{chloride}}}{CH_3Cl} \xrightarrow[-HCl]{Cl_2/Sunlight} \underset{\substack{\text{Methylene} \\ \text{chloride}}}{CH_2.Cl_2}$$

$$\xrightarrow[-HCl]{Cl_2/Sunlight} \underset{\text{Chloroform}}{CHCl_3} \xrightarrow[-HCl]{Cl_2/Sunlight} \underset{\substack{\text{Carbon} \\ \text{tetrachloride}}}{CCl_4}$$

Halogenation of alkanes proceeds by the free radical mechanism.

2. **Addition of hydrogen halides to alkenes:** An alkene is converted into the corresponding alkyl halides by the addition of hydrogen halides. Addition of hydrogen halides to symmetrical alkenes is as usual and primary alkyl halides are formed but the unsymmetrical alkenes react with the acid according to Markownikov's rule to produce secondary and tertiary alkyl halides. The reaction proceeds via electrophilic addition mechanism.

$$\underset{\text{Ethene}}{CH_2 = CH_2} + HX \longrightarrow \underset{\substack{\text{Primary ethyl} \\ \text{halide}}}{CH_3.CH_2.X} \qquad HX = HCl, HBr, HI$$

$$\underset{\text{Propene}}{CH_3.CH = CH_2} + HX \longrightarrow \underset{\substack{| \\ X \\ \text{Isopropyl halide}}}{CH_3.CH.CH_3}$$

$$\underset{\text{Dimethyl ethene}}{(CH_3)_2.C = CH_2} + HX \longrightarrow \underset{\text{tert-Butyl halide}}{(CH_3)_3.C - X}$$

However, if the reaction is conducted in the presence of peroxide, the condensation takes place according to anti-Markownikov's rule yielding mainly primary halides (via free-radical mechanism).

$$\underset{\text{1-Butene}}{CH_3.CH_2.CH = CH_2} + HBr \xrightarrow{\text{Peroxide}} \underset{\text{1-Bromobutane}}{CH_3.CH_2.CH_2.CH_2.Br}$$

3. **From alcohols:** Alcohols are widely used for the preparation of alkyl halides by the replacement of hydroxyl group with a halogen atom. Generally halogen acids, phosphorus halides and thionyl halides are used for this purpose.

(i) **Reaction of alcohols with halogen acids:** Halogen acids are the most common reagents used with alcohol under different reaction conditions. The reaction is carried out either by passing the dry hydrogen halide gas into the alcohol, or by heating alcohol with the concentrated aqueous acid.

$$R.OH + HX \xrightarrow{\text{Heat}} R.X + H_2O$$

Hydrogen chloride reacts with primary and secondary alcohols in the presence of zinc chloride, but tertiary alcohols and allyl alcohol readily react with aqueous concentrated hydrochloric acid without catalyst and at moderate temperatures:

$$CH_3.CH_2.CH_2.OH \xrightarrow[\text{130–150°C}]{\text{HCl + ZnCl}_2} CH_3.CH_2.CH_2.Cl$$
n-Propyl alcohol   n-Propyl chloride

$$(CH_3)_3C.OH \xrightarrow[\text{room temp.}]{\text{Conc. HCl}} (CH_3)_3C.Cl$$
tert-Butyl alcohol   tert-Butyl chloride

$$CH_2 = CH.CH_2.OH \xrightarrow[\text{100°C}]{\text{Conc. HCl}} CH_2 = CH.CH_2.Cl$$
Allyl alcohol   Allyl chloride

If concentrated sulphuric acid is added to the reaction mixture, then the formation of halides is sped up. The alkyl group in the halide does not always have the same structure as the alkyl group in the starting alcohol e.g.:

$$(CH_3)_2CH.CH.CH_3 \qquad\qquad (CH_3)_2C-CH_2.CH_3$$
$$\overset{|}{OH} \qquad\qquad\qquad\qquad\qquad \overset{|}{Cl}$$
3-Methyl-2-butanol   3-Chloro-3-methylbutane

Alkyl bromides are formed when the mixture of primary alcohol and hydrobromic acid is refluxed in the presence of concentrated sulphuric acid catalyst. Reaction of secondary and tertiary alcohols under these conditions produces alkenes by dehydration.

The alkyl iodides are generally prepared by refluxing a mixture of hydriodic acid and alcohols without the use of sulphuric acid. The order of reactivity of alcohols towards hydrogen halides is:

$$3^0 > 2^0 > 1^0 > CH_3$$

(ii) **Reaction of alcohols with phosphorus halides:** Alkyl halides are prepared from alcohols by use of phosphorus halides under reflux. For example, alkyl chlorides are prepared as follows:

$$C_2H_5.OH + PCl_5 \longrightarrow C_2H_5Cl + POCl_3 + HCl$$
Ethyl
chloride

$$3CH_3.OH + PCl_3 \longrightarrow 3CH_3.Cl + H_3PO_3$$

Similarly alkyl bromides or iodides are prepared satisfactorily by the action of phosphorus tribromide or triodide on alcohols.

$$3C_2H_5.OH + PBr_3 \longrightarrow 3C_2H_5.Br + H_3PO_3$$

$$CH_3.CH_2.CH_2.OH + PI_3 \longrightarrow CH_3CH_2.CH_2.I$$
n-Propyl alcohol   n-Propyl iodide

(iii) **Reaction of alcohols with thionyl chloride:** When alcohols are treated with thionyl chloride in the presence of pyridine, alkyl chlorides are obtained.

$$C_2H_5.OH + SOCl_2 \xrightarrow{\text{Pyridine}} CH_2.H_5.Cl + HCl + SO_2$$

In this process pure alkyl chlorides are obtained because the by-products formed are gases and thus get easily separated from the alkyl chlorides. The excess of thionyl chloride is easily removed by distillation due to its low boiling point.

(iv) **Reaction of alcohols with halogens in the presence of triphenyl phosphate:** Treatment of an alcohol with halogen in the presence of triphenyl phosphate yields the corresponding alkyl halides.

$$C_2H_5.OH + Br_2 + (C_6H_5O)_3P \longrightarrow C_2H_5.Br + (C_6H_5O)_2POBr + C_6H_5OH$$

4. **Reaction on silver salts of fatty acids with halogens:** When silver salts of fatty acids are reacted with halogens in carbon tetrachloride, alkyl halides are obtained.

$$CH_3.COOAg + Br_2 \longrightarrow CH_3.Br + CO_2 + AgBr$$

The order of formation of alkyl halides is: Primary > secondary > tertiary. Bromine gives better results than chlorine. The reaction proceeds through the following free radical mechanism:

$$R.CO_2Ag + Br_2 \longrightarrow R.COO.Br + AgBr$$

$$R.COO.Br \longrightarrow \overset{\cdot}{Br} + R\overset{\cdot}{COO} \longrightarrow \overset{\cdot}{R} + CO_2$$

$$\overset{\cdot}{R} + Br_2 \longrightarrow R.Br + \overset{\cdot}{Br}$$

$$\overset{\cdot}{R} + R.COO\,Br \longrightarrow R.Br + R\overset{\cdot}{COO}, \text{ etc.}$$

In another method alkyl bromide has been prepared by adding bromine to the solution of acid in carbon tetrachloride in the presence of an excess of red mercuric oxide.

$$2R.CO_2H + 3Br_2 + HgO \longrightarrow 2RBr + 2CO_2 + HgBr_2 + 2HBr$$

5. **Halide exchange method:** An alkyl iodide is generally prepared from the corresponding bromide or chloride by treatment with a solution of sodium iodide in acetone. Alkyl bromides are also obtained from the alkyl chlorides when they are reacted with sodium bromide.

$$R.Cl + NaBr \longrightarrow R.Br + NaCl$$

$$R.Cl + KI \longrightarrow R.I + KCl$$

$$R.Br + NaI \longrightarrow R.I + NaBr$$

General Physical Properties

1. The lower members like methyl chloride, methyl bromide and ethyl chloride are gases. Methyl iodide and some of the higher members are colourless sweet smelling liquids or solids.

2. Like alkane they are insoluble in water and soluble in organic solvents like alcohol, ether etc. Alkyl bromides and iodides are heavier than water.

3. Most of the alkyl halides burn with a green-edged flame. The boiling points increase in the order for a given alkyl group: iodide > bromide > chloride > fluoride for halogens. For isomeric halides the order of boiling points is:

Primary > Secondary > Tertiary

4. Their densities also increase with increase in atomic weight of the halogen. The order is: Fluoride < chloride < bromide < iodide for a given alkyl group and decreases with increase of the size of alkyl group.

5. Alkyl iodides liberate iodine due to decomposition in the presence of light and so they become violet or brown in colour on standing.

6. They are toxic compounds and cause general anaesthesia on inhalation in large amounts.

Table 11.1. Physical constants of alkyl halides

Name	Chloride		Bromide		Iodide	
(Alkyl group)	B.P. ^oC	Density at 20^oC	B.P. ^oC	Density at 20^oC	B.P. ^oC	Density at 20^oC
Methyl	−24	0.920	5	0.732	43	2.279
Ethyl	12.5	0.910	38	1.430	72	1.933
n-Propyl	47	0.890	71	1.335	102	1.747
n-Butyl	78.5	0.884	102	1.276	130	1.617
n-Pentyl	108	0.883	130	1.223	157	1.517
n-Hexyl	134	0.882	156	1.173	180	1.441
n-Heptyl	160	0.880	180	–	204	1.401
n-Octyl	185	0.879	202	–	222.5	–
Isopropyl	36.5	0.859	60	1.310	89.5	1.705
sec-Butyl	68	0.871	91	1.258	119	1.595
tert-Butyl	51	0.840	73	1.222	100	–
Cyclohexyl	142.5	1.000	165	–	–	–
Vinyl (Halo ethane)	−14	–	16	1.517	56	–
Allyl	45	0.938	71	1.398	103	1.848
Crotyl	84	–	–	–	132	–
Propargyl	65	–	90	1.520	115	–

General Chemical Reactions of Alkyl Halides

A halide ion is a weak base and is readily displaced by stronger bases. These bases possess an unshared pair of electrons. They react at the positive site of the molecule, i.e., they share their electrons with the nucleus. Such reagents are called nucleophilic reagents (Greek: nucleus-loving) and the reactions are referred to as **Nucleophilic substitution**.

$$R:X + :Z \longrightarrow R:Z + X^-$$
Nucleophile   Leaving group

The weakly basic halide group, which is replaced, is known as 'leaving group'. The order of ease of displacement of these groups is not fixed. It depends on the nature of the R group and on the reaction conditions. However, the order found for various alkyl halides is: iodides > bromides > chlorides > fluorides for a particular alkyl group, and tertiary > secondary > primary alkyl groups for a given halogen. The order of reactivity amongst the primary alkyl halides is $CH_3X > C_2H_5X >$ n-C_3H_7X > n-C_4H_9X, etc.

The carbon-halogen bond in alkyl halides is highly polarized covalent linkage due to the involvement of two dissimilar atoms. The halogen is more electronegative than carbon and tends to pull the electron towards itself from carbon. Due to this alkyl halides are dipolar molecules having halogen end negative and carbon as positive of the dipole. Halogen atom containing negative charge is replaced easily by the strong nucleophile like hydroxide, alkoxide, cyanide, ammonia, water, etc. Their characteristic feature is that these reagents contain an unshared pair of electrons.

The positive charge at carbon is propagated through the series of carbon atoms by inductive effect. Proton is removed usually from the β-carbon atom. This effect gives rise to **elimination reactions**. In this way alkyl halides show two types of reactions which are represented as following:

$$R.X + Nu^- \longrightarrow R - Nu + X^- \text{ (Nucleophilic substitution)}$$

$$R.X \xrightarrow[\text{Slow}]{-X^-} R^{(+)} \xrightarrow{Nu^-} R - Nu \text{ (SN}_1 \text{ reaction)}$$

$$Nu^- + R - X \xrightarrow{\text{Slow}} (\overset{\sigma-}{Nu}....R....\overset{\delta-}{X}) \rightarrow Nu - R + \overline{X} \text{ (SN}_2 \text{ reaction)}$$

$$R.CH_2.CH_2X \xrightarrow[\text{Slow}]{-X^-} R.CH_2.CH_2^{(+)} \xrightarrow[\text{Fast}]{-H^{(+)}} R.CH = CH_2 \text{ (E}_1 \text{ reaction)}$$

$$R.CH_2.CH_2X \xrightarrow[-HX]{Nu^-} RCH = CH_2 \text{ (Elimination)}$$

$$Nu^- + H - \overset{\overset{\displaystyle R}{|}}{C}H - CH_2 - X \rightarrow (Nu ...... H ...... \overset{\overset{\displaystyle R}{|}}{C}H - CH_2 ...... X^-)$$
$$\rightarrow R.CH = CH_2 + NuH + X^{(-)} \text{ (E}_2 \text{ reaction)}$$

Bond energy in alkyl halides increases with increase in dipole moment or electronegativity of the halogen. In alkyl iodides, iodine is replaced easily due to less bond energy. In the same way alkyl chlorides are less reactive due to high bond energy as shown below:

Carbon-halogen bond	C–I	C–Br	C–Cl
Bond energy (kcal/mole)	45.5	54	66.5

Alkyl groups attached to the halogen also effect the carbon halogen bond polarity. These groups exhibit + I (inductive) effect, i.e., they donate electrons to which they are attached. When the greater number of alkyl groups are attached to carbon atom, the greater will be polarity and, therefore, greater will be the reactivity, e.g.

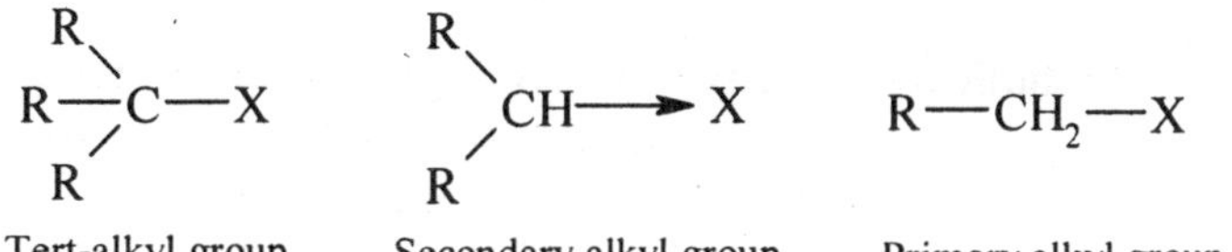

Tert-alkyl group   Secondary alkyl group   Primary alkyl group

The highest reactivity of tertiary alkyl halides is due to this effect.

The presence of bulky groups in the molecules effect the reactivity of alkyl halides due to steric hindrance. A molecule undergoes chemical reaction via a transition state. Steric hindrance is caused in the transition state due to the presence of bulky groups. Therefore, the order of reactivity is:

$$CH_3.X > C_2H_5.X > C_3H_7.X, \text{ etc.}$$

The reaction in tertiary alkyl halides is favoured by structural features stabilizing the intermediate carbonium ion. The secondary alkyl halides undergo reactions either by SN_1 or SN_2 or both of these mechanisms depending on the structure of alkyl halide and the nature of the reagents.

Both elimination and substitution reactions are brought about by basic reagents and there is always a competition between the two reactions. This competition is effected by such factors as the structure of halides or the nucleophilic reagents used.

Alkyl groups are made up of a halogen and alkyl group and, therefore, alkyl halides show the reactions of the both. Their important chemical reactions are given below:

NUCLEOPHILIC SUBSTITUTION REACTIONS:

1. **Reactions with aqueous alkalis (OH^-):** Hydrolysis of alkyl halides takes place to the corresponding alcohols by the action of moist silver oxide (AgOH) or aqueous alkalis like KOH or NaOH.

$$\underset{\text{Ethyl bromide}}{C_2H_5.Br} + NaOH \longrightarrow \underset{\text{Ethanol}}{C_3H_5.OH} + NaBr$$

2. **Reaction with dry silver oxide or alkoxide (OR^-):** Alkyl halides when allowed to react with dry silver oxide (Ag_2O) or sodium alkoxides form ethers (Williamson's synthesis).

$$2C_2H_5.Br + Ag_2O \longrightarrow \underset{\text{Diethyl ether}}{C_2H_5.O.C_2H_5} + 2AgBr$$

$$C_2H_5.I + NaOC_2H_5 \longrightarrow C_2H_5.O.C_2H_5 + NaI$$

3. **Reaction with potassium or sodium hydrosulphide (SH^-):** Treatment of alkyl halides with hydrosulphide converts them into mercaptans or thioalcohols.

$$C_2H_5.Cl + \underset{\substack{\text{Sodium} \\ \text{hydrosulphate}}}{NaSH} \longrightarrow \underset{\substack{\text{Ethyl} \\ \text{mercaptan}}}{C_2H_5.SH} + NaCl$$

4. **Reaction with potassium of sodium sulphide (S^{-2}):** Thioethers are obtained when alkyl halides react with sodium sulphide or sodium mercaptides (sodium thioalkoxide).

$$2C_2H_5.Br + Na_2S \longrightarrow C_2H_5.S.C_2H_5 + 2NaBr$$

$$C_2H_5.I + \underset{\substack{\text{Sodium} \\ \text{thiomethoxide}}}{NaS.CH_3} \longrightarrow \underset{\substack{\text{Ethyl} \\ \text{methylthioether}}}{C_2H_5.S.CH_3} + NaI$$

5. **Reaction with alcoholic potassium and silver cyanides (CN^-):** Alkyl cyanides or nitriles are formed by the treatment of alkyl halides with potassium or sodium cyanide at room temperature in a solvent that will dissolve both reactants.

$$C_2H_5.Cl + KCN \longrightarrow \underset{\text{Ethyl cyanide}}{C_2H_5.C \equiv N} + KCl$$

However, when these are heated with silver cyanide instead of potassium cyanide, alkyl isocyanides or carbylamines are obtained.

$$C_2H_5.I + AgCN \longrightarrow C_2H_5.N \equiv C + AgBr$$
Ethyl isocyanide

6. **Reaction with silver salts of carboxylic acids (RCOO⁻):** Esters are obtained when silver salts of fatty acids are heated with alkyl halides.

$$C_2H_5.I + Ag.O.OC.CH_3 \longrightarrow C_2H_5.O.CO.CH_3 + Ag.I$$
Silver acetate   Ethyl acetate

7. **Reaction with potassium and silver nitrites (NO₂):** Treatment of alkyl halides with alcoholic potassium nitrite affords alkyl nitrites whereas silver nitrite yields a nitroalkane in addition to alkyl nitrites.

$$C_2H_5.Br + KNO_2 \longrightarrow C_2H_5.O.NO + KBr$$
Ethyl nitrite

$$C_2H_5.Br + 2AgNO_2 \longrightarrow C_2H_5.O.NO + C_2H_5.NO + AgBr$$

The formation of alkyl nitrite and nitroalkane in the latter case is due to existing silver nitrite into two tautomeric form.

$$Ag-O-N=O \rightleftharpoons Ag-N\underset{O}{\overset{O}{\big<}}$$

8. **Reaction with sodium alkanides (CH $\equiv$ C⁻):** Higher alkynes are synthesized when alkyl halides are reacted with sodium alkanides in an inert solvent.

$$C_2H_5.Br + Na.C \equiv CH \longrightarrow C_2H_5.C \equiv CH + NaBr$$
Sodium acetylide   1-Butyne

9. **Reaction with alcoholic ammonia (NH₃):** Halogen is displaced by amino group when alkyl halides are reacted with alcoholic ammonia under pressure and primary amines are formed. The amines further react with alkyl halides to form quaternary ammonium salts, since amines act as nucleophilic reagents due to the presence of lone pair of electrons on nitrogen.

$$C_2H_5.Br + NH_3 \xrightarrow[-HBr]{Alcohol} C_2H_5.NH_2 \xrightarrow[-HBr]{C_2H_5Br} (C_2H_5)_2NH \xrightarrow[-HBr]{C_2H_5Br}$$

$$(C_2H_5)_3N \xrightarrow{C_2H_5.Br} (C_2H_5)_4N^+Br^-$$
Tetraethyl ammonium bromide

10. **Reaction with halides (X⁻):** Reaction of alkyl chloride with sodium bromide or iodide affords alkyl bromide or iodide. Similarly, alkyl bromide reacts with sodium or potassium iodide in acetone or methanol to form alkyl iodides.

$$C_2H_5.Cl + NaBr \xrightarrow[-NaCl]{} C_2H_5.Br \xrightarrow[-KBr]{KI} C_2H_5.I$$

11. **Reaction with sodium and zinc (Na, Zn):** When alkyl halides are heated with sodium metal in ether solution, higher alkanes are obtained (Wurtz reaction).

$$C_2H_5.I + 2Na + IC_2H_5 \rightarrow C_2H_5.C_2H_5 + 2NaI$$
n-Butane

Similarly, heating of alkyl halides with zinc in an inert solvent results in the formation of higher alkanes (Frankland's method).

$$C_2H_5.Br + Zn + Br.C_2H_5 \longrightarrow C_2H_5.C_2H_5 + ZnBr_2$$
n-Butane

12. **Reaction with malonic and acetoacetic esters $[CH(CO.O.C_2H_5)_2]^-$ $[CH_3COCH-COOC_2H_5)]^-$:** When sodium derivatives of malonic and acetoacetic esters are treated with alkyl halides, substituted esters are formed.

$$CH_2(CO.OC_2H_5)_2 \xrightarrow{NaOC_2H_5} NaCH(CO.OC_2H_5)_2 \xrightarrow{C_2H_5Br} C_2H_5.CH(CO.OC_2H_5)_2$$
Malonic ester   Sodium derivative   Ethyl malonic ester

$$CH_3CO.CH_2.CO.OC_2H_5 \xrightarrow{Na.OC_2H_5} CH_3.CO.\underset{\underset{Na}{|}}{CH}-CO-OC_2H_5 \xrightarrow[-NaBr]{C_2H_5Br} CH_3.CO.\underset{\underset{C_2H_5}{|}}{CH}.CO.OC_2H_5$$
Acetoacetic ester   Sodium derivative   Ethyl acetoacetic ester

ELIMINATION REACTIONS:

13. **Reaction with alcoholic alkalis:** Alkyl halides on boiling with alcoholic potassium hydroxide are converted into alkenes by dehydrohalogenation i.e. elimination of hydrogen halides.

$$CH_3-CH_2.Br + KOH \xrightarrow{C_2H_5.OH} CH_2=CH_2 + KBr + H_2O$$

$$CH_3.CH_2.\underset{\underset{Cl}{|}}{CH}.CH_3 + KOH \xrightarrow{C_2H_5.OH} CH_3.CH=CH.CH_3 + CH_3.CH_2CH=CH_2$$
sec-Butyl chloride   2-Butene (80%)   1-Butene (20%)

Mechanism: Hydroxide ion abstracts a hydrogen ion from carbon, simultaneously the double bond is formed when halide ion separates.

$$KOH \rightleftharpoons K^+ + OH^-$$

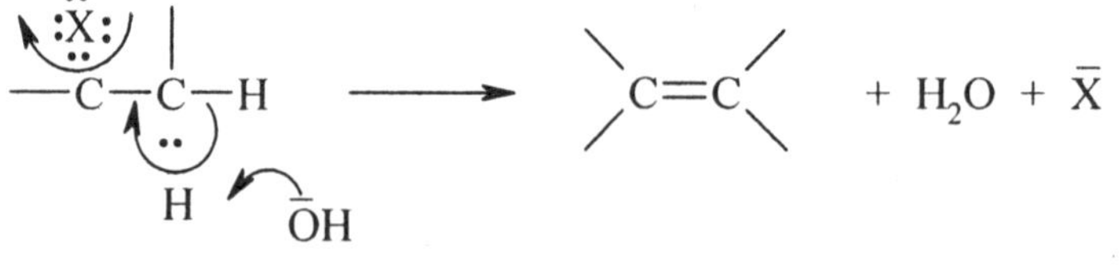

Similarly,

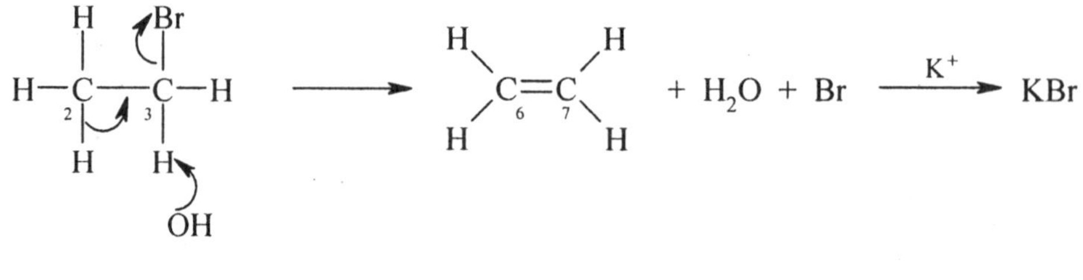

14. **Action of heat:** Heating of alkyl halides above 300°C affords the formation of alkenes by elimination of hydrogen halide.

$$CH_3.CH_2.Br \xrightarrow{300°C} CH_2 = CH_2 + HBr$$
$$\text{Ethene}$$

OTHER REACTIONS:

15. **Reduction:** Formation of alkanes takes place when alkyl halides are reduced either catalytically or chemically. Chemical reduction may be done by a variety of metal-acid combinations like tin (or zinc) and hydrochloric acid, zinc-copper couple or sodium and alcohol. Catalytic reduction is brought about by hydrogen gas and catalyst like Raney nickel, palladium, carbon, etc.

$$C_2H_5.Br + 2H \xrightarrow{Zn-HCl} C_2H_6 + HBr$$
$$C_2H_5.Cl + H_2 \xrightarrow{Ni} C_2H_6 + HCl$$

Reduction of alkyl halides is also carried out by heating them with hydriodic acid in the presence of red phosphorus.

$$C_2H_5.I + HI \xrightarrow{\Delta, P} C_2H_6 + I_2$$

16. **Reaction with magnesium:** When a solution of an alkyl halide in dry ether is allowed to react with magnesium turnings, a vigorous reaction takes place and alkyl magnesium halides, known as Grignard reagents, are obtained. The Grignard reagents are organometallic compounds having the general formula RMgX in which the carbon magnesium bond is considered to be covalent and highly polar. These reagents are useful intermediates for the synthesis of large number of organic compounds.

$$C_2H_5Br + Mg \xrightarrow{Ether} C_2H_5.MgBr$$
$$\text{Ethyl magnesium} \\ \text{bromide}$$

17. **Reaction with other metals:** Organometallic compounds may also be prepared by reacting alkyl halides with other metals. For example, treatment of alkyl halides with zinc powder yields dialkyl zinc compounds known **Frankland's reagents**, with lead-sodium alloy gives tetraalkyl lead, with lithium in inert solvents like pentane form alkyl lithium compounds and with sodium amalgam produces dialkyl mercury derivatives.

$$2C_2H_5.Br + 2Zn \xrightarrow{Ether} C_2H_5.Zn.C_2H_5 + ZnBr_2$$
$$\text{Diethyl zinc}$$

$$4C_2H_5Cl + 4Pb(Na) \longrightarrow (C_2H_5)_4PB + 4NaCl + 3Pb$$
$$\text{Lead sodium} \qquad \text{Tetraethyl lead}$$

$$C_4H_9.Br + 2Li \xrightarrow{C_5H_{12}} C_4H_9.Li + Li.Br$$
$$\text{n-Butyl} \qquad\qquad \text{n-Butyl} \\ \text{bromide} \qquad\qquad \text{lithium}$$

$$C_2H_5.Br + Hg(Na) \longrightarrow C_2H_5.Hg.C_2H_5 + NaBr$$

Sodium   Diethyl mercury
amalgam

18. **Reaction with halogens:** Further halogenation of alkyl halides takes place in the presence of sunlight and polyhalogen derivatives of alkanes are obtained. For example, chlorination of methyl chloride yields the following compounds.

$$CH_3Cl \xrightarrow[\substack{Sunlight \\ -HCl}]{Cl_2} CH_2Cl_2 \xrightarrow[\substack{Sunlight \\ -HCl}]{Cl_2} CHCl_3 \xrightarrow[\substack{Sunlight \\ -HCl}]{Cl_2} CCl_4$$

Methyl   Methylene   Chloroform   Carbon
chloride   chloride   tetrachloride

19. **Rearrangement:** When higher alkyl halides are heated either at 300°C or at a lower temperature in the presence of aluminium chloride catalyst, they undergo molecular rearrangement to yield isomeric alkyl halides. For example:

$$CH_3.CH_2.CH_2.CH_2.Cl \xrightarrow{300°C} \underset{\underset{Cl}{|}}{CH_3.CH_2.CH.CH_3.}$$

1-Chlorobutane   2-Chlorobutane

If there is no hydrogen atom on the carbon adjacent to that carbon on which a halogen is attached, then alkyl group migrates as in case of neopentyl chloride.

$$(CH_3)_3C.CH_2Cl \xrightarrow{\Delta} \underset{\underset{Cl}{|}}{(CH_3)_2.C - CH_2CH_3.}$$

Neopentyl chloride   2-Chloro-2-methylbutane

GRIGNARD REAGENTS

Victor Grignard who received Nobel Prize in 1912 for the discovery of most useful and versatile reagents, alkyl magnesium halides, began to work on organometallic compounds in 1899 with his teacher, Barbier. These compounds, known as Grignard reagents after the name of the discoverer, have the general formula R–Mg–X, where R is a hydrocarbon radical, e.g. $CH_3^-, C_2H_5^-$, $CH_2 = CH - CH_2^-$, $CH \equiv C - CH_2^-, C_6H_5^-, C_6H_5CH_2^-$, etc. and X may be Cl, Br or I. The carbon-magnesium bond present in such molecule is covalent and highly polar. However, magnesium halide bond is ionic in character.

$$R : Mg^+ X^-$$

Preparation

For the preparation of a Grignard reagent an alkyl halides is allowed to react with turnings of metallic magnesium in alcohol-free dry ether. The reaction takes place vigorously, mixture becomes cloudly and begins to boil. The metallic magnesium gradually disappears due to combination with the halide.

$$RX + Mg \xrightarrow{Ether} R.Mg.X$$

Alkyl   Magnesium   Alkyl magnesium
halide   halide or Grignard reagent

$$C_2H_5.Br + Mg \xrightarrow{Ether} C_2H_5.Mg.Br$$

Ethyl magnesium bromide

Besides diethyl ether other ethers like butyl ether, dimethyl ether of glycol (diglyme), tertiary amines and tetrahydrofuran are employed as a solvent. Various alkyl halides having the same group react with magnesium in the order iodides > bromides > chlorides, but the yields obtained are in the reverse order. For a given halogen the alkyl halides form Grignard reagent in the order $CH_3 > C_2H_5$ > C_3H_7, etc. Thus as the number of carbon atom increases, the formation of the reagent becomes difficult.

Precautions:

1. Magnesium turnings are treated with dilute acid to remove magnesium oxide deposited on the surface of the metal, washed with water, and alcohol and then dried at once.

2. Diethyl ether is washed with water to remove alcoholic impurities and then dried over anhydrous calcium chloride for few days to remove moisture. After it, the ether is purified by distilling it over metallic sodium and phosphorus pentoxide to remove the remaining alcohol and water.

3. Dried alkyl halide is used which is obtained by keeping it over anhydrous calcium chloride and then distilling over phosphorus pentoxide.

4. The apparatus should be cleaned and well dried.

For the preparation of Grignard reagents in laboratory pure and dry magnesium turnings in one atomic proportion are kept in alcohol-free dry ether (10 times that of magnesium) in a round bottom flask. A water condenser carrying a calcium chloride tube is fitted at the top as shown in Fig. 11.1. Alkyl halide (1 gm mole for every 1 gm atom of Mg) is added slowly and with stirring through the condenser after removing the $CaCl_2$ tube.

When the reagents are combined, a vigorous reaction takes place and the mixture becomes warm. Sometimes the reaction starts when the flask is warmed or few crystals of iodine or few drops of ethylene bromide are added as a catalyst. Once the reaction starts, the solution turns cloudly. It is necessary sometimes to control the reaction by cooling the flask, the reaction mixture is warmed on a steam bath to complete the reaction. It is generally unnecessary to isolate the Grignard reagents in solid state. The solution is used as such for most preparative purposes.

The formation of Grignard reagents takes place via free radial mechanism. Magnesium turnings absorb alkyl halides which then transfer an electron to halogen. The insertion of magnesium between an alkyl group and halogen gives alkyl magnesium halide.

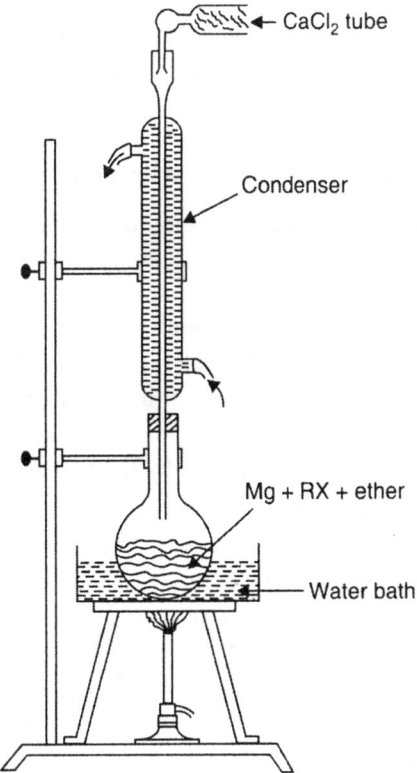

Fig. 11.1. Preparation of Grignard reagent.

The various structures of Grignard reagents suggested are given below.

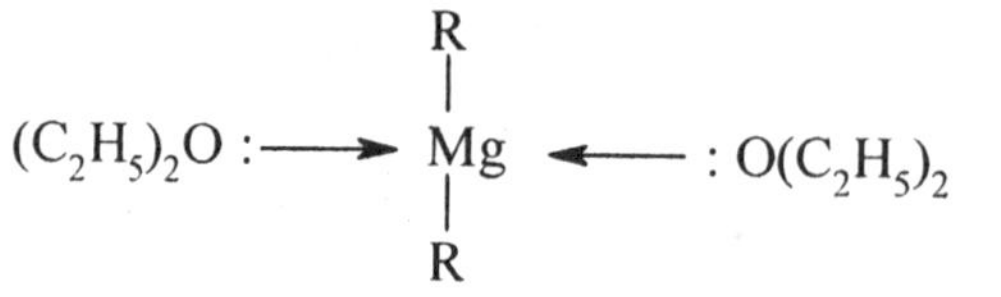

$$(C_2H_5)_2O : \longrightarrow \overset{\overset{R}{|}}{\underset{\underset{R}{|}}{Mg}} \longleftarrow : O(C_2H_5)_2 \qquad \bigg| \qquad R_2Mg.MgX_2$$

Dimer structure of Grignard

Ubbelohde's structure
(1955)

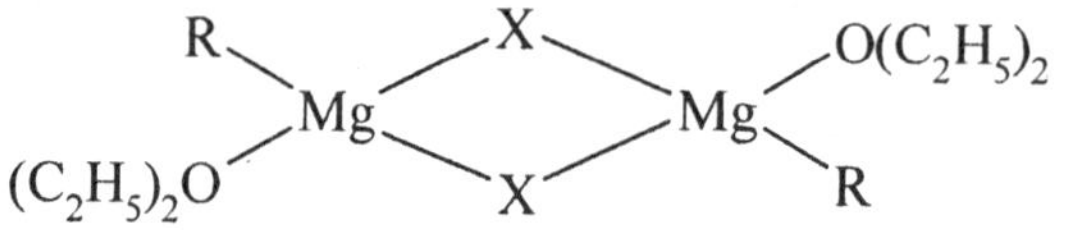

Complex structure exists in solution

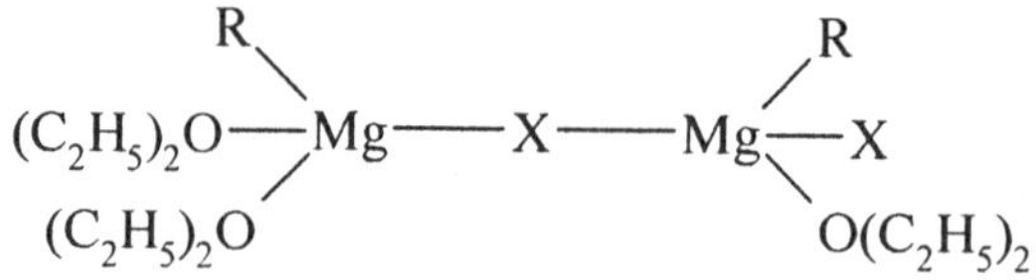

Trimer structure

In this text, Grignard reagent is represented as RMgX. In ether solutions it is accurately illustrated as $RMgX.(OC_2H_5)_2$.

General Properties and Synthetic Uses of Grignard Reagents

Grignard reagents, obtained by evaporation of ether in solid form, are colourless and hygroscopic products. They are seldom in solid form for synthetic purposes. They are unstable in moist air, react with wide variety of compounds and are used as synthetic tool in the synthesis of numerous organic compounds due to high reactivity and high selectivity. Generally they do not react with carbon-carbon double bond but react with organic compounds containing carbon-oxygen, carbon-sulphur double bonds and carbon nitrogen triple bond as well as inorganic compounds like water, CO_2, O_2, etc. An intermediate products formed due to the addition of Grignard reagents with the substrate which is decomposed by the action of acid to give the desired organic product.

Addition of the alkyl group of Grignard reagent to a compound containing a multiple-bond takes place at the less electronegative centre whereas the MgX group is added to the more electronegative atom. The reaction of Grignard reagent with compounds containing an active hydrogen atom (hydrogen atom joined to oxygen, nitrogen or sulphur) form hydrocarbons in the quantitative yield.

Some important synthetic uses of Grignard reagents are discussed below:

A. Nucleophilic Substitution Reaction

1. **Formation of hydrocarbons with active hydrogen compounds:** Compounds containing active hydrogen such as alcohol, water, ammonia, amines, enols, acetylene, etc. react with Grignard

reagents and form a hydrocarbons corresponding to the alkyl group of the reagents by double decomposition.

$$C_2H_5.MgBr + H.OH \longrightarrow C_2H_6 + Mg\big\langle{}^{Br}_{OH}$$

Ethyl magnesium bromide   Ethane

$$C_2H_5.MgCl + HO.C_2H_5 \longrightarrow C_2H_6 + Mg\big\langle{}^{Cl}_{OH}$$

Ethyl magnesium chloride   Ethanol   Ethane

$$CH_2 = CH.MgBr + H.NH_2 \longrightarrow CH_2 = CH_2 + Mg\big\langle{}^{Br}_{NH_2}$$

Vinyl magnesium chloride   Ammonia   Ethene

$$C_2H_5.MgBr + CH \equiv CH \longrightarrow C_2H_6 + HC \equiv C.MgBr$$

Ethyne

$$\downarrow C_2H_5.MgBr$$

$$BrMg.C \equiv C.MgBr + C_2H_6$$

Ethynyl bis-magnesium bromide

In these reactions the hydrocarbons are obtained in quantitative yield. This reaction is, however, used for the determination of active hydrogen atoms in a compounds containing such hydrogens as in case of OH, NH_2, SH, etc. This method of estimation is called as **Zerewitinoff active hydrogen determination**. Methyl magnesium iodide is usually employed as the Grignard reagent and methane liberated by the action of active hydrogen is measured. One molecule of methane is equivalent to one active hydrogen.

2. **Formation of hydrocarbon with halogen derivatives:** Treatment of Grignard reagent with halogen derivatives such as alkyl, alkenyl and alkynyl halides yields saturated and unsaturated hydrocarbons by double decomposition. For example:

$$C_2H_5.MgBr + Br.C_2H_5 \longrightarrow C_2H_5.C_2H_5 + MgBr_2$$

Ethyl bromide   n-Butane

$$C_2H_5.MgBr + Br.CH_2.CH = CH_2 \longrightarrow C_2H_5.CH_2CH = CH_2 + MgBr_2$$

Allyl bromide   1-Pentene

$$C_2H_5.MgI + I.CH_2.C \equiv CH \longrightarrow C_2H_5.CH_2.C \equiv CH + MgI_2$$

Propargyl iodide   1-Pentyne

Alkynes are also obtained by reacting alkynyl magnesium halide with an alkyl halide.

$$CH_3.C \equiv C.MgBr + CH_3.Br \longrightarrow CH_3.C \equiv C.CH_3 + MgBr_2$$

Propynyl magnesium bromide   2-Butyne

3. **Formation of higher ethers with monohaloethers:** Higher ethers are formed by double decomposition when Grignard reagents combine with monohaloethers.

$$C_2H_5.MgBr + Cl.CH_2.CH_2.O.CH_3 \longrightarrow C_2H_5.CH_2CH_2.O.CH_3 + Mg \begin{matrix} Cl \\ Br \end{matrix}$$

Monochloroethyl   Butyl methyl ether
methyl ether

4. **Formation of ketones with acid halides:** Under selective conditions acid halides react with Grignard reagents in equimolecular proportion to produce ketones.

$$C_2H_5.MgBr + Cl.CO.CH_3 \longrightarrow C_2H_5.CO.CH_3 + Mg \begin{matrix} Cl \\ Br \end{matrix}$$

Ethyl methyl
ketone

5. **Formation of organometallic compounds with inorganic halides:** Various organometallic compounds are synthesized by reacting Grignard reagents with inorganic halides.

$$4C_2H_5.MgBr + 2PbCl_2 \longrightarrow (C_2H_5)_4Pb + 4Mg \begin{matrix} Cl \\ Br \end{matrix} + Pb$$

Tetraethyl
lead

$$2C_2H_5.MgBr + 2HgCl \longrightarrow (C_2H_5)_2Hg + 2Mg \begin{matrix} Cl \\ Br \end{matrix}$$

Diethyl
mercury

6. **Formation of esters with chloroformic esters:** Formation of higher esters takes place when Grignard reagent is allowed to react with chloroformic ester in equimolar proportion.

$$C_2H_5.MgBr + Cl.CO.O.C_2H_5 \longrightarrow C_2H_5CO.O.C_2H_5 + Mg \begin{matrix} Br \\ Cl \end{matrix}$$

Ethyl   Ethyl propionate
chloroformate

7. **Formation of primary amines with chloramine or O-methyl hydroxylamine:** Primary amines are conveniently prepared by the action of Grignard reagent with chloramine or hydroxylamine derivatives.

$$C_2H_5.MgBr + ClNH_2 \longrightarrow C_2H_5NH_2 + Mg \begin{matrix} Br \\ Cl \end{matrix}$$

Chloramine   Ethyl amine

$$C_2H_5.MgBr + CH_3.O.NH_2 \longrightarrow C_2H_5.NH_2 + Mg(OCH_3)Cl$$

O-Methyl
hydroxylamine

8. **Formation of cyanides with cyanogen chloride:** The reaction of cyanogen chloride (1 mole) with Grignard reagent (1 mole) yields alkyl cyanides. If excess of the Grignard reagent is taken, it will combine with the cyanide formed to afford ketones and then tertiary alcohols.

$$C_2H_5.MgBr + ClCN \longrightarrow C_2H_5.CN + Mg\begin{smallmatrix} Cl \\ Br \end{smallmatrix}$$

Cyanogen Ethyl
chloride cyanide

Alkyl cyanides are also obtained when Grignard reagent is reacted with cyanogen.

$$R.MgBr + (CN)_2 \longrightarrow R.CN + Mg\begin{smallmatrix} CN \\ Br \end{smallmatrix}$$

Cyanogen

B. Nucleophilic Addition Reactions

Grignard reactions add to a compound containing a multiple bond group such as C = O, C ≡ N, C = S, N = O and S = O which are hydrolyzed to yield numerous compounds. In Grignard reagents an unsymmetrical or heterolytic cleavage of carbon-magnesium takes place to give a carbanion and cationic magnesium. The carbanion possesses an unshared pair of electrons and behaves as a nucleophile. The reactions, in which such carbanions are involved, are referred as nucleophilic addition reactions.

$$R - Mg - X \longrightarrow R\overset{..}{:}{}^- + \overset{+}{M}gX$$

The following mechanism may be demonstrated for the nucleophilic addition of Grignard reagents.

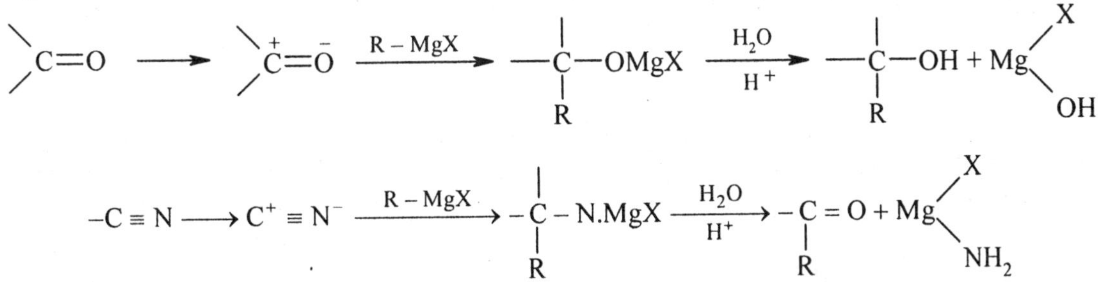

1. **Formation of alcohol with carbonyl compounds:** All types of alcohols, i.e., primary, secondary and tertiary may be prepared when Grignard reagents are allowed to react with carbonyl compounds: formaldehyde (H.CHO) yields primary alcohol; other aldehydes (R.CHO) yield secondary alcohols, and ketones (R$_2$CO) yield tertiary alcohols.

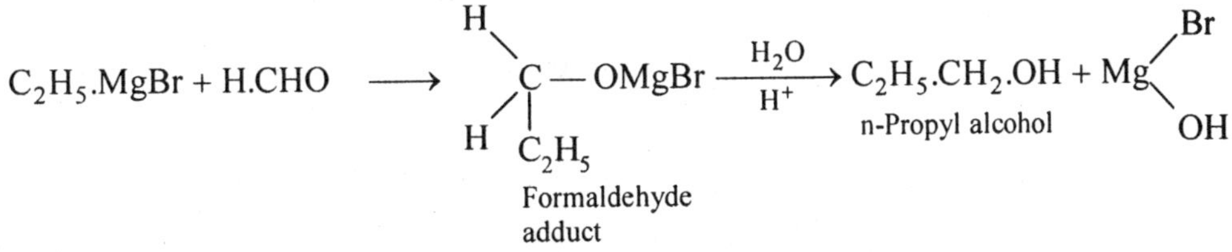

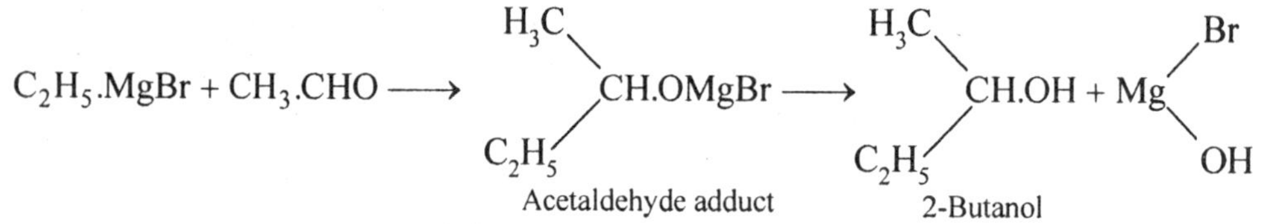

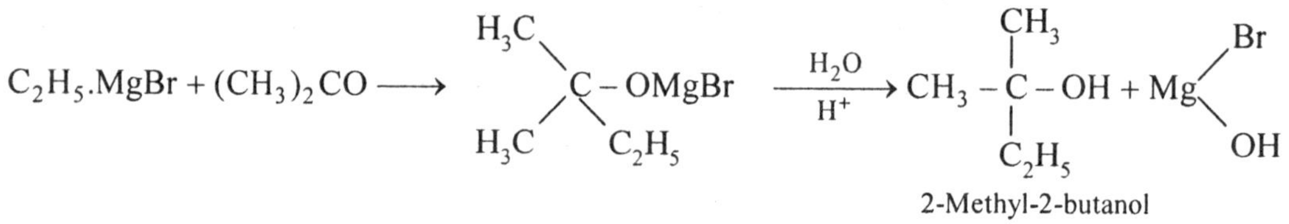

$$C_2H_5.MgBr + CH_3.CHO \longrightarrow \underset{\text{Acetaldehyde adduct}}{\overset{H_3C}{\underset{C_2H_5}{>}}CH.OMgBr} \longrightarrow \underset{\text{2-Butanol}}{\overset{H_3C}{\underset{C_2H_5}{>}}CH.OH} + Mg\overset{Br}{\underset{OH}{<}}$$

$$C_2H_5.MgBr + (CH_3)_2CO \longrightarrow \overset{H_3C}{\underset{H_3C}{>}}\underset{C_2H_5}{C} - OMgBr \xrightarrow[H^+]{H_2O} CH_3 - \underset{\underset{C_2H_5}{|}}{\overset{\overset{CH_3}{|}}{C}} - OH + Mg\overset{Br}{\underset{OH}{<}}$$

$$\text{2-Methyl-2-butanol}$$

Tertiary alcohols are also obtained when a Grignard reagent (3 molecules) is treated with ethyl carbonate (1 molecule).

$$3C_2H_5.MgBr + (C_2H_5O)_2CO \longrightarrow (C_2H_5)_3C.OMgBr + 2Mg(OC_2H_5)Br$$

$$\downarrow H_2O$$

$$(C_2H_5)_3.C.OH$$
$$\text{3-Ethyl-3-pentanol}$$

2. **Formation of primary alcohols with ethylene oxide:** Primary alcohols are also obtained when Grignard reagents are reacted with ethylene oxide, carbon-oxygen bond of ethylene oxide is broken to yield an adduct which on hydrolysis leads to the formation of the alcohol.

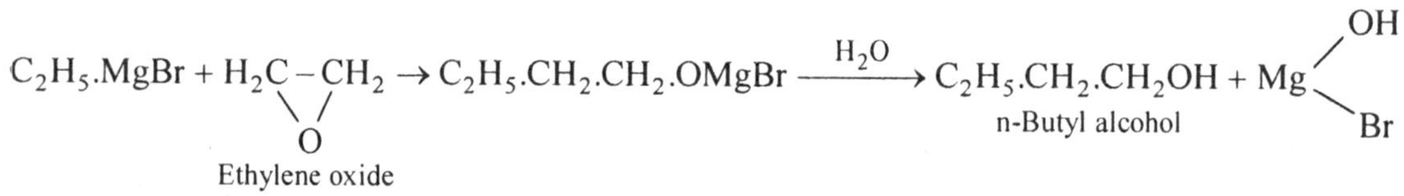

$$C_2H_5.MgBr + \underset{\underset{O}{\diagdown\diagup}}{H_2C-CH_2} \rightarrow C_2H_5.CH_2.CH_2.OMgBr \xrightarrow{H_2O} \underset{\text{n-Butyl alcohol}}{C_2H_5.CH_2.CH_2OH} + Mg\overset{OH}{\underset{Br}{<}}$$

$$\text{Ethylene oxide}$$

3. **Formation of primary alcohols with oxygen:** Grignard reagent adds to dry oxygen at −80°C to yield the condensation products, halomagnesium salt of hydroperoxide, which further reacts with excess of Grignard reagent at room temperature to form halomagnesium alcoholate.

Hydrolysis of these adducts gives alcohols as usual.

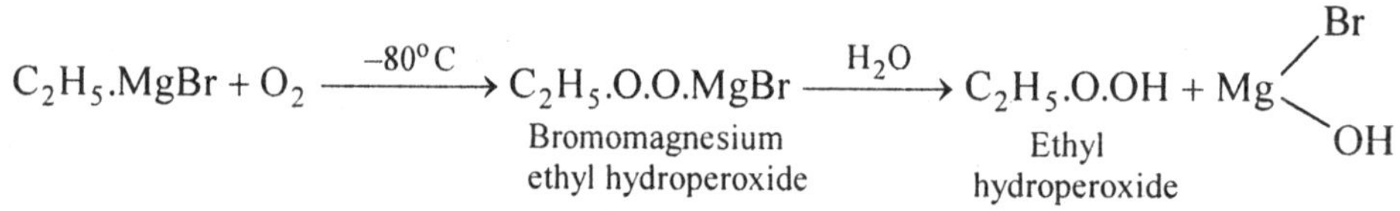

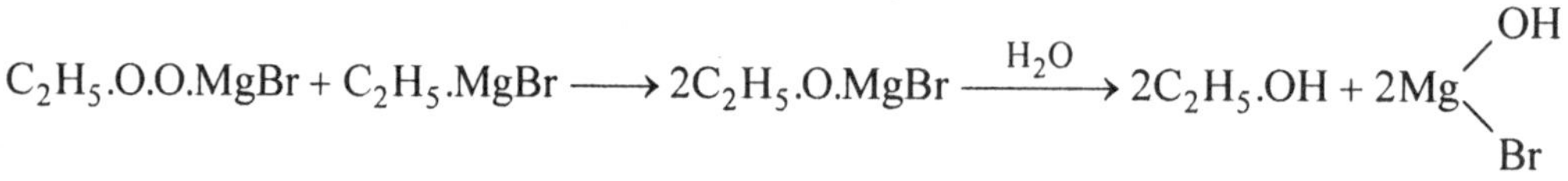

$$C_2H_5.MgBr + O_2 \xrightarrow{-80°C} \underset{\substack{\text{Bromomagnesium} \\ \text{ethyl hydroperoxide}}}{C_2H_5.O.O.MgBr} \xrightarrow{H_2O} \underset{\substack{\text{Ethyl} \\ \text{hydroperoxide}}}{C_2H_5.O.OH} + Mg\overset{Br}{\underset{OH}{<}}$$

$$C_2H_5.O.O.MgBr + C_2H_5.MgBr \longrightarrow 2C_2H_5.O.MgBr \xrightarrow{H_2O} 2C_2H_5.OH + 2Mg\overset{OH}{\underset{Br}{<}}$$

4. **Formation of carboxylic acids with carbon dioxide:** The treatment of Grignard reagent with carbon dioxide in equimolar proportion gives carboxylic acid.

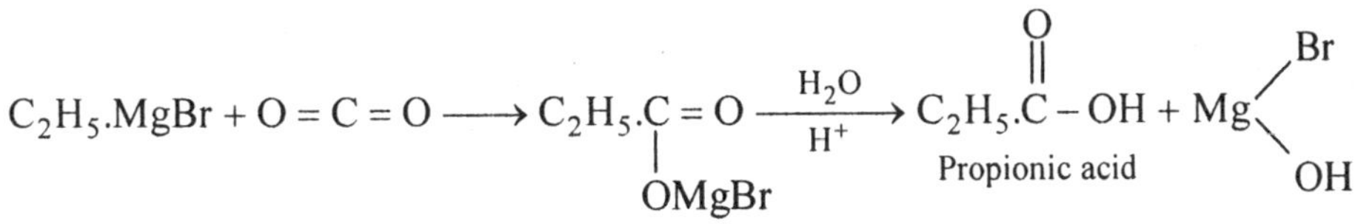

$$C_2H_5.MgBr + O = C = O \longrightarrow C_2H_5.\underset{\underset{OMgBr}{|}}{C} = O \xrightarrow[H^+]{H_2O} C_2H_5.\overset{\overset{O}{||}}{C} - OH + Mg\overset{Br}{\underset{OH}{\diagdown}}$$

Propionic acid

5. **Formation of aldehydes with formic esters:** Equimolar amounts of Grignard reagent and formic ester affords aldehydes. However, if excess of Grignard reagent is used, aldehydes further combines to produce alcohols.

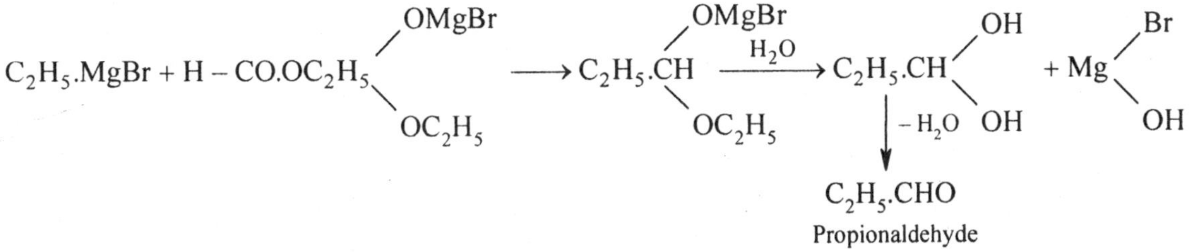

$$C_2H_5.MgBr + H - CO.OC_2H_5\overset{OMgBr}{\underset{OC_2H_5}{\diagdown}} \longrightarrow C_2H_5.CH\overset{OMgBr}{\underset{OC_2H_5}{\diagup}} \xrightarrow{H_2O} C_2H_5.CH\overset{OH}{\underset{OH}{\diagup}} + Mg\overset{Br}{\underset{OH}{\diagdown}}$$

$$\downarrow -H_2O$$

$C_2H_5.CHO$

Propionaldehyde

6. **Formation of ketones with esters other than formic esters:** Reaction of Grignard reagent with esters in equimolar amount yields ketones. Grignard reagent, if present in excess, further reacts with ketone to give tertiary alcohol.

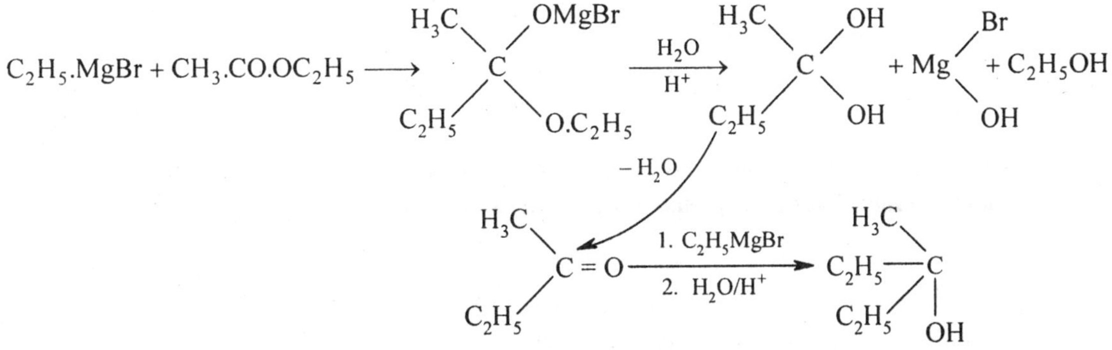

$$C_2H_5.MgBr + CH_3.CO.OC_2H_5 \longrightarrow \overset{H_3C}{\underset{C_2H_5}{\diagup}}C\overset{OMgBr}{\underset{O.C_2H_5}{\diagdown}} \xrightarrow[H^+]{H_2O} \overset{H_3C}{\underset{C_2H_5}{\diagup}}C\overset{OH}{\underset{OH}{\diagdown}} + Mg\overset{Br}{\underset{OH}{\diagdown}} + C_2H_5OH$$

$$-H_2O$$

$$\overset{H_3C}{\underset{C_2H_5}{\diagup}}C = O \xrightarrow[\text{2. } H_2O/H^+]{\text{1. } C_2H_5MgBr} \overset{H_3C}{\underset{C_2H_5}{\diagup}}\underset{\underset{OH}{|}}{C}{-}C_2H_5$$

7. **Formation of ketones from cyanides:** In another synthetic procedure of ketones equimolar amounts of Grignard reagents are allowed to react with alkyl cyanides. Excess of Grignard reagent gives tertiary alcohol as the final product.

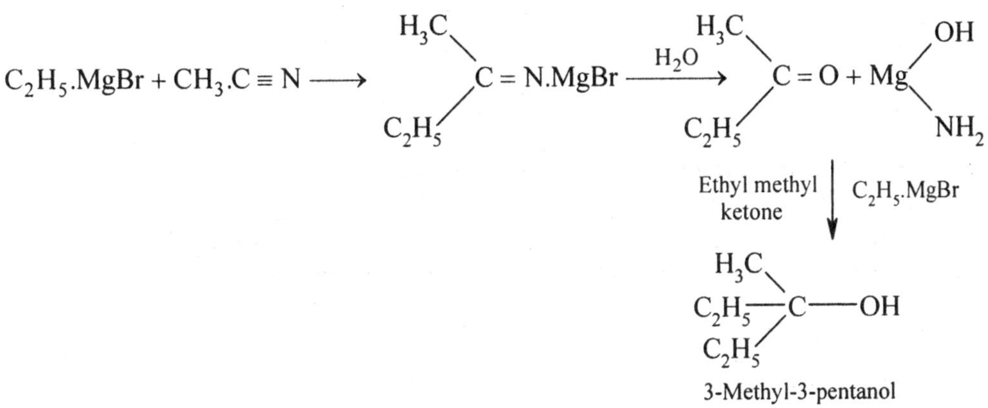

$$C_2H_5.MgBr + CH_3.C \equiv N \longrightarrow \overset{H_3C}{\underset{C_2H_5}{\diagup}}C = N.MgBr \xrightarrow{H_2O} \overset{H_3C}{\underset{C_2H_5}{\diagup}}C = O + Mg\overset{OH}{\underset{NH_2}{\diagdown}}$$

Ethyl methyl ketone $\Big| C_2H_5.MgBr$

$\downarrow$

$\overset{H_3C}{\underset{C_2H_5}{\diagup}}\underset{C_2H_5}{\overset{}{}}C{-}OH$

3-Methyl-3-pentanol

Formation of ketones also takes place by the reaction between a Grignard reagent and acyl chloride in equimolar proportion.

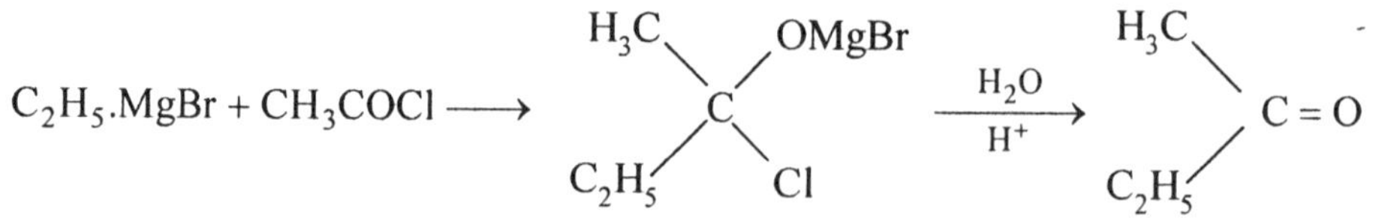

$$C_2H_5.MgBr + CH_3COCl \longrightarrow$$

$$\underset{C_2H_5}{\overset{H_3C}{>}}C\underset{Cl}{\overset{OMgBr}{<}} \xrightarrow[H^+]{H_2O} \underset{C_2H_5}{\overset{H_3C}{>}}C = O$$

Ethyl methyl ketone

8. **Formation of dithioic acids with carbon dioxide:** Likewise carbon dioxide, carbon disulphide adds to the Grignard reagents to give dithioic acids.

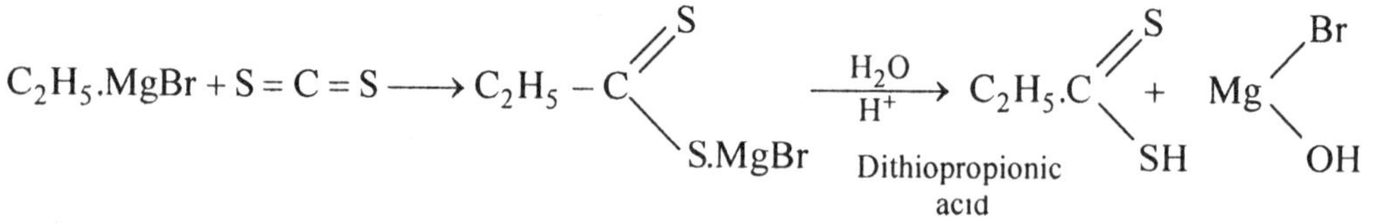

$$C_2H_5.MgBr + S = C = S \longrightarrow C_2H_5 - C\underset{S.MgBr}{\overset{S}{<}} \xrightarrow[H^+]{H_2O} C_2H_5.C\underset{SH}{\overset{S}{<}} + Mg\underset{OH}{\overset{Br}{<}}$$

Dithiopropionic acid

9. **Formation of sulphinic acids with sulphur dioxide:** Conversion of sulphur dioxide into sulphinic acid takes place when it is reacted with Grignard reagent.

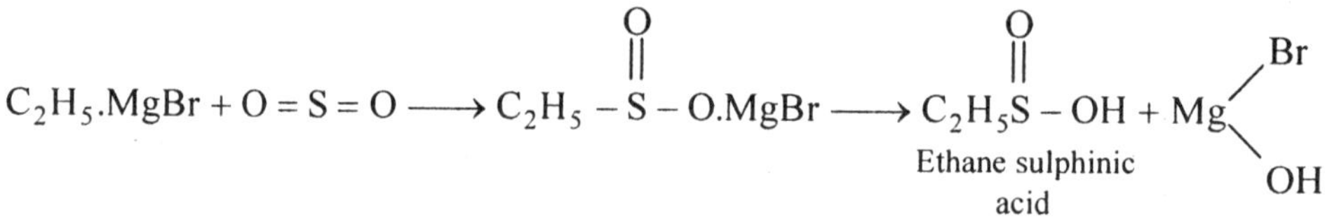

$$C_2H_5.MgBr + O = S = O \longrightarrow C_2H_5 - \overset{O}{\overset{||}{S}} - O.MgBr \longrightarrow C_2H_5\overset{O}{\overset{||}{S}} - OH + Mg\underset{OH}{\overset{Br}{<}}$$

Ethane sulphinic acid

10. **Formation of thio alcohols with sulphur:** Grignard reagents combine with sulphur to yield thioalcohols via hydrolysis of the condensed product.

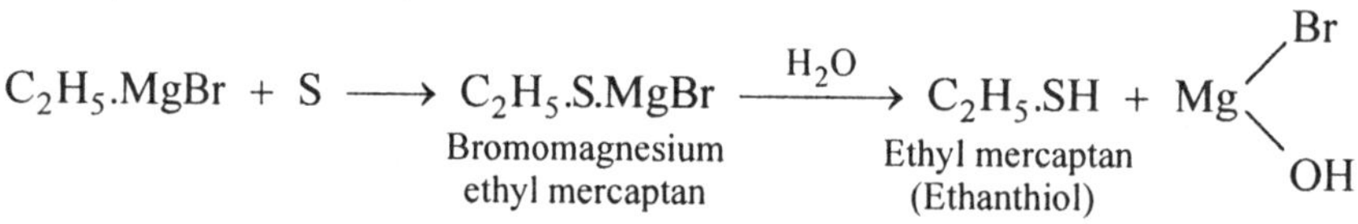

$$C_2H_5.MgBr + S \longrightarrow C_2H_5.S.MgBr \xrightarrow{H_2O} C_2H_5.SH + Mg\underset{OH}{\overset{Br}{<}}$$

Bromomagnesium   Ethyl mercaptan
ethyl mercaptan   (Ethanthiol)

11. **Formation of alkyl halides with halogens:** Reaction of halogen with Grignard reagent gives the corresponding alkyl halide.

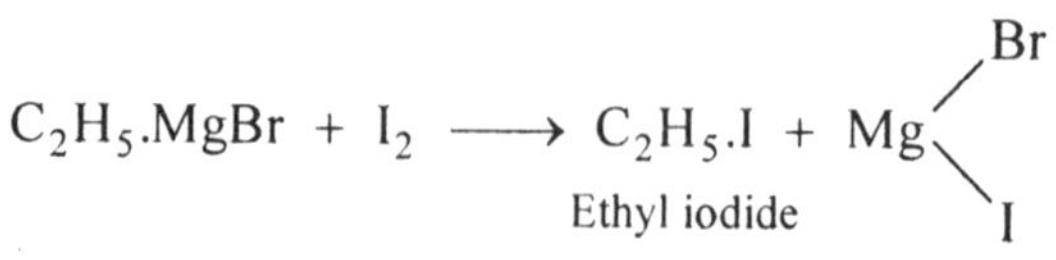

$$C_2H_5.MgBr + I_2 \longrightarrow C_2H_5.I + Mg\underset{I}{\overset{Br}{<}}$$

Ethyl iodide

12. **Formation of new Grignard reagents with alkenes:** Addition of Grignard reagents to double bond does not take place due to less reactivity of the double bond towards nucleophile R^- obtained from R.Mg.X. However, exchange of olefin with Grignard reagents takes place in the presence of titanium tetrachloride to yield new Grignard reagents.

$$R.CH = CH_2 + C_2H_5.MgBr \xrightarrow{TiCl_4} R.CH_2CH_2.MgBr + CH_2 = CH_2$$

Alkene   New Grignard reagent

OFFICIAL COMPOUNDS
CHLOROFORM

Mol. Form.: $CHCl_3$ Mol Wt.: 119.4

Chloroform is trichloromethane. It contains 1–2 per cent v/v ethyl alcohol, which is added to it.

Alcohol-free chloroform can be prepared by extracting alcohol with water, drying it over sodium sulphate and distilling it. For chromatographic work alcohol can be removed by filtering chloroform over activated aluminium oxide (Al_2O_3).

Preparation: It was in 1831 that chloroform was first prepared simultaneously by two scientists, namely Sicbig and Soubeiran independently. The method is still being used. In this, ethanol is converted into chloroform with calcium hydroxide, which acts as an oxidizing, chlorinating and hydrolyzing agent, as follows:

$$CH_3CH_2.OH + Cl_2 \xrightarrow{\text{Oxidation}} CH_3.CHO + 2HCl$$

$$3Cl_2 \downarrow \text{Chlorination}$$

$$2Cl_3CH + Ca(OOCH)_2 \xleftarrow[\text{Hydrolysis}]{Ca(OH)_2} CCl_3.CHO + 3HCl$$

1. In the laboratory, it is obtained by the action of ethyl alcohol or acetone on bleaching powder through a complicated reaction.

$$2CH_3.CH_2.OH + 8Cl_2 + Ca(OH)_2 \longrightarrow 2CHCl_3 + (H.CO.O)_2Ca + 10HCl$$

$$2CH_3.CO.CH_3 + 6Cl_2 + Ca(OH)_2 \longrightarrow 2CHCl_3 + (CH_3.CO.O)_2Ca + 6HCl$$

In this reaction bleaching powder acts as a source of chlorine and gives mild alkali calcium hydroxide. The different steps involved in the conversion of alcohol to chloroform are:

(1) Oxidation of alcohol to trichloroacetaldehyde with chlorine.

(2) Chlorination of acetaldehyde to chloral.

(3) Hydrolysis of chloral to chloroform and formic acid by free calcium hydroxide present in the bleaching powder.

(i) $CH_3.CH_2.OH + Cl_2 \longrightarrow CH_3.CHO + 2HCl$
  Ethanol   Acetaldehyde

(ii) $CH_3.CHO + 3Cl_2 \longrightarrow CCl_3.CHO + 3H_2O$
                        Chloral

(iii) $CCl_3.CHO + Ca(OH)_2 \longrightarrow 2CH.Cl_3 + (HCOO)_2Ca$

When acetone is used, its chlorination gives trichloroacetone, which on hydrolysis by calcium hydroxide gives chloroform.

(i) $CH_3.CO.CH_3 + 3Cl_2 \longrightarrow CCl_3.COCH_3 + 3HCl$
                        Trichloroacetone

(ii) $CCl_3.CO.CH_3 + Ca(OH)_2 \longrightarrow 2CHCl_3 + (CH_3.COO)_2Ca$

2. Reduction of carbon tetrachloride with iron fillings and water produces chloroform.

$$CCl_3 + 2(H) \xrightarrow{Fe/H_2O} CHCl_3 + HCl$$

3. Pure chloroform is prepared by the action of aqueous sodium hydroxide on chloral hydrate.

$$CCl_3.CH(OH)_2 + NaOH \longrightarrow CHCl_3 + H.COONa + H_2O$$
Chloral hydrate

For preparing chloroform in the laboratory one litre round-bottomed flask placed on a tripod and wire gauze is connected to a condenser. 100 g of bleaching powder is suspended in 200–300 ml of water along with 25 ml of acetone or ethyl alcohol. On heating the flask continuously, a vigorous reaction sets up and chloroform distils over. When the reaction has subsided the flask is further heated to get the distillate which is free from chloroform and collected separately (Fig. 11.2).

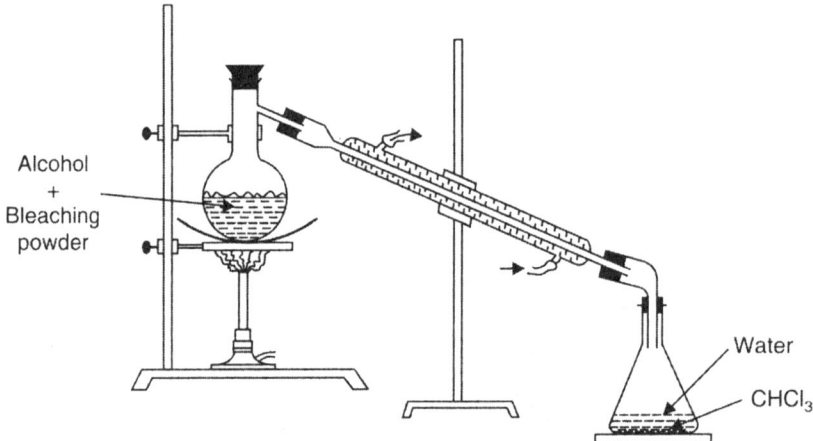

Alcohol + Bleaching powder

Water

CHCl$_3$

Fig. 11.2. Laboratory preparation of chloroform.

The heavy layer of the distillate is separated by a separating funnel and washed with dilute alkali and water successively. After drying it over anhydrous calcium chloride, it is distilled between 60–65°C for obtaining pure substance.

Physical Properties

Chloroform is a colourless, heavy, pleasant smelling, volatile liquid, b.p. 61°C, sp. gr. 1.485. It has sweet pungent taste and is insoluble in water. It is soluble in alcohol and either and is itself a good solvent for many natural products like oils and fats. It is non-inflammable but its vapours may be ignited with a green flame.

Temporary unconsciousness is caused when vapours of chloroform are inhaled.

Description: Chloroform is a colourless, volatile liquid with characteristic odour and sweet and burning taste.

Solubility: It is slightly soluble in water, freely miscible with ethyl alcohol and solvent ether.

Chemical Properties

1. **Oxidation:** In the presence of air and sunlight chloroform is oxidized slowly to form a highly poisonous substance phosgene.

$$CHCl_3 + \tfrac{1}{2}O_2 \xrightarrow{\text{Air/Sunlight}} \underset{\text{Phosgene}}{COCl_2} + HCl$$

2. **Reduction:** When chloroform is reduced with zinc and hydrogen chloride in alcohol, methylene dichloride is obtained. However, reduction with zinc and water gives methane.

$$CHCl_3 + 2(H) \xrightarrow{Zn/HCl} CH_2Cl_2 + HCl$$

$$CHCl_3 + 6(H) \xrightarrow{Zn/H_2O} CH_4 + 3HCl$$

3. **Hydrolysis:** Alkaline hydrolysis of chloroform produces an unstable compound with three –OH groups attached to the same carbon atom which loses a molecule of water to give formic acid.

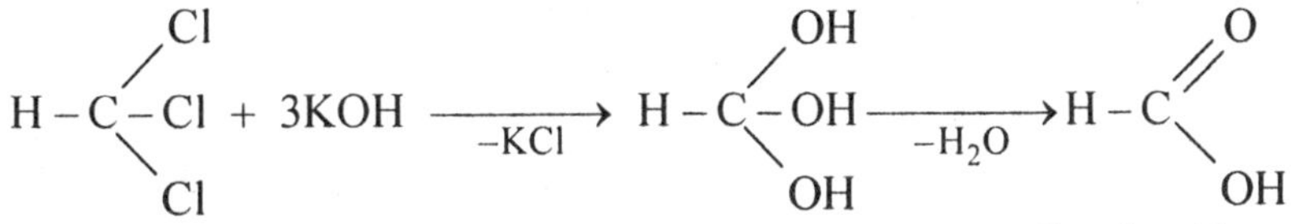

Formic acid

4. **Nitration:** When chloroform is reacted with concentrated acid, nitration takes place and it is transformed into chloropicrin or nitrochloroform.

$$CHCl_3 + \underset{\text{Nitric acid}}{HO.NO_2} \longrightarrow \underset{\text{Chloropicrin (b.p. 112°C)}}{C.Cl_3.NO_2} + H_2O$$

5. **Chlorination:** Formation of carbon tetrachloride takes place when chlorine is passed through chloroform in sunlight.

$$CHCl_3 + Cl_2 \longrightarrow CCl_4 + HCl$$

6. **Condensation with ketones:** Chloroform condenses with ketone in the presence of potassium hydroxide to yield chlorohydroxy addition products. With acetone it produces a colourless, crystalline solid chloretone (m.p. 97°C).

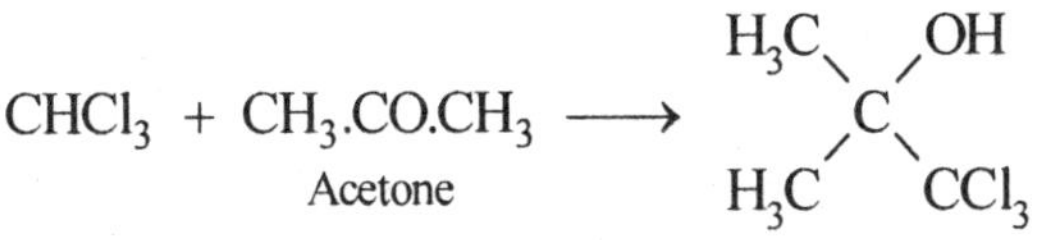

$$CHCl_3 + \underset{\text{Acetone}}{CH_3.CO.CH_3} \longrightarrow$$

Chloretone

7. **Heating with silver:** When chloroform is heated with silver powder acetylene is obtained.

$$2CHCl_3 + 6Ag \longrightarrow CH \equiv CH + 6AgCl$$

8. **Carbylamine reaction:** On heating chloroform with a primary amine and alcoholic potassium hydroxide, an unpleasant smell of carbylamine or isocyanide is obtained. The reaction is used for the detection of primary amines (isocyanide test).

$$CHCl_3 + 3KOH + C_6H_5NH_2 \longrightarrow C_6H_5NC + 3KCl + 3H_2O$$

Phenyl
isocyanide

9. **Reaction with secondary amines:** When chloroform is boiled with a secondary amine in the presence of potassium tert-butoxide, substituted formamides are formed.

$$CHCl_3 + (C_2H_5)_2NH \xrightarrow{(CH_3)_3CO.K} HCO.N(C_2H_5)_2$$

Diethylamine   N,N-Diethylformamide

10. **Reaction with phenol and alkali:** Treatment of chloroform with a solution of phenol in sodium hydroxide leads to the formation of salicylaldehyde (Reimer-Tiemann reaction).

$$C_6H_5OH + CHCl_3 + 3NaOH \longrightarrow C_6H_4 \begin{matrix} OH \\ CHO \end{matrix} + 3NaCl + H_2O$$

Salicylaldehyde

Tests for identity: (1) It is not inflammable. The vapour when introduced into a Bunsen flame produces a green colour and gives rise to noxious vapours having a characteristic odour.

(2) When 2 drops of chloroform are warmed with a drop of aniline and of solution of sodium hydroxide, phenylisocyanide is produced.

Test for purity: It is tested for Wt. per ml, Boiling range; Acidity; Chloride; Free chlorine; Aldehyde; Ethanol; Decomposition products; Foreign organic matter; Foreign chlorine compounds; Foreign odour and non-volatile matter (I.P. p. 912).

Chloroform which is required to be used as an anaesthetic has to pass strict purity tests.

Foreign organic matter is tested by shaking with concentrated sulphuric acid. In the case of anaesthetic chloroform, formaldehyde is added to the sulphuric acid.

The presence of **phosgene** in the anaesthetic chloroform is tested by adding benzidine. The chloroform should not show lemon-yellow colour or turbidity.

$$2H_2N-\langle\text{benzene}\rangle-\langle\text{benzene}\rangle-NH_2 + COCl_2 \longrightarrow (H_2N-\langle\text{benzene}\rangle-\langle\text{benzene}\rangle-NH)_2CO + 2HCl$$

Benzidine   Phosgene

When chloroform is stored in brown bottle filled upto the neck to which about 1% ethanol is added, it remains stable. Alcohol is believed to act as stabilizer and preservative. Any phosgene which ultimately results gets converted into the nonotoxic diethyl carbonate.

$$COCl_2 + 2C_2H_5OH \longrightarrow (C_2H_5.O)_2CO + 2HCl$$

All the tests for purity are detailed in I.P. to which reference may be made.

Storage: Chloroform should be preserved in a well-closed glass-stoppered bottles, protected from light.

Uses: It is used as a general anaesthetic and as a pharmaceutical aid.

As an anaesthetic, it is about five times more potent than ether. These days chloroform is seldom used as a narcotic. Its advantages are its inflammability and quick onset of narcotic action, without much sign of excitation. Its disadvantages are its toxicity which is very dangerous to heart, circulatory system, liver and kidney. Chloroform lowers the blood pressure. In concentration of 1 vol % of chloroform in the inhaling air, full narcotic action is achieved. Concentrations from 1.5 to 1.8 vol % prove lethal.

In the USA, the use of chloroform in drugs and cosmetics is lessened, as it has been found through animal experiments that chloroform acts as carcinogenic.

Preparations: (1) Chloroform spirit and (2) Chloroform water.

These preparations are official in I.P. (85) and are used as pharmaceutical aids.

ETHYL CHLORIDE
Chloroethane

Mol. Form.: $C_2H_5.Cl$ Mol. Wt.: 64.52

Ethyl chloride contains not less than the equivalent of 99.5 per cent w/w of $C_2H_5.Cl$.

Preparation: Ethyl chloride may be prepared by the action of hydrogen chloride on ethyl alcohol or on industrial methylated spirit. Industrially ethyl chloride is prepared as following:

1. By passing dry halogen chloride gas into alcohol containing anhydrous zinc chloride catalyst.

$$C_2H_5.OH + HCl \xrightarrow{ZnCl_2} C_2H_5.Cl + H_2O$$

2. By reacting hydrogen chloride with ethene in the presence of anhydrous aluminium chloride.

$$CH_2 = CH_2 + HCl \xrightarrow{AlCl_3} CH_3.CH_2.Cl + H_2O$$

Properties: It is colourless inflammable gas containing pleasant ethereal smell. It liquefies at 12^oC which has density 0.91. It burns with green and smoky flame and forms hydrogen chloride. On alkaline hydrolysis, it yields ethanol and chloride. It gives all the general chemical reactions of alkyl halides mentioned earlier.

Description: Gaseous at ordinary temperatures and pressures. It is usually compressed and supplied as a colourless, very volatile and inflammable liquid; odour pleasant and ethereal and taste burning.

Solubility: Slightly soluble in water, freely soluble in alcohol and in solvent ether.

Tests for identity: To 50 ml add solution of sodium hydroxide and heat under reflux for a few minutes, the solution obtained after hydrolysis yields the reaction characteristic of chloride. Add solution of iodine and warm, crystals of iodoform are deposited.

Distillation range: Fit a rubber bung carrying a short exit tube to dry 100 ml cylinder. The internal diameter of the tube is not less than 6 mm and the bung also carries an accurately standardised short bulb thermometer covering the range –20 to +30°C and graduated in tenths of a degree. Cover the bulb with a piece of very fine muslin, free from sizing materials and grease, in such a manner that one end hang 1 cm below the bulb. Cool the cylinder and the sample separately in ice-water and transfer 100 ml of the cooled sample to the cylinder. Insert the bung and adjust the thermometer in such a manner that the hanging end of the muslin dips into the liquid and the bulb is above the surface. Replace the ice-water around the cylinder with water between 24°C and 26°C and observe the temperature when 5 ml of sample has evaporated and when 5 ml remains. Lower the thermometer continuously to maintain its position relative to the liquid surface throughout the test. Correct the apparent temperatures by adding or subtracting $0.035^{\circ}C$ for every 1 mm the barometric pressure is below or above 760 mm respectively. The corrected distillation range temperatures so obtained are between 12.0° and $12.5^{\circ}C$.

Weight per ml: 0.918 to 0.923 g, determined by the following method. In a silvered Dewar flask having two clear side slits place a sufficient quantity and insert a specific gravity hydrometer caliberated at $15^{\circ}C$, cool to $0^{\circ}C$ and note the reading on the hydrometer.

Reaction, ionisable chloride, ethyl alcohol: To 10 ml add 10 ml of ice-cold water and allow the ethyl chloride to evaporate spontaneously, the residual liquid complies with the following tests.

Reaction: It is neutral to solution of litmus.

Ionisable chlorides: 5 ml yields no turbidity with solution of silver nitrate.

Ethyl alcohol: To 5 ml add solution of iodine and sodium carbonate; no iodoform is produced.

Other organic compounds: Evaporate 25 ml spontaneously from a shallow dish, no foreign odour is detectable at any stage of the evaporation.

Non-volatile matter: Evaporate and dry to constant weight at $105^{\circ}C$ and not more than 0.01 per cent w/w is left as residue.

Assay: Introduce quickly about 1.5 g into a tared glass ampoule provided with a long neck, containing 25 ml of 2 N alcoholic potassium hydroxide. Surround the ampoule with freezing mixture and seal the neck hermetically, weigh accurately after bringing the ampoule to room temperature, and heat in a water bath for two hours. Cool, and carefully break the neck of the ampoule and dilute the contents to 100 ml and titrate with 2 N hydrochloric acid, using solution of phenolphthalein as indicator.

Each ml of 2 N alcoholic potassium hydroxide is equivalent to 0.12904 g of C_2H_5Cl.

Storage: Ethyl chloride is preserved in a hermetically closed container, protected from light. It is stored away from fire in a cool place.

Uses: It is used as a general anaesthetic and acts as a local anaesthetic by freezing. Earlier ethyl chloride was only used as an external local anaesthetic (Freezing anaesthetic). For quite some time now, it is also used as a short narcotic and for inducing rapid anaesthesia. For full and prolonged narcotic action it cannot be used, as it has a weaker narcotic action than the chloroform. Surgical anaesthesia can be induced with 4 volume per cent of vapour. It produces liver damage and cardiac arrhythmia and it can be lethal in small doses. Externally, it is used as a spray on undamaged skin. It is also used as a solvent, refrigerant, ethylating agent and in the preparation of tetra-ethyl lead and diethyl mercury.

TETRACHLOROETHYLENE[1]

Mol. Form.: $CCl_2 : CCl_2$ Mol. Wt.: 165.8

Tetrachloroethylene contains not less than 99.0 per cent and not more than 99.5 per cent of C_2Cl_4. It contains 0.01 per cent w/w of thymol.

---

1. The compound has been deleted from I.P. 2007. However, it is retained here, being still useful and official in other official books and pharmacopoeias.

Description: It is a colourless, mobile liquid, odour characteristic, not inflammable.

Solubility: It is insoluble in water, soluble in alcohol (95 per cent), miscible with solvent ether, chloroform, benzene and with fixed and volatile oils.

Tests for identity: (1) Boil a few drops with 5 ml of 2 N sodium hydroxide for one minute, cool and add 10 ml of dilute nitric acid and 5 drops of solution of silver nitrate, a white precipitate is formed which dissolves in dilute ammonia solution.

(2) Shake 2 ml with 2 ml of solution of bromine, the brownish colour disappears within a few minutes when the solution is exposed to sunlight slowly in diffused light (distinction of chloroform from carbon tetrachloride).

Tests for purity: Wt. per ml, Boiling range; Acetylenic compounds; Thymol; Chloride; Free acid; Sulphur compounds; Free chlorine; Readily carbonisable substances; Phosgene and non-volatile matter.

Wt. per ml at 25°C is 1.597 to 1.6099 (App. I), indicating not less than 99.0 per cent and not more than 99.5 per cent of C_2Cl_4.

Boiling range: It distils within a range of 1.5 (App. II).

Acetylenic compounds: Place 5 ml in a stoppered cylinder, add 2 ml of ammonical solution of copper nitrate and 5 ml ethyl alcohol, mix, add 0.1 g of hydroxylamine hydrochloride, agitate gently and set aside in the dark for fifteen minutes, no orange-red colour is produced.

Thymol: Place 0.5 ml in a dry 25 ml stoppered cylinder (A). Dilute exactly 10 ml of a 0.193 per cent w/v solution of thymol in carbon tetrachloride to 100 ml with carbon tetrachloride and place 0.5 ml of this dilute solution in a second 25 ml stoppered cylinder (B). Dilute exactly 10 ml of the 0.193 per cent solution of thymol in carbon tetrachloride to 150 ml with carbon tetrachloride and place 0.5 ml of this diluted solution in a third 25 ml stoppered cylinder (C). To the cylinders add 5 ml of carbon tetrachloride and 5 ml of solution of titanium dioxide, shake vigorously for thirty seconds and allow to stand until the layer in cylinder (A) lies between those of the corresponding acid layers in the cylinders (B) and (C), indicating 0.008 to 0.012 per cent w/w of thymol.

Chloride: Shake 25 ml with an equal volume of water for five minutes and allow to separate quickly. To 10 ml of the aqueous layer add 5 drops of solution of silver nitrate and 1 drop of nitric acid. No turbidity is produced.

Free acid: Shake 25 ml with 25 ml of water for a few minutes, allow the liquid to separate completely and reject the lower layer, filter the aqueous liquid. To 10 ml of the filtrate add 5 drops of solution of phenol red, a yellow colour is produced which changes to red on the addition of 0.05 ml of 0.01 N sodium hydroxide.

Sulphur compounds: Boil 10 ml for fifteen minutes under a reflux condenser with 1 ml of ethyl alcohol and 3 ml of solution of potassium plumbite, and set aside for five minutes, the aqueous layer remains colourless.

Free chlorine: Shake 5 ml with a solution of 0.1 g of potassium iodide in 5 ml of water and a few drops of solution of starch for one minute, and allow the liquids to separate completely, both layers are colourless or nearly colourless.

Readily carbonisable substances: Place 20 ml in a glass-stoppered cylinder which has been previously moistened with sulphuric acid. Add 5 ml of sulphuric acid (having from 94.5 to 95.5%

of H_2SO_4), shake vigorously for five minutes and allow the two liquids to separate completely. The acid layer is colourless.

Phosgene: Place 20 ml in a glass-stoppered container and add 0.1 g of benzidine. Stopper the container and allow to stand in the dark for twenty-four hours. The solution shows no turbidity or flocculence.

Non-volatile matter: 50 ml leaves, on evaporation and drying at 105°C, not more than 0.002 g of residue.

Storage: Tetrachloroethylene should be kept in a well-closed container, protected from light.

Uses: As an anthelmintic used in the treatment of hookworm infection.

Dose: 1 to 3 ml, as a single dose.

Preparation: Tetrachloroethylene capsule.

TRICHLOROETHYLENE[2]

Mol. Form.: $CHCl : CCl_2$ Mol. Wt.: 131.4

Trichloroethylene contains not less than 99.5 per cent of C_2HCl_3. It contains 0.01 per cent w/w of thymol as a preservative. A suitable blue colour upto 0.001 per cent w/w (as per Drugs and Cosmetics Act, 1940) may also be added. Blue colour helps in identification.

Preparation: $ClCH = CCl_2$ is prepared by converting acetylene in the presence of antimony pentachloride (additive which makes the reaction less dangerous and safer) with chlorine into tetrachloroethane, which in presence of calcium hydroxide loses HCl to give $ClCH = CCl_2$.

$$HC \equiv CH + 2Cl_2 \xrightarrow{\text{SbCl}_5} Cl_2HC - CHCl_2 \xrightarrow{\text{Ca(OH)}_2} ClHC = CCl_2$$

Description: Almost insoluble in water, miscible with dehydrated ethyl alcohol, with solvent ether, with chloroform and with fixed and volatile oils.

Tests for identity: Transfer 5 ml to a glass-stoppered cylinder, add 5 ml of solution of bromine and shake the mixture vigorously at intervals of fifteen minutes, at the end of one hour a white turbid solution forms in the lower layer (chloroform and carbon tetrachloride remain clear).

Tests for purity: It is tested for Distillation range. Wt. per ml, Acidity or Alkalinity; Non-volatile matter; Chloride; Free chlorine; Phosgene; Acetylenic compounds, and Thymol.

Acidity is tested with bromocresol purple (pH range 5.2–6.8).

Chloride is tested with silver nitrate solution.

Free chlorine is tested with cadmium iodide and starch.

For details of the above tests, I.P. may be consulted. Also see Tetrachloroethylene (above).

Storage: Preserve trichloroethylene in a tight container protected from light and store in a cool place. It is slowly decomposed on exposure to bright light in the presence of air.

Labeling: The label bears, in a prominent place, the word "Warning: Trichloroethylene must not be used in any closed-rebreathing system utilising soda lime or other alkali because phosgene or other toxic products may be formed."

---

2. The compound has been deleted from I.P. 2007. It is retained here. Its anaesthetic use is now almost fully curtailed. It is still official in other official books.

Uses: It is used as a general anaesthetic and analgesic. It is often used in midwifery. It was first in 1935 that trichloroethylene was introduced as an inhalation analgesic for small surgical operations. Trichloroethylene is commonly used as a solvent. It is not inflammable.

CARBON TETRACHLORIDE

Mol. Form.: CCl_4 Mol. Wt.: 197.4

It is included in App. in I.P. and is an important agent/chemical used mainly as a solvent. It is less narcotic but more toxic than chloroform. Its use earlier as anthelmintic is no more valid. 2–5 ml of CCl_4/kg body wt. can be lethal. It is known to damage liver after it is inhaled a few times.

HALOTHANE

Mol. Form.: $CHBrCl.CF_3$ Mol. Wt.: 197.4

Halothane (Fluothane) is not official in I.P. but has been official in B.P. and U.S.P. It is 2-bromo-2-chloro-1,1,1-trifluoroethane. It was introduced in 1956 as a general anaesthetic and has an estimated potency 4 times that of ether.

It is manufactured from trichloroethylene (see above) as follows:

$$CCl_2:CHCl \xrightarrow{+\,HCl} CCl_3.CH_2Cl \xrightarrow{HF} CF_3.CH_2Cl \xrightarrow{Br_2} CF_3.CHBrCl$$

Official halothane contains 0.01 per cent w/w of thymol as a stabilizer. It is a colourless mobile volatile heavy liquid with characteristic chloroform-like odour and sweet burning taste. It is non-inflammable. It is used as a general anaesthetic. Its induction period is very rapid, being 2–10 minutes and recovery is equally quick and complete. Its side effects are comparable to chloroform and carbon tetrachloride.

Alcohols

Introduction: An alcohol is an organic compound having one or more hydroxyl (OH) functional groups. They may be considered as hydroxyl derivatives of parafinic hydrocarbons or as alkyl derivatives of water since they are obtained by substituting one or more atoms of a hydrocarbon by hydroxyl group or by replacing one hydrogen of water by an alkyl group.

$$R.H \xrightarrow[-OH]{H} R.OH \xleftarrow[-R]{H} H.OH$$

Hydrocarbon $\quad\quad\quad$ Alcohol

Classification: Alcohols are classified according to the number of hydroxyl groups present in the molecule. Thus they are mono-, di-, tri- or poly-hydric alcohols containing one, two, three or more hydroxyl groups.

$$CH_3.CH_2.OH$$

Ethyl alcohol
(Monohydric)

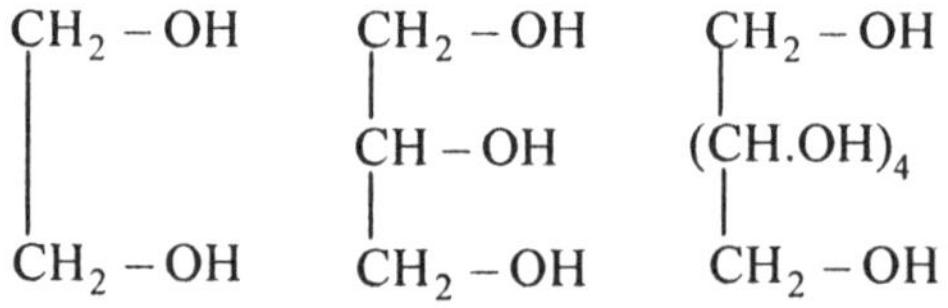

$$\begin{array}{c} CH_2 - OH \\ | \\ CH_2 - OH \end{array}$$

Ethylene glycol
(Dihydric)

$$\begin{array}{c} CH_2 - OH \\ | \\ CH - OH \\ | \\ CH_2 - OH \end{array}$$

Glycerol
(Trihydric)

$$\begin{array}{c} CH_2 - OH \\ | \\ (CH.OH)_4 \\ | \\ CH_2 - OH \end{array}$$

Sorbitol
(Polyhydric)

Monohydric alcohols are the members of a homologous series having general formula $C_nH_{2n+2}.O$. The general formula of alcohols is usually represented as $C_nH_{2n+1}.OH$ or R.OH since they have hydroxyl functional group.

On the basis of the kind of carbon atom attached to hydroxy group they may also be classified as primary, secondary and tertiary alcohols.

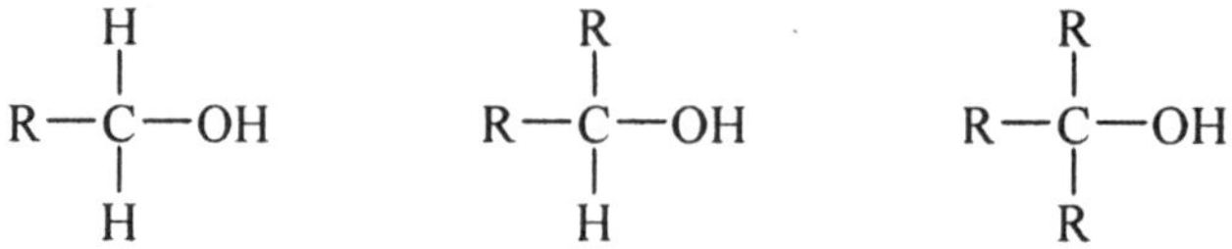

$$\begin{array}{c} H \\ | \\ R-C-OH \\ | \\ H \end{array}$$

Primary
(1°)

$$\begin{array}{c} R \\ | \\ R-C-OH \\ | \\ H \end{array}$$

Secondary
(2°)

$$\begin{array}{c} R \\ | \\ R-C-OH \\ | \\ R \end{array}$$

Tertiary
(3°)

The group attached may be open chain (alkyl alcohols), cyclic (alicyclic alcohols), unsaturated chain (alkenyl and alkynyl alcohols), groups containing a halogen atom (chlorohydrins) or an aromatic ring (aromatic alcohols). For example:

$(CH_3)_2.CH.OH$ $H_2C = CH.CH_2.OH$ Cyclohexanol (OH on cyclohexane ring) $CH_2.CH_2.OH$ with Cl $CH_2.OH$ (on benzene ring)

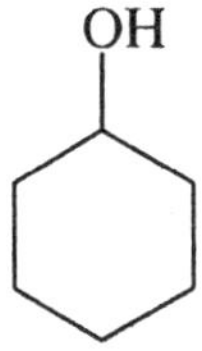

Isopropyl alcohol   Allyl alcohol   Cyclohexanol   Ethylene chlorohydrin   Benzyl alcohol

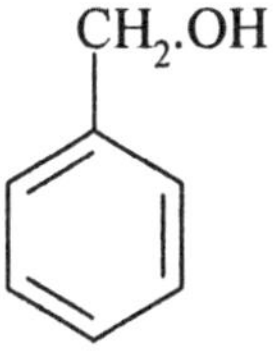

Nomenclature: The following three systems are used for naming alcohols.

Common system: The alcohols are named based on the alkyl group attached to the hydroxyl group. The common name is thus alkyl alcohol. The simplest alcohol $CH_3.OH$ is known as methyl alcohol.

Carbinol system: The simplest monohydric alcohol $CH_3.OH$ is known as carbinol. For example, $C_2H_5.OH$ is known as methyl carbinol, $C_3H_7.OH$ is known as ethyl carbinol, $C_4H_9.OH$ as propyl carbinol and so on.

IUPAC system: In this system the common name of alcohols is alkanols. The name of particular member is obtained by dropping the final 'e' of the parent alkane and adding the classes suffix 'ol'. For example, ethanol ($C_2H_5.OH$), propanol ($C_3H_7.OH$), butanol ($C_4H_9.OH$), etc.

Isomerism: The following three types of isomerism have been shown by monohydric alcohols.

Chain isomerism: Different carbon chains may be written for a given formula. For instance, $C_4H_9.OH$ shows two chain isomeric forms:

$CH_3.CH_2.CH_2.CH_2.OH$ and $\begin{array}{c} H_3C \\ \diagdown \\ CH.CH_2.OH \\ \diagup \\ H_3C \end{array}$

n-Butyl alcohol   Isobutyl alcohol

Position isomerism: For a given carbon chain different position of hydroxyl group may be represented as:

$CH_3.CH_2.CH_2.OH$ $CH_3.CH(OH).CH_3$

1-Propanol   2-Propanol

Functional isomerism: Saturated monohydric alcohols are isomeric forms with ethers. Since alcohols and ethers have different functional groups, therefore, the isomerism which is different in the functional group is called functional isomerism. For example, ethanol ($C_2H_5.OH$) and dimethyl ether ($CH_3.O.CH_3$) are the isomeric structures of the formula C_2H_6O.

Optical isomerism: Alcohols having a symmetric carbon atom such as butanol-2 show this type of isomerism:

$$\begin{array}{c} C_2H_5 \\ | \\ H-C-OH \\ | \\ CH_3 \end{array} \qquad \begin{array}{c} C_2H_5 \\ | \\ HO-C-H \\ | \\ CH_3 \end{array}$$

d-Butan-2-ol   l-Butan-2-ol

Methods of preparation: Alcohols may be prepared by any general method described below:

1. **Hydrolysis of alkyl halides:** Hydrolysis of alkyl halides with aqueous alkalis or moist silver oxide affords alcohols.

$$C_2H_5.Br + AgOH \longrightarrow C_2H_5.OH + AgBr$$

Ethyl bromide   Ethanol

2. **Hydrolysis of esters:** Esters on hydrolysis with alkalis or mineral acids yield alcohols and carboxylic acids.

$$CH_3.CO.OC_2H_5 + KOH \longrightarrow CH_3COOK + C_2H_5.OH$$

Ethyl acetate   Potassium acetate   Ethanol

In the hydrolysis of esters the cleavage of acyl-oxygen bond $\left(R.\overset{\overset{\displaystyle O}{||}}{C} - OR' \right)$ occurs.

3. **Hydration of alkenes:** Conversion of alkenes into alcohols takes place by the addition of water in the presence of alumina, manganese phosphate etc. as catalysts.

$$R.CH = CH_2 + H_2O \xrightarrow[\Delta\,/\,Press.]{Al_2O_3} R.\underset{\underset{\displaystyle OH}{|}}{CH} - CH_3$$

Acids may be used as catalysts for hydration. The addition to unsymmetrical alkenes is according to Markownikov's rule.

Indirectly, hydration of alkenes occurs when they are first reacted with concentrated sulphuric acid. The alkyl hydrogen sulphate formed is hydrolysed with water to yield alcohol.

$$CH_2 = CH_2 + H_2SO_4 \longrightarrow CH_3.CH_2.OSO_3H \longrightarrow CH_3.CH_2.OH + H_2SO_4$$

Ethene   Ethyl hydrogen sulphate   Ethanol

Alcohols can be prepared from alkenes by **hydroboration-oxidation**. With diborane alkenes undergo hydroboration to produce alkylboranes which on oxidation give alcohols. For example:

$$(BH_3)_2 + CH_2 = CH_2 \longrightarrow CH_3.CH_2.BH_2 \xrightarrow{CH_2 = CH_2} (CH_3.CH_2)_2 BH$$

Diborane   Ethyl borane   Diethyl borane

$$\xrightarrow{CH_2 = CH_2} (CH_3.CH_2)_3 B \xrightarrow[{[O]}]{H_2O_2\,/\,OH} 3CH_3.CH_2.OH + B(OH)_3$$

    Triethyl borane   Ethanol   Boric acid

4. **Hydrolysis of ethers:** Ethers are hydrolysed to alcohols when they are heated with dilute sulphuric acid.

$$C_2H_5.O.C_2H_5 \xrightarrow[H_2O]{H_2SO_4} 2C_2H_5.OH$$

Diethyl ether   Ethanol

5. **Reduction of carbonyl compounds:** Reduction of aldehydes and ketones either by catalytic hydrogenation or by chemical reduction using sodium borohydride, lithium aluminium hydride produces primary and secondary alcohols. Many catalysts like Ni, Pt, Pd, Rh, Ru, $CuCrO_4$ and $CuBaCrO_3$ are used in the hydrogenation.

$$CH_3.CHO + H_2 \xrightarrow{Ni} CH_3.CH_2.OH$$

Acetaldehyde   Ethanol
                                   (1° alcohol)

$$\begin{array}{c} H_3C \\ \diagdown \\ \diagup \quad C = O \ + H_2 \longrightarrow \\ H_3C \end{array} \qquad \begin{array}{c} H_3C \\ \diagdown \\ \quad CH.OH \\ \diagup \\ H_3C \end{array}$$

Acetone   Isopropyl alcohol
                                     (2° alcohol)

Sodium borohydride ($NaBH_4$) which is insoluble in ether but soluble in water without decomposition can be used for effecting reduction in water or methanol of aldehydes and ketones.

$$CH_3.CH = CH.CHO \xrightarrow[H^+]{NaBH_4} CH_3.CH = CH.CH_2.OH$$

Crotonaldehyde   2-Buten-1-ol

Lithium aluminium hydride reacts at room temperature with a carbonyl compound to form an alcoholate, which on hydrolysis yields the alcohol in ether:

$$CH_3.CO.CH_2.CH_3 \xrightarrow[H^+]{LiAlH_4} CH_3.\underset{\underset{OH}{|}}{CH}.CH_2.CH_3$$

Butanone   2-Butanol

Carbon-carbon double bond is not reduced by sodium borohydride. Thus unsaturated alcohols can be obtained by reduction of unsaturated carbonyl compounds by this reagent. Lithium aluminium hydride also does not reduce the double bond and along with carbonyl group this reagent reduces **carboxylic functional group** to the primary alcohol.

Carbonyl group may also be reduced by a metal-solvent combination of sodium and ethanol (Bouveault-Blanc reduction) as given hereunder:

$$CH_3.CH_2.CH_2.CHO + 2H \xrightarrow{Na/C_2H_5OH} CH_3.CH_2.CH_2.CH_2.OH$$

Butyraldehyde   1-Butanol

6. **Reduction of acids and esters:** Lithium aluminium hydride reduces acids and esters to alcohols. In acids the initial product is an alkoxide from which alcohol is achieved on hydrolysis.

$$4R.COOH + 3LiAlH_4 \longrightarrow 4H_2 + 2LiAlO_2 + (RCH_2O)_4.AlLi$$

$$\downarrow H_2O$$

$$4R.CH_2.OH$$

1° alcohol

Esters may be reduced by catalytic hydrogenation using a mixture of oxides as copper chromite ($CuO.CuCr_2O_4$) as a catalyst or chemical reduction employing metal and alcohol.

$$CH_3.(CH_2)_{10}.COOCH_3 \xrightarrow[150^\circ C,\ 5000\ lb/in^2]{H_2,\ CuO.CuCr_2O_4} CH_3.(CH_2)_{10}.CH_2.OH + CH_3OH$$

Methyl laurate   Lauryl alcohol

$$CH_3.(CH_2)_{14}.COO.C_2H_5 \xrightarrow[[H]]{NaC_2H_5.OH} CH_3.(CH_2)_{14}.CH_2.OH + C_2H_5.OH$$

Ethyl palmitate   1-Hexadecanol

7. **Aldol condensation:** Two molecules of an aldehyde or ketone containing hydrogen atom at α-carbon may combine in the presence of dilute acids or bases to form a β-hydroxy compound. This reaction is termed as aldol condensation. The products are very easily dehydrated producing carbon-carbon double bond between the α- and β-carbon atoms. Catalytic hydrogenation of these unsaturated carbonyl compounds yields the desired saturated alcohols.

$$2CH_3.CHO \xrightarrow{OH^-} \underset{\text{Aldol product}}{CH_3.\overset{\overset{\displaystyle OH}{|}}{CH}.CH_2.CHO} \xrightarrow{-H_2O} \underset{\text{Crotonaldehyde}}{CH_3.CH = CH.CHO}$$

$$\downarrow H_2,\ Ni$$

$$\underset{\text{n-Butyl alcohol}}{CH_3.CH_2.CH_2.CH_2.OH}$$

8. **From Grignard reagent:** All types of alcohols may be prepared by the action of Grignard reagent, RMgX, the most important reagent. Reaction of formaldehyde, epoxide or oxygen with alkyl magnesium halides yields primary alcohols. The essential step consists in the addition of an alkyl magnesium to the carbonyl group of the second component followed by hydrolysis.

$$\underset{\text{Formaldehyde}}{H-\overset{\overset{\displaystyle O}{\|}}{C}-H} + \underset{\substack{\text{Methyl} \\ \text{magnesium iodide}}}{CH_3.Mg.I} \longrightarrow \underset{\substack{CH_3 \\ \text{Adduct}}}{H-\overset{\overset{\displaystyle O.MgI}{|}}{\underset{\displaystyle |}{C}}-H} \xrightarrow{H_2O/H^+} \underset{\text{Ethanol}}{CH_3.CH_2.OH} + MgOHI$$

$$\underset{\text{Ethylene oxide}}{\overset{\overset{\displaystyle O}{\diagup \diagdown}}{H_2C-CH_2}} + \underset{\substack{\text{Ethyl magnesium} \\ \text{bromide}}}{C_2H_5.MgBr} \longrightarrow \underset{\text{Adduct}}{C_2H_5.CH_2.CH_2.OMgBr} \xrightarrow{H_2O/H^+} \underset{\text{n-Butanol}}{C_2H_5.CH_2.CH_2.OH} + MgBrOH$$

$$\tfrac{1}{2}O_2 + \underset{\substack{\text{Ethyl magnesium} \\ \text{iodide}}}{C_2H_5.MgI} \longrightarrow \underset{\text{Adduct}}{C_2H_5.O.MgI} \xrightarrow{H_2O/H^+} \underset{\text{Ethanol}}{C_2H_5.OH} + MgOHI$$

Secondary alcohols may be obtained by the reaction of Grignard reagent with aldehydes other than formaldehyde or with alkyl acetate.

$$\underset{\text{Acetaldehyde}}{CH_3CHO} + CH_3.MgBr \longrightarrow \underset{\text{Adduct}}{CH_3.\overset{\overset{\displaystyle CH_3}{|}}{CH}.O.MgBr} \xrightarrow{H_2O/H^+} \underset{\text{2-Propanol}}{CH_3.\overset{\overset{\displaystyle CH_3}{|}}{CH}.OH} + MgBrOH$$

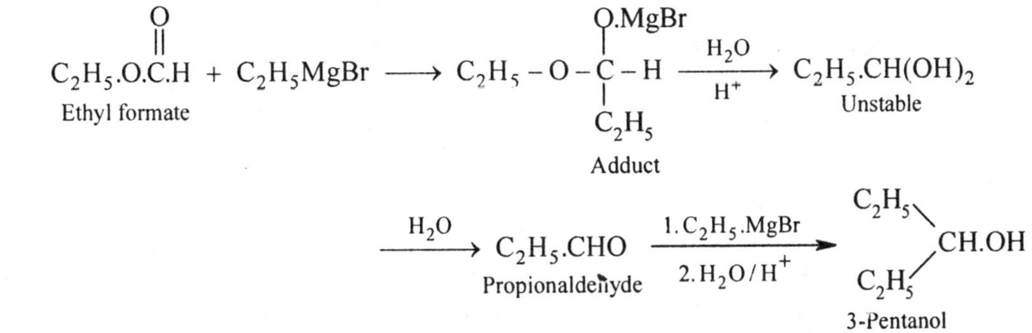

$$C_2H_5.O.\overset{\overset{\displaystyle O}{\|}}{C}.H + C_2H_5MgBr \longrightarrow C_2H_5-O-\overset{\overset{\displaystyle O.MgBr}{|}}{\underset{\underset{\displaystyle C_2H_5}{|}}{C}}-H \xrightarrow[H^+]{H_2O} C_2H_5.CH(OH)_2$$

Ethyl formate — Adduct — Unstable

$$\xrightarrow{H_2O} C_2H_5.CHO \xrightarrow[2.H_2O/H^+]{1.C_2H_5.MgBr} \begin{matrix} C_2H_5 \\ \diagdown \\ CH.OH \\ \diagup \\ C_2H_5 \end{matrix}$$

Propionaldehyde — 3-Pentanol

Treatment of Grignard reagents with ketones, esters other than formal ester or acid halides yields tertiary alcohols.

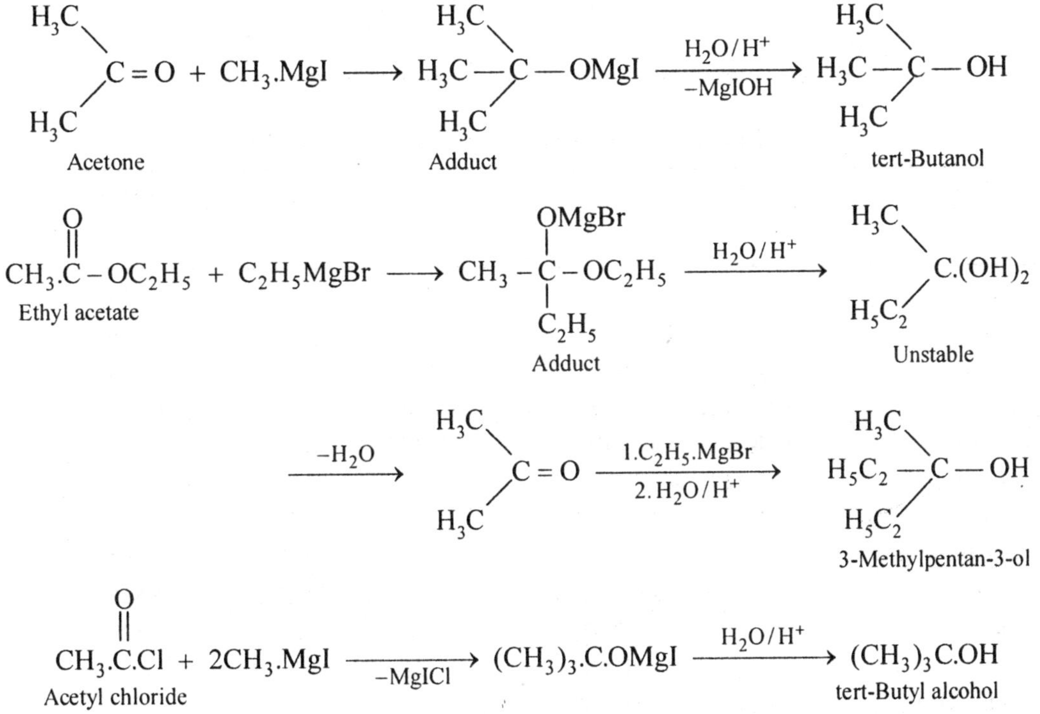

$$\begin{matrix} H_3C \\ \diagdown \\ C=O \\ \diagup \\ H_3C \end{matrix} + CH_3.MgI \longrightarrow \begin{matrix} H_3C \\ \diagdown \\ H_3C-C-OMgI \\ \diagup \\ H_3C \end{matrix} \xrightarrow[-MgIOH]{H_2O/H^+} \begin{matrix} H_3C \\ \diagdown \\ H_3C-C-OH \\ \diagup \\ H_3C \end{matrix}$$

Acetone — Adduct — tert-Butanol

$$CH_3.\overset{\overset{\displaystyle O}{\|}}{C}-OC_2H_5 + C_2H_5MgBr \longrightarrow CH_3-\overset{\overset{\displaystyle OMgBr}{|}}{\underset{\underset{\displaystyle C_2H_5}{|}}{C}}-OC_2H_5 \xrightarrow{H_2O/H^+} \begin{matrix} H_3C \\ \diagdown \\ C.(OH)_2 \\ \diagup \\ H_5C_2 \end{matrix}$$

Ethyl acetate — Adduct — Unstable

$$\xrightarrow{-H_2O} \begin{matrix} H_3C \\ \diagdown \\ C=O \\ \diagup \\ H_3C \end{matrix} \xrightarrow[2.H_2O/H^+]{1.C_2H_5.MgBr} \begin{matrix} H_3C \\ \diagdown \\ H_5C_2-C-OH \\ \diagup \\ H_5C_2 \end{matrix}$$

3-Methylpentan-3-ol

$$CH_3.\overset{\overset{\displaystyle O}{\|}}{C}.Cl + 2CH_3.MgI \xrightarrow{-MgICl} (CH_3)_3.C.OMgI \xrightarrow{H_2O/H^+} (CH_3)_3C.OH$$

Acetyl chloride — tert-Butyl alcohol

9. **From primary amines:** Primary amines except methylamine react with nitrous acid to give primary alcohols. Methylamine yields methyl nitrite in this reaction.

$$\underset{\substack{\text{Primary} \\ \text{amine}}}{R.NH_2} + HO.N=O \longrightarrow \underset{\text{Alcohol}}{R.OH} + N_2 + H_2O$$

$$\underset{\text{Methylamine}}{CH_3.NH_2} + HO.NO \longrightarrow \underset{\text{Methyl nitrite}}{CH_3.O.NO} + NH_3$$

10. **Fermentation of carbohydrates:** Carbohydrates decompose to yield alcohols in the presence of suitable microorganisms. The process is known as fermentation.

$$C_6H_{12}O_6 \xrightarrow{\text{Yeast}} 2C_2H_5.OH + 2CO_2$$

$$\underset{\text{Glucose}}{\phantom{C_6H_{12}O_6}} \qquad \underset{\text{Ethanol}}{}$$

General Physical Properties

1. The lower members are liquids with a distinctive smell and burning taste. The higher members are odourless solids.
2. The lower members are highly soluble in water but the solubility decreases with the rise of molecular weight. The solubility is due to the formation of hydrogen bonds with water molecules. In the lower alcohols the hydroxy group is the main part, whereas in higher homologues hydrocarbon character of the molecules increases due to increase in the molecular weight. So higher members are not soluble in water.

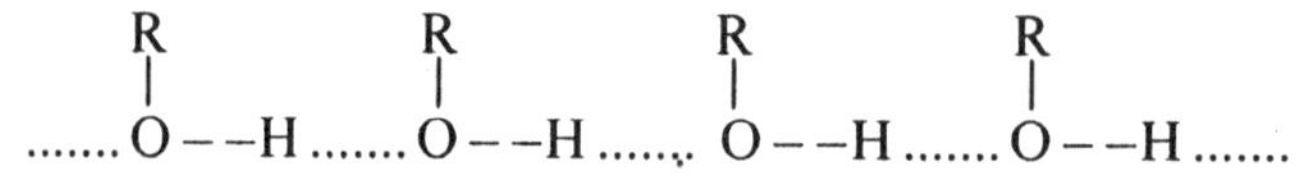

$$\begin{array}{cccc} R & R & R & R \\ | & | & | & | \\ \cdots O--H \cdots O--H \cdots, O--H \cdots O--H \cdots \end{array}$$

3. Alcohols are toxic compounds and toxic character increases with increase in molecular weight.

Table 12.1. Physical constants of monohydric alcohols

Compound	Formula	M.P. °C	B.P. °C	Density at 20°C	Solubilities g/100 g of H_2O
Methyl	$CH_3.OH$	−97	65.5	0.793	−
Ethyl	$CH_3.CH_2.OH$	−115	78.3	0.789	−
n-Propyl	$CH_3.CH_2.CH_2.OH$	−126	97	0.804	−
n-Butyl	$CH_3.(CH_2)_2.CH_2.OH$	−90	118	0.810	7.9
n-Pentyl	$CH_3.(CH_2)_3CH_2.OH$	−78.5	138	0.817	2.3
n-Hexyl	$CH_3.(CH_2)_4CH_2.OH$	−52	156.5	0.819	0.6
n-Heptyl	$CH_3.(CH_2)_5CH_2.OH$	−34	176	0.822	0.2
Cyclohexyl	$C_6H_{11}.OH$	−24	161.5	0.962	−
n-Octyl	$CH_3.(CH_2)_6.CH_2.OH$	−15	195	0.825	0.05
n-Decyl	$CH_3.(CH_2)_8.CH_2.OH$	6	228	0.829	−
n-Dodecyl (Lauryl)	$CH_3.(CH_2)_{10}.CH_2.OH$	24	−	−	−
n-Tetradecyl	$CH_3.(CH_2)_{12}.CH_2.OH$	38	−	−	−
n-Hexadecyl (Cetyl)	$CH_3.(CH_2)_{14}.CH_2.OH$	49	−	−	−
n-Octadecyl	$CH_3.(CH_2)_{16}.CH_2.OH$	58.5	−	−	−
Isopropyl	$CH_3.CH(OH).CH_3$	−86	82.5	0.789	−
Isobutyl	$(CH_3)_2CH.CH_2.OH$	−108	108	0.802	10.0
sec-Butyl	$CH_3.CH_2.CH(OH).CH_3$	−114	99.5	0.806	12.5
tert-Butyl	$(CH_3)_3.C.OH$	25.5	83	0.789	−
Isopentyl	$(CH_3)_2.CH.CH_2.CH_2.OH$	−117	132	0.813	2
Allyl	$CH_2 = CH.CH_2.OH$	−129	97	0.855	−
Crotyl	$CH_3.OH = CH.CH_2.OH$	−	118	0.853	16.6

4. The boiling and melting points of alcohols are higher than the corresponding alkanes. Their boiling and melting points and the specific gravity increase with increase in molecular weights as tabulated.

General Chemical Properties

The chemical properties of alcohols are due to the presence of hydroxyl functional group. Reaction of an alcohol can involve the breaking of either C–OH bond, with the removal of –OH group; or the O–H bond, with the removal of –H. The substitution reactions, involved by removal of –OH or –H, or the elimination reactions forming a double bond generally take place in alcohols.

(A) Reactions Involving O–H Bond Cleavage

1. **Action of metals:** Strongly electropositive metals like K, Na, Mg, Al, Zn react with alcohols to form alkoxides.

$$2C_2H_5.OH + 2Na \longrightarrow 2C_2H_5.ONa + H_2$$

Ethanol $\qquad\qquad$ Sodium ethoxide

$$6(CH_3)_2.CH.OH + 2Al \longrightarrow 2[(CH_3)_2.CO.O]_3Al + 3H_2$$

Isopropyl alcohol $\qquad\qquad$ Aluminium isopropoxide

2. **Ester formation:** The reaction between an alcohol and acid to form an ester is called as **esterification**. The reaction is reversible and is carried out in the presence of acid catalysts.

$$CH_3.COOH + HO.C_2H_5 \rightleftharpoons CH_3.CO.OC_2H_5 + H_2O$$

Acetic acid $\qquad$ Ethanol $\qquad\qquad$ Ethyl acetate

Inorganic acids except the halo acids also react with alcohols to form the inorganic esters.

$$R.OH + HO.NO_2 \rightleftharpoons R.O.NO_2 + H_2O$$

Nitric acid $\qquad\qquad$ Alkyl nitrate

$$R.OH + HO.SO_3H \underset{-H_2O}{\rightleftharpoons} R.O.SO_3H \xrightarrow[-H_2O]{R.OH} R.O.SO_2.O.R$$

Sulphuric acid $\qquad$ Alkyl hydrogen $\qquad\qquad$ Dialkyl sulphate
$\qquad\qquad\qquad\quad$ sulphate

The same catalyst H^+ ion, catalyzes the forward reaction as well as the reverse hydrolysis reaction.

The presence of bulky groups near the functional group, whether in the alcohol or in the acid, slows down esterification. The order of formation of ester is as follows:

Alcohols: Methyl alcohol > Primary > Secondary > Tertiary alcohols.

Acids: H.COOH > CH_3.COOH > R.CH_2.COOH > R_2CH.COOH > R_3C.COOH.

Mechanism:

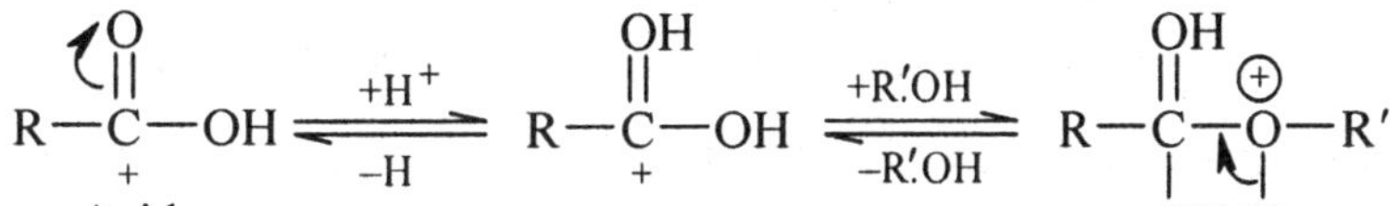

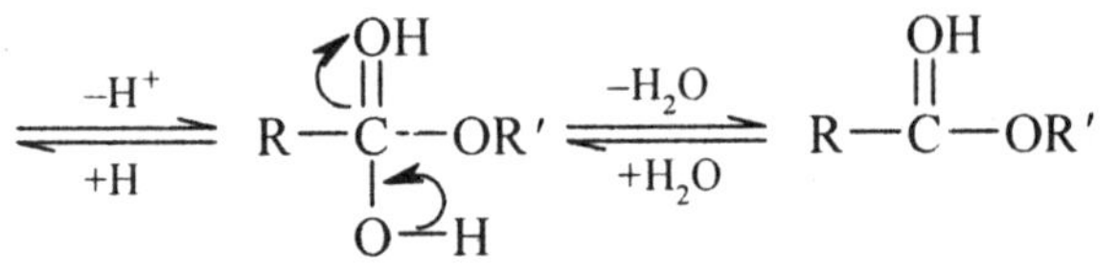

$$\xrightarrow[+H]{-H^+} \quad R-\underset{\underset{O-H}{|}}{\overset{\overset{OH}{||}}{C}}-OR' \xrightleftharpoons[+H_2O]{-H_2O} \quad R-\underset{\overset{OH}{|}}{\overset{\overset{OH}{||}}{C}}-OR'$$

Esterification also takes place when alcohols react with acid chlorides or acid anhydrides. The hydrogen atom of the hydroxyl group is replaced by an acyl group (RCO–) and the reaction is also known as acylation.

$$C_2H_5.OH + Cl.CO.CH_3 \longrightarrow C_2H_5.O.CO.CH_3 + HCl$$

Acetyl chloride   Ethyl acetate

$$C_2H_5.OH + (CH_3CO)_2O \longrightarrow C_2H_5.O.CO.CH_3 + CH_3.COOH$$

Acetic anhydride   Ethyl acetate   Acetic acid

3. **Alkylation:** Alcohols react with dialkyl sulphates to form the corresponding alkyl derivatives of ethers. Hydrogen of –OH group is replaced by an alkyl group and the reaction is used for the protection of hydroxyl group of alcohols.

$$C_2H_5.OH + (CH_3)_2SO_4 \longrightarrow C_2H_5.O.CH_3 + CH_3.HSO_4$$

Dimethyl   Ethyl methyl   Methyl hydrogen
sulphate   ether   sulphate

4. **Reaction with Grignard reagent:** The reaction of alcohols with Grignard reagents forms alkanes. For example.

$$C_2H_5.OH + CH_3.MgI \longrightarrow CH_4 + Mg(OC_2H_5)I$$

Methane

(B) Reactions Involving C–OH Bond Cleavage

In these reactions hydroxyl group of alcohols is replaced by other groups.

5. **Reaction with halo acids:** Alcohols react with hydrogen halides to yield alkyl halides and water. The reactivity of halo acids is in the order of HI > HBr > HCl. The reaction is conducted either by passing the dry halo acid gas into the alcohol or by heating the mixture of concentrated aqueous acid.

$$C_2H_5.OH + HBr \xrightarrow[\text{anhydrous}]{ZnCl_2} C_2H_5Br + H_2O$$

Ethanol   Ethyl bromide

$$CH_3.CH_2.CH_2.OH + HCl \xrightarrow[\text{Heat}]{ZnCl_2} CH_3.CH_2.CH_2.Cl + H_2O$$

n-Propyl alcohol   n-Propyl chloride

$$(CH_3)_3C.OH \xrightarrow[\text{Room temperature}]{\text{Conc. HCl}} (CH_3)_3C-Cl$$

tert-Butyl alcohol   tert-Butyl chloride

Hydrochloric acid is the least reactive and requires the presence of zinc chloride. The order of reactivity of alcohols towards HX is allyl, benzyl > 3° > 2° > 1° > CH_3.

6. **Dehydration:** Dehydration of alcohols, i.e. elimination of a molecule of water is a valuable path to alkenes and is carried out in the presence of acid catalysts at high temperature or by passing the vapours over heated alumina.

$$CH_3.CH_2.OH \xrightarrow[\text{or } Al_2O_3/\text{heat}]{H_2SO_4/\text{heat}} CH_2 = CH_2 + H_2O$$

Ethanol   Alkene

The ease of dehydration of alcohols is $3^\circ > 2^\circ > 1^\circ$ and the difference in reactivity is illustrated in the following examples:

$$CH_3.CH_2.CH_2.CH_2.OH \xrightarrow[140^\circ]{7.5\% H_2SO_4} CH_3.CH = CH.CH_3$$

n-Butyl alcohol   2-Butene (main product)

$$CH_3.CH_2.CH(OH).CH_3 \xrightarrow[100^\circ C]{60\% H_2SO_4} CH_3.CH = CH.CH_3$$

sec-Butanol   2-Butene (main product)

$$(CH_3)_3.C - OH \xrightarrow[85-90^\circ C]{20\% H_2SO_4} \begin{matrix} H_3C \\ \diagdown \\ \diagup \\ H_3C \end{matrix} C = CH_2$$

tert-Butyl alcohol   Isobutylene

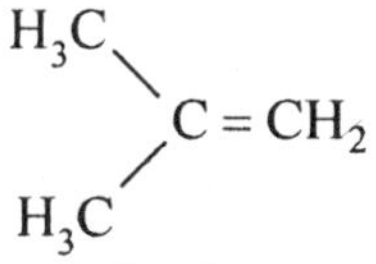

The mechanism of dehydration (e.g., in case of ethanol) is given below:

$$CH_3.CH_2.OH + H^+ \rightleftharpoons CH_3.CH_2.O^+H_2$$

Ethanol   Protonated alcohol

$$CH_3.CH_2 : \overset{+}{O}H_2 \rightleftharpoons CH_3.\overset{+}{C}H_2 + H_2O$$

Carbonium ion

$$H - \overset{H}{\underset{H}{C}} : \overset{+}{C} - H \rightleftharpoons H - \overset{|}{\underset{H}{C}} = \overset{|}{\underset{H}{C}} - H + H^+$$

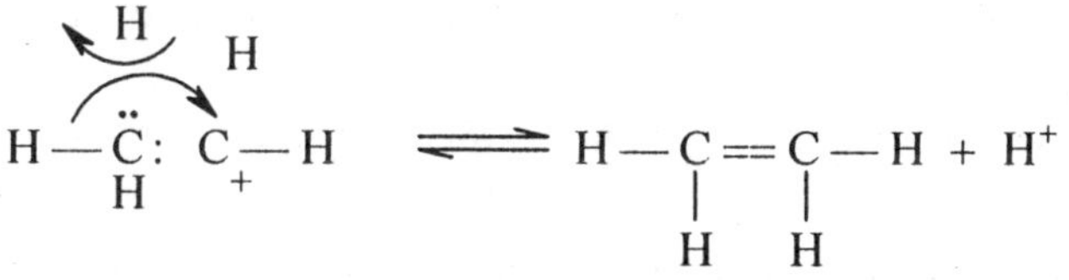

Ethene

7. **Reaction with phosphorus halides:** Alcohols give alkyl halides when they are treated with phosphorus halides. For instance:

$$3 C_2H_5.OH + POCl_3 \longrightarrow 3 C_2H_5.Cl + H_3PO_4$$

$$C_2H_5.OH + PCl_5 \longrightarrow C_2H_5.Cl + POCl_3 + HCl$$

Ethyl chloride

8. **Reaction with thionyl halides:** Alkyl halides are also prepared by treating alcohols with thionyl halides in pyridine.

$$C_2H_5.OH + SOCl_2/SOBr_2 \xrightarrow[-HCl/HBr]{Pyridine} C_2H_5.Cl/C_2H_5.Br + SO_2$$

9. **Action with ammonia:** Alcohols and ammonia form a mixture of primary, secondary and tertiary amines when their vapours are passed over heated alumina at high temperature.

$$C_2H_5.OH + NH_3 \xrightarrow[-H_2O]{Al_2O_3/360^0} C_2H_5.NH_2 \xrightarrow[-H_2O/360^0]{C_2H_5.OH/Al_2O_3} (C_2H_5)_2.NH$$

Ethyl amine   Diethyl amine

$$\xrightarrow[-H_2O/360^0]{C_2H_5.OH/Al_2O_3} (C_2H_5)_3.N + H_2O$$

Triethyl amine

(C) Other Reactions

10. **Dehydrogenation:** Dehydrogenation of primary and secondary alcohols, by passing their vapours over faintly reduced copper at 300°C, yields aldehydes and ketones respectively.

$$R.CH_2OH \xrightarrow{Cu/300^0C} R.CHO + H_2$$

Primary alcohol   Aldehyde

$$R_2.CH.OH \xrightarrow{Cu/300^0C} R.CO.R + H_2$$

Secondary alcohol   Ketone

$$R_2.C.OH \atop | \atop CH_2.R \quad \xrightarrow{Cu/300^0C} R_2.C = CH.R + H_2O$$

Alkene

Tertiary

Alcohol can be differentiated by this procedure.

11. **Oxidation:** Under different oxidising conditions, different alcohols afford different products.

(i) Primary alcohols are highly susceptible to oxidation and can be oxidized easily to aldehydes and then to carboxylic acids in the presence of aqueous $KMnO_4$.

$$CH_3.CH_2.OH \xrightarrow[KMnO_4]{[O]} CH_3.CHO \xrightarrow[KMnO_4]{[O]} CH_3.COOH$$

Ethanol   Acetaldehyde   Acetic acid

Both aldehyde and acid contain the same number of carbon atoms as the original alcohol.

(ii) Secondary alcohols are oxidized to ketones either by potassium permanganate or by chromic acid in aqueous glacial acetic acid or in pyridine. On further oxidation carboxylic acids are formed.

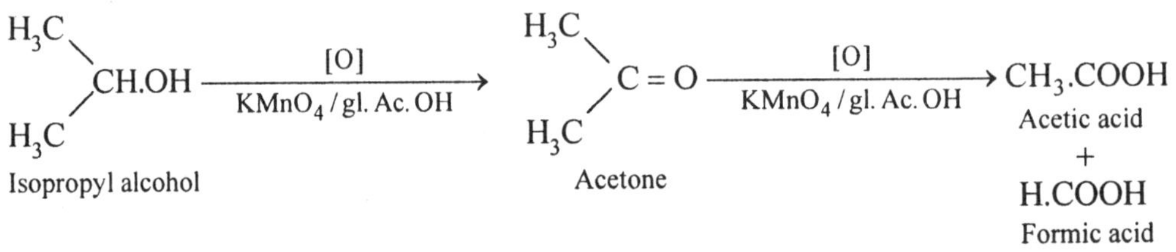

$$\begin{matrix} H_3C \\ \diagdown \\ \diagup \\ H_3C \end{matrix} CH.OH \xrightarrow[KMnO_4/gl. Ac. OH]{[O]} \begin{matrix} H_3C \\ \diagdown \\ \diagup \\ H_3C \end{matrix} C=O \xrightarrow[KMnO_4/gl. Ac. OH]{[O]} \begin{matrix} CH_3.COOH \\ \text{Acetic acid} \\ + \\ H.COOH \end{matrix}$$

Isopropyl alcohol   Acetone   Formic acid

The ketone has the same number of carbon atoms as the original alcohol whereas each acid contains fewer carbon atoms than the starting alcohols.

(iii) The tertiary alcohols are not oxidized at all under neutral or alkaline conditions, but are readily oxidized by acid oxidizing agents to a mixture of aldehydes and ketones and then into acids, each having the fewer carbon atoms than the original alcohols.

$$(CH_3)_3.OH \xrightarrow{[O]} (CH_3)_2.CO + H.CHO \xrightarrow{[O]} CH_3.COOH + H.COOH$$

tert Butyl alcohol   Acetone   Formaldehyde

This procedure is also employed for differentiating primary, secondary and tertiary alcohols.

12. **Reaction with halogens:** Alcohols are first oxidized to carbonyl compounds with halogens and then halogenation of the oxidized product takes place. Thus:

$$CH_3.CH_2.OH \xrightarrow[Cl_2]{[O]} CH_3.CHO \xrightarrow{Cl_2} CCl_3.CHO$$

Ethanol   Acetaldehyde   Trichloro acetaldehyde

$$CH_3.CH(OH)CH_3 \xrightarrow[Br_2]{[O]} CH_3.CO.CH_3 \xrightarrow{Br_2} CBr_3.CO.CH_3$$

Isopropyl alcohol   Acetone   Tribromoacetone

FERMENTATION

Fermentation is the oldest and most important method for the manufacture of alcohols, beer, wine, brandy etc. Fermentation is the slow decomposition of complex organic compounds into simpler molecules in the presence of enzymes, e.g. souring of milk, putrefaction of meat or food, formation of vinegar or wine, etc.

Pasteur (1860) showed that fermentation is a physiological process carried out by living micro-organism like bacteria or yeast. Oxygen and energy are required for their growth. They utilize energy and oxygen liberated during decomposition and breathe out carbon dioxide. Liebig pointed out that fermentation is purely a chemical change. However, Buchner (1897) suggested that the fermentation is brought about by enzymes which are complex nitrogenous substances present in the living organisms and not by the living organisms themselves. Their action may be linked to that of inorganic catalysts.

Fermentation is carried out generally at 25–35°C in the presence of air or oxygen and certain inorganic salt solutions like ammonium sulphate, ammonium phosphate, etc. The solution used for fermentation should be dilute (8–10%), as the living organisms become inactive at high concentration.

The enzymes or biocatalysts are non-living, complex, soluble, proteinous substances. They catalyze the reactions taking place in living organisms. They occur in plant cells and are responsible for bringing about most of the chemical changes associated with animal and plant life. They contain high molecular weight and are highly selective and specific, i.e., a particular enzyme can bring about one particular type of reaction. They are nitrogenous complexes and living organic compounds and bring about the conversion of highly complex organic compounds into simpler ones. A small quantity of an enzyme can bring about chemical change in a large amount of material.

Substances like boric acid, sodium benzoate, hydrochloric acid and mercuric salts destroy the enzymes. Some substances increase their activity which are known as co-enzymes.

Enzymes can bring about the hydrolysis, oxidation, and reduction. They are described as hydrolyses, oxidases, reductases according to the type of reaction in which they are involved. The names of all specific enzymes end in 'ase'. This is added at the end of that substance of substrate upon which they act; thus maltase hydrolyzes maltose, amylase hydrolyzes starch (Latin amylym = starch), and so on. Yeast is a unicellular plant which contains three important enzymes: maltase which ferments maltose into glucose; invertase or sucrase which converts sucrose into a mixture of glucose and fructose; and zymase which converts glucose and fructose into alcohol and carbon dioxide.

Alcohol is usually manufactured by the fermentation of sugars such as sucrose and glucose in the presence of yeast. In this process only two enzymes, invertase and zymase take part in the conversion.

$$\underset{\text{Sucrose}}{C_{12}H_{22}O_{11}} + H_2O \xrightarrow[\text{(Yeast)}]{\text{Invertase}} \underset{\text{Glucose}}{C_6H_{12}O_6} + \underset{\text{Fructose}}{C_6H_{12}O_6} \xrightarrow[\text{(Yeast)}]{\text{Zymase}} \underset{\text{Ethanol}}{2C_2H_5.OH} + 2CO_2$$

Manufacture of ethyl alcohol

Alcohol occurs in wine, bears and spirits and is obtained on technical scale by the fermentation of sugars, such as cane sugar (sucrose) and glucose in the presence of yeast. The sugars are obtained either from fruit juice and molasses or by the hydrolysis of starchy materials like potatoes, barley, maize and cellulosic saw dust.

(I) **From molasses:** Ethyl alcohol is prepared on large scale from molasses which is a dark brown mother liquor left after the crystallization of cane sugar from the concentrated juice. A 50% mixture of sucrose, glucose and fructose is present in it. The separation of these sugars is uneconomical and, therefore, molasses is the cheap raw material for the alcohol industry in sugar producing countries like India. The following steps are involved in the manufacture of alcohol from molasses:

(i) **Dilution:** The high percentage of sugars in molasses is not suitable for the fermentation reaction. Therefore, water is added to molasses to obtain the sugars in 8–10 per cent. The solution is acidified to a suitable pH with dilute sulphuric acid to check the bacterial growth.

(ii) **Fermentation:** The dilute solution is then taken in a fermentation tank. A small quantity of some nutrients like ammonium sulphate and ammonium phosphate are added alongwith some yeast. The mixture is kept at 25–30°C for 2–3 days. The fermentation takes place and the enzymes invertase and zymase present in yeast cell decompose sugars into ethyl alcohol. Carbon dioxide gas is evolved during the process. Then the yeast is filtered off and the filtrate containing about 6–10% ethanol is subjected to distillation (see reaction above).

(iii) **Distillation:** The fermented liquor known as wash or wort, is a mixture of alcohol, acetaldehyde, glycerol, higher alcohols and argol (potassium hydrogen tartrate). A specially designed continuous plant known as Coffey still is employed for its distillation. The plant consists of two fractionating columns, analyzer and rectifier, possessing a number of perforated plates with valves opening upwards (Fig. 12.1).

The wash is heated and flowed down the analyzer from the top. The steam is passed up the analyzer which takes away the alcohol vapours from the down coming dilute alcohol to the rectifier from the top end of the analyzer. Steam is condensed in the analyzer and the alcohol vapours leave the rectifier at the top. The distillate contains only 90 per cent alcohol which is subjected to further distillation known as rectification. The residue left in the still is used as cattle feed.

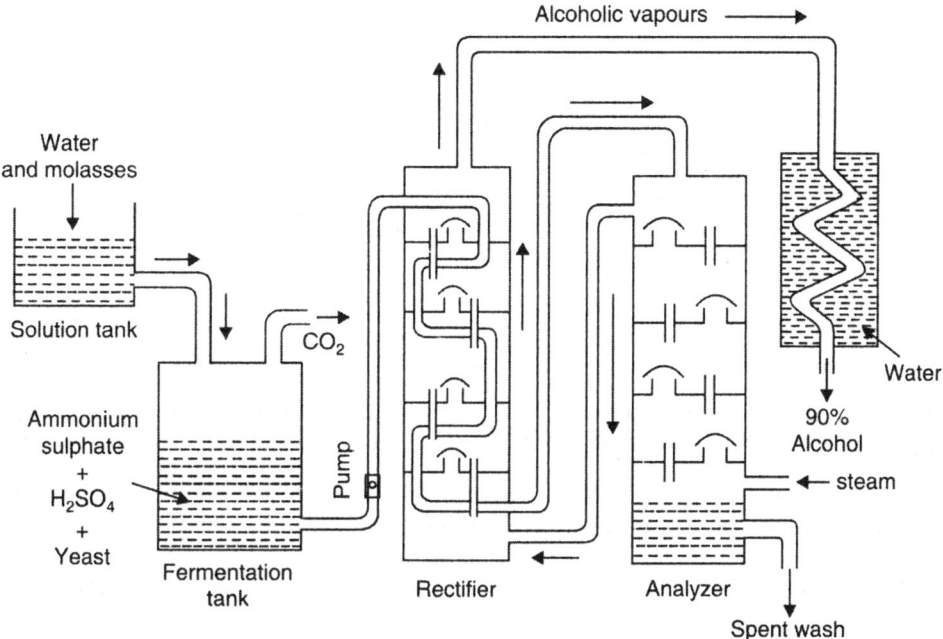

Fig. 12.1. Manufacture of alcohol by fermentation of molasses.

(iv) **Rectification:** Three important fractions are obtained from the rectification of 90 per cent alcohol. The first fraction contains mainly the low volatile liquids like acetaldehyde. The second running contains 93–95 per cent alcohol (w/w). This alcohol is called rectified spirit or industrial alcohol. The last fraction contains water and fused oil. Fused oil is a mixture of n-propyl, n-butyl, isobutyl, n-amyl, isoamyl, and optically active amyl alcohols which distil at 125–140°C.

(II) **From starch:** The following steps are involved in the manufacture of alcohol from starchy materials like potatoes, barley, maize, etc.

(a) **Saccharification:** In this process the starch is first converted into maltose by the following steps:

(i) **Malting:** Moist barley is allowed to germinate in dark at 15°C. The germinated barley known as malt is heated to 60°C to stop its further growth. These seeds are crushed in water and filtrate known as malt extract contains enzyme diastase.

(ii) **Mashing:** Mashing is a process in which starch is liberated from the starchy materials. For the separation of starch the substances like potatoes, maize, barley, etc. are crushed and distilled with superheated steam under pressure. The starch which forms a paste-like mass is called mash.

(iii) **Hydrolysis:** Malt extract is now added to the mash at 50–60°C. The enzyme diastase hydrolyzes the starch to maltose in about half an hour.

$$2(C_6H_{10}O_5)_n + H_2O \xrightarrow[\text{50–60°C}]{\text{Diastase}} nC_{12}H_{22}O_{11}$$

Starch   Maltose

Starch is also hydrolysed to glucose with dilute sulphuric acid or hydrochloric acid at higher temperature. The excess of acid is neutralized with lime.

$$(C_6H_{10}O_5)_n + H_2O \xrightarrow{\text{Acid}} nC_6H_{12}O_6$$
$$\text{Starch} \qquad\qquad\qquad \text{Glucose}$$

(b) **Fermentation:** The hydrolyzed product maltose or glucose is then fermented with yeast at 30°C for 2–3 days. The enzyme maltase present in yeast hydrolyzes maltose to glucose. Zymase, another enzyme of yeast, converts glucose to ethanol.

$$C_{12}H_{22}O_{11} + H_2O \xrightarrow[\text{(Yeast)}]{\text{Maltase}} 2C_6H_{12}O_6 \xrightarrow[\text{(Yeast)}]{\text{Zymase}} 2C_2H_5.OH + CO_2$$
$$\text{Maltose} \qquad\qquad\qquad \text{Glucose} \qquad\qquad\qquad \text{Ethanol}$$

The fermented solution is known as wort which contains about 10 per cent alcohol. The distillation and rectification of wort are carried out in a Coffey still as discussed in the case of molasses.

(III) From sugars: Manufacture of alcohol from sugars is the earliest method. Sugars like glucose and sucrose are transformed into ethanol by fermentation in the presence of yeast cell as:

$$C_{12}H_{22}O_{11} + H_2O \xrightarrow[\text{(Yeast)}]{\text{Invertase}} C_6H_{12}O_6 + C_6H_{12}O_6 \xrightarrow[\text{(Yeast)}]{\text{Zymase}} 2C_2H_5.OH + CO_2$$
$$\text{Sucrose} \qquad\qquad\qquad \text{Glucose} \quad \text{Fructose} \qquad\qquad\qquad \text{Ethanol}$$

(IV) From cellulose (Schroller process): Saw dust is cheap cellulose raw material which is hydrolyzed to glucose with dilute sulphuric acid and steam at a pressure of 6–7 atmospheres. Lime is added to neutralize excess of sulphuric acid. To the resulting solution yeast cells are mixed to convert glucose into ethanol by enzyme zymase.

$$(C_6H_{10}O_5)_n + H_2O \xrightarrow[\text{H}_2\text{SO}_4]{\Delta} nC_6H_{12}O_6 \xrightarrow[\text{(Yeast)}]{\text{Zymase}} 2C_2H_5.OH + CO_2$$

In the industry, alcohol is not obtained through glucose. It is rather manufactured from starch containing materials, like potatoes, molasses, rice or maize through malt enzyme, diastase. The following consolidated scheme shows the conversion of starch to ethanol and carbon dioxide.

$$2(C_6H_{10}O_5)_n + nH_2O \xrightarrow{\text{Diastase}} nC_{12}H_{22}O_{11}$$
$$\text{Starch} \qquad\qquad\qquad\qquad \text{Maltose}$$

$$C_{12}H_{22}O_{11} + H_2O \xrightarrow{\text{Maltose}} 2C_6H_{12}O_6$$
$$\text{Maltose} \qquad\qquad\qquad\qquad \text{Glucose}$$

$$C_6H_{12}O_6 \longrightarrow 2C_2H_5OH + 2CO_2$$
$$\text{Glucose}$$

Fig. 11.2. Process of alcohol fermentation.

The fermentation process has been researched in detail by quite a few scientists, of whom the outstanding ones are *Liebig, Pasteur* and *Edward Buchner. Buchner* of the University of Tubingen, Germany, received the Nobel Prize of chemistry in 1907 for his work on fermentation.

By-Products of Alcoholic Fermentation

The following important by-products are obtained during the alcoholic fermentation:

(a) **Carbon dioxide gas:** Large amount of carbon dioxide gas evolved during fermentation is liquefied and then solidified. The solid carbon dioxide, known as dry ice, is used as refrigerant.

(b) **Potassium hydrogen tartate or argol:** Fruit juices, such as grape juice, give brown-red coloured solid substance which is called as argol. It is used in the preparation of tartaric acid and Rochelle salt (sodium potassium tartarate).

(c) **Fused oil:** The final runnings of the wash distillation give a mixture of high boiling alcohols, known as fusel oil. Mainly amyl alcohols are present in the fusel oil which are separated and used as solvents.

(d) **Acetaldehyde:** The first running of the wort distillation contains acetaldehyde which is used in the preparation of dyes, drugs and insecticides.

(e) **Spent wash:** It is liquid left after the distillation of alcohol from the wort. It contains all the nutritive ingredients like protein, fats etc. which are present in the starting materials. The spent wash is used as a cattle feed.

Other Examples of Fermentation

Alcoholic beverages, known as wines, are prepared by fermented fruit juices. Fermentation of sugar solutions by yeast in the presence of sodium sulphite gives glycerol. Citric acid is manufactured from molasses or glucose by the addition of enzyme *Aspergillus niger* or *Citromyces prefferians*. Butyl alcohol and acetone are industrially prepared by fermenting the starch by *Clostridium acetobutylicum*. Acetic acid is obtained commercially by the fermentation of sugars on starch with yeast in the presence of *Mycoderma aceti*. Sugars like lactose, sucrose, maltose or glucose on fermentation afford lactic acid by the action of *Lacto bacilli*. Urea is decomposed into ammonia and carbon dioxide by the action of enzyme urease present in the air.

PROOF SPIRIT

Proof spirit, a spirit that at a temperature of 51°F has a weight 12/13th of the weight of an equal measure of distilled water, is a dilute alcohol having a specific gravity of 0.91976 at 15°C. In British Pharmacopoeia this was official under the title of *spiritus tenuior* upto 1885.

Proof spirit contains 57.10 per cent by volume or 49.28 per cent by weight of ethyl alcohol. When the alcohol of this concentration is poured onto the gunpowder, the powder would lit and catch fire. If there is more water in the spirit, i.e., dilute alcohol, the powder is too wet to burn when the alcohol is poured over it.

Since heavy excise duty is levied on alcohol and its preparations, the term Under-proof (U.P.) for weaker spirit and Over-proof (O.P.) for stronger spirits are used for the determination of the amount of alcohol in a sample ready for excise purpose. '25 Degrees over-proof' means that 100 volumes of the alcohol are diluted with water to give 125 volumes of the proof spirit. '25 Degree under proof' indicates that there are 75 volumes of proof spirit in the alcohol. For determining the strength of alcohol solutions the specific gravity is found out by means of a hydrometer or a specific gravity bottle. This process of determining the percentage of alcohol in a given sample is termed as alcoholmetry. The chemical methods of analysis take time. Therefore, hydrometer is used for determining the specific gravity of the sample. The strength is calculated by knowing the specific gravity and it is compared by reading the percentage of alcohol against it from a standard reference table.

DENATURED SPIRIT OR METHYLATED SPIRIT

Ethyl alcohol in the form of alcoholic beverages is generally used for drinking which is a social evil. Therefore, the manufacture and supply of alcohol is controlled by the government all over the world. To diminish the use of ethyl alcohol, it is heavily taxed in the form of excise duty. To prevent the misuse of industrial alcohol and in order to make it unfit for drinking, it is denatured by mixing poisonous substances like methanol, pyridine, petroleum, etc. For industrial and pharmaceutical purposes this type of alcohol may be obtained from licensed persons and free from excise duty.

The alcohol denatured by the addition of about 5–10 per cent methanol (Wood naphtha or Wood spirit) and some amount of pyridine and acetone is known as methylated spirit. In India, a mixture of light caoutchoucine and pyridine base is used to denature the ethanol which is known as denatured spirit. It is used for the preparation of paints, varnishes, tinctures and as a solvent.

For pharmaceutical purpose, industrial methylated spirit, i.e., alcohol denatured with methanol only, may be used. These spirits may be consumed for the preparation of certain liquids for external use. A highly denatured spirit called mineralized methylated spirit has the following composition:

Alcohol	90 parts by volume
Methanol (Wood naphtha)	9½ ” ” ”
Crude pyridine	½ ” ” ”
Petroleum (Mineral naphtha)	3/8 of a gal. per 100 gal.
Methyl violet	0.025 oz. per 100 gal.

The methyl violet is added for colouring the spirit and other substances give the spirit a highly disagreeable taste. This spirit has been mainly used for burning purposes in spirit lamps.

GLYCOLS

The compounds containing two hydroxyl groups are known as dihydric alcohols or glycols. They are derived from the alkanes by substitution of two –OH groups for hydrogen atoms. Because of their sweet taste they are also known as glycols (Greek, glykys = sweet). The two hydroxyl groups must be attached to two different carbon atoms because the compounds having two hydroxyl groups on the same carbon atoms are usually unstable. They show the same chemical reactions as that of monohydric alcohols, i.e., they react with acids to give esters; the hydrogen atoms of –OH group are replaceable by electropositive metals; on oxidation the $-CH_2.OH$ groups are converted into –CHO and –COOH groups.

They are classified according to the relative positions of the two hydroxyl groups, that is, 1 : 2-glycols are referred as α; 1 : 3-glycols as β; and 1 : 4 glycols as γ and so on.

Nomenclature

1. **Common system:** In this system α-glycols are named after the alkane from which they are obtained by direct hydroxylation, while β- and γ-glycols are called as polymethylene glycols.
2. **IUPAC system:** The suffix 'diol' is added after the name of parent alkane to obtain the systematic names of dihydric alcohols. The position of the groups and side chain, if any, is indicated by numbers. The names of some dihydric alcohols in both the systems are given below:

Formula	Common name	IUPAC name
$CH_2(OH).CH_2.OH$	Ethylene glycol	Ethane-1,2-diol
$CH_3.CH(OH).CH_2.OH$	Propylene glycol	Propane-1,2-diol
$CH_2(OH).CH_2CH_2.OH$	Trimethylene glycol	Propane-1,3-diol
$CH_3.CH_2.CH(OH).CH_2.OH$	Butylene glycol	Butane-1,2-diol
$(CH_3)_2.C(OH).CH_2.OH$	Isobutylene glycol	2-Methyl propane-1,2-diol
$CH_3.CH(OH).CH_2.CH_2.OH$	Butylene glycol	Butane-1,3-diol
$CH_2(OH).CH_2.CH_2.CH_2.OH$	Tetramethylene glycol	Butane-1,4-diol

Isomerism: Dihydric alcohols, represented by a general formula $C_nH_{2n+2}.O_2^{\bullet}$, may exhibit position isomerism among themselves and functional isomerism with ethers. Thus four isomeric compounds containing the general formula $C_3H_8O_2$ are represented as:

Compound	Formula	Isomers
Propane-1,2-diol	$CH_3.CH(OH).CH_2OH$	Position isomers
Propane-1,3-diol	$CH_2(OH).CH_2CH_2.OH$	
Dimethoxymethane	$CH_3O.CH_2.O.CH_3$	Functional isomers
2-Methoxyethanol	$\cdot CH_3O.CH_2.CH_2.OH$	

Ethyl Glycol or Ethane-1,2-diol: $CH_2(OH).CH_2.OH$

Preparation: This is the simplest dihydric alcohol and is prepared by one of the methods outline below:

1. **From ethylene:** Three different methods are employed for the preparation of ethylene glycol:
   (i) By treating ethylene with cold, dilute alkaline potassium permanganate solution. Hydroxylation of ethylene takes place to give the glycol.

   $$CH_2 = CH_2 + H_2O + [O] \xrightarrow{\text{Alk. KMnO}_4} CH_2(OH).CH_2OH$$

   (ii) Ethylene is first converted to ethylene oxide by passing a mixture of ethylene and air over hot silver catalyst under pressure or by treating ethylene with a per acid. The oxide formed is then hydrolyzed with dilute hydrochloric acid to yield ethylene glycol.

   $$CH_2 = CH_2 + \tfrac{1}{2}O_2 \xrightarrow[250^\circ C]{Ag} \underset{\text{Ethylene oxide}}{H_2C \!-\! CH_2 \atop \diagdown\!O\!\diagup} \xrightarrow{H_2O} {H_2C \!-\! CH_2 \atop HO \quad OH}$$

   Ethylene

   $$CH_2 = CH_2 + H.COO.OH \longrightarrow \underset{\text{Performic acid}}{H_2C \!-\! CH_2 \atop \diagdown\!O\!\diagup} \xrightarrow[H^+]{H_2O} {H_2C \!-\! CH_2 \atop HO \quad OH}$$

   (iii) Ethylene is treated with hydrochlorous acid to form ethylene chlorohydrin which is hydrolyzed with milk of lime to produce ethylene glycol (industrial process).

   $$CH_2 = CH_2 + HOCl \longrightarrow \underset{\text{Ethylene chlorohydrin}}{CH_2(OH).CH_2Cl} \xrightarrow[-CaCl_2]{Ca(OH)} CH_2(OH).CH_2.OH$$

2. **Hydrolysis of halides:** Hydrolysis of ethylene bromide with moist silver oxide or aqueous solution of sodium carbonate gives ethylene glycol.

$$CH_2(Br).CH_2.Br + H_2O \xrightarrow[\substack{\text{or } Na_2CO_3 \\ \text{Heat}}]{Ag_2O} CH_2(OH).CH_2.OH$$

Ethylene glycol is extracted with ether-alcohol mixture from the reaction mixture which on distillation yields glycol in poor yield.

Strong alkalis like KOH and NaOH when reacted with ethylenedibromide result in the formation of vinyl bromide and other side products.

To obtain high yield, ethylene bromide is first converted to glycol diacetate by the reaction with sodium or silver acetate which on hydrolysis with dilute alkalies gives ethylene glycol.

$$\begin{array}{c} CH_2.Br \\ | \\ CH_2.Br \end{array} + 2Ag.O.CO.CH_3 \xrightarrow[-2AgBr]{} \begin{array}{c} CH_2.O.CO.CH_3 \\ | \\ CH_2.O.CO.CH_3 \end{array} \xrightarrow[-2CH_3.COONa]{2NaOH/H^+} \begin{array}{c} CH_2.OH \\ | \\ CH_2.OH \end{array}$$

3. **From oxalic ester, glyoxal or glycolic aldehyde:** These compounds on reduction with sodium and alcohol give ethylene glycol.

$$\begin{array}{c} CO.O.C_2H_5 \\ | \\ CO.O.C_2H_5 \\ \text{Diethyl oxalate} \end{array} \searrow \quad \begin{array}{c} CH_2.OH \\ | \\ CH_2.OH \end{array} \xleftarrow{2H} \begin{array}{c} CHO \\ | \\ CH_2.OH \\ \text{Glycolic} \\ \text{aldehyde} \end{array}$$

$$\begin{array}{c} CHO \\ | \\ CHO \\ \text{Glyoxal} \end{array} \nearrow$$

4. **From ethylene diamine:** Diamine when reacted with nitrous acid gives glycol.

$$\begin{array}{c} CH_2.NH_2 \\ | \\ CH_2.NH_2 \end{array} \xrightarrow[-2N_2]{2HNO_2} \begin{array}{c} CH_2.OH \\ | \\ CH_2.OH \end{array} + 2H_2O$$

5. **Biomolecular reduction of carbonyl compound:** Bimolecular reduction of aldehydes and ketones gives dihydric alcohols. For example, acetone when reduced with magnesium in benzene and then hydrolyzed produces pinacol, a substituted ethylene glycol.

$$2(CH_3)_2CO \xrightarrow{Mg,\ benzene} \begin{array}{c} (CH_3)_2.C — C.(CH_3)_2 \\ |\quad\quad | \\ O\quad\ O \\ \diagdown\ \diagup \\ Mg \end{array}$$

$$\downarrow H_2O$$

$$\begin{array}{c} (CH_3)_2C — C.(CH_3)_2 \\ |\quad\quad\ | \\ OH\ \ OH \\ \text{Pinacol} \end{array}$$

Physical properties: Ethylene glycol is a colourless, viscous liquid, having m.p. $-11.5°C$, b.p. $197°C$ and sp. gr. 1.11 at $20°C$. It is hygroscopic in nature having a sweet taste. It is miscible with water and ethanol in all proportions but insoluble in ether. It has toxic effect and forms low freezing mixture water.

Chemical properties: The two primary alcoholic groups are attached in the molecule and it shows the reaction of monohydric primary alcohol. However, in most of the reactions both these groups are not equally reactive, one group generally reacts completely before the other is attacked. The two groups may undergo two different types of reactions.

1. **Reaction with sodium:** Electropositive metals like sodium react with ethylene glycol at 50°C to form monosodium glycolate while disodium derivatives are achieved at 160°C.

$$\underset{}{\overset{CH_2.OH}{\underset{CH_2.OH}{|}}} \xrightarrow[50°C]{Na} \underset{\substack{Monosodium \\ glycolate}}{\overset{CH_2.ONa}{\underset{CH_2.ONa}{|}}} \xrightarrow[160°C]{Na} \underset{\substack{Disodium \\ glycolate}}{\overset{CH_2.ONa}{\underset{CH_2.ONa}{|}}}$$

2. **Reaction with acids:** Ethylene glycol reacts with inorganic and organic acids to afford various types of products. With hydrogen chloride gas it forms ethylene chlorohydrin at 160°C and ethylene chloride at 200°C.

$$\underset{}{\overset{CH_2.OH}{\underset{CH_2.OH}{|}}} \xrightarrow[-H_2O]{HCl/160°C} \underset{}{\overset{CH_2.Cl}{\underset{CH_2.OH}{|}}} \xrightarrow[-H_2O]{HCl/200°C} \underset{}{\overset{CH_2.Cl}{\underset{CH_2.Cl}{|}}}$$

Ethylene dinitrite is obtained from ethylene glycol when it is allowed to react with conc. nitric acid in the presence of conc. sulphuric acid.

$$\underset{}{\overset{CH_2.OH}{\underset{CH_2.OH}{|}}} + 2HNO_3 \xrightarrow[Heat]{H_2SO_4} \underset{\substack{Ethylene\ dinitrate \\ (highly\ explosive\ liquid)}}{\overset{CH_2.O.NO_2}{\underset{CH_2.O.NO_2}{|}}} + H_2O$$

Reaction with fatty acids like acetic acid (or acetic anhydride, acetyl chloride) gives first glycol monoacetate and then diacetate derivative.

$$\underset{}{\overset{CH_2.OH}{\underset{CH_2.OH}{|}}} + CH_3.COOH \xrightarrow[-H_2O]{H_2SO_4} \underset{\substack{Glycol\ monoacetate}}{\overset{CH_2.O.CO.CH_3}{\underset{CH_2.OH}{|}}} \xrightarrow[H_2SO_4]{CH_3.COOH} \underset{\substack{Glycol\ diacetate}}{\overset{CH_2.O.CO.CH_3}{\underset{CH_2.O.CO.CH_3}{|}}}$$

On heating with dibasic acids ethylene glycol forms a condensation polymer. With terephthalic acid it forms a polymer terylene or dacron used as synthetic fibre.

$$nHOCH_2.CH_2.OH + n\underset{\text{Terephthalic acid}}{HOOC.C_6H_4.COOH}$$

$$\downarrow H_2O$$

$$\underset{\text{Dacron}}{HO.CH_2.CH_2.O[OC.C_6H_4.CO.O.CH_2.CH_2.O]_{n-1}OC.C_6H_5 - COOH}$$

3. **Acylation:** Reaction of ethylene glycol with acid chlorides and acid anhydrides is the same as the formation of ester with acetic acid. Two types of esters are formed as shown earlier.

$$\underset{\overset{|}{CH_2.OH}}{\overset{CH_2.OH}{|}} \xrightarrow[\text{–}CH_3.COOH]{(CH_3.CO)_2O} \underset{\overset{|}{CH_2.OH}}{\overset{CH_2.O.CO.CH_3}{|}} \xrightarrow[\text{–}CH_3.COOH]{(CH_3.CO)_2O} \underset{\overset{|}{CH_2.O.CO.CH_3}}{\overset{CH_2.O.CO.CH_3}{|}}$$

Glycol monoacetate   Glycol diacetate

4. **Oxidation:** Depending on the nature of oxidizing agents and the number of alcoholic groups involved in oxidation different products are obtained on oxidation of ethylene glycol. With dilute nitric acid or alkaline potassium permanganate the following compounds are produced on oxidation.

$$\underset{\overset{|}{CH_2.OH}}{\overset{CH_2.OH}{|}} \xrightarrow{[O]} \underset{\overset{|}{CH_2.OH}}{\overset{CHO}{|}} \xrightarrow{[O]} \underset{\overset{|}{CH_2.OH}}{\overset{COOH}{|}} \xrightarrow{[O]} \underset{\overset{|}{CHO}}{\overset{COOH}{|}} \xrightarrow{[O]} \underset{\overset{|}{COOH}}{\overset{COOH}{|}}$$

                 Glycolic   Glycolic   Glyoxalic   Oxalic
                 aldehyde   acid   acid   acid

$$\downarrow [O]$$

$$\underset{\overset{|}{CHO}}{\overset{CHO}{|}} \xrightarrow{[O]}$$

Glyoxal

Oxidation with periodic acid or lead tetraacetate breaks the carbon-carbon bond and formaldehyde is produced.

$$\underset{\overset{|}{CH_2.OH}}{\overset{CH_2.OH}{|}} \xrightarrow[HIO_4]{[O]} \underset{H.CHO}{\overset{H.CHO}{+}} + H_2O$$

Cleavage of carbon-carbon bond also takes place when acidic potassium permanganate or potassium dichromate is used as the oxidizing agent.

$$\underset{\overset{|}{CH_2.OH}}{\overset{CH_2.OH}{|}} \xrightarrow[\substack{KMnO_4 \text{ or} \\ K_2Cr_2O_7 \text{ in} \\ H_2SO_4}]{[O]} \underset{H.COOH}{\overset{H.COOH}{+}} + H_2O$$

5. **Reaction with phosphorus halides:** With phosphorus tri- or penta-chlorides and bromides ethylene glycol first gives halohydrin and then dihalides. However, with phosphorus tri-iodide it first forms unstable ethylene iodide which yields ethene on decomposition.

$$\underset{\overset{|}{CH_2.OH}}{\overset{CH_2.OH}{|}} \begin{cases} \xrightarrow{PCl_5} \underset{\overset{|}{CH_2.Cl}}{\overset{CH_2.OH}{|}} \xrightarrow{PCl_5} \underset{\overset{|}{CH_2.Cl}}{\overset{CH_2.Cl}{|}} & \text{Ethylene dichloride} \\ \xrightarrow{PBr_3} \underset{\overset{|}{CH_2.OH}}{\overset{CH_2.Br}{|}} \xrightarrow{PBr_3} \underset{\overset{|}{CH_2.Br}}{\overset{CH_2.Br}{|}} & \text{Ethylene dibromide} \\ \xrightarrow{PI_3} \underset{\overset{|}{CH_2.I}}{\overset{CH_2.I}{|}} \xrightarrow{-I_2} \underset{\overset{||}{CH_2}}{\overset{CH_2}{|}} & \text{Ethene} \end{cases}$$

6. **Condensation with carbonyl compounds:** Condensation of glycol with aldehydes and ketones in the presence of mineral acids as catalyst gives cyclic acetals and ketals respectively.

$$\begin{array}{c} CH_2.OH \\ | \\ CH_2.OH \end{array} + O{=}C\begin{array}{c} H \\ \diagdown \\ CH_3 \end{array} \xrightarrow[Heat]{H^+} \begin{array}{c} CH_2{-}O \\ | \qquad \diagup C \diagdown \\ CH_2{-}O \qquad CH_3 \end{array}{\scriptstyle H} + H_2O$$

Acetaldehyde   Glycol acetal

7. **Dehydration:** Ethylene glycol yields the following different products on dehydration under different conditions.

$$\begin{array}{c} CH_2.OH \\ | \\ CH_2.OH \end{array} + O{=}C\begin{array}{c} CH_3 \\ \diagdown \\ CH_3 \end{array} \xrightarrow[Heat]{H^+} \begin{array}{c} CH_2{-}O \\ | \qquad \diagup C \diagdown \\ CH_2{-}O \qquad CH_3 \end{array}{\scriptstyle CH_3} + H_2O$$

Acetone   Glycol ketal

$$\begin{array}{c} CH_2.OH \\ | \\ CH_2.OH \end{array}$$

$\xrightarrow[-H_2O]{500°C}$ $\underset{O}{H_2C{-}CH_2}$ (triangle) Ethylene oxide

$\xrightarrow[-H_2O]{Anhyd.\ ZnCl_2}$ $\left[\begin{array}{c} CH_2 \\ \| \\ CH{-}OH \end{array} \right]$ $\xrightarrow{Rearrangement}$ $\begin{array}{c} CH_3 \\ | \\ CHO \end{array}$

Unstable   Acetaldehyde

$\xrightarrow[Heat/-H_2O]{Conc.\ H_3PO_4}$ $\begin{array}{c} HO.CH_2.CH_2 \\ \diagdown \\ HO.CH_2.CH_2 \diagup \end{array} O$ Diethylene glycol

$\xrightarrow[Heat]{Conc.\ H_2SO_4}$ $O\begin{array}{c} \diagup CH_2.CH_2 \diagdown \\ \diagdown CH_2.CH_2 \diagup \end{array} O$ 1,4-Dioxane

Uses: Ethylene glycol is used:
1. As an antifreeze in automobile radiators due to formation of low freezing mixture with water.
2. In the manufacture of synthetic polyesters, fibre, terylene and in making low freezing dynamite.
3. As a coolant for aeroplane engines and for preventing the deposition and formation of ice on aeroplane wings.
4. As a solvent, preservative and dielectric in electrical condensers.
5. In the preparation of various organic compounds such as dioxane, diethylene glycol (used as solvent) ethylene dinitrate (used as explosive) and glycol stearate (used as lubricant for springs).

Glycerol or Propane-1,2,3-triol

$HO.CH_2.CH(OH).CH_2.OH$ (see also under Official Compounds, p. 213)

Glycol was first discovered by Scheele in 1779 who obtained it by hydrolysis of olive oil. It may be considered as a trihydric derivative of propane which is obtained by the replacement of three hydrogen atoms from different carbon atoms by three hydroxyl groups.

It is related with fats and in nature it occurs in combined state as glycerol ester of higher fatty acids present in vegetable and animal oils and fats. The esters of higher fatty acids like palmitic ($C_{15}H_{31}.COOH$), oleic, ($C_{17}H_{33}.COOH$) and stearic ($C_{17}.H_{35}.COOH$) acids with glycerol are known as glycerides. For example:

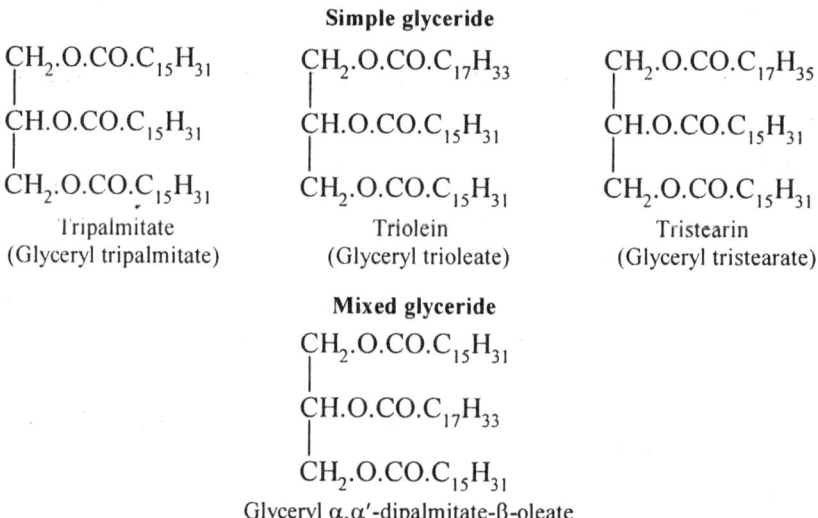

Simple glyceride

$CH_2.O.CO.C_{15}H_{31}$
$CH.O.CO.C_{15}H_{31}$
$CH_2.O.CO.C_{15}H_{31}$
Tripalmitate
(Glyceryl tripalmitate)

$CH_2.O.CO.C_{17}H_{33}$
$CH.O.CO.C_{15}H_{31}$
$CH_2.O.CO.C_{15}H_{31}$
Triolein
(Glyceryl trioleate)

$CH_2.O.CO.C_{17}H_{35}$
$CH.O.CO.C_{15}H_{31}$
$CH_2.O.CO.C_{15}H_{31}$
Tristearin
(Glyceryl tristearate)

Mixed glyceride

$CH_2.O.CO.C_{15}H_{31}$
$CH.O.CO.C_{17}H_{33}$
$CH_2.O.CO.C_{15}H_{31}$
Glyceryl α,α'-dipalmitate-β-oleate

Preparation: Different methods used for the preparation of glycerol are:

1. **From oils and fats:** Hydrolysis of fats and oils gives glycerol and the fatty acids. Either alkalies or superheated steam is used as the hydrolyzing agent.

   In the soap industry, fats and oils are hydrolyzed with caustic alkali solution known as lye to salts of higher fatty acids and glycerol. This hydrolysis in which the formation of soap takes place is termed as saponification. Soap is precipitated by the addition of sodium chloride and the filtrate, known as spent lye, containing glycerol (3–5%) is separated out.

$$CH_2.O.CO.R$$
$$CH.O.CO.R \quad + 3NaOH \longrightarrow$$
$$CH_2.O.CO.R$$
Glyceride

$$CH_2.OH,$$
$$CH.OH \quad + 3R.COONa$$
$$CH_2.OH \qquad\qquad Soap$$

2. **By fermentation of sugars:** When sugars are fermented for alcohols then glycerol is obtained as a by-product. If sodium sulphate is added in the fermented mixture, the yield of glycerol is increased upto 25 per cent. The fermented liquids give glycerol on subjection to fractional distillation.

$$C_{12}H_{22}O_{11} \xrightarrow[+ H_2O]{Yeast} 2C_6H_{12}O_6 \xrightarrow[Yeast]{Na_2SO_3} HO.CH_2.CH(OH).CH_2OH + CH_3.CHO + CO_2 + H_2O$$

Sucrose   Glucose and fructose   Glycerol

3. **Synthetic methods:**

(i) **From propylene** (Industrial procedure):

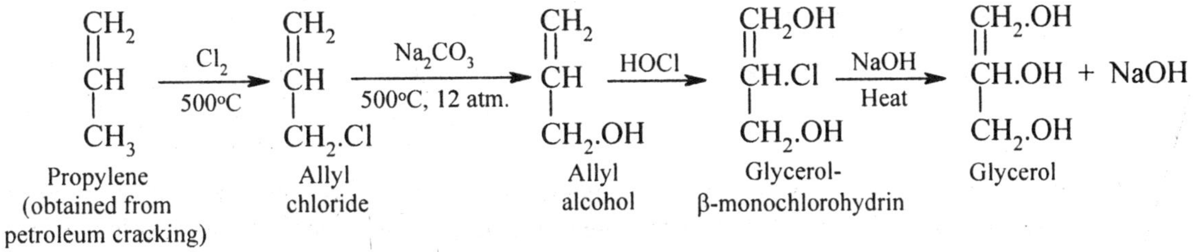

$$
\underset{\substack{\text{Propylene} \\ \text{(obtained from} \\ \text{petroleum cracking)}}}{\begin{array}{c} CH_2 \\ \| \\ CH \\ | \\ CH_3 \end{array}}
\xrightarrow[\text{500°C}]{Cl_2}
\underset{\substack{\text{Allyl} \\ \text{chloride}}}{\begin{array}{c} CH_2 \\ \| \\ CH \\ | \\ CH_2.Cl \end{array}}
\xrightarrow[\text{500°C, 12 atm.}]{Na_2CO_3}
\underset{\substack{\text{Allyl} \\ \text{alcohol}}}{\begin{array}{c} CH_2 \\ \| \\ CH \\ | \\ CH_2.OH \end{array}}
\xrightarrow{HOCl}
\underset{\substack{\text{Glycerol-} \\ \beta\text{-monochlorohydrin}}}{\begin{array}{c} CH_2OH \\ \| \\ CH.Cl \\ | \\ CH_2.OH \end{array}}
\xrightarrow[\text{Heat}]{NaOH}
\underset{\text{Glycerol}}{\begin{array}{c} CH_2.OH \\ \| \\ CH.OH \\ | \\ CH_2.OH \end{array}} + NaOH
$$

(ii) **From allyl chloride and hypochlorous acid:**

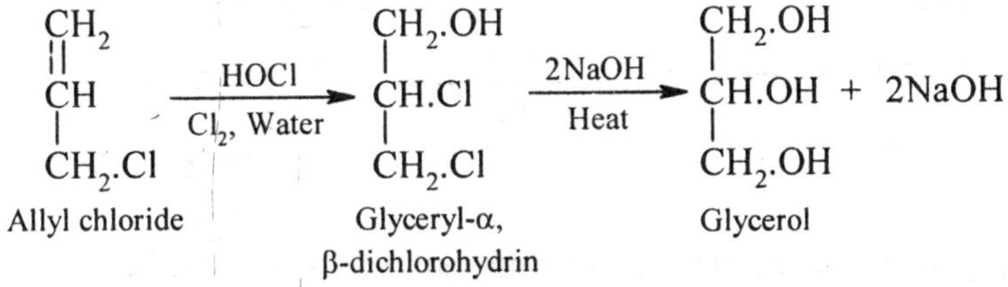

$$
\underset{\text{Allyl chloride}}{\begin{array}{c} CH_2 \\ \| \\ CH \\ | \\ CH_2.Cl \end{array}}
\xrightarrow[\text{Cl}_2, \text{ Water}]{HOCl}
\underset{\substack{\text{Glyceryl-}\alpha, \\ \beta\text{-dichlorohydrin}}}{\begin{array}{c} CH_2.OH \\ | \\ CH.Cl \\ | \\ CH_2.Cl \end{array}}
\xrightarrow[\text{Heat}]{2NaOH}
\underset{\text{Glycerol}}{\begin{array}{c} CH_2.OH \\ | \\ CH.OH \\ | \\ CH_2.OH \end{array}} + 2NaOH
$$

Physical properties: Glycerol is a colourless, odourless, viscous and hygroscopic liquid having b.p. 290°C and sp. gr. 1.265 at 20°C. It has a sweet taste (Gr. Glykys = sweet) and is miscible with water and alcohol in all proportions. It is almost insoluble in solvents like ether, benzene and chloroform. On cooling at 17°C it gives transparent crystals which are very hygroscopic. On absorbing a small amount of water from the air the crystals are converted into the ordinary syrupy liquid. It decomposes on heating at its b.p. It dissolves readily many substances such as tannic acid and phenol, which are much less soluble in water and thus it is used for galenical preparations.

Chemical properties: In chemical reactions glycerol is very similar to the monohydric alcohols. It contains two primary and one secondary alcoholic groups. The primary alcoholic group is more reactive. Therefore, it gives the reactions of two types of groups as shown below:

1. **Reaction with sodium:** The primary alcoholic groups of glycerol react with sodium to give solid monosodium glycerolate at room temperature with the evolution of hydrogen.

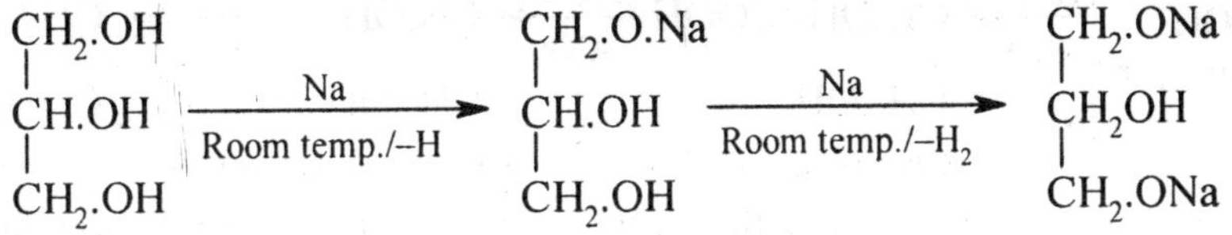

$$
\begin{array}{c} CH_2.OH \\ | \\ CH.OH \\ | \\ CH_2.OH \end{array}
\xrightarrow[\text{Room temp./–H}]{Na}
\begin{array}{c} CH_2.O.Na \\ | \\ CH.OH \\ | \\ CH_2.OH \end{array}
\xrightarrow[\text{Room temp./–H}_2]{Na}
\begin{array}{c} CH_2.ONa \\ | \\ CH_2OH \\ | \\ CH_2.ONa \end{array}
$$

2. **Reaction with acids:**

(i) Reaction with hydrochloric acid at 110°C gives a mixture of two mono derivatives.

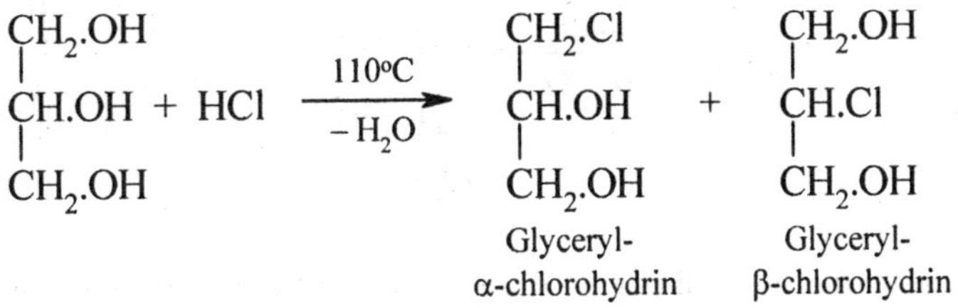

$$
\begin{array}{c} CH_2.OH \\ | \\ CH.OH \\ | \\ CH_2.OH \end{array} + HCl
\xrightarrow[\text{– H}_2\text{O}]{110°C}
\underset{\substack{\text{Glyceryl-} \\ \alpha\text{-chlorohydrin}}}{\begin{array}{c} CH_2.Cl \\ | \\ CH.OH \\ | \\ CH_2.OH \end{array}} +
\underset{\substack{\text{Glyceryl-} \\ \beta\text{-chlorohydrin}}}{\begin{array}{c} CH_2.OH \\ | \\ CH.Cl \\ | \\ CH_2.OH \end{array}}
$$

If the reaction is continued the following products are obtained:

$$
\begin{array}{ccc}
\underset{\substack{| \\ \text{CH.OH} \\ | \\ \text{CH}_2.\text{OH}}}{\text{CH}_2.\text{OH}} \quad \text{or} \quad
\underset{\substack{| \\ \text{CH.Cl} \\ | \\ \text{CH}_2.\text{OH}}}{\text{CH}_2.\text{OH}}
\xrightarrow[\text{110°C}]{\text{HCl (excess)}}
\underset{\substack{| \\ \text{CH.OH} \\ | \\ \text{CH}_2.\text{Cl}}}{\text{CH}_2.\text{Cl}} +
\underset{\substack{| \\ \text{CH.Cl} \\ | \\ \text{CH}_2.\text{OH}}}{\text{CH}_2.\text{Cl}}
\end{array}
$$

Glycerol-α,α′-dichlorohydrin   Glycerol-α,β-dichlorohydrin

(ii)   With concentrated nitric acid at low temperature and in the presence of sulphuric acid as catalyst glycerol gives glyceryl trinitrate or nitroglycerine which is highly explosive and is used in the preparation of dynamite.

$$
\underset{\substack{| \\ \text{CH.OH} \\ | \\ \text{CH}_2.\text{OH}}}{\text{CH}_2.\text{OH}} + 3\text{HO.NO}_2
\xrightarrow[\text{Heat}]{\text{H}_2\text{SO}_4}
\underset{\substack{| \\ \text{CH.O.NO}_2 \\ | \\ \text{CH}_2.\text{O.NO}_2}}{\text{CH}_2.\text{O.NO}_2} + 3\text{H}_2\text{O}
$$

Glyceryl trinitrate[1]

With fatty acids like acetic acid it forms mono-, di- and tri-esters.

$$
\underset{\substack{| \\ \text{CH.OH} \\ | \\ \text{CH}_2.\text{OH}}}{\text{CH}_2.\text{OH}}
\xrightarrow{\text{CH}_3\text{COOH}}
\underset{\substack{| \\ \text{CH.OH} \\ | \\ \text{CH}_2.\text{OH}}}{\text{CH}_2.\text{O.CO.CH}_3}
\xrightarrow{\text{CH}_3\text{COOH}}
\underset{\substack{| \\ \text{CH.OH} \\ | \\ \text{CH}_2.\text{O.CO.CH}_3}}{\text{CH}_2.\text{O.CO.CH}_3}
\xrightarrow{\text{CH}_3\text{COOH}}
\underset{\substack{| \\ \text{CH.O.CO.CH}_3 \\ | \\ \text{CH}_2.\text{O.CO.CH}_3}}{\text{CH}_2.\text{O.CO.CH}_3}
$$

Glyceryl-α-monoacetate   Glyceryl-α-α′-diacetate   Glyceryl triacetate

With a dibasic acids like oxalic acid it forms different products under different reaction conditions. At 110°C it first forms glycerol monoxalate and then yields glycerol monoformate on decomposition. Hydrolysis of the monoformate leads to the formation of formic acid.

$$
\underset{\substack{| \\ \text{CH.OH} \\ | \\ \text{CH}_2.\text{OH}}}{\text{CH}_2.\text{OH}} +
\underset{\substack{| \\ \text{COOH} \\ \text{Oxalic acid}}}{\text{COOH}}
\xrightarrow[-\text{H}_2\text{O}]{\text{110°C}}
\underset{\substack{| \\ \text{CH.OH} \\ | \\ \text{CH}_2.\text{OH}}}{\text{CH}_2.\text{O.OC}}\;\text{COOH}
\xrightarrow[-\text{CO}_2]{\text{110°C}}
\underset{\substack{| \\ \text{CH.OH} \\ | \\ \text{CH}_2.\text{OH}}}{\text{CH}_2.\text{O.OCH}}
\xrightarrow[\text{110°C}]{+\text{H}_2\text{O}}
\underset{\substack{| \\ \text{CH.OH} \\ | \\ \text{CH}_2.\text{OH}}}{\text{CH}_2.\text{OH}} + \text{H.COOH}
$$

Glycerol monoxalate   Glycerol monoformate   Glycerol   Formic acid

At 260°C glycerol reacts with oxalic acid to form glycerol dioxalate which then decomposes to produce allyl alcohol.

$$
\underset{\substack{| \\ \text{CH.OH} \\ | \\ \text{CH}_2.\text{OH} \\ \text{Glycerol}}}{\text{CH}_2.\text{OH}} +
\underset{\substack{| \\ \text{COOH}}}{\text{COOH}}
\xrightarrow[-2\text{H}_2\text{O}]{\text{260°C}}
\underset{\substack{| \\ \text{CH.O.OC} \\ | \\ \text{CH}_2.\text{OH} \\ \text{Glycerol dioxalate}}}{\text{CH}_2.\text{O.OC}}
\xrightarrow[-2\text{CO}_2]{\text{260°C}}
\underset{\substack{\| \\ \text{CH} \\ | \\ \text{CH}_2.\text{OH} \\ \text{Allyl alcohol}}}{\text{CH}_2}
$$

---

1. Glyceryl trinitrate is also official (as tablets in I.P.). See under Official Compounds (p. 215).

When glycerol is reacted with small amount of concentrated hydriodic acid glyceryl tri-iodide is formed. This compound is highly unstable, it further reacts with allyl iodide to yield di-iodopropane which also decomposes to form propylene. Propylene then reacts with hydriodic acid to form isopropyl iodide.

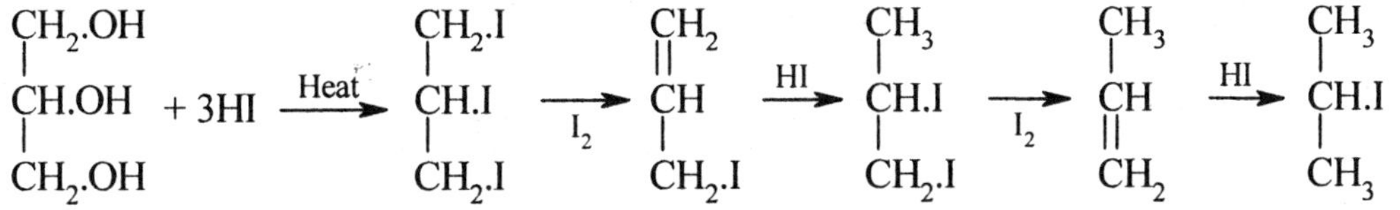

$$
\begin{array}{c}
CH_2.OH \\
| \\
CH.OH \\
| \\
CH_2.OH
\end{array}
+ 3HI \xrightarrow{\text{Heat}}
\begin{array}{c}
CH_2.I \\
| \\
CH.I \\
| \\
CH_2.I
\end{array}
\xrightarrow{I_2}
\begin{array}{c}
CH_2 \\
|| \\
CH \\
| \\
CH_2.I
\end{array}
\xrightarrow{HI}
\begin{array}{c}
CH_3 \\
| \\
CH.I \\
| \\
CH_2.I
\end{array}
\xrightarrow{I_2}
\begin{array}{c}
CH_3 \\
| \\
CH \\
|| \\
CH_2
\end{array}
\xrightarrow{HI}
\begin{array}{c}
CH_3 \\
| \\
CH.I \\
| \\
CH_3
\end{array}
$$

Glycerol   Glyceryl tri-oxide (unstable)   Allyl iodide   1,2-Diiodo-propane (unstable)   Propylene   Isopropyl iodide

3. **Acylation:** When glycerol is heated with acid chloride or acid anhydrides three types of acyl derivatives (esters) are formed.

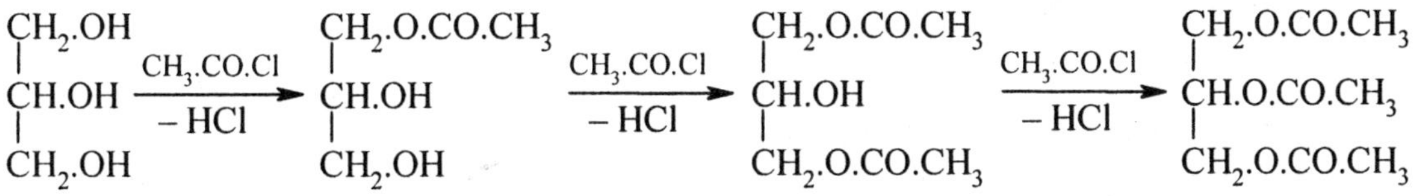

$$
\begin{array}{c}
CH_2.OH \\
| \\
CH.OH \\
| \\
CH_2.OH
\end{array}
\xrightarrow[-HCl]{CH_3.CO.Cl}
\begin{array}{c}
CH_2.O.CO.CH_3 \\
| \\
CH.OH \\
| \\
CH_2.OH
\end{array}
\xrightarrow[-HCl]{CH_3.CO.Cl}
\begin{array}{c}
CH_2.O.CO.CH_3 \\
| \\
CH.OH \\
| \\
CH_2.O.CO.CH_3
\end{array}
\xrightarrow[-HCl]{CH_3.CO.Cl}
\begin{array}{c}
CH_2.O.CO.CH_3 \\
| \\
CH.O.CO.CH_3 \\
| \\
CH_2.O.CO.CH_3
\end{array}
$$

4. **Reaction with phosphorus halides:** Phosphorus pentachloride or phosphorus trichloride reacts with glycerol to form trichloride.

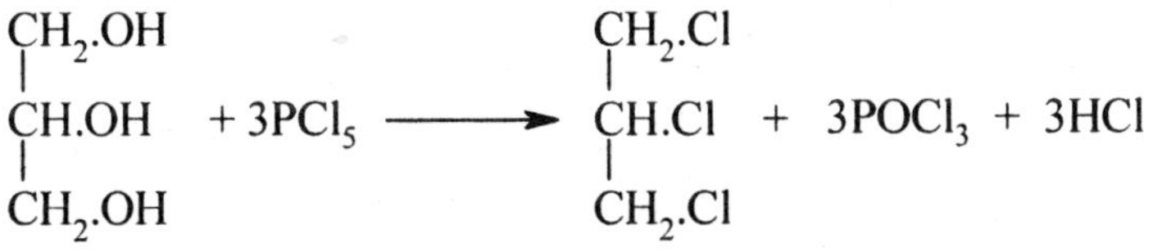

$$
\begin{array}{c}
CH_2.OH \\
| \\
CH.OH \\
| \\
CH_2.OH
\end{array}
+ 3PCl_5 \longrightarrow
\begin{array}{c}
CH_2.Cl \\
| \\
CH.Cl \\
| \\
CH_2.Cl
\end{array}
+ 3POCl_3 + 3HCl
$$

Glyceryl trichloride

Phosphorus penta- or tribromide reacts similarly. However, phosphorus tri-iodide on reaction with it forms allyl iodide via the formation of glyceryl tri-iodide. With excess of phosphorus tri-iodide it forms isopropyl iodide as shown above.

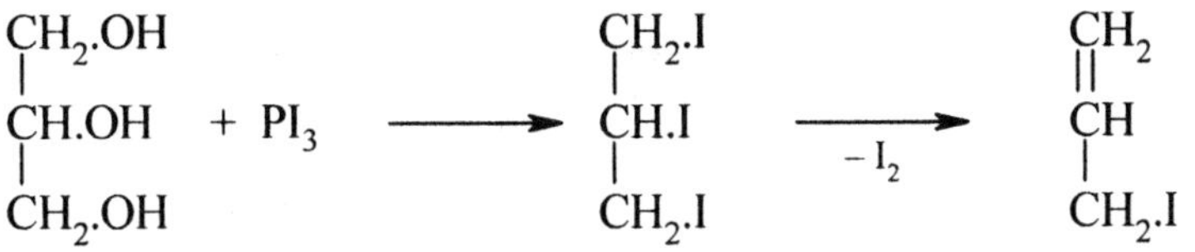

$$
\begin{array}{c}
CH_2.OH \\
| \\
CH.OH \\
| \\
CH_2.OH
\end{array}
+ PI_3 \longrightarrow
\begin{array}{c}
CH_2.I \\
| \\
CH.I \\
| \\
CH_2.I
\end{array}
\xrightarrow{-I_2}
\begin{array}{c}
CH_2 \\
|| \\
CH \\
| \\
CH_2.I
\end{array}
$$

                         Unstable   Allyl iodide

5. **Oxidation:** Due to the presence of primary and secondary alcoholic groups glycerol forms a large number of oxidation products under different oxidizing conditions. Dilute nitric acid gives glyceric acid, concentrated nitric acid gives glyceric and tartonic acids, bismuth and sodium nitrate form mesoxalic acid. Fenton's reagent (H_2O_2 + $FeSO_4$) or sodium hypobromide yields glyceraldehyde and dihydroxy acetone, bromine water produces glyceraldehyde and dihydroxy acetone and potassium permanganate oxidizes glycerol to oxalic acid.

$$
\begin{array}{c}
CH_2.OH \\
| \\
CH.OH \\
| \\
CH_2.OH
\end{array}
$$

(starting material branches via [O])

Upper branch:

$$
\xrightarrow{[O]}
\begin{array}{c}
CHO \\
| \\
CH.OH \\
| \\
CH_2.OH \\
\text{Glyceraldehyde}
\end{array}
\xrightarrow{[O]}
\begin{array}{c}
COOH \\
| \\
CH.OH \\
| \\
CH_2.OH \\
\text{Glyceric acid}
\end{array}
\xrightarrow{[O]}
\begin{array}{c}
COOH \\
| \\
CH.OH \\
| \\
COOH \\
\text{Tartronic acid}
\end{array}
$$

Lower branch:

$$
\xrightarrow{[O]}
\begin{array}{c}
CH_2.OH \\
| \\
CO \\
| \\
CH_2.OH \\
\text{Dihydroxy} \\
\text{acetone}
\end{array}
\xrightarrow{[O]}
\begin{array}{c}
COOH \\
| \\
CO \\
| \\
CH_2.OH \\
\text{Hydroxy} \\
\text{pyruvic acid}
\end{array}
\xrightarrow{[O]}
\begin{array}{c}
COOH \\
| \\
CO \\
| \\
COOH \\
\text{Mesoxalic} \\
\text{acid}
\end{array}
\xrightarrow{[O]}
\begin{array}{c}
COOH \\
| \\
COOH \\
\text{Oxalic} \\
\text{acid}
\end{array}
$$

6. **Dehydration:** Dehydration of glycerol takes place when it is heated alone or in the presence of dehydrating agents like conc. sulphuric acid, phosphorus pentoxide, potassium hydrogen sulphate etc. to yield acrylic aldehyde.

$$
\begin{array}{c}
HO \quad H \quad OH \\
| \quad | \quad | \\
H-C-C-C-H \\
| \quad | \quad | \\
H \quad OH \quad H
\end{array}
\xrightarrow[-2H_2O]{P_2O_5/heat}
\underset{\text{Unstable}}{CH_2 = C = CHOH}
\xrightarrow{\text{Rearrangement}}
\begin{array}{c}
CH_2 \\
|| \\
CH \\
| \\
CHO \\
\text{Acrolein}
\end{array}
$$

7. **Condensation with carbonyl compounds:** It forms five- and six-membered cyclic acetals with acetaldehyde and ketals with ketones in the presence of hydrogen chloride gas.

$$
\begin{array}{c}
CH_2.OH \\
| \\
CH.OH \\
| \\
CH_2.OH
\end{array}
$$

$$
\xrightarrow[HCl]{CH_3.CHO}
\begin{array}{c}
CH_2\!\!-\!\!O \\
| \quad\quad\ \diagdown \\
\quad\quad\quad CH.CH_3 + H_2O \\
| \quad\quad\ \diagup \\
CH\!\!-\!\!O \\
| \\
CH_2.OH \\
\text{Cyclic acetal} \\
\text{(5-membered)}
\end{array}
$$

$$
\xrightarrow[HCl]{(CH_3)_2.CO}
\begin{array}{c}
CH_2\!\!-\!\!O \\
| \quad\quad\ \diagdown \\
CH.OH \quad C.(CH_3)_2 \\
| \quad\quad\ \diagup \\
CH_2\!\!-\!\!O \\
\text{Ketal (6-membered)}
\end{array}
$$

8. **Reaction with aniline:** Glycerol reacts with aniline in the presence of nitrobenzene, conc. H_2SO_4 and ferrous sulphate to yield quinoline.

$$
\underset{\text{Aniline}}{\text{C}_6\text{H}_5\text{-NH}_2} +
\begin{array}{c}
CH_2.OH \\
| \\
CH.OH \\
| \\
CH_2.OH
\end{array}
+ C_6H_5.NO_2
\xrightarrow[FeSO_4/heat/-H_2O]{H_2SO_4}
\underset{\text{Quinoline}}{\text{(quinoline)}} + C_6H_5NH_2
$$

Uses: Glycerol is used as a sweetening agent in confectionary, beverages and medicines, as a preservative, as an antifreeze in automobile radiators, as a plasticizer for cellophane, lubricant in watches, moisture conditioner for tobacco products and in the preparation of soaps, cosmetics, non-drying inks, stamp pad inks, allyl resins, esterifying resins, acid-proof cements and various organic compounds like formic acid, allyl alcohol, acrolein, etc.

OFFICIAL COMPOUNDS

Ethanol (95%) / Alcohol (95%)

Alcohol is a mixture of ethyl alcohol and water. It is also known as ethanol and wine spirit and is commonly considered to contain 95 per cent of ethyl alcohol. Alcohol of I.P. contains not less than 94.7 per cent v/v or 92.0 per cent w/w and not more than 95.2 per cent v/v or 92.7 per cent w/w of C_2H_6O at 15.56°C.

Preparation: It is easily obtained from fermented liquors, and as a fermented product of carbohydrates, a common source these days being molasses. Other cheap industrial materials rich in starch are potatoes, rice or maize. Starch gets changed to glucose, which under the influence of zymase is changed to ethanol and carbon dioxide (see also previous pages). It is also prepared synthetically.

$$KOH + CH_3CH_2Br \longrightarrow CH_3CH_2OH + KBr$$

Description: Alcohol is a colourless, transparent, mobile and volatile liquid with a characteristic odour and spirituous burning taste. It is inflammable and burns with a blue smokeless flame.

Solubility: It is miscible in all proportions with water, chloroform and solvent ether. When alcohol is mixed with water, it contracts in volume and produces heat, e.g. 52 vol. ethanol with 48 vol. water does not give 100 vol. but 96.3 vol. of the mixture. The contraction is the greatest in equal volume. The contents of alcohol in a mixture cannot be calculated easily. It is done by knowing the specific weight (sp. gr.) and then calculating the content from a table. It is, therefore, desired to work with the knowledge of weight-percent of alcohol. The content of alcohol in the liquid pharmaceutical preparation is attained by following the I.P. method through the determination of sp. gr. of the distillate.

Test for identity: To about 10 ml of a 0.5 percent v/v solution, add 2 ml of a 4 percent w/v solution of sodium hydroxide and add slowly 4 ml of a solution of iodine, a yellow precipitate is produced and the odour of iodoform is perceptible.

I.P. 2007 describes another test by treating the alcoholic solution in potassium permanganate and dilute sulphuric acid and filtering the mixed solution through moistened filter paper with aqueous solution of sodium nitroprusside and piperazine hydrate. An intense blue colour becoming lighter later is produced.

Tests for purity: It is tested for specific gravity, acidity or alkalinity, aldehydes, fusel oil constituents, ketones, isopropyl alcohol and tertiary butyl alcohol, methyl alcohol, oily and resinous substances, and non-volatile matter and benzene and related substances (Appendix VII).

Specific gravity: At 25°C, 0.808–0.810 (Appendix III).

Refractive index: At 20°C, 1.3637 to 1.3639.

Acidity or alkalinity: To 50 ml add water to produce 100 ml, titrate with 0.02 N sodium hydroxide using solution of phenolphthalein as an indicator; not more than 0.9 ml of 0.02 N sodium hydroxide is required (I.P. 07 has modified a little the test).

Non-volatile matter: Leaves not more than 5 mg of residue when 100 ml evaporated and dried to constant weight at 105°.

Storage: Alcohol is preserved in a tightly closed contained away from fire.

Uses: It is an important pharmaceutical aid and necessity. Alcohol behaves basically as a narcotic, only the narcosis stage, which could cause paralysis, is different from the actual narcotics. Thus the action of alcohols is characterized through a long excitation stage (Haze) and through a short span between the onset of narcosis and death. With ether, however, the excitation stage is relatively short but the narcotic stage is long as shown below.

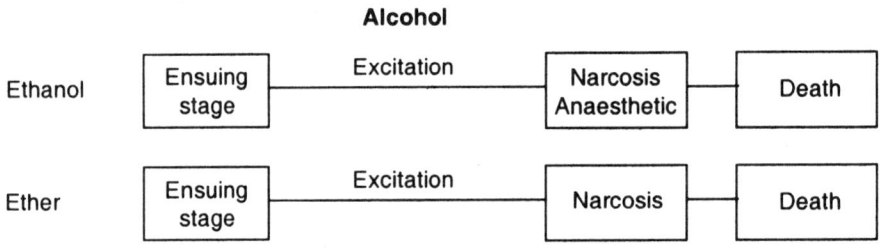

Alcohol is quickly absorbed from stomach and alimentary canal and is degraded through oxidation in liver. 0.1 g per kg of body weight of alcohol burns in one hour. One g of alcohol gives rise to 7.1 kcal. If the blood concentration of alcohol reaches 0.1% one loses balance and self-control. With concentration of 0.4–0.5% one becomes unconscious and endangers life through impairment of respiration.

DILUTE ALCOHOLS

Alcohol is diluted with water to produce Dilute Alcohols. They are prepared as described in the following paragraphs. Their specific gravity and refractive index are measured at 15.56° and 20° respectively.

1. Alcohol (90 per cent v/v) (limits 89.6 to 90.5% v/v).
   Dilute 947 ml of alcohol to 1000 ml with water. Specific gravity 0.832 to 0.835; refractive index 1.3645 to 1.3647.
2. Alcohol (80 per cent v/v) (limit 79.5 to 80.3% v/v).
   Dilute 842 ml of alcohol to 1000 ml with water.
   Specific gravity 0.863 to 0.865; refractive index 1.3648 to 1.3649.
3. Alcohol (70 per cent v/v) (limit 69.5 to 70.2% v/v).
   Dilute 737 ml of alcohol to 1000 ml with water.
   Specific gravity 0.899 to 0.891.
   Refractive index 1.3636 to 1.3638.
4. Alcohol (60 per cent v/v) (limit 59.7 to 60.2% v/v).
   Dilute 642 ml of alcohol to 1000 ml of water.
   Specific gravity 0.913 to 0.914.
   Refractive index 1.3617 to 1.3618.

5. Alcohol (50 per cent v/v) (limit 49.6 to 50.2% v/v).
   Dilute 526 ml of alcohol to 1000 ml with water.
   Specific gravity 0.934 to 0.935.
   Refractive index 1.3567 to 1.3589.

6. Alcohol (45 per cent v/v) (limit 44.7 to 45.3% v/v).
   Dilute 474 ml of alcohol to 1000 ml with water.
   Specific gravity 0.943 to 0.999.
   Refractive index 1.3576 to 1.3572.

7. Alcohol (25 per cent v/v) (limit 24.6 to 25.4% v/v).
   Dilute 263 ml of alcohol to 1000 ml with water.
   Specific gravity 0.9705 to 0.9713.
   Refractive index 1.3468 to 1.3472.

8. Alcohol (20 per cent v/v) (limit 19.5 to 20.5% v/v).
   Dilute 210 ml of alcohol to 1000 ml with water.
   Specific gravity 0.9755 to 0.9765.
   Refractive index 1.3436 to 1.3442.

Tests for purity: It is tested for acidity and alkalinity, aldehyde, fusel oil constituents, ketones, isopropyl alcohol and tertiary butyl alcohol, oil or resinous substances. Non-volatile matter complies with the requirements described under Alcohol and Methyl alcohol. The tests comply with the requirement described under Alcohol. For Methyl alcohol 5 ml diluted solution, diluted to about 10 per cent v/v of alcohol, is used for test, which should comply with the test for Methyl alcohol, described under Alcohol; commencing with the word add 2.0 ml of solution of potassium permanganate.

ETHYL ALCOHOL
Dehydrated alcohol, Absolute alcohol

Mol. Form.: C_2H_5OH Mol. Wt. 46.1

Ethyl alcohol contains not less than 99.5 per cent v/v or 99.0 per cent w/w of C_2H_6O.

Preparation: It is prepared from the constant-boiling mixture obtained by distilling the dilute alcohols by azotropic distillation with benzene or by distillation over quick lime.

Description: It is a very hygroscopic, colourless, transparent mobile, volatile liquid, odour characteristic and spirituous. It burns with a blue smokeless flame.

Solubility: It is soluble with water, with chloroform and with solvent ether.

Specific gravity: At 25° not above 0.7900 indicating not less than 99.5 per cent v/v of C_2H_6O (Appendix III).

Refractive index: At 20°, 1.3614 to 1.3618.

Tests for purity: It is tested for acidity and alkalinity, aldehyde, fusel oil constituents, methyl alcohol oily or resinous substances, non-volatile matter and benzene and related substances (complies with the requirements described under alcohol).

Test for water: Shake 10 ml in a well-closed vessel with about 0.5 g of anhydrous copper sulphate; the latter does not assume a blue colour.

Storage: Preserve Ethyl Alcohol in a tightly-closed container away from fire.

SPECIALLY DENATURED SPIRIT

Specially denatured spirit is a mixture of 19 volumes of alcohol and 1 volume of approved wood naphtha. It is not official in I.P.

Description: Complies with the description given under alcohol but having in addition the odour of wood naphtha.

Tests for identity: Dilute 0.5 ml to 5 ml with water and carry out the test for methyl alcohol under alcohol. A deep violet colour is produced.

Tests for purity: It is tested for specific gravity (at 25° 0.816 to 0.824), acidity, alkalinity, oily and resinous substances, and non-volatile matters.

Acidity: 20 ml requires not more than 0.2 ml of 0.1 N sodium hydroxide to give a pink colour with solution of phenolphthalein.

Alkalinity: 20 ml requires not more than 0.3 ml of 0.1 N hydrochloric acid to render it neutral to methyl red.

Oily or resinous substances: When mixed with water in any proportion, the solution remains clear.

Non-volatile matter: Leaves not more than 0.01 per cent w/v of residue when evaporated and dried at 105°.

Uses: This alcohol is made unfit for drinking use. It is used as an important chemical solvent for industrial and pharmaceutical purposes.

ISOPROPYL ALCOHOL
2-Propanol, Propane-2-ol

Mol. Form.: C_3H_8O Mol. Wt.: 60.1

Isopropyl alcohol, which is an isomer of propanol, is official in I.P. 2007. It is a clear colourless liquid which possesses a characteristic spirituous odour and is flammable.

Tests for identity: (A) Heat, just to boiling, a 10% v/v solution mixed with 2 ml of mercuric sulphate solution. White or yellowish white precipitate is produced.

(B) Heat gently 1 ml with 4 ml of dil. potassium dichromate sol. and 1 ml of sulphuric acid and note the acetone odour.

Tests for purity: It is tested for acidity and alkalinity; distillation range (Appendix VI); refractive index (Appendix VIII); weight per ml (Appendix III); aldehydes and ketones; benzene and related substances (Appendix VII); non-volatile matter; water insoluble matter and water (Appendix IX).

Most of the tests for purity are the same as in absolute alcohol and ethanol 95 per cent monographs.

Uses: Isopropyl alcohol is widely used as a solvent, especially for lipophilic materials, mostly oils. It is relatively non-toxic and evaporates rapidly. It is a very popular cleansing material in all kinds of electronic devices.

Biologically isopropyl alcohol is a safe non-toxic preservative and has proved to be a good alternative to formaldehyde and other synthetic preservatives. In the industry and other technical houses it is used as a solvent.

It causes headache, nausea, vomiting and CNS depression.

It should be kept away from heat and open flame and handled carefully.

STEARYL ALCOHOL
Octadecyl alcohol, 1-Octadecenol

Stearyl alcohol is a mixture of solid alcohols consisting chiefly of l-octadecanol, $C_{18}H_{38}O$.

Preparation: It can be prepared by catalytic hydrogenation of stearic acid.

Description: It is a white unctuous mass whitish flakes or granules. It has faint characteristic odour.

Tests for identity: A. Its solution, 0.5 g in 20 ml of ethanol (95%), yields a clear solution on being heated to boiling followed by cooling.

Tests for purity: It is tested for melting range, 55 to 60°C (Appendix I); acid value, not more than 2.0; hydroxyl value, 195 to 220; iodine value, not more than 2.0, saponification value, not more than 2.0, determined on 19.0 g.

Storage: Stearyl alcohol is to be stored well protected from moisture.

Uses: Its inclusion in latest I.P. should be because of its continued widespread use in pharmaceutical and cosmetic industries, as an emollient, emulcifier and as a thickener in ointments, as also its utility in shampoos and hair conditioners. It is used as an ingredient in perfumes, resins and lubricants.

CETOSTEARYL ALCOHOL

Cetostearyl alcohol is a mixture of solid aliphatic alcohol consisting chiefly of stearyl and cetyl alcohol. It may be obtained from the sperm oil, which contains the alcohols or by the reduction of the appropriate fatty acids, i.e., mixture of stearic and palmitic acids of the natural fats.

Description: It is a white or cream-coloured unctuous mass or almost white flakes or granules or cubes or castings, when heated it melts to a clear colourless or pale yellow liquid free from cloudiness or suspended matter, odour faint and characteristic, taste blend.

Solubility: Practically insoluble in water, less soluble in alcohol and in light petroleum.

Tests for purity: It is tested for Acetyl value (180 to 194), Acidity, Melting range (not below 43°), Iodine value (not greater than 3.0), Saponification value (not greater than 1.0, using about 20 g), Hydroxyl value, water, lower alcohols and hydrocarbons.

Acidity: Weigh accurately in a flask about 20 g and add 250 ml of alcohol previously neutralised to solution of phenolphthalein. Heat on a water-bath and triturate the hot solution with 0.02 N sodium hydroxide vigorously and keeping the temperature as high as possible until a pink colour persists for at least fifteen seconds. Not more than 0.25 ml of 0.02 N sodium hydroxide is required for each g of the substance taken.

Water and lower alcohols: When distilled in a boiling point apparatus not more than traces of water are present and the initial boiling point is not lower than 300°.

Hydrocarbons: Weigh accurately about 2 g and dissolve in 100 ml of petroleum ether (b.p. 40° to 60°), warming lightly on a water bath if necessary. Transfer the solution to an alumina column of about 20 cm long and 1 cm in diameter and elute successively with two portions, each of 50 ml of petroleum ether (b.p. 40° to 60°). Filter in a flask and remove the light petroleum and dry to a constant weight at 80°. The residue weighs not more than 30 mg.

Uses: It is an important pharmaceutical aid and is used in the preparation of emulsifying wax and is an ingredient of paraffin ointment and Simple ointment.

CHLOROBUTOL
Chlorbutanol, Chloretone

Mol. Form.: $CCl_3.C(CH_3)_2.OH$, $\frac{1}{2}H_2O$ Mol. Wt.: 186.5

Chlorbutol is trichloro-tert-butyl alcohol with half a molecule of water of crystallization (hemihydrate of 1,1,1-trichloro-2-methyl propanol). It contains not less than 98.0 per cent and not more than the equivalent of 101.0 per cent of $C_4H_7OCl_3$, $\frac{1}{2}H_2O$.

Preparation: It is prepared by treating alcohol with chloroform in the presence of solid potassium hydroxide.

Description: It is a fine, white to greyish-white, or yellowish-white needle-like crystals or elongated plates, odourless, taste bitter.

Solubility: Soluble in about 400 parts of water; freely soluble in alcohol; slightly soluble in chloroform and in solvent ether.

Tests for identity: (1) Dissolve 10 mg in 1 ml of alcohol (50 per cent) and add 3 ml of a 1 per cent w/v solution of calcium chloride. Add 50 mg of zinc powder and heat on a water-bath for ten minutes. Decant the clear supernatant liquid into a test tube, add 0.1 g of anhydrous sodium acetate and 2 drops of calcium chloride and, if necessary, add sufficient dilute hydrochloric acid to produce a clear solution. A red-violet to purple colour is produced. Repeat the test with the same quantities of the same reagents in the same manner but omitting zinc powder. The colour is produced.

(2) To 5 ml of a 0.1 per cent w/v solution add a few drops of solution of silver nitrate, no precipitate is produced. I.P. 2007 gives three modified tests (p. 904).

Test for purity: It is tested for reaction; melting range (not lower than 77°); chloride and sulphated ash.

Assay: Weigh accurately about 0.1 g and dissolve in 20 ml of alcohol, add 10 ml of 2 N sodium hydroxide, and heat on a water bath for five minutes. Cool, add 2.0 ml of nitric acid and 25 ml of 0.1 N silver nitrate, mix well and shake the mixture vigorously with 3 ml of nitrobenzene to coagulate the precipitate. Add 2 ml of solution of ferric ammonium thiocyanate until a permanent reddish brown colour appears which does not fade within five minutes. I.P. 2007 gives same, but a little modified assay (p. 904).

$$C_4H_7Cl_3O \longrightarrow 3NaCl$$
$$AgNO_3 + NaCl = AgCl + NaNO_3$$

Each ml of 0.1 N silver nitrate is equivalent to 0.006211 g of $C_4H_7O.Cl_3$, $\frac{1}{2}H_2O$.

Uses: Chlorbutol is used for its sedative and hypnotic properties. It was earlier used as a popular preventive for sea-sickness. Its sedative and hypnotic action resembles that of chloral hydrate. It is said to possess local anaesthetic action as well. This property is made use for making powders for topical use. As a bacteriostatic agent chlorbutol is used in pharmaceutical preparations, like injections and for ophthalmic use or for intranasal administration.

GLYCERIN
Glycerol

Mol. Form.: $CH_2(OH).CH(OH).CH_2OH$ (= $C_3H_8O_3$)   Mol. Wt.: 92.1

Glycerin is a trihydric alcohol. It contains not less than 98.0 per cent of $C_3H_8O_3$.

The European Pharmacopoeia mentions two types of products: Glycerolum 85% (with wt. per ml 1.221–1.232) and Glycerolum about 98% (with wt. per ml 1.258–1.263).

Glycerin was first discovered in 1783 by Scheele by saponification of olive oil and lead oxide. Even today large quantities of glycerins are obtained through the sponification of fats and oils. A technically important synthetic method consists in using propylene as starting material.

Preparation: Previously described under glycerol.

Description: It is a clear, colourless liquid of syrupy consistency, odourless, tastes sweet, followed by a sensation of warmth. It is hygroscopic.

Solubility: It is soluble in water and in alcohol, practically insoluble in chloroform, in solvent ether and in fixed oils.

Tests for identity: (1) Heat a few drops with 0.5 g of potassium bisulphate, acrolein is evolved which is recognised by its characteristic pungent odour.

(2) Heat in a Bunsen flame on a borax bead, it produces a green flame.

(3). I.P. 2007 gives new tests: A. It determines the identification by infrared absorption spectrophotometry (2.4.6). Spectrums with that obtained with glycerin (85%) RS or with the reference spectrum (85%) are compared. B. In this 1 ml of glycerin sample is mixed with 0.5 ml of nitric acid and this mixture is superimposed with 5 ml of potassium dichromate solution. The blue ring which develops at the interface of the two liquids should not diffuse the blue colour into the lower layer when allowed to stand for 10 minutes. C. On heating 1 ml of glycerin with 2 g of potassium hydrogen sulphate in an evaporating dish, irritant vapours are evolved which blacken the filter paper moistened with alkaline potassium mercuric iodide solution. D. Glycerin's refractive index at 20°C should be 1.470 to 1.475 (2.4.27).

Tests for purity: It is tested for colour, reaction, wt. per ml., arsenic, copper, iron, heavy metals, sulphate, chloride, acraldehyde and glucose, certain reducing substances, fatty acids and ester, water, ash, ethylene glycol, diethylene glycol and related substances.

Colour: When viewed downward against a white surface in a 50 ml Nessler tube the colour of the sample is not darker than the colour of a standard solution made by diluting 0.40 ml of ferric chloride. T.S. with water to 50 ml and similarly viewed in a Nessler tube of approximately the same diameter and colour as that containing the sample.

Reaction: A 10 per cent w/v solution is neutral to solution of litmus.

Wt. per ml: At 25°, 1.252 to 1.257 g corresponding to 98.0 to 100.0 per cent of $C_2H_8O_3$ (Appendix III).

Arsenic: Not more than 2 parts per million.

Copper: To 10 ml add 30 ml of water, mix, add 1 ml of dilute hydrochloric acid and 10 ml of a solution of hydrogen sulphide, no colour is produced.

Iron: 10 g complies with the limit test for iron.

Heavy metals: Mix 5 g with 2 ml of 0.1 N hydrochloric acid, add water to make 25 ml, the limit of heavy metals is 1.5 parts per million.

Sulphate: 1 ml complies with the limit test for sulphates.

Chloride: 1 ml complies with the limit test for chlorides.

Acraldehyde and glucose: Heat strongly, it assumes not more than a faint yellow and not pink colour. Heat further, it burns with little or no charring and with an odour of burnt sugar.

Certain reducing substances: To 5 ml in a Nessler cylinder add 5 ml of dilute solution of ammonia. Mix well and heat at 60° for five minutes. Quickly add 0.5 ml of a solution of silver nitrate from a pipette keeping the tip of the pipette above the mouth of the cylinder and allowing the reagent to fall directly into the solution without touching the sides of the cylinder. Mix thoroughly and keep in the dark for five minutes. Repeat the experiment with the same quantities of the same reagents in the same manner omitting glycerin but using 5 ml of water. Compare the turbidities/colours of the two solutions in normal daylight viewing them from the top of the cylinders preferably against a white background. The turbidity or the darkening in the sample is not greater than that of the blank.

Fatty acids and esters: Mix 50 g with 100 ml of freshly boiled water, add 1 ml of solution of phenolphthalein and neutralize, if alkaline, with 0.2 N sulphuric acid. Add 15 ml of 0.2 N sodium hydroxide, boil under a reflux condenser for five minutes, and wash down the condenser with a little water, disconnect the flask, titrate with 0.2 N sulphuric acid. Repeat the experiment with the same quantities of the same reagents in the same manner omitting glycerin and using 240 ml of water. The difference between the titrations is not more than 1.5 ml.

Sulphated ash: Ignite 50 g and allow to burn. Cool the residue, moisten with sulphuric acid, ignite, cool, moisten again with sulphuric acid and ignite to constant weight, the residue weighs not more than 5 mg (Appendix II).

Ethylene glycol, diethylene glycol and related substances: These are determined by gas chromatography (2.4.13 and Appendix VII).

Water: Not more than 2.0%, when determined on 1.5 g (Appendix IX).

Assay: I.P. 2007 describes an assay method also (p. 1170) based on titrimetry.

Storage: Glycerin is kept in a well-closed container.

Uses: Glycerin has manyfold uses. It finds large scale use in industries, including tobacco industry, as moisture holding material. It is used for nitroglycerine and for preparing cosmetic preparations. As such it is an important pharmaceutical necessity, being also used as an emollient and demulcent. It is no stranger to the body as it is regular intermediary metabolic product. Orally glycerin acts as a diuretic and if given as suppositories, it increases the parastaltic movements of the alimentary canal and acts as a mild laxative. Its use in cosmetic preparation depends upon its hygroscopic nature. It draws water from the tissues and renders the outer skin smooth and shining. It is not irritant to the skin and is an ingredient of kaolin, poultice and zinc gelatin.

Preparations: Glycerin suppositories.

Ethylene glycol [$CH_2(OH).CH_2OH$]: It is official in German Pharmacopoeia. It has been industrially manufactured in large quantities since 1928 and is used as an antifreeze material for motor radiators. Medically it was tried as a substitute for glycerin. A few deaths had resulted obviously due to use of technical grade of ethylene glycol. It is, however, considered to be not more toxic than glycerin.

Propylene glycol [$CH_3.CH(OH).CH_2OH$]: It is now official in I.P. and in B.P., DAB and USP. It is synthetically made from propene by oxidation to propene oxide, followed by acid catalyzed hydrolysis. Like glycerin it is miscible with water and is insoluble in fatty oils. It is considered to be a substitute for glycerin. Pharmaceutically its use is limited (as a solvent in the preparation of dimenhydrinate injection).

Assay: I.P. 2007 describes an assay method also based on titrimetry.

An accurately weighed amount of glycerin, about 0.1 g, is mixed with 45 ml of water and to the solution is added 25.0 ml of 2.14% w/v solution of sodium periodate and 1.0 ml of 1 M sulphuric acid. The mixture is allowed to stand for 15 minutes protected from light, followed by the addition of a 50% w/v solution of ethylene glycol and allowed to stand for another period of 20 minutes, protected from light. The solution is titrated with 0.1 M sodium hydroxide using 0.5 ml of phenolphthalein solution as an indicator. The procedure is repeated without glycerin. The difference between the two titrations represents the amount of sodium hydroxide required by glycerin.

1 ml of 0.1 M sodium hydroxide is equivalent to 0.00921 g of glycerin.

GLYCERYL TRINITRATE TABLETS
Nitroglycerin tablets; Trinitrin tablets

Nitroglycerin is actually the glyceride of nitric acid. It has been official in B.P. and other pharmacopoeias and has now been included in the latest I.P. 2007. The tablets of nitroglycerin contain not less than 85.0% and not more than 115.0% of the stated amount of glyceryl trinitrate, $C_3H_5N_3O_9$.

Preparation: Its preparation is given on p. 204 with reactions. Thus it is prepared by slowly adding glycerin to an ice-cooled mixture of conc. sulphuric acid (4 parts) and conc. nitric acid (1 part). Nitroglycerin is obtained separated as heavy oil which is purified by washing repeatedly with cold water (see reaction on p. 201).

Description: Nitroglycerin is a heavy, colourless oily liquid, practically insoluble in water and in alcohol, but it is readily soluble in ether. It has a sweetish taste. Nitroglycerin as such is a very dangerous substance to handle, and if impure it is likely to explode spontaneously. Also on being heated and/or struck with a hammer it explodes dangerously.

Tests for identity: (A) Determined by use of TLC, using silica gel G with toluene as a mobile phase (2.4.17) and p. 1712.

(B) Extract an amount equivalent to 3 mg of nitroglycerin from the powdered tablets with 5 ml of ether and filter. Evaporate the ether and dissolve the residue in 0.2 ml of sulphuric acid containing a trace of diphenylamine and note the intense blue colour produced.

Other tests relate to the tablets and should comply with the tests stated under tablets. Such tests include uniformity of content, disintegration test, etc. (p. 1173).

Assay: Since the official preparation is tablets, usual method is taking 20 tablets, making them powder and taking the powder in an amount which represents 1 mg of glyceryl trinitrate is taken for the assay, which consists of simple spectrophotometric measurement of absorbance at about 405 nm (2.4.7) (p. 1173).

Storage: Nitroglycerin tablets should be stored well protected from light and moisture in glass containers containing not more than 100 tablets and at a temperature not exceeding 30°C.

The label should state that the tablets should be dissolved slowly in the mouth.

Uses: Glyceryl trinitrate (GTN) or nitroglycerin is used to treat angina and heart failure for the last about one and a half century. In medical and pharmacy fields it is also referred to as "nitro". It is used in preventing angina attacks rather than reversing them once they have commenced. In pharmaceutical outlets transdermal patches of glyceryl trinitrate with long activity duration are also available. GTN is also indicated for AMI and pulmonary oedema. It is usually given as a sublingual dose in the form of a tablet placed under the tongue or a spray into the mouth for the treatment of an angina attack.

The principal action of glyceryl trinitrate is relaxation of vascular smooth muscle producing a vasodilator effect on both peripheral arteries and veins. Dilation of the post-capillary vessels, including large veins, promotes peripheral pooling of blood and decreases venous return to the heart, thereby reducing left ventricular end-diastolic pressure (preload). Arteriolar relaxation reduces systemic vascular resistance and arterial pressure (afterload). Myocardial oxygen consumption or demand for a given level of exercise is decreased by both the arterial and venous effects of nitroglycerin. Dilatation of the large epicardial coronary arteries by nitroglycerin contributes to the relief of exertional angina.

DIMECAPROL (B.A.L.)

$$HO \diagup \diagdown OH$$
$$SH$$

Mol. Form.: $C_3H_8OS_2$ Mol. Wt. 124.2

Dimercaprol is (RS)-2,3-dimercaptopropanol and it is a sulphur equivalent of glycerol. It contains not less than 98.5 % ant not more than 101.5% w/w of $C_3H_8OS_2$.

Preparation: It is prepared from allyl alcohol, as follows:

Description: It is a liquid, which is clear, colourless or slightly yellowish and has strong alliaceous odour, reminding of organic thiols.

Tests for identity: (A) 2 ml solution of 0.1 ml dimercaprol in 4 ml of water on the addition of lead acetate solution gives a yellow precipitate.

(B) To the other 2 ml solution of dimercaprol (from the test A above) add 1 ml of 0.05 M iodine. The colour of iodine is immediately discharged.

Tests for purity: It is tested for appearance of solution; pH, 5.0 to 6.5 (Appendix X); refractive index, 1.568 to 1.574 at 20°C (Appendix VIII); weight per ml, 1.238 to 1.240 (Appendix III); iron (2.3.14) and halides (1043).

Assay: An accurately weighed quantity (about 0.1 g) is dissolved in methanol (40 ml), to which is added 0.1 M hydrochloric acid (20 ml) and 0.05 M iodine (50.0 ml). The solution is allowed to stand for 10 minutes and titrated with 0.1 M sodium thiosulphate. A blank titration is repeated without dimercaprol. The difference between the titrations represents the amount of iodine required by the substance.

1 ml of 0.05 M iodine is equivalent to 0.00621 g of $C_3H_8OS_2$.

Storage: Dimercaprol should be stored in well filled containers protected from light in refrigerator, below 8°C.

Uses: Dimercaprol has been formerly called **British Anti-Lewisite (BAL)**, a name which is still retained as a short name. It is a heavy-metal antagonist and as such it is used as a chelating agent in the treatment of heavy metal poisoning. The drug forms a relatively stable compound with arsenic, mercury, gold and certain other metals, thus protecting the vital enzyme systems of the cells against the effects of the metals. Dimercaprol is used to treat poisoning with arsenic, gold or mercury. It is also used together with another chemical agent called edetate disodium (EDTA) to treat lead poisoning. In veterinary medicine it is used in treating intoxication caused by arsenical compounds. Dimercaprol is contraindicated in patients with impaired hepatic function. The drug is also contraindicated in iron, cadmium, and selenium poisoning as the chelated complex can be more toxic than the metal alone.

- **Dimercaprol** or **British Anti-Lewisite (BAL)** was developed by British biochemists at Oxford University during World War II. It was developed secretly as an antidote for Lewisite, the now-obsolete arsenic-based chemical warfare agent. Today, it is used medically in the treatment of arsenic, mercury, gold and lead, and other toxic metals poisoning. In addition, it has in the past been used for the treatment of Wilson's disease, a genetic disorder in which the body tends to retain copper.

- Arsenic and some other heavy metals act by chemically reacting with adjacent sulfhydryl residues on metabolic enzymes, creating a chelate complex that inhibits the affected enzyme's activity. Dimercaprol competes with the sulfhydryl groups for binding the metal ion, which is then excreted in the urine.

- Dimercaprol is itself toxic, with a narrow therapeutic range and a tendency to concentrate arsenic in some organs. Other drawbacks include the need to administer it by painful intramuscular injection.

PROPYLENE GLYCOL
1,2-Propanediol

$$\underset{H_3C}{}\overset{OH}{\diagup}\diagdown OH$$

Mol. Form.: $C_3H_8O_2$ Mol. Wt.: 75.1

Propylene glycol is (RS)-propane-1,2-diol.

Propylene glycol now forms a full-fledged official monograph in I.P. Earlier it has been official in B.P., U.S.P. and DAB.

Preparation: It is synthetically made from propene by oxidation to propene oxide, followed by acid catalysed hydrolysis.

Description: Like glycerin it is a clear colourless viscous liquid, miscible with water and insoluble in fatty oils.

Tests for identity: (A) Cool in ice 0.5 ml of 0.01% w/v solution and add to it 5 ml of a cooled mixture of 10 ml of water and 90 ml of sulphuric acid. Heat the mixture for 10 minutes at 70°C on a water bath. Add to the cool solution 0.2% of a 3% w/v of ninhydrin in a 2.5% w/v solution of sodium metabisulphite and note the violet colour, which slowly appears.

(B) On heating 0.15 ml with 0.1 g of boric acid a pleasant odour is developed.

(C) When1 ml is added to 0.5 g of potassium bisulphate and heated gently, a fruity odour develops; and when the solution is heated to dryness, no sharp acrid smell of acrolein is perceptible.

Tests for purity: It is tested for appearance of solution; acidity; boiling range (184–189°C); relative density (1.035–1.040); refractive index (1.431–1.433); heavy metals; oxidising substances; reducing substances; ethylene glycol and diethylene glycol; sulphated ash and water.

N.B.: These tests for purity are mostly common for official compounds of this chapter and they can be gone through in different appendices of this book as well as the I.P. appendices referred to here and I.P. itself.

Uses: Propylene glycol has long been considered a substitute for glycerin. It is used as a solvent in pharmaceutical industry in preparations required to be used as topical (ointments), oral and injectable formulations. It is equally important in food industry. Also it is utilized as a carrier for fragrant oils, massage oils, antibacterial lotions and saline solutions.

It is also utilized in other technical products and preparations like food colour, deodorant and moisturizer in medicines and cosmetics, tooth pastes, mouth washes, tobacco products and as an emulsifying agent. Propylene glycol has been approved by the USA's Food and Drug Administration (FDA) for its use in foods and drugs. In fact more recently FDA's experts have found that propylene glycol can be safely used in cosmetic preparations up to an amount of 50%.

Ethers

Ethers are compounds of the general formula $C_nH_{2n+2}O$ and are isomeric with monohydric alcohols. They are represented by the general structure R–O–R and they may be regarded as alkyl oxides or more appropriately as the anhydrides of the alcohols from which they are prepared. They may also be considered as the dialkyl derivatives of water.

H.O.H.	R.O.H.	R.O.R.
Water	Alcohol	Ether

When the two alkyl groups in the ether are the same, the ether is said to be symmetrical or simple, e.g. diethyl ether, $C_2H_5.O.C_2H_5$. When the two alkyl groups are different the ether is said to be unsymmetrical or mixed, e.g. ethyl methyl ether, $CH_3.O.C_2H_5$. They are also classified as open chain, cyclic, saturated, unsaturated and aromatic ethers depending on the nature of the attached groups.

Nomenclature: Two systems are used for naming ethers:

1. **Common system:** In this system, the common name is used as alkyl ether, and the individuals are named according to the alkyl group attached to the oxygen atom, e.g. $CH_3.O.CH_3$, dimethyl ether, $CH_3.O(CH_3)_2$ methyl isopropyl ether; cyclic ethers $H_2C\!\!-\!\!-\!\!CH_2$ are named

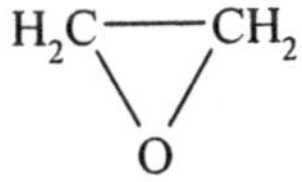

   $$\overset{H_2C-CH_2}{\underset{O}{\diagdown\diagup}}$$

   as oxides or epoxy compounds.

2. **IUPAC system:** In IUPAC system, ethers are regarded as alkoxy derivatives of alkanes and are named as alkoxy alkanes. The larger group is chosen as the alkane, e.g. $CH_3.O.CH_3$ methoxymethane, $CH_3.O.C_2H_5$ methoxyethane, $C_2H_5O.C_3H_7$ ethoxypropane and so on.

Isomerism: Ethers exhibit the structural isomerism as follows:

1. **Functional isomerism:** As stated above, ethers are isomeric with monohydric alcohols as both have the same general formula $(C_nH_{2n+2}O)$ and different functional groups. For example:

Formula:	C_2H_5O	$CH_3.O.CH_3$	C_2H_5OH
		Dimethyl ether	Ethyl alcohol
	C_3H_8O	$CH_3.O.C_2H_5$	$CH_3CH_2CH_2OH$
		Methyl ethyl ether	Propyl alcohol

2. **Metamerism:** Ethers having the same molecular formula exhibit metamerism due to the difference in the nature of alkyl group attached to oxygen atom. For example, the formula $C_4H_{10}O$ represents the isomeric ethers as given below:

$$CH_3.O.CH_2.CH_2.CH_3 \qquad CH_3.O.CH\Big\langle {\overset{\displaystyle CH_3}{\underset{\displaystyle CH_3}{}}} \qquad C_2H_5.O.C_2H_5$$

Methyl-n-propyl ether Methyl isopropyl ether Diethyl ether

GENERAL METHODS OF PREPARATION

1. **Dehydration of alcohols:** Simple ethers are prepared by the reactions of the corresponding alcohols with sulphuric or phosphoric acid at high temperature. Since a molecule of water is lost for every pair of alcohol molecules, such reaction is termed as dehydration, e.g.

$$C_2H_5.OH + HO.C_2H_5 \xrightarrow[150^\circ C]{H_2SO_4} C_2H_5.O.C_2H_5 + H_2O$$

Diethyl ether

Nucleophilic substitution reaction is involved in the preparation of ethers. The protonated alcohol acts as a substitute and a second molecule of alcohol as nucleophile. The reaction proceeds by either SN^1 or SN^2 mechanism depending whether the protonated alcohol loses the water before or simultaneously with attack by the second alcohol molecule.

$$ROH + H^+ \rightleftharpoons ROH_2^+$$

$$R^+ \xrightarrow{ROH} R\overset{\displaystyle +}{\underset{\displaystyle |}{-O}}{-}R \longrightarrow H^+ + ROR \qquad SN^1 \text{ reaction}$$

$$ROH_2^+ \quad ROH \quad \left[\underset{\displaystyle RO}{\overset{\displaystyle \delta}{}} - \underset{\displaystyle R}{\overset{\displaystyle H}{}} - \underset{\displaystyle OH_2}{\overset{\displaystyle \delta+}{}} \right] \longrightarrow \underset{\displaystyle +}{ROR} + H_2O \rightleftharpoons H^+ + ROR + H_2O$$

$$SN^2 \text{ mechanism}$$

Generally secondary and tertiary alcohols follow the SN^1 pattern. Dehydration of primary alcohols may also be effected by passing alcohol vapours over heated catalysts like thorium alumina and aluminium phosphate under high pressure and high temperature.

$$R.OH + HO.R \xrightarrow[250^\circ C/Press.]{Al_2O_3} R.O.R. + H_2O$$

Alkenes are formed when secondary and tertiary alcohols are dehydrated under these conditions.

2. **Williamson synthesis:** This method can be used for the preparation of simple as well as mixed ethers and aryl alkyl as well as dialkyl ethers. In this synthesis an alkyl halide is interacted with sodium alkoxide.

$$CH_3.O.K + BrC_2H_5 \longrightarrow CH_3.O.C_2H_5 + KBr$$

Potassium
methoxide

$$C_2H_5ONa + Cl.C_2H_5 \longrightarrow C_2H_5.O.C_2H_5 + NaCl$$

Sodium   Ethyl   Diethyl ether
ethoxide   chloride

This reaction involves SN^2 mechanism and involves the attack of alkoxide ion on the polar carbon hydrogen bond of alkyl halide.

$$R.ONa \rightleftharpoons RO^- + Na^+$$

$$RO^- + R'-X \text{ Slow } (R-O.......R'.......X^-) \xrightarrow{\text{Fast}} ROR + X^-$$

$$Na^+ + X' \rightleftharpoons NaX$$

3. **Heating alkyl halides with dry silver oxide:** Ethers are prepared by heating alkyl halides with dry silver oxide (Ag_2O). Mixed ethers can be prepared by taking different alkyl halides in equimolecular ratio.

$$2C_2H_5.Br + Ag_2O \longrightarrow C_2H_5.O.C_2H_5 + 2AgI$$

Ethyl bromide

$$CH_3I + Ag_2O + I.C_2H_5 \longrightarrow CH_3.O.C_2H_5 + 2AgI$$

4. **Reaction of lower halogenated ethers with Grignard reagents:** Grignard reagents react with lower halogenated ethers to form higher homologues of ethers.

$$CH_3.O.CH_2Cl + Br.Mg.C_2H_5 \longrightarrow CH_3.O.CH_2.C_2H_5$$

Chloromethyl   Ethyl magnesium   Methyl propyl
ether   bromide   ether

5. **Action of diazomethane on alcohols:** Ethers may be prepared by the action of diazomethane on alcohols in the presence of boron trifluoride or aluminium alkoxide as a catalyst.

$$C_2H_5OH + CH_2N_2 \xrightarrow{BF_3} C_2H_5.O.CH_3 + N_2$$

Diazomethane   Ethyl methyl ether

General Physical Properties

1. The lower members dimethyl ether and methyl ethyl ether are gases while higher members are colourless, low boiling, volatile liquids having pleasant smell.
2. All ethers are lighter than water in which they are less soluble. The solubility in water increases in the presence of small amount of alcohol. They are readily soluble in organic solvents such as benzene, chloroform, etc. Ethers themselves are very good solvents. Diethyl ether is an excellent extraction medium because it is a good solvent for organic compounds and it is not miscible with water and separates as a discrete upper layer.
3. The boiling points are much lower than those of alcohols containing the same number of carbon atoms due to the absence of hydrogen bonding. Their physical constants like boiling points, melting points and specific gravity increase with increase in molecular weight as given in the table overleaf.
4. Lower ethers show anaesthetic properties and their vapours are highly inflammable. Ether was first used as surgical anaesthesia by Long in Georgia in 1842.
5. Since C–O–C bond angle is not $180°$, the dipole moments of the two C–O bonds do not cancel each other and, therefore, ethers possess a net dipole moment (e.g. 1.18 D for diethyl ether). The C–O–C valency angle in dimethyl ethers is $111°$, while it is $118°$ in diethyl ether.

Physical constants of ether

Compound	Name	B.P. $^{\circ}$C	M.P. $^{\circ}$C	Sp. gr. at 20°C
$CH_3.O.CH_3$	Dimethyl ether	−24.9	−140	0.661
$CH_3.O.C_2H_5$	Ethyl methyl ether	7–9	–	0.697
$C_2H_5.O.C_2H_5$	Diethyl ether	35	−116	0.714
$C_3H_7.O.C_3H_7$	Di-n-propyl ether	91	−122	0.736
$C_4H_9.O.C_4H_9$	Di-n-butyl ether	142	−95	0.784

General Chemical Properties

Ethers are comparatively unreactive compounds because of their structure. There is no active hydrogen attached to oxygen as present in alcohols. The ether linkage is quite stable towards bases, oxidising agents and reducing agents. They show the reactions due to the presence of:

(i) **Alkyl group:** Substitution reactions occur on alkyl radicals as in case of saturated hydrocarbons.

(ii) **Ethereal oxygen:** The oxygen atom present in ether molecule donates electron to the electron deficient molecules or Lewis acids.

(iii) **Carbon oxygen linkage:** The carbon oxygen bond in ethers is a stable bond but not so stable as carbon-carbon linkage. So ether linkage is cleaved by acids under quite vigorous conditions, i.e. with concentrated acids at high temperature.

The following are the general chemical properties of ethers:

1. **Chemical inertness:** Ethers do not react with alkalis, dilute acids, metals, phosphorous halides in cold. They do not show the oxidation and reduction properties. The lack of reactivity is due to the absence of active group in ether molecule.

2. **Reaction of alkyl group (substitution reactions):**

   (i) **Halogenation:** When ethers are treated with chlorine or bromine they undergo substitution of alkyl radicals depending on the condition. In the dark usually the hydrogen joined to the carbon directly attached to the oxygen atom is most readily replaced, e.g. diethyl ether reacts with chlorine in the dark to form 1,1-dichlorodiethyl ether:

$$CH_3.CH_2.O.CH_2.CH_3 + Cl_2 \xrightarrow[-HCl]{} CH_3.CH(Cl).O.CH_2CH_3 \xrightarrow[-HCl]{Cl_2} CH_3.CCl_2.O.CH_2.CH_3$$

   In the presence of light, perdichlordiethyl ether is formed when all the hydrogens of ethers are substituted with chlorine atoms.

$$C_2H_5.O.C_2H_5 + 10Cl_2 \xrightarrow{Light} C_2Cl_5.O.C_2Cl_5 + 10HCl$$

   (ii) **Combustion:** Ethers are highly volatile and inflammable. They burn in air to give carbon dioxide and water.

$$C_2H_5.O.C_2H_5 + 4O_2 \longrightarrow 4CO_2 + 5H_2O$$

3. **Reaction of ethereal oxygen:** Ethers behave as Lewis bases due to the presence of two unshared lone pair of electrons on oxygen atom. Therefore, they react with Lewis acids or electron deficient species. The following reactions of ethereal oxygen are observed.

   (i) **Formation of oxonium salts:** Concentrated mineral acids form stable oxonium salts with ethers at low temperature. Thus diethyl ether combines with hydrogen chloride by attachment of a proton to oxygen by one of the unshared electron pairs to produce a cation that is bonded to chloride ion by electrostatic forces.

$$C_2H_5.O.C_2H_5 + HCl \longrightarrow (C_2H_5)_2OH^+Cl^- \longrightarrow (C_2H_5)_2O + HCl$$

Diethyl oxonium salt

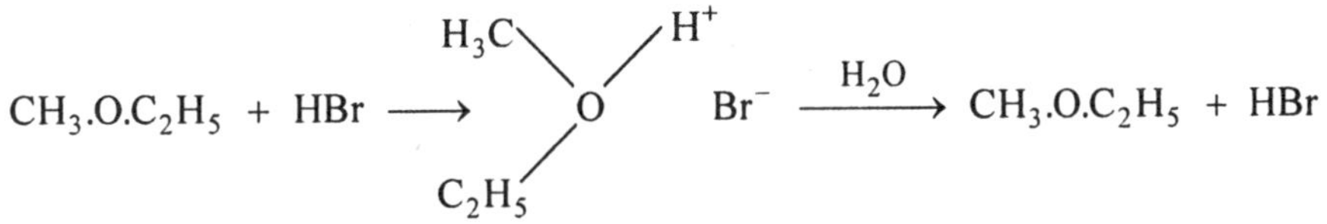

$$CH_3.O.C_2H_5 + HBr \longrightarrow$$

Ethyl methyl
oxonium salt

Ethers also readily form coordination complexes called etherates with Lewis acids like BF_3, $AlCl_3$, $RMgX$, etc.

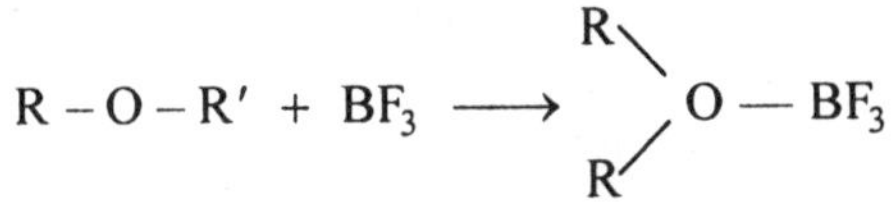

$$R-O-R' + BF_3 \longrightarrow$$

Boron trifluoride etherate

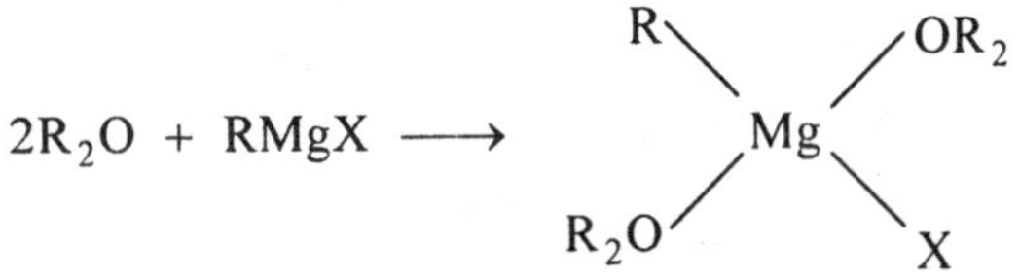

$$2R_2O + RMgX \longrightarrow$$

Ether complex of
Grignard reagent

(ii) **Formation of peroxides:** Formation of peroxides takes place when ethers react with atmospheric oxygen or ozonized oxygen due to formation of coordinate bond with one lone pair of the ethereal oxygen and that of another atom.

$$C_2H_5 - O - C_2H_5 + O \longrightarrow C_2H_5 - O - C_2H_5$$

O
Peroxide

These peroxides are unstable compounds and decompose violently when they are heated. It is, therefore, necessary to remove the peroxide by washing with alkaline $KMnO_4$ or $FeSO_4$ solutions before distilling the long-stored ether.

(iii) **Dehydration:** The ethereal oxygen can be eliminated in the form of water when vapours of ethers are passed over heated aluminium to produce alkenes.

$$C_2H_5.O.C_2H_5 \xrightarrow[360°C]{Al_2O_3} 2CH_2 = CH_2 + H_2O$$

4. **Reaction of ether linkage:**

(i) **Hydrolysis:** Hydrolysis of ethers is carried out either by boiling water or with steam to form alcohols in the presence of dilute acids as catalysts.

$$C_2H_5 - O - C_2H_5 + H_2O \longrightarrow 2C_2H_5OH$$

(ii) **Action of hydrobromic or hydroiodic acids:** Ethers react with hydrobromic or hydroiodic acids in cold and the ether linkage between hydrocarbon residues is split producing alcohols and alkyl halides. When mixed ethers are treated with these acids the halogen attaches itself to the smaller of the two alkyl groups of ether, e.g.:

$$CH_3.O.C_2H_5 + HI \longrightarrow \underset{\substack{\text{Methyl} \\ \text{iodide}}}{CH_3I} + \underset{\substack{\text{Ethyl} \\ \text{alcohol}}}{C_2H_5.OH}$$

When the reaction is carried out under hot conditions only alkyl halides are formed.

$$C_2H_5.O.C_2H_5 + 2HI \longrightarrow 2C_2H_5I + H_2O$$

$$CH_3.O.C_2H_5 + 2HBr \longrightarrow CH_3Br + C_2H_5Br + H_2O$$

The order of reactivity of the halogen acids is HI > HBr > HCl. This reaction is used for the detection and estimation of alkoxy group in ethers and is referred as Zeivel's method. A weighed sample of ether is heated with approximately 57 percent HI. The alkyl halide formed is isolated and absorbed in an alcoholic solution of silver nitrate when the precipitate of silver iodide is obtained. This is filtered, washed, dried and weighed. Thus $AgI \equiv R. I \equiv OR$ and the number and amount of –OR groups can be calculated from the weights of silver iodide and the compound.

The mechanism involved in this reaction is either SN^1 (for secondary and tertiary alkyl groups) or SN^2 (for primary alkyl groups).

$$R.O.R' + H^+ \longrightarrow \overset{\overset{\displaystyle H}{|}}{\underset{+}{R.O.R}}$$

SN^1 mechanism:

$$\underset{+}{\overset{\overset{\displaystyle H}{|}}{R - O - R}} \xrightarrow{\text{Slow}} R^+ + R'OH$$

$$R^+ + X^- \xrightarrow{\text{Fast}} R - X$$

SN^2 mechanism:

$$X^- + \underset{+}{\overset{\overset{\displaystyle H}{|}}{R - O - R}} \longrightarrow (H ....R........ \overset{\overset{\displaystyle H}{|}}{O - R'}) \longrightarrow R - X + R'OH$$

(iii) **Action of sulphuric acid:** Ethers form oxonium salts with cold sulphuric acid. With hot sulphuric acid the ether linkage is broken to form alcohol and alkyl hydrogen sulphate.

$$C_2H_5.O.C_2H_5 + H_2SO_4 \text{ (Conc.)} \longrightarrow C_2H_5.OH + C_2H_5.HSO_4$$

Ethanol   Ethyl hydrogen
sulphate

(iv) **Action of acid chlorides or anhydrides:** Ethers react with acid derivatives in the presence of catalysts like anhydrous aluminium chloride or zinc chloride to give esters.

$$C_2H_5.O.C_2H_5 + (CH_3.CO)_2O \longrightarrow 2CH_3.CO.OC_2H_5$$

Acetic anhydride   Ethyl acetate

(v) **Reaction with carbon monoxide:** When treated with carbon monoxide at 125–180°C and at a pressure of 500 atmosphere in the presence of boron trifluoride and a little water, ethers yield esters.

$$C_2H_5.O.C_2H_5 + CO \xrightarrow[\text{500 atm., } H_2O]{BF_3/150°C} C_2H_5.CO.OC_2H_5$$

Ethyl propionate

5. **Other reactions:**

(i) **Oxidation:** Ethers are oxidized with strong oxidising agents like acidic potassium dichromate to form aldehydes or acids:

$$C_2H_5.O.C_2H_5 \xrightarrow[-H_2O]{K_2Cr_2O_7/H^+} 2CH_3.CHO \xrightarrow{(O)} 2CH_3.COOH$$

Acetaldehyde   Acetic acid

(ii) **Reaction with alkali metals:** Most of the ethers react with strong bases like alkali metals and sodamide, e.g. ethyl sodium, being a very strong base, abstracts one hydrogen from ether.

$$NaC_2H_5 + H-CH_2-CH_2-O-C_2H_5 \longrightarrow C_2H_6 + C_2H_4 + C_2H_5ONa$$

Ethane   Ethene   Sodium
ethoxide

Uses: Diethyl ether is used as a general anaesthetic, as refrigerant and as solvent for extraction of organic compounds in perfumery and acts as a denaturant of alcohols. It provides an inert medium for various organic reactions such as Wurtz's reaction. Grignard reagents, lithium aluminium hydride reduction, etc.

ANAESTHETIC ETHER

Anaesthetic ether is the purified diethyl ether containing a suitable stabilizer in a proportion of about 0.002 percent w/w and 4 percent of ethanol and water.

When ether is kept in contact with air and light, it partly decomposes with formation of non-volatile unstable oxidizing substances called ethyl peroxide. Clover (1922) suggested the oxidizing product as a derivative of hydrogen peroxide of formula $CH_3.CH_2.O.CH.(CH_3).O.OH$, while Wieland and Wingler (1923) considered it as a dihydroxydiethyl peroxide of formula $CH_3.CH(OH).O.CH(OH).CH_3$. The oxidizing properties of impure ether are due to the presence of this organic peroxide. The peroxide may explode violently in a distillation carried to dryness with consequent overheating.

The stabilizers added to the anaesthetic ether are the reducing agents and prevent the formation of peroxides. Generally di- or polyhydric phenols or propyl gallate are used as stabilizers.

The small proportion of ethanol and water present in the ether raises the boiling point and prevents frosting on the anaesthetic mask in open anaesthesia resulting from the rapid evaporation of the ether.

The bottles containing Anaesthetic ether, if closed by ordinary corks, extracts matter from the cork. So the cork should be coated with foil to prevent the extraction.

THIO-ETHERS (R₂S)

They are either sulphur analogues of the ethers or dialkyl derivatives of hydrogen sulphides, just as ethers are the dialkyl derivatives of water.

$$R.O.R. \xrightarrow[+S]{-O} R.S.R. \xleftarrow[+2R]{-2H} H.S.H$$

Ether   Thioether   Hydrogen
                                            sulphide

The two alkyls may be the same or different. The common as well as systematic names are given in the chapter of nomenclature.

General Methods of Preparation

(i) **From alkyl halides:** They are prepared by heating alkyl halides with potassium sulphide, e.g.:

$$2C_2H_5I + K_2S \longrightarrow C_2H_5.S.C_2H_5 + 2KI$$

Ethyl iodide   Diethyl thio ether
                           or diethyl sulphide

Thioethers are also formed when alkyl halides are heated with sodium mercaptide.

$$C_2H_5Cl + Na.S.C_2H_5 \longrightarrow C_2H_5.S.C_2H_5 + NaCl$$

Sodium ethyl
mercaptide

(ii) **From ethers:** Formation of thioethers takes place when ethers are heated with phosphorous pentasulphide.

$$5RO.R + P_2S_5 \longrightarrow 5R.S.R. + P_2O_5$$

$$5C_2H_5.O.C_2H_5 + P_2S_5 \longrightarrow 5C_2H_5.S.C_2H_5 + P_2O_5$$

(iii) **From thioalcohols:** When a thiol is passed over heated catalyst like alumina or zinc sulphide at 300° thioethers are produced.

$$2C_2H_5SH \xrightarrow[300°C]{Al_2O_3/ZnS} C_2H_5.S.C_2H_5 + H_2S$$

Thioethers are also formed by the addition of thiol to an alkene in the presence of peroxides.

$$CH_3.CH = CH_2 + C_2H_5.SH \xrightarrow{Benzyl\ peroxide} CH_3.CH_2.CH_2.S.C_2H_5$$

$$CH_2 = CH_2 + C_2H_5.SH \xrightarrow{Peroxide} C_2H_5.S.C_2H_5$$

Ethene

(iv) **From mercaptides:** The mercaptides decompose on heating to yield thioethers. For example:

$$(C_2H_5S)Pb \longrightarrow C_2H_5.S.C_2H_5 + PbS$$

Lead diethyl   Diethyl sulphide
mercaptide

General physical properties: Thioethers are colourless, volatile, unpleasant oils. They have higher boiling points than those of the corresponding ethers. They are insoluble in water but soluble in organic solvents. The C–S–C bond angle in thioethers is about 105°.

General chemical properties: They resemble ethers in their chemical properties. Since the nine pairs of electrons present on sulphur atom are somewhat far away from the nucleus in comparison to ethers, therefore, sulphur has a greater tendency to act as an electron pair donor or base and they undergo addition reactions much more readily than ethers.

1. **Addition of halogens:** Thioethers add with halogens easily to give dihalo derivatives.

$$C_2H_5.S.C_2H_5 + Br_2 \longrightarrow$$

Diethyl sulphide

$$\begin{matrix} C_2H_5 & & Br \\ & \diagdown \diagup & \\ & S & \\ & \diagup \diagdown & \\ C_2H_5 & & Br \end{matrix}$$

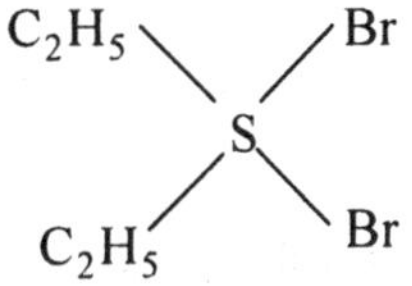

Diethyl sulphide
dibromide

2. **Addition of alkyl halides:** They add with alkyl halides to form sulphonium salts which are similar to oxonium salts formed in case of ethers.

$$C_2H_5.S.C_2H_5Br \longrightarrow (C_2H_5)_3 : S.Br$$

Triethyl sulphonium
bromide

These sulphonium salts form sulphonium hydroxides when they are treated with moist silver oxide. Sulphonium hydroxides decompose on heating to form thioethers and alkenes.

$$(C_2H_5)_3.S:I + AgOH \longrightarrow (C_2H_5)_3.S:OH$$

Triethyl sulphonium
hydroxide

$\downarrow \Delta$

$$(C_2H_5)_2.S + CH_2 = CH_2 + H_2O$$

Diethylthioether   Ethene

3. **Addition of metal salts:** Thioethers react with metal salts to give coordination compounds in the precipitated form, e.g.:

$$C_2H_5.S.C_2H_5 + HgCl_2 \longrightarrow (C_2H_5)_2.S \longrightarrow HgCl_2$$

Diethyl sulphide   Mercuric chloride

4. **Addition with sulphuric acid:** With concentrated sulphuric acid they give sulphonium salts like ethers.

$$C_2H_5.S.C_2H_5 + H_2SO_4 \longrightarrow (C_2H_5.SH)_2.HSO_4$$

5. **Hydrolysis:** They are hydrolyzed with alkalis to yield alcohols.

$$C_2H_5.S.C_2H_5 + H_2O \xrightarrow{\text{NaOH}} 2C_2H_5.OH + H_2S$$

6. **Oxidation:** With mild oxidizing agents like hydrogen peroxide, chlorine water etc. they are oxidized to sulphoxides and then to sulphones.

$$C_2H_5.S.C_2H_5 \xrightarrow{H_2O_2 + CH_3.COOH} [(C_2H_5)_2.S \longrightarrow O] \longrightarrow (C_2H_5)_2.S \overset{O}{\underset{O}{\lessgtr}}$$

Diethyl sulphoxide

Diethyl sulphone

With strong oxidizing agents like concentrated nitric acid or potassium permanganate they directly give sulphones on oxidation.

$$(C_2H_5)S \xrightarrow[2[O]]{\text{HNO}_3} (C_2H_5)_2.S \overset{O}{\underset{O}{\lessgtr}}$$

Uses: They are used for the preparation of sulphoxide (used as solvent, e.g. dimethyl sulphoxide), sulphine (crystalline solids used to characterize thioethers), mustard gas (used as a poison gas in war) and sulphonium salts (useful in the study of sulphur chemistry).

VINYL ETHER (CH$_2$ = CH)$_2$O

Divinyl ether or vinyl ether or vinesthene is an unsaturated ether. It is prepared from ethylene chlorohydrin which is dehydrated by concentrated sulph.ric acid to give 2,2-dichlorodiethyl ether. This product when treated with solid potassium hydroxide yields divinyl ether by dehalogenation reaction.

$$\begin{array}{c} CH_2Cl.CH_2OH \\ + \\ CH_2Cl.CH_2OH \end{array} \xrightarrow[-H_2O]{H_2SO_4} \begin{array}{c} CH_2Cl.CH_2 \\ \diagdown \\ O \\ \diagup \\ CH_2Cl.CH_2 \end{array} \xrightarrow[-2HCl]{2KOH} \begin{array}{c} CH_2 = CH \\ \diagdown \\ O \\ \diagup \\ CH_2 = CH \end{array}$$

Two moles of
ethylene chlorohydrin

2, 2-Dichloro-
diethyl ether

Divinyl ether

Divinyl ether is a colourless, inflammable, highly volatile liquid which boils at 28.3°C.

It is similar to ether and ethene in chemical characteristics and shows the general reactions of both. Due to unsaturation, it immediately decolourises bromine water.

Vinyl ether contains about 4 percent v/v dehydrated alcohol, 0.01 percent w/v of N-phenyl-α-naphthylamine as a stabilizer. The small portion of alcohol raises the boiling point and prevents frosting on the anaesthetic mask as in case of anaesthetic ether. The phenyl-α-naphthylamine added to the ether acts as an antioxidant. Due to the presence of this stabilizer vinyl ether often contains purple fluorescence. It is unstable in air and light.

Vinyl ether is used by inhalation for short anaesthesia and for inducing anaesthesia. It is considered to do better than diethyl ether because of its rapid recovery from the anaesthesia.

OFFICIAL COMPOUNDS

ANAESTHETIC ETHER
(CH₃CH₂OCH₂CH₃)

Mol. Form: $(C_2H_5)_2O$ Mol. Wt.: 74.12

Anaesthetic ether is purified diethyl ether. It contains a suitable stabilizer in a proportion not greater than 0.002 per cent w/v.

It is a grade of ether which is specially prepared for use as an anaesthetic. The use of stabilizer in ether is intended to prevent the development of peroxides. The reducing agents used in ether are di- or polyhydric phenols and propyl gallate. The decomposition of ether takes place through the formation of hydroperoxides by the action of oxygen of the air as:

$$CH_3-CH_2-O-CH_2-CH_3 + O_2 \longrightarrow CH_3-CH-O-CH_2-CH_3$$

$$\underset{\underset{CH_3-CH-O-CH_2-CH_3}{|}}{H-O-O} \longrightarrow H_2O_2 + CH_2=CH-O-CH_2-CH_3$$

$$\underset{CH_3-CH-O-O-HC-CH_3}{\overset{OH\quad\quad OH}{|\qquad\quad|}} \xleftarrow{\;\;H_2O_2\;\;} CH_3-CHO + HOH_2C-CH_3$$

The pharmacopoeia prescribes the test for aldehyde with Nessler's reagent when no colour or turbidity should result in five minutes (only very faint opalescence). The ether peroxides can decompose with explosion if ether is heated. Hence ether should be tested for peroxide only before its distillation (boiling range). The peroxides are tested by use of potassium iodide and starch. If peroxides are present, the potassium iodide (reducing agent) gets its iodide ion oxidised to free elemental iodine, which gives colour with starch.

Preparation: See previous pages.

Description: A colourless, transparent, very mobile liquid; odour characteristic, taste sweet and burning, very volatile and inflammable; mixture of its vapour with oxygen air or nitrous oxide in certain concentrations are explosive.

Solubility: Soluble in 12 parts of water, miscible with alcohol, with chloroform and with fixed and volatile oils.

Boiling range: 34 to 35° (App. VI). It is dangerous to determine the boiling range, if the sample does not comply with the test for peroxides.

Tests for purity: It is tested for wt. per ml (at 20°, 0.714 to 0.716) (App. IV), acetone and aldehyde; foreign odour; methyl alcohol; peroxides; sulphurous acid and other free acids; non-volatile matters and water (not more than 0.2% in 20 ml) (App. IX).

Acetone and aldehyde: Place 2 ml of alkaline solution of potassium mercuric iodide in a stoppered tube of about 12 ml capacity and about 1.5 cm diameter and fill the tube with Anaesthetic ether, insert the stopper, shake vigorously for fifteen seconds and set aside for five minutes; no colour or turbidity is produced; ig colour or turbidity is produced, distill carefully the Anaesthetic ether in a fractionating column and repeat the test on the distillate; no colour or turbidity is produced.

A very faint opalescence may sometimes be produced but there shall be no colouration or colouration followed by turbidity.

Foreign odour: Pour 10 ml in successive portions on to a clean filter paper and allow to evaporate spontaneously; no foreign odour is detectable at any stage of the evaporation.

Methyl alcohol: To 10 ml, add 5 ml of alcohol (20 percent) and 5 ml of water, in a separator, shake vigorously, set aside and allow the mixture to separate and draw off the lower layer. To 5 ml of lower layer add 2.0 ml of solution of potassium permanganate and phosphoric acid, set aside for ten minutes and add 2.0 ml of solution of oxalic and sulphuric acids, to the colourless solution add 5 ml of decolourised solution of magenta and set aside for thirty minutes; no colour is produced.

Peroxides: Place in a stoppered tube of about 12 ml capacity and about 1.5 cm in diameter 8 ml of solution of potassium iodide and starch, fill to the brim with the sample of Anaesthetic ether and place the stopper in position so that no air bubble is enclosed, shake vigorously and set aside in the dark for thirty minutes; no brown or reddish colour is produced.

Sulphurous acid and other free acids: Place 10 ml of alcohol (80 percent) in a 50 ml glass stoppered flask, add 0.5 ml of solution of phenolphthalein and just sufficient 0.02 N sodium hydroxide to produce a pink colour which persists after gently shaking the mixture for thirty seconds. Add a further quantity of 0.2 ml of 0.02 N sodium hydroxide and 25 ml of Anaesthetic ether. Stopper the cylinder, mix and shake gently for thirty seconds; the pink colour is not discharged.

Non-volatile matter: 50 ml when evaporated and dried to constant weight at 105° leaves not more than 1 mg of residue. It is dangerous to perform this test if the sample does not comply with the test for peroxides.

Storage: Preserve Anaesthetic ether in a dry bottle protected from light, or in a copper container or container copper plated internally and store in a cool place. The bottle shall be closed with a well fitting screw cap or with velvet cork covered with tin foil.

Note: It is absolutely essential that a preservative of the type of sodium pyrogallate, hydroquinone or propyl gallate in suitable concentrations shall be added in Anaesthetic ether intended for use in tropical climates unless the Anaesthetic ether is stored in a copper container or in a container copper plated internally. The preservative used and its concentration shall be declared on the label.

Labelling: The label also states (1) very inflammable; do not use near an open flame or other source of heat which may cause ignition; (2) the name and proportion of any stabilizer added.

Uses: Ether is used as a general anaesthetic and as such it was first used in 1842 for its narcotic action in surgical operation. In a concentration of 7 vol. percent in the inspired air, full narcosis is achieved in about 20 minutes. Since concentration of 7 vol. percent is the maximum tolerated, the long indication time is avoided by using initially rapidly acting narcotics, like ethyl chloride, nitrous oxide etc. and then maintaining the narcosis with 4.5 vol. percent of ether. For an adult for full narcosis about 50 to 60 ml of ether is required. Ninety percent of ether is eliminated through respiration. In overdoses of ether respiratory centre is paralysed. In contrast to chloroform, which may stop the heart, ether has no undesirable action on heart. Ether's inflammability and explosive nature (by forming explosive mixture with air) are the disadvantages which speak in its disfavour as an ideal anaesthetic. Besides, it has local irritant effect. It is contraindicated in patients suffering from diabetes, pneumonia and certain thorax diseases. With the modern technical operations the lethal cases by use of ether as a narcotic are only 1 in 30,000.

Preparation: Spirit of ether: It is prepared by shaking 330 ml of anaesthetic ether and mixing it with alcohol (90%) sufficient to produce 1000 ml. It is used as a pharmaceutical aid.

Dose: 1 to 4 ml.

Like most of other preparations of compounds, spirit of ether is also not included in I.P. any more.

SOLVENT ETHER
(Ethyl oxide)

Mol. Form: $(C_2H_5)_2O$ Mol. Wt.: 74.12

Solvent ether is diethyl ether. For description and solubility see under anaesthetic ether above.

Tests for purity: It is tested for wt. per ml (at $20°$ is 0.714 to 0.718 g), boiling range ($34°$ to $36°$), methyl alcohol (same as in anaesthetic ether), acetone and aldehyde; peroxides; sulphurous acid and other free acids (same as in anaesthetic ether using 0.4 ml in place of 0.02 N sodium hydroxide); and non-volatile matter (same as under anaesthetic ether).

Peroxides: Place in a stoppered tube of about 12 ml capacity and about 1.5 cm in diameter, 8 ml of a freshly prepared solution of potassium iodide and starch and fill to the brim with the solvent ether being tested. Place the stopper in position so that no air bubble is enclosed; shake vigorously and set aside in the dark for thirty minutes. If any yellow colour is produced, it is not deeper than that of 0.5 ml of 0.001 N iodine diluted with 8 ml of solution of potassium iodide and starch.

Storage: Preserve solvent ether in a well closed container in a cool place, protected from light.

Uses: It is used as a pharmaceutical aid.

VINYL ETHER
(Divinyl ether, Divinyl oxide, Vinethene, Ethnoxyethene)

Mol. Form.: $(CH_2 : CH)_2O$ Mol. Wt.: 70.09

Vinyl ether is divinyl ether to which has been added about 4 percent v/v of Ethyl alcohol and not more than 0.01 percent w/v of phenyl-α-naphthylamine or other stabiliser. It is not official now in I.P. though it continues to be so in other official books.

Preparation: Vinyl ether is prepared from ethylene chlorohydrin, which on dehydration by sulphuric acid gives 2,2-dichlorodiethyl ether. The 2,2-dichlorodiethyl ether is then treated with solid potassium hydroxide to yield divinyl ether as follows:

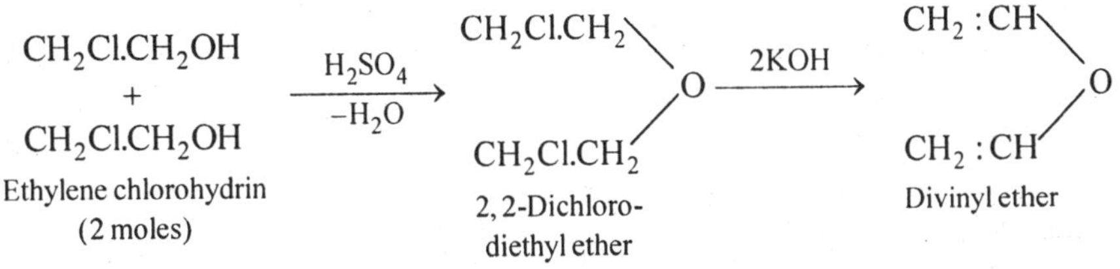

Description: A clear colourless, inflammable liquid, often with a purplish fluorescence derived from the stabiliser, odour characteristic.

Solubility: Sparingly soluble in water. Miscible with alcohol, with solvent ether and with chloroform.

Tests for identity: (1) Warm 2 ml with 2 ml of dilute sulphuric acid; acetaldehyde is evolved.

(2) Shake 2 ml with 2 ml of solution of bromine; the colour is immediately discharged.

Tests for purity: It is tested for the following:

Boiling range: 28° to 31° (App. VI).

Reaction: Shake 5 ml with 2 ml of water for two minutes; the aqueous layer is neutral to solution of litmus.

Wt. per ml: At 25°, 0.767 to 0.771 g (App. III).

Aldehydes: Add 2 ml previously cooled to 0° to a mixture of 1 ml of a 10 percent v/v solution of sodium hydroxide and 1 ml of solution of silver ammonium nitrate previously cooled to 0°. Shake the mixture for ten seconds, then allow to stand for thirty minutes in the dark at 0°. Shake again and allow the aqueous layer to separate. The aqueous layer is not darker than that of a standard prepared by shaking 2 ml of benzene with 2 ml of a solution prepared by diluting to 100 ml of a mixture of 2 ml of a solution of cobalt chloride, and 2 ml of a 2.70 percent w/v solution of ferric chloride.

Chlorinated compounds: Mix 25 ml with 20 ml of amyl alcohol in a flask fitted with a reflux condenser and add 2 g of sodium in small pieces. Heat on a water bath until evolution of hydrogen ceases; then boil gently under a reflux condenser until all the sodium has dissolved; continue the heating for a further twenty minutes. Cool, add 15 ml of nitric acid, 1 ml of nitrobenzene and 10 ml of 0.02 N silver nitrate. Add 20 ml of water, shake well and titrate using solution of ferric ammonium sulphate as indicator. Repeat the experiment with the same quantities of the same reagents in the same manner omitting vinyl ether; the difference in the volumes of 0.02 N ammonium thiocyanate required does not exceed 4 ml.

Non-volatile matter: Leaves not more than 0.01 percent w/v of residue when evaporated spontaneously and dried to constant weight at 105°.

Foreign odour: Pour 10 ml in successive portions on a clean paper and allow to evaporate spontaneously; no foreign odour is detectable at any stage of the evaporation.

Storage: Preserve Vinyl ether in a well closed container of not more than 200 ml capacity and store in a cool place protected from light. It should not be used if the original container has been opened for a period longer than forty hours.

Labelling: The label on the container must state very inflammable. Do not use near an open flame or other source of heat which may cause ignition. The name and proportion of any stabiliser added must be stated.

Uses: It is used as a general anaesthetic. It acts stronger than ether and induces full anaesthesia quickly. The elimination is also quick. It has the disadvantage of damaging liver and other organs. Besides, it is less stable chemically.

Vinyl ether is, as a matter of fact, a potent anaesthetic with a large safety margin. The ratio of the anaesthetic to lethal dose for vinyl ether is 1 to 2.4, while that of ethyl ether is 1 : 1.5. This potency was, however, found to be difficult to control with simplistic equipment. Besides warm temperatures increase the volatility of vinyl ether, making it hard to regulate it through open drop technique. Its only strengths over ethyl ether are its favourable induction and recovery, as stated above.

Aldehydes and Ketones

Aldehydes and ketones have the general formula $C_nH_{2n}O$ and contain the same functional group, carbonyl group (C=O). When one valency of this group is satisfied by hydrogen atom then the group is called a formyl group (–CHO). The compounds possessing the carbonyl group are often referred to as carbonyl compounds. It is the carbonyl group that largely determines the chemistry of aldehydes and ketones. The name 'aldehyde' is derived from the fact that they are obtainable by dehydrogenation of alcohol (alcohol dehydrogenation), and the well known name ketone is derived from that of the simplest member of the series, acetone.

In aldehydes the remaining two valencies of the carbon atom of carbonyl group are satisfied by a hydrogen atom and a hydrocarbon group. Formaldehyde is exceptional in which two hydrogen atoms are attached to the carbonyl carbon and no alkyl substituents are present; and it exhibits certain unique properties. In ketones both these valencies are satisfied by the same or different hydrocarbon groups. This difference in structure affects their properties in two ways: (a) aldehydes are easily oxidised, whereas ketones are oxidized with difficulty, (b) aldehydes are usually more reactive than ketones towards nucleophilic addition reaction.

$$
\begin{array}{ccccc}
& \overset{\displaystyle H}{\overset{\displaystyle |}{}} & \overset{\displaystyle R}{\overset{\displaystyle |}{}} & \overset{\displaystyle R}{\overset{\displaystyle |}{}} & \overset{\displaystyle R'}{\overset{\displaystyle |}{}} \\
-\text{C}=\text{O} & \text{H}-\text{C}=\text{O} & \text{H}-\text{C}=\text{O} & \text{R}-\text{C}=\text{O} & \text{R}-\text{C}=\text{O} \\
\text{Carbonyl group} & \text{Formaldehyde} & \text{An Aldehyde} & \text{Simple Ketone} & \text{Mixed Ketone}
\end{array}
$$

Ketones may be of two types: Simple ketones when both the alkyl groups are the same (e.g., acetone) and mixed when both groups are different (e.g. ethyl methyl ketone).

Carbonyl carbon is attached to other atoms by σ bonds. Since these bonds utilize sp^2 orbitals, they lie in a plane having bond angle of 120°. The remaining p orbital of the carbon overlaps a p orbital of oxygen to form a π-bond. Thus carbon and oxygen atoms are joined by a double bond. The double bond between carbon and oxygen atoms contains σ-bond and a π-bond. The carbonyl group holds together atoms of different electronegativity and, therefore, the electrons are not equally shared. The mobile electrons are pulled towards the more electronegative oxygen atom. Hence, the bond is about 40 to 50 per cent ionic in character and, therefore, has high dipole moment and high boiling point as compared to the corresponding hydrocarbons.

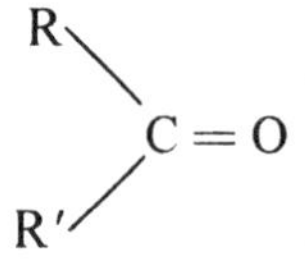

Flat carbonyl group

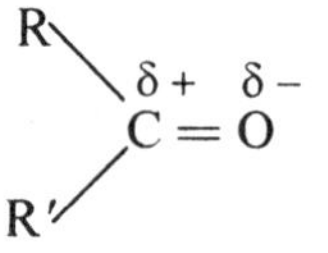

Polarity of carbonyl group

Nomenclature

Aldehydes: The common names of aldehydes are derived from the names of the corresponding carboxyl acids by replacing -ic of acid by -aldehyde. Thus the aldehyde which on oxidation gives formic acid is called as formaldehyde and the one which gives acetic acid as acetaldehyde.

In IUPAC system the longest chain carrying the –CHO group is considered the parent structure and is named by replacing the -e of the corresponding alkane by -al. The position of a substituent is indicated by a number, the carbonyl carbon always being considered as C-1. Thus:

Formula of aldehyde	Corresponding acid	Common name	IUPAC name
H.CHO	H.COOH (Formic acid)	Formaldehyde	Methanal
CH_3.CHO	CH_3.COOH (Acetic acid)	Acetaldehyde	Ethanal
C_2H_5.CHO	C_2H_5.COOH (Propionic acid)	Propionaldehyde	Propanal
C_3H_7.CHO	C_3H_7.COOH (Butyric acid)	Butyraldehyde	Butanal
C_4H_9.CHO	C_4H_9.COOH (Valeric acid)	Valeraldehyde	Pentanal
CH_3.CH.CH_2.CHO | OH	CH_3.CH.CH_2.COOH | OH (β-Hydroxy) - butyric acid)	β-Hydroxybutyraldehyde	2-Hydroxy butanal
CH_3.CH_2.CH.CH_2.CHO | CH_3	CH_3.CH_2.CH.CH_2.COOH | CH_3 (β-Methylvaleric acid)	β-Methylvaleraldehyde	3-Methyl pentanal
CH_3.CH.CH_2.CH_2.CHO | CH_3	CH_3.CH.CH_2.CH_2.COOH | CH_3 (γ-Methylvaleric acid)	Isocaproaldehyde	4-Methyl pentanal

Ketones: The common name of the simplest aliphatic ketone is acetone. For naming other aliphatic ketones two groups are named attached to carbonyl carbon following these names by the word ketone.

According to the IUPAC system the longest chain carrying the carbonyl group is considered the parent structure, and is named replacing the -e of the corresponding alkane with -one. The positions of various groups are indicated by numbers, the carbonyl carbon being given the lowest possible number, e.g.:

Formula	Common name	IUPAC
$CH_3.CO.CH_3$	Acetone	Propanone
$CH_3.CH_2.COCH_3$	Ethyl methyl ketone	Butanone
$CH_3.CH_2.CH_2.CO.CH_3$	Methyl-n-propyl ketone	2-Pentanone
$CH_3.CH_2.CO.CH_2CH_3$	di-Ethyl ketone	3-Pentanone
$(CH_3)_2.CH.CO.CH_3$	Methylisopropyl ketone	3-Methyl-2-butanone

Isomerism: Aldehydes exhibit chain isomerism amongst themselves and functional isomerism with ketones, cyclic ethers and unsaturated alcohols. Ketones show chain isomerism and metamerism.

(i) Chain isomerism:

$CH_3.CH_2.CH_2.CHO$ n-Butyraldehyde $(CH_3)_2.CH.CHO$ Isobutyraldehyde

$CH_3.CH_2CH_2.COCH_3$ Methyl propyl ketone $(CH_3)_2.CH.CO.CH_3$ Methyl isopropyl ketone

(ii) Functional isomerism:

$CH_3.CH_2.CHO$ Propanal $CH_3.COCH_3$ Acetone $CH_2 = CH.CH_2.OH$ Allyl alcohol

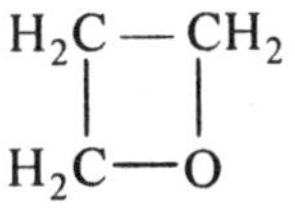

α,γ-Propylene oxide α,β-Propylene oxide

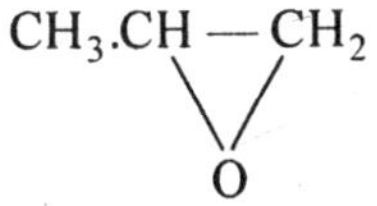

(iii) Metamarism:

$CH_3.CH_2.CO.CH_2.CH_3$ 3-Pentanone $CH_3.CH_2CH_2.CO.CH_3$ 2-Pentanone

General methods of preparation: The aldehydes and ketones can be prepared by the following analogous methods:

1. **From alcohols:** A primary alcohol on oxidation with acidic potassium dichromate, manganese dioxide or chromic acid in glacial acetic acid or in pyridine gives aldehydes as the initial product and this is convertible on further oxidation. The aldehyde so obtained is more susceptible to oxidation than the starting material. Secondary alcohols, however, under these conditions readily yield ketones which are more stable to oxidation than aldehydes.

$$CH_3.CH_2.OH + [O] \longrightarrow CH_3.CHO + H_2O$$
Ethanol   Acetaldehyde

$$(CH_3)_2CH.OH + [O] \longrightarrow CH_3.CO.CH_3 + H_2O$$
Isopropyl alcohol   Acetone

In an alternate experimental procedure conversion of an alcohol to the corresponding carbonyl compounds takes place when the vapourized substance is passed over heated copper in the temperature range 200–300°. The carbon-oxygen double bond is formed by elimination of two atoms of hydrogen as a molecule of H_2; hence the process is usually referred as dehydrogenation.

$$CH_3.CH_2.OH \xrightarrow[200-300°C]{Cu} CH_3.CHO + H_2$$

$$(CH_3)_2.CHOH \xrightarrow[200-300°C]{Cu} CH_3.COCH_3 + H_2$$

Aluminium tert-butroxide oxidizes secondary alcohols to ketones in the presence of acetone. The reaction is called as Oppenauer oxidation (1937), and is useful for oxidizing unsaturated secondary alcohols.

$$\begin{matrix} R \\ \diagdown \\ CH.OH \\ \diagup \\ R' \end{matrix} + CH_3.CO.CH_3 \xrightarrow{[(CH_3)_3C.O]_3-Al} \begin{matrix} R \\ \diagdown \\ C=O \\ \diagup \\ R' \end{matrix} + (CH_3)_2CH.OH$$

2. **From fatty acids: (i) Pyrolysis of calcium salts:** This elegant method consists of heating the calcium salts of fatty acids alone at high temperature; the net result is the pyrolysis of the salts. Thus formaldehyde is achieved when calcium formate is subjected to pyrolysis.

$$\underset{\text{Calcium formate}}{(H.COO)_2Ca} \xrightarrow{\text{Heat}} CaCO_3 + \underset{\text{Formaldehyde}}{H.CHO}$$

Other aldehydes are obtained by heating a mixture of the calcium salts of formic acid and any one of its homologues, e.g.

$$\underset{\text{Calcium acetate}}{(CH_3.COO)_2Ca} + (H.COO)_2Ca \xrightarrow{\text{Heat}} 2CaCO_3 + \underset{\text{Acetaldehyde}}{2CH_3.CHO}$$

Heating the calcium salts of any monocarboxylic acid other than formic acid leads to the formation of ketones. The barium, thorium, and manganese salts are also used in place of calcium salts.

$$(CH_3.COO)_2Ca \xrightarrow{\text{Heat}} CaCO_3 + \underset{\text{Acetone}}{CH_3.CO.CH_3}$$

A mixed ketone is produced by heating together a mixture of calcium salts of different fatty acids. However, the yield achieved is poor due to side reactions.

$$\underset{\text{Calcium acetate}}{(CH_3.COO)_2Ca} + \underset{\text{Calcium propionate}}{(C_2H_5.COO)_2Ca} \xrightarrow{\text{Heat}} 2CaCO_3 + \underset{\text{Methyl ethyl ketone}}{CH_3.CO.C_2H_5}$$

(ii) **Catalytic decomposition of fatty acids:** In this process aldehydes are formed when a mixture of formic acid and any other carboxylic acid in vapourized form are passed over thorium (350°), alumina (440°) or manganese oxide (500°).

$$CH_3.COOH + H.COOH \xrightarrow[400°C]{Al_2O_3} \underset{60°}{CH_3.CHO} + H_2O + CO_2$$

A ketone is achieved when vapours of fatty acids are passed alone over these catalysts at high temperature.

$$CH_3COOH \xrightarrow[500°C]{MnO_2} CH_3.CO.CH_3 + H_2O + CO_2$$

Mixed ketones are also formed when a mixture of vapours of different fatty acids other than formic acid is subjected to this reaction.

3. **From acid chlorides:** A useful procedure transforming an acid into an aldehyde having the same carbon chain is the reduction of acid chlorides with hydrogen in the presence of

palladium catalyst supported on barium sulphate in boiling xylene (Rosemund's reduction, 1918).

$$R.CO.Cl + H_2 \xrightarrow[\text{Xylene}]{Pd/BaSO_4} R.CHO + HCl$$

Use of barium sulphate prevents further reduction of aldehydes to alcohols. Ketones cannot be synthesized by this method. However, they can be prepared by the use of organocadmium compounds.

Grignard reagents react with dry cadmium chloride to yield the corresponding organo-cadmium compounds which react with acid chlorides to yield ketones:

$$2R'.MgX + CdCl_2 \longrightarrow R'_2.Cd + 2MgXCl$$

Alkyl magnesium   Dialkyl
halide   cadmium

$$R_2.Cd + 2R.CO.Cl \longrightarrow 2R.CO.R' + CaCl$$

Ketone

4. **From dihalides:** A convenient route for the preparation of carbonyl compounds is the hydrolysis of dihalides. Terminal halides containing two halogens on the same carbon atom are hydrolyzed with mild alkalies such as barium hydroxide to yield aldehydes. However, hydrolysis of dihalides containing two halogens on middle carbon atom results in the formation of a ketone.

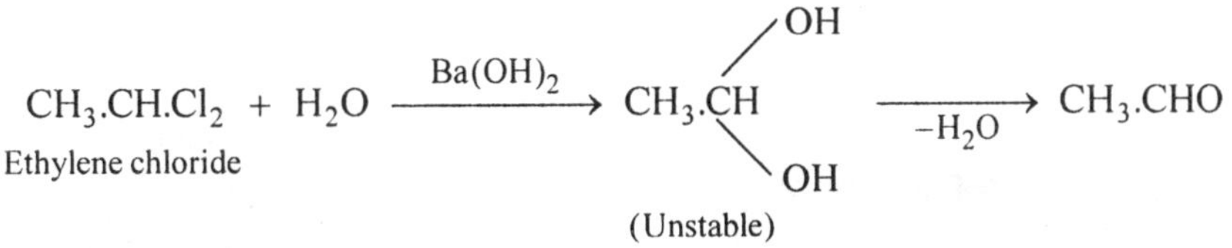

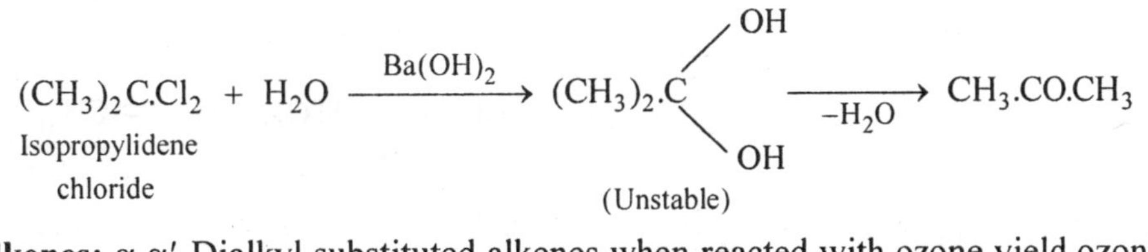

$$CH_3.CH.Cl_2 + H_2O \xrightarrow{Ba(OH)_2} CH_3.CH \Big\langle {}^{OH}_{OH} \xrightarrow[-H_2O]{} CH_3.CHO$$

Ethylene chloride   (Unstable)

$$(CH_3)_2C.Cl_2 + H_2O \xrightarrow{Ba(OH)_2} (CH_3)_2.C \Big\langle {}^{OH}_{OH} \xrightarrow[-H_2O]{} CH_3.CO.CH_3$$

Isopropylidene
chloride   (Unstable)

5. **From alkenes:** α,α'-Dialkyl substituted alkenes when reacted with ozone yield ozonides which when subjected to hydrolysis or catalytic hydrogenation produce aldehydes.

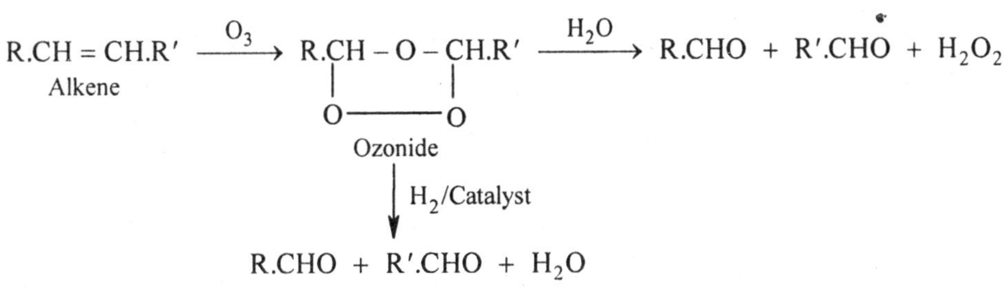

$$R.CH = CH.R' \xrightarrow{O_3} R.CH - O - CH.R' \xrightarrow{H_2O} R.CHO + R'.CHO + H_2O_2$$

Alkene

$$\begin{array}{c} | \qquad\qquad | \\ O \underline{\qquad\qquad} O \end{array}$$

Ozonide

$$\Big\downarrow H_2/\text{Catalyst}$$

$$R.CHO + R'.CHO + H_2O$$

With tetra substituted alkenes at carbon-carbon double bond ozonolysis gives ketones.

$$R_2C = CR'_2 \xrightarrow{O_3} R_2.C - O - CR'_2 \xrightarrow{H_2O} R_2C = O + R'_2.C = O + H_2O_2$$

Alkene (with the $O - O$ bridge below)

$$\downarrow H_2/Catalyst$$

$$R_2.C = O + R'_2.C = O + H_2O$$

Aldehydes are also prepared by the hydroformylation of alkenes. In this process, developed in Germany (1943) and investigated further by Adkins (1948–49), aldehydes are obtained when a mixture of alkene, carbon monoxide and hydrogen is passed over dicobalt octa-carbonyl catalyst at 125° under high pressure (600–1000 lbs/sq. in.).

$$R.CH = CH_2 + CO + H_2 \xrightarrow[125°/(1000\,lbs/sq.\,in.)]{[Co(CO)_4]_2} R.CH_2.CH_2.CHO + R.CH_2CH_3 + R.CH.CH_3$$
$$|$$
$$CHO$$

A mixture of two possible aldehydes results, but the primary aldehyde generally predominates.

6. **From glycols:** Oxidation of secondary and tertiary glycols with lead tetraacetate or periodic acid leads to the formation of aldehydes and ketones, respectively.

$$\begin{array}{c} R.CH.OH \\ | \\ R.CH.OH \end{array} + [O] \xrightarrow{(CH_3.COO)_4 Pb} 2R.CHO + H_2O$$

$$\begin{array}{c} R_2C.OH \\ | \\ R'_2C.OH \end{array} + [O] \xrightarrow{HIO_4} 2R_2C = O + H_2O$$

7. **From alkynes:** Acetylene, when passed into hot dilute sulphuric acid under the catalytic influence of mercuric sulphate, is converted into acetaldehyde.

$$CH \equiv CH + H_2O \xrightarrow[HgSO_4]{H_2SO_4} [CH_2 = CH.OH] \rightleftharpoons CH_3.CHO$$
Ethyne $\qquad\qquad\qquad\qquad$ Unstable $\qquad$ Acetaldehyde

Other alkynes such as propyne when treated in the same manner yield ketones.

$$CH_3CH \equiv CH + H_2O \longrightarrow CH_3.C(OH) = CH_2 \rightleftharpoons CH_3.CO.CH_3$$
Propyne $\qquad\qquad\qquad$ Unstable $\qquad\qquad$ Acetone

On the other hand, terminal and non-terminal alkynes give aldehydes and ketones respectively, by hydroboration and disiamyl borane followed by oxidation.

$$R.C = C.H + \xrightarrow{Si\,\alpha_2BH} R.CH = CH.BSi\,\alpha_2 \xrightarrow{H_2O} [R.CH = CH.OH]$$
$$\downarrow$$
$$R.CH_2.CHO$$

8. **From cyanides:** Grignard reagent reacts with hydrogen cyanide and alkyl cyanides to form adducts which on hydrolysis produce the carbonyl compounds.

$$HC \equiv N + R.MgBr \longrightarrow R.CH = NMgBr \xrightarrow{H_2O} R.CHO + NH_3 + Mg(OH).Br$$

Hydrogen   Grignard   Adduct   Aldehyde
cyanide   reagent

$$CH_3.C \equiv N + R.MgX \longrightarrow \underset{H_3C}{\overset{R}{\diagdown}} C = N.MgBr \xrightarrow{H_2O} \underset{H_3C}{\overset{R}{\diagdown}} C = O + NH_3 + Mg(OH).Br$$

Methyl cyanide   Ketone

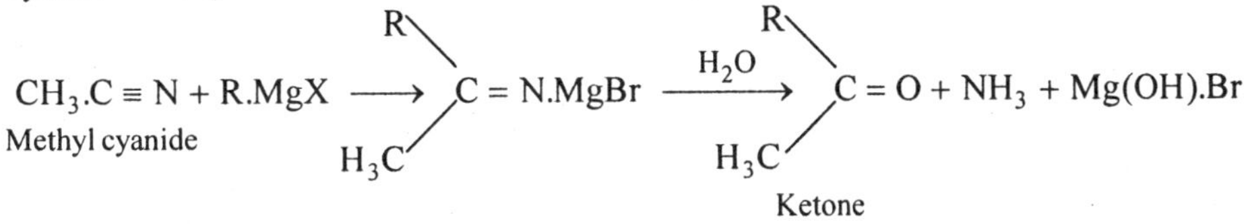

Aldehydes may be obtained by reducing a nitrile dissolved in ether with stannous chloride and hydrochloric acid following the hydrolysis of aldimine stannic chloride so obtained (Stephen's method). An aldehyde is also obtained when alkyl cyanide is reduced with lithium aluminium hydride following the hydrolysis of the resultant product.

$$CH_3C \equiv N \xrightarrow{HCl} [CH_3.C \equiv \overset{+}{N}H]\,\overset{-}{C}l \xrightarrow{SnCl_2/HCl} [CH_3.CH = NH_2]\,SnCl_6$$

Methyl cyanide   Imino chloride   Aldimine stannic chloride

$$\xrightarrow{H_2O} 2CH_3.CHO + 2NH_4Cl + SnCl_4$$

9. **From esters:** Reaction of Grignard reagent with equimolar amounts of formic ester gives aldehydes. However, ketones are obtained when esters other than formic esters are treated with Grignard reagent in the same proportion.

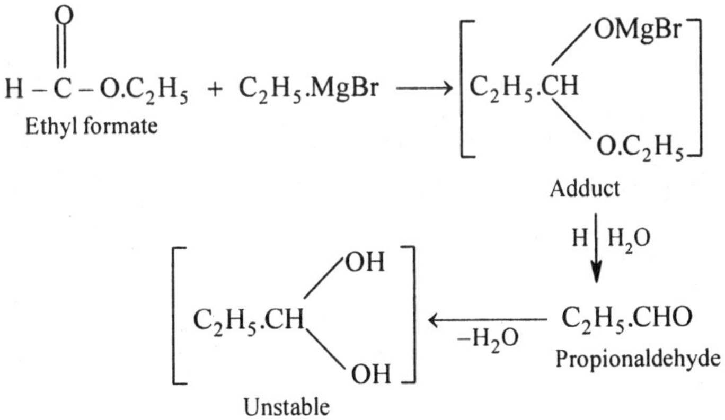

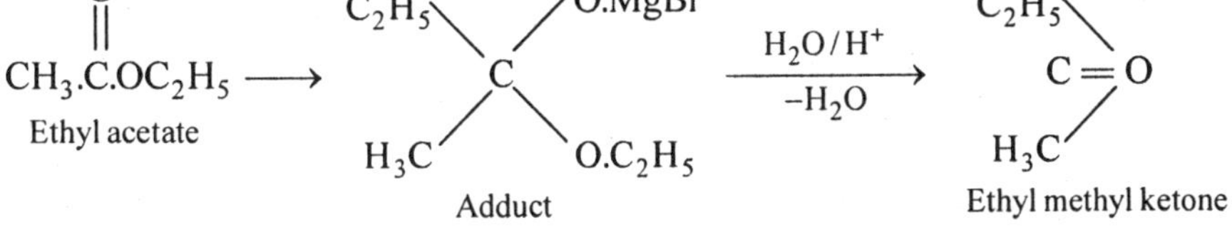

H–C–O.C$_2$H$_5$ + C$_2$H$_5$.MgBr $\longrightarrow$ Adduct

Ethyl formate

$$C_2H_5.CH\diagup^{OH}_{\diagdown OH} \xleftarrow[-H_2O]{} C_2H_5.CHO$$

Unstable   Propionaldehyde

CH$_3$.C.OC$_2$H$_5$ $\longrightarrow$

Ethyl acetate   Adduct   Ethyl methyl ketone

10. **From acetoacetic ester:** Acetoacetic ester is converted by sodium ethoxide into the sodioacetoacetic ester which is then allowed to react with an alkyl halide to form an alkyl acetoacetic ester. The alkylation can be repeated to yield a dialkyl acetoacetic ester. When hydrolyzed by dilute aqueous alkali or acid, these mono- or dialkyl acetoacetic esters yield the corresponding acids which on decarboxylation form ketones.

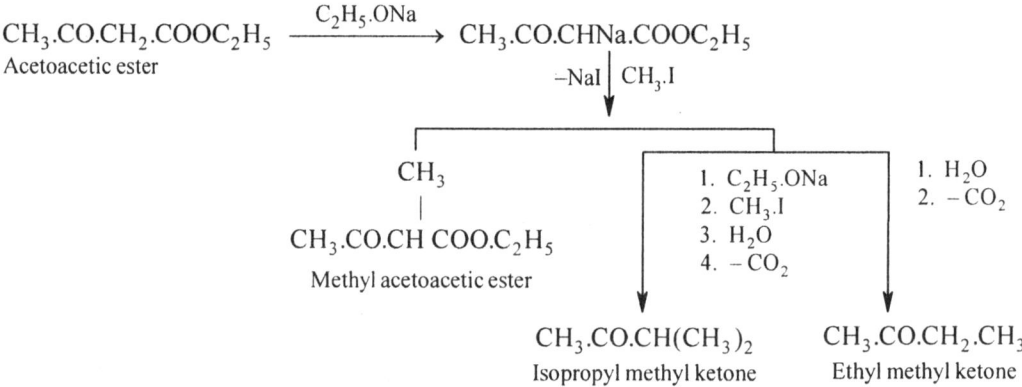

Acetaldehyde cannot be prepared by this method.

General Physical Properties

Formaldehyde is the first member of the aldehyde series which is a gas. The next ten aldehydes are colourless volatile liquids. Lower ketones having upto ten carbon atoms are also colourless volatile liquids. The higher members of these carbonyl compounds are solids.

The lower aldehydes have unpleasant odour and ketone members have fruity smell. Ketones possess pleasant odour.

The polar carbonyl group makes aldehydes and ketones polar compounds, and hence they have higher boiling points than non-polar compounds of comparable molecular weight. They contain hydrogen bonded only to carbon and so they do not have intermolecular hydrogen bonding. As a result they have lower boiling points than comparable alcohols or carboxylic acids. Boiling points increase with increase in molecular weight.

The lower members upto five carbons of aldehydes and ketones are freely soluble in water but the solubility decreases rapidly with rise in the molecular weight. However, they dissolve freely in organic solvents like alcohol and ether. Their physical contents are tabulated below

Physical constants of aldehydes and ketones

Formula	Name	B.P. (°C)	M.P. (°C)	Sp. gr.	Solubility g/100 g H_2O
Aldehydes					
H.CHO	Formaldehyde	–21	–92	0.815	v. sol.
CH_3.CHO	Acetaldehyde	20	–121	0.795	–
$CH_3.CH_2CHO$	Propionaldehyde	49	–81	0.797	16
$CH_3(CH_2)_2CHO$	n-Butyraldehyde	76	–99	0.817	7
$(CH_3)_2.CH.CHO$	Isobutyraldehyde	64	–66	0.794	–
$CH_3.(CH_2)_3.CHO$	n-Valeraldehyde	93	–51	0.819	sl. vol.
$CH_3.(CH_2)_4.CHO$	n-Caproicaldehyde	131	–56	0.834	sl. vol.
$CH_3.(CH_2)_5.CHO$	Heptaldehyde	155	–42	–	0.1

(Contd.)

Formula	Name	B.P. (°C)	M.P. (°C)	Sp. gr.	Solubility g/100 g H_2O
$CH_2 = CH.CHO$	Acrylicaldehyde	53	–87	0.814	–
$CH_3.CH = CH.CHO$	Crotonaldehyde	104	–69	0.858	–
Ketones					
$CH_3.CO.CH_3$	Acetone	56	–94	0.790	–
$CH_3.CO.C_2H_5$	Methyl ethyl ketone	80	–86	0.805	26
$C_2H_5.CO.C_2H_5$	Diethyl ketone	101	–39	–	5
$CH_3.CO.C_3H_7$	Methyl propyl ketone	102	–78	–	6.3
$C_2H_5.CO.C_3H_7$	Ethyl propyl ketone	124	–	0.818	sl. sol.
$CH_3.CO.C_4H_9$	Methyl butyl ketone	150	–35	–	2.0
$CH_3.CO.CH(CH_3)_2$	Methyl isosropyl ketone	119	–85	1.9	–
$CH_3.CO.C.(CH_3)_3$	t-Butyl methyl ketone	106	–53	–	–
$CH_3.CO.CH = C(CH_3)_2$	Mesityl oxide	130	–53	0.865	–
$CH_3.CO.CH_2.CO.CH_3$	Acetylacetone	138	–23	0.972	–
$CH_3.CO.CO.CH_3$	Biacetyl	88	–	0.990	–

General Chemical Properties

The reactions of aldehydes and ketones are due to the presence of carbonyl group, C=O. This carbonyl group governs the reactions in two ways: (a) by providing a site for nucleophilic addition; and (b) by increasing the acidity of the hydrogen atoms attached to the α-carbon.

The carbonyl group contains a carbon-oxygen double bond. Oxygen attracts the mobile electrons strongly, carbonyl carbon is electron deficient and carbonyl oxygen is electron rich. Due to this unequal distribution of electrons, the carbon is positive and oxygen is negative. The nucleophilic reagents, or electron rich species, will attack the carbonyl groups at the electron deficient carbon. Therefore, the typical reaction of aldehydes and ketones is nucleophilic addition, the mechanism is demonstrated below:

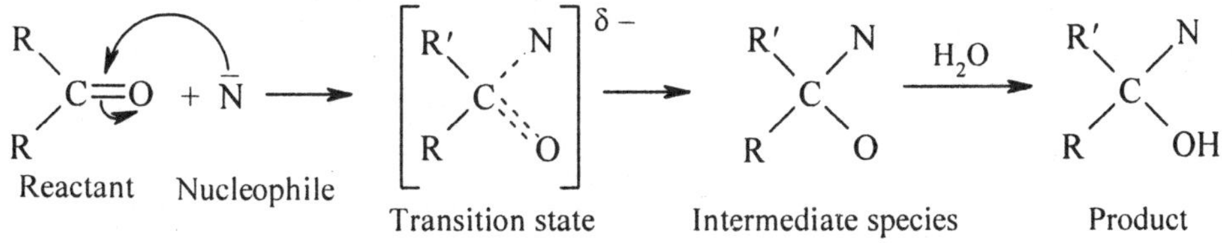

When a nucleophile approaches the carbonyl carbon, the electrons are shifted towards oxygen atom by electrometric shift and the carbon atom becomes electron deficient. The nucleophile then combines with this carbon to yield an anion which then reacts with a proton or an electrophile to give the product.

In the transition state oxygen has gained negative charge and acquired the electrons. It is the tendency of oxygen to acquire electrons as well as its ability to carry a negative charge that is the real cause of the reactivity of the carbonyl group towards nucleophiles.

Aldehydes generally undergo nucleophilic addition reaction more readily than ketones because in ketones +I effect due to two alkyl groups will decrease the electron density at carbonyl carbon to a greater extent than the one alkyl group present in aldehydes. The other factor is the steric hindrance. A second alkyl group of a ketone is larger than the hydrogen of an aldehyde, and resists more strongly the crowding together in the transition state. For the same reason formaldehyde will be more reactive than any other aldehyde.

If α-hydrogen of the alkyl group is replaced by a group causing strong inductive effect like halogen and nitro groups then the reactivity of carbonyl group increases.

The hydrogen atoms attached to α-carbon are acidic. When this hydrogen is released carbanion is formed which is resonance stabilized. This release is facilitated by strong bases which accept these protons.

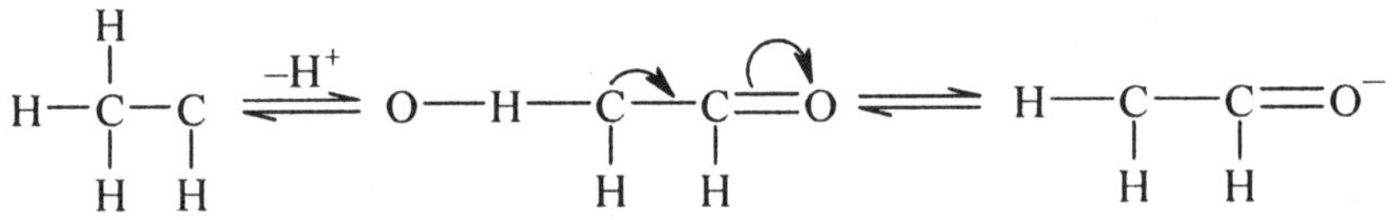

The reaction sites in aldehydes and ketones are the carbonyl group and α-alkyl groups which are common in both of them. Therefore, the reactions involving these parts are more or less similar. However, the attachment of a hydrogen to the carbonyl group in aldehydes gives some different properties from that of ketones.

REACTIONS COMMON TO ALDEHYDES AND KETONES

1. **Reduction:** Most aldehydes and ketones can be readily reduced to primary and secondary alcohols respectively, either by catalytic hydrogenation or by use of chemical reducing agents like, sodium borohydride etc.

$$CH_3.CHO + H_2 \xrightarrow{\text{Ni}} CH_3.CH_2.OH$$

Acetaldehyde   Ethanol

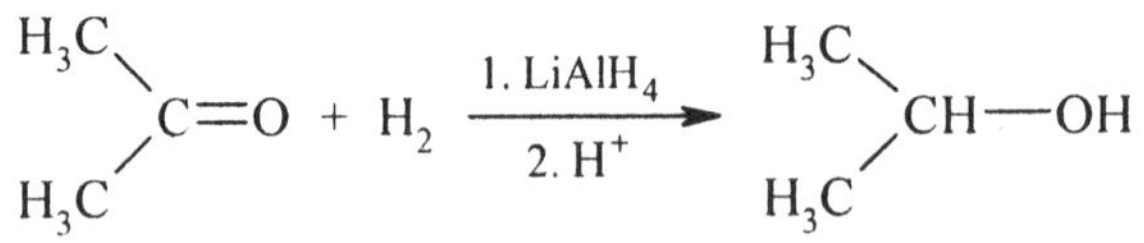

Acetone   Isopropyl alcohol

$$CH_3.CH = CH.CHO + 2[H] \xrightarrow[\text{2. H}^+]{\text{1. NaBH}_4} CH_3.CH = CH.CH_2.OH$$

Crotonaldehyde   2-Buten-1-ol

The carbonyl compounds on reduction with amalgamated zinc and concentrated hydrochloric acid or with red phosphorus and hydriodic acid result in the formation of alkanes (Clemmensen reduction).

$$R'.CO.R \xrightarrow[\text{Zn–Hg/HCl}]{\text{H}^+} R.CH_2.R$$

Ketone   Alkane

A process for reduction of the aldehydes and ketones is the Meerwein-Ponndorf procedure (1925–26) which consists of heating a compound in benzene or toluene with aluminium isopropoxide and distilling the acetone from the mixture so obtained.

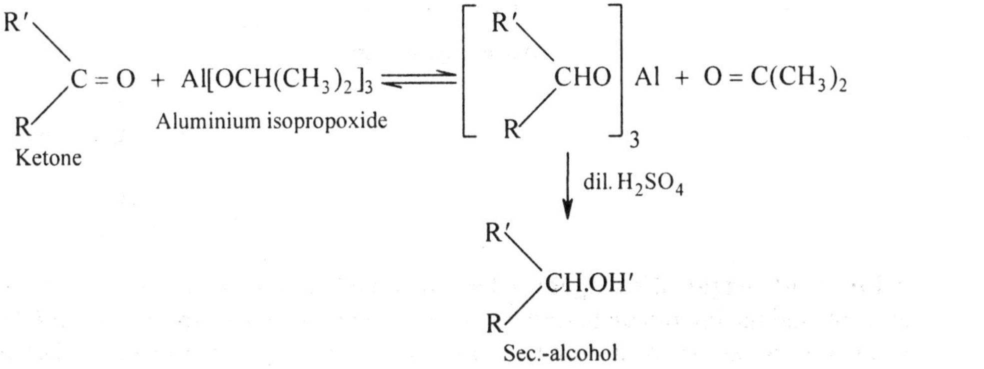

$$\underset{\substack{\text{Ketone}}}{\underset{R}{\overset{R'}{\diagdown}}C=O} + Al[OCH(CH_3)_2]_3 \rightleftharpoons \left[\underset{R}{\overset{R'}{\diagdown}}CHO\right]_3 Al + O=C(CH_3)_2$$

Aluminium isopropoxide

$$\downarrow \text{dil. } H_2SO_4$$

$$\underset{\substack{\text{Sec.-alcohol}}}{\underset{R}{\overset{R'}{\diagdown}}CH.OH'}$$

2. **Addition of sodium bisulphite:** Aldehydes and ketones add on sodium bisulphite to form crystalline bisulphite compounds.

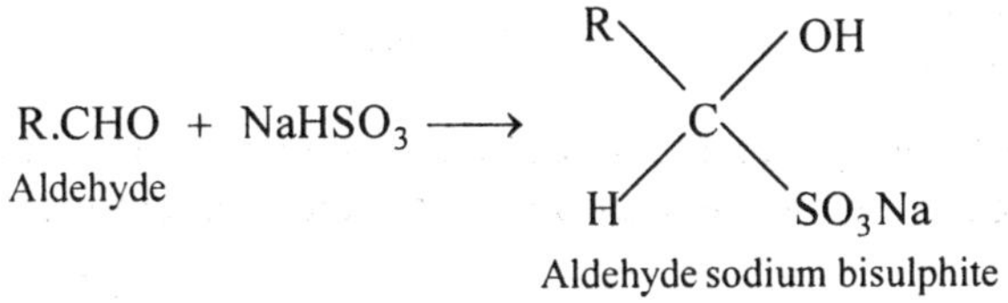

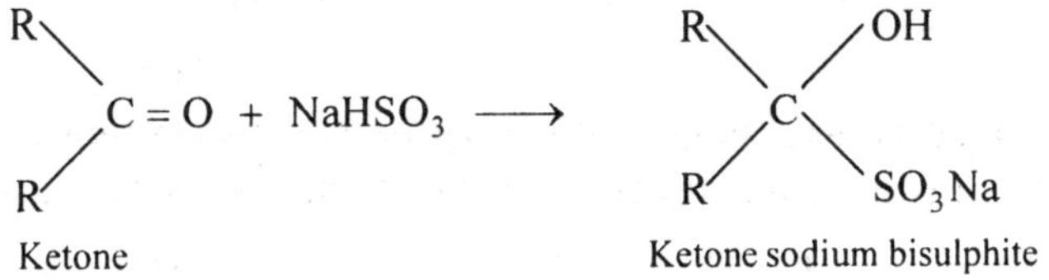

$$\underset{\substack{\text{Aldehyde}}}{R.CHO} + NaHSO_3 \longrightarrow \underset{\substack{\text{Aldehyde sodium bisulphite}}}{\overset{R}{\underset{H}{\diagup}}\overset{OH}{\underset{C}{\diagdown}}\overset{}{\underset{SO_3Na}{}}}$$

$$\underset{\substack{\text{Ketone}}}{\underset{R}{\overset{R}{\diagdown}}C=O} + NaHSO_3 \longrightarrow \underset{\substack{\text{Ketone sodium bisulphite}}}{\overset{R}{\underset{R}{\diagup}}\overset{OH}{\underset{C}{\diagdown}}\overset{}{\underset{SO_3Na}{}}}$$

These sulphites are hydroxysulphuric acid salts in which the sulphur is directly attached to the carbon atom. They reproduce the carbonyl compounds when heated with dilute acid or sodium bicarbonate. Hence this reaction is generally used for separating carbonyl compounds from non-carbonyl compounds.

3. **Addition of hydrogen cyanide:** Aldehydes and ketones add on hydrogen cyanide to yield cyanohydrin products. The reaction is often carried out by adding dilute sulphuric acid into a mixture of carbonyl compound and aqueous sodium cyanide. Cyanohydrins are important compounds in organic synthesis since they are easily converted to α-hydroxy acids.

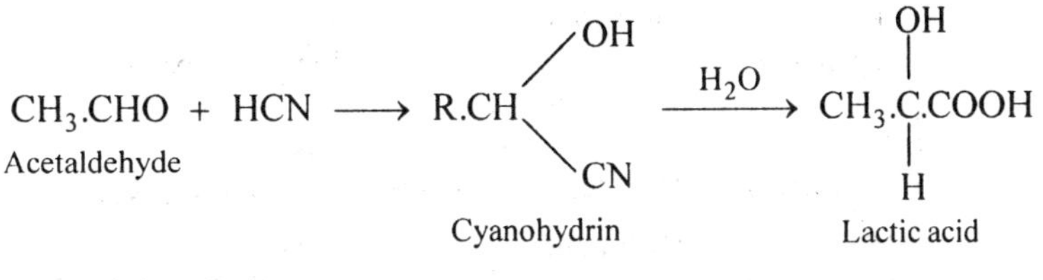

$$\underset{\substack{\text{Acetaldehyde}}}{CH_3.CHO} + HCN \longrightarrow \underset{\substack{\text{Cyanohydrin}}}{R.CH{\overset{OH}{\underset{CN}{\diagdown}}}} \xrightarrow{H_2O} \underset{\substack{\text{Lactic acid}}}{CH_3.\overset{OH}{\underset{H}{C}}.COOH}$$

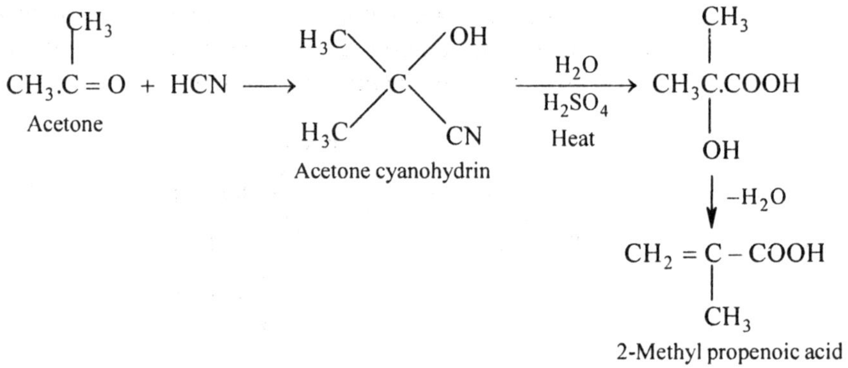

$$CH_3.C=O + HCN \longrightarrow$$

Acetone

Acetone cyanohydrin

$$\xrightarrow[\text{Heat}]{\underset{H_2SO_4}{H_2O}} CH_3C.COOH$$

$$\downarrow -H_2O$$

$$CH_2 = C - COOH$$

2-Methyl propenoic acid

4. **Addition of Grignard's reagent:** Aldehydes and ketones are added to a molecule of Grignard reagent, and the intermediate formed gives secondary alcohol from an aldehyde and a tertiary alcohol from a ketone on decomposition. Formaldehyde gives primary alcohol in this reaction.

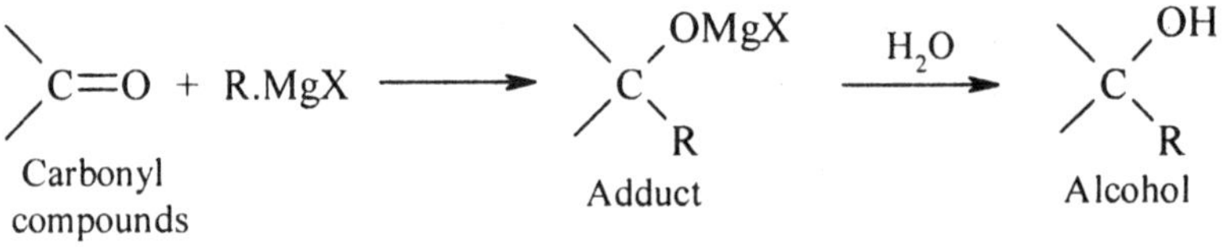

$$\text{C}=O + R.MgX \longrightarrow$$

Carbonyl compounds

Adduct

$$\xrightarrow{H_2O}$$

Alcohol

5. **Addition of water:** Aldehydes add on water as such while an acid or base catalyst is required in a case of ketones since carbonyl-carbon is less electron deficient.

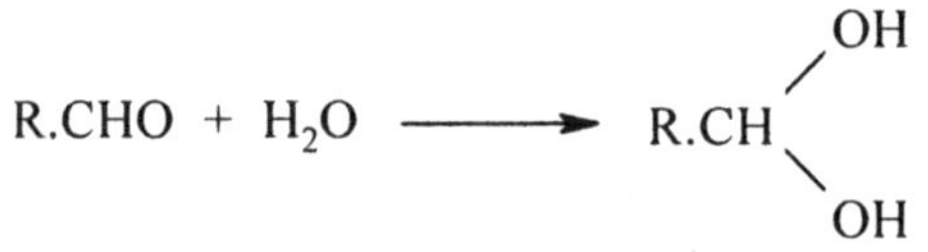

$$R.CHO + H_2O \longrightarrow R.CH$$

The hydrate so formed is less stable and cannot be isolated except in those cases where a strong electron withdrawing substituent is attached to the carbonyl carbon, e.g.:

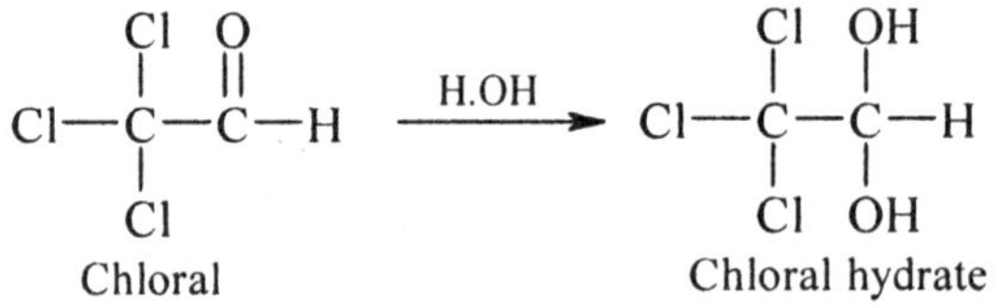

$$Cl-C-C-H \xrightarrow{H.OH} Cl-C-C-H$$

Chloral

Chloral hydrate

6. **Addition of derivatives of ammonia:** Aldehydes and ketones add to certain compounds related to ammonia like hydroxylamine, hydrazine, phenylhydrazine, and semicarbazide to form well defined crystalline products which are used to identify carbonyl compounds. Thus:

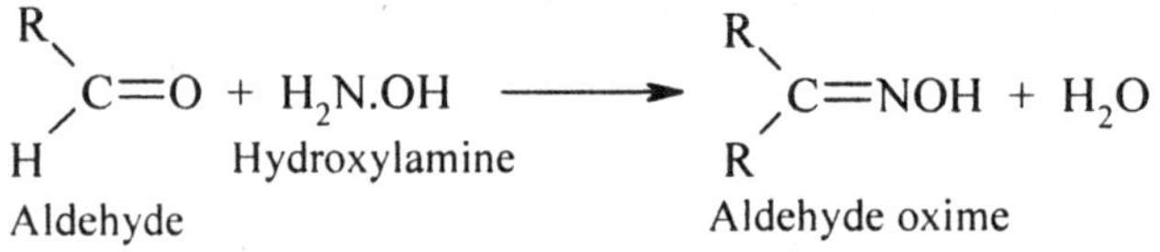

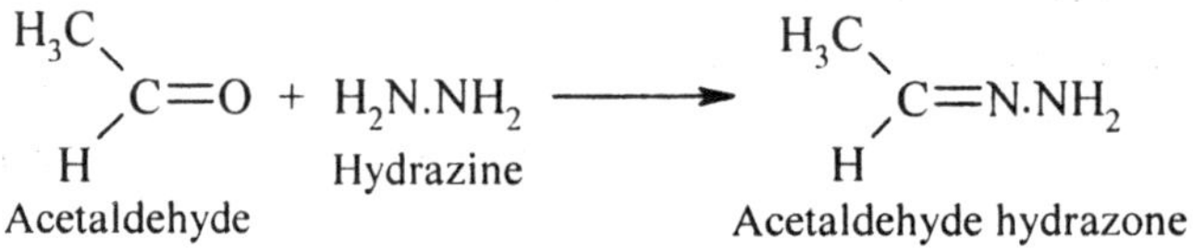

$$\text{C}=O + H_2N.OH \longrightarrow \text{C}=NOH + H_2O$$

Aldehyde   Hydroxylamine   Aldehyde oxime

$$\text{C}=O + H_2N.NH_2 \longrightarrow \text{C}=N.NH_2$$

Acetaldehyde   Hydrazine   Acetaldehyde hydrazone

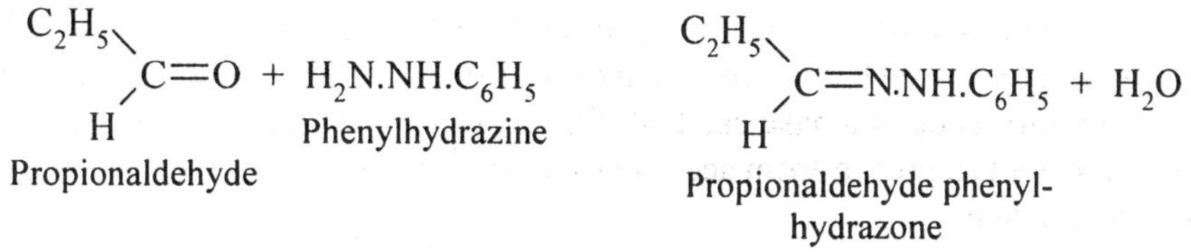

$$\begin{array}{c} C_2H_5 \\ \diagdown \\ \diagup \\ H \end{array} C{=}O \ + \ H_2N.NH.C_6H_5$$

Propionaldehyde   Phenylhydrazine

$$\begin{array}{c} C_2H_5 \\ \diagdown \\ \diagup \\ H \end{array} C{=}N.NH.C_6H_5 \ + \ H_2O$$

Propionaldehyde phenyl-
hydrazone

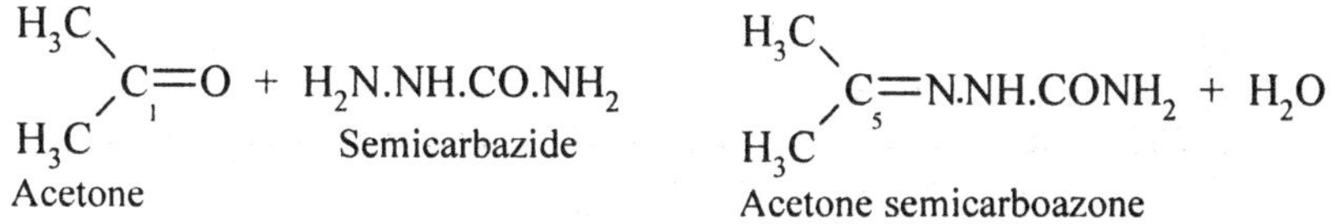

$$\begin{array}{c} H_3C \\ \diagdown \\ \diagup \\ H_3C \end{array} C{=}O \ + \ H_2N.NH.CO.NH_2$$

Acetone   Semicarbazide

$$\begin{array}{c} H_3C \\ \diagdown \\ \diagup \\ H_3C \end{array} C{=}N.NH.CONH_2 \ + \ H_2O$$

Acetone semicarboazone

The products contain carbon-nitrogen double bond resulting from elimination of a molecule of water from the initial addition products. Oximes and hydrazones regenerate the carbonyl compounds when refluxed with dilute hydrochloric acid.

7. **Addition of thio alcohols:** Aldehydes and ketones condense with thioalcohols (mercaptans), in the presence of hydrochloric acid to yield mercaptals and mercaptols, respectively.

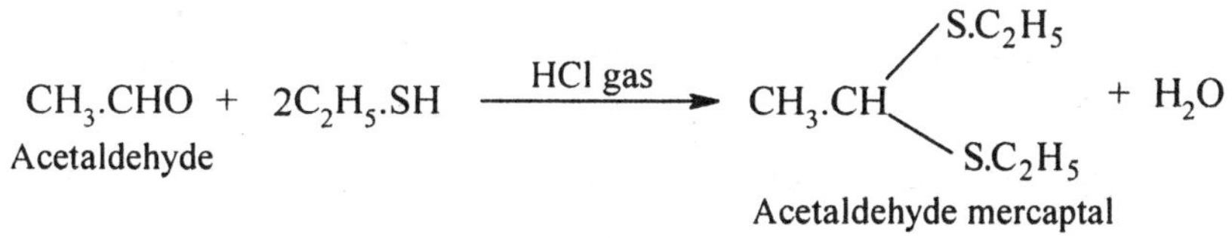

$$CH_3.CHO \ + \ 2C_2H_5.SH \ \xrightarrow{\text{HCl gas}} \ CH_3.CH \begin{array}{c} \diagup S.C_2H_5 \\ \\ \diagdown S.C_2H_5 \end{array} \ + \ H_2O$$

Acetaldehyde   Acetaldehyde mercaptal

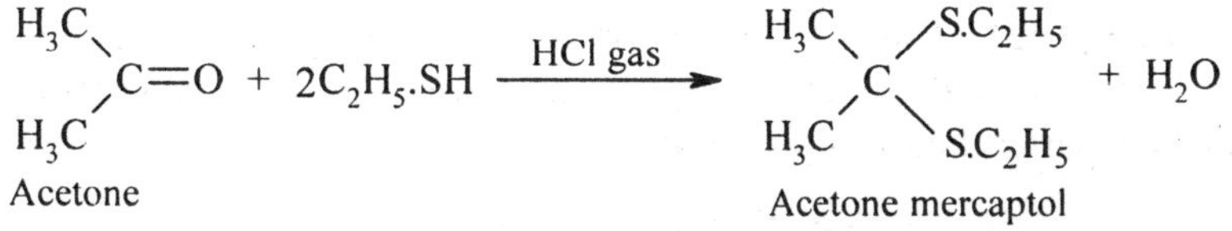

$$\begin{array}{c} H_3C \\ \diagdown \\ \diagup \\ H_3C \end{array} C{=}O \ + \ 2C_2H_5.SH \ \xrightarrow{\text{HCl gas}} \ \begin{array}{c} H_3C \\ \diagdown \\ \diagup \\ H_3C \end{array} C \begin{array}{c} \diagup S.C_2H_5 \\ \\ \diagdown S.C_2H_5 \end{array} \ + \ H_2O$$

Acetone   Acetone mercaptol

8. **Reaction with phosphorus pentachlorides:** Aldehydes and ketones produce dichloro compounds when they are allowed to react with phosphorus pentachloride.

$$CH_3.CHO \ + \ PCl_5 \ \longrightarrow \ CH_3.CH.Cl_2 \ + \ POCl_3$$

Ethylidene dichloride

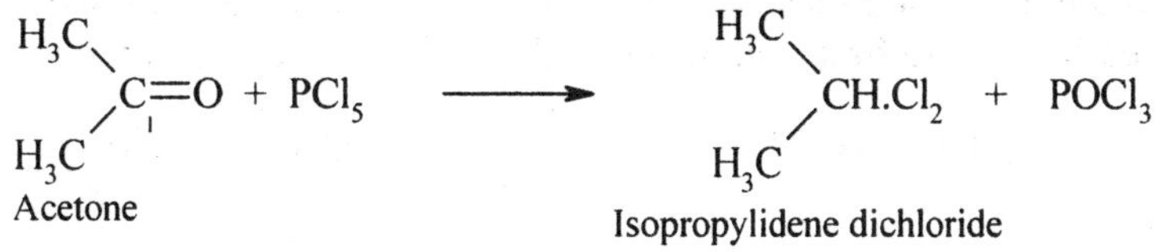

$$\begin{array}{c} H_3C \\ \diagdown \\ \diagup \\ H_3C \end{array} C{=}O \ + \ PCl_5 \ \longrightarrow \ \begin{array}{c} H_3C \\ \diagdown \\ \diagup \\ H_3C \end{array} CH.Cl_2 \ + \ POCl_3$$

Acetone   Isopropylidene dichloride

9. **Reactions of alkyl group:**

(i) **Halogenation:** Chlorine or bromine replaces one or more α-hydrogen atoms in aldehydes and ketones in the presence of an acid or a base as catalyst.

$$CH_3.CHO \ + \ 3Cl_2 \ \xrightarrow{CH_3.COOH} \ CCl_3.CHO \ + \ 3HCl$$

Acetaldehyde   Trichloro-acetaldehyde
or Chloral

$$CH_3.CO.CH_3 \ + \ Br_2 \ \xrightarrow{CH_3.COO.Na} \ CBr_3.CO.CH_3 \ + \ 3HBr$$

Acetone   Tribromoacetone

Kinetic studies indicate that the rate of reaction depends upon the concentration of acetone and of catalyst used but independent of bromine concentration. In case of bromination of acetone influence of a base catalyst, the following mechanism can be demonstrated. The base abstracts a proton from acetone to form carbanion which then reacts readily to yield bromoacetone.

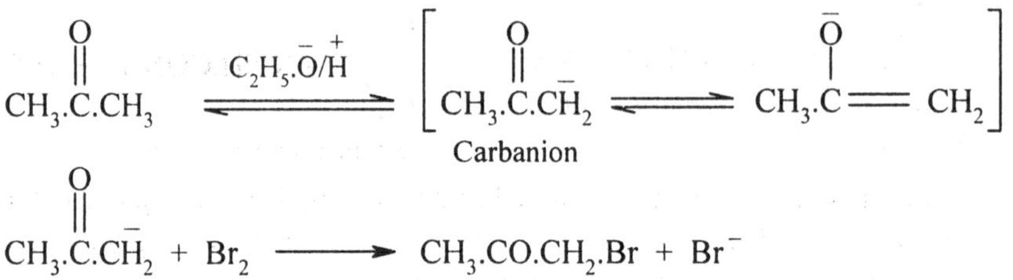

$$CH_3.C.CH_3 \xrightarrow{C_2H_5.\bar{O}/\overset{+}{H}} \left[CH_3.\overset{O}{\overset{\|}{C}}.\bar{C}H_2 \rightleftharpoons CH_3.\overset{\bar{O}}{\overset{|}{C}} = CH_2 \right]$$
Carbanion

$$CH_3.\overset{O}{\overset{\|}{C}}.\bar{C}H_2 + Br_2 \longrightarrow CH_3.CO.CH_2.Br + Br^-$$

(ii) **Oxidation by selenium dioxide:** Aldehydes and ketones with a methyl or methylene group adjacent to the carbonyl group are oxidized by selenium dioxide at room temperature to dicarbonyl compounds, e.g.:

$$\underset{\text{Acetaldehyde}}{CH_3.CHO} + SeO_2 \longrightarrow \underset{\text{Glyoxal}}{OCH.CHO} + Se + H_2O$$

$$\underset{\text{Acetone}}{CH_3.CO.CH_3} + SeO_2 \longrightarrow \underset{\text{Methyl glyoxal}}{CH_3.CO.CHO} + Se + H_2O$$

10. **Schmidt reaction (1924):** Carbonyl compounds react with hydrazoic acid in the presence of concentrated sulphuric acid. Aldehydes give a mixture of cyanide and formyl derivatives of primary amines, whereas ketones give amide.

$$R.CHO + HN_3 \xrightarrow{H_2SO_4} R.CN + RNH.CHO + N_2$$

$$R.CO.R + HN_3 \xrightarrow{H_2SO_4} R.CO.NH.R + N_2$$

11. **Aldol condensation:** Two molecules of an aldehyde or ketone may combine to afford a β-hydroxyaldehyde or β-hydroxyketone with or without the elimination of water under the influence of dilute acids or bases. This reaction is called the aldol condensation. In every product the α-carbon of the first is attached to the carbonyl carbon of the second.

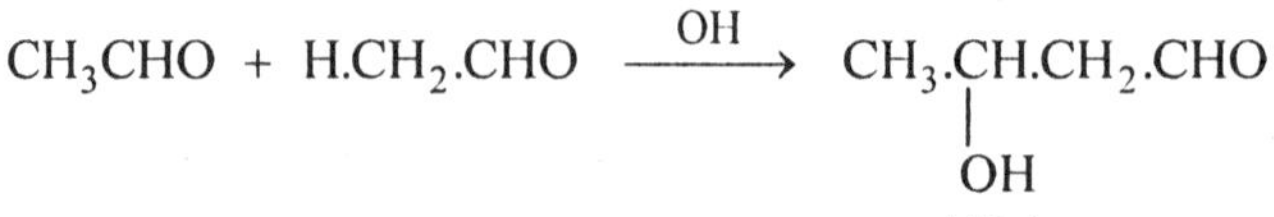

$$CH_3CHO + H.CH_2.CHO \xrightarrow{OH} CH_3.\underset{\underset{OH}{|}}{CH}.CH_2.CHO$$
Aldol
3-Hydroxybutanal

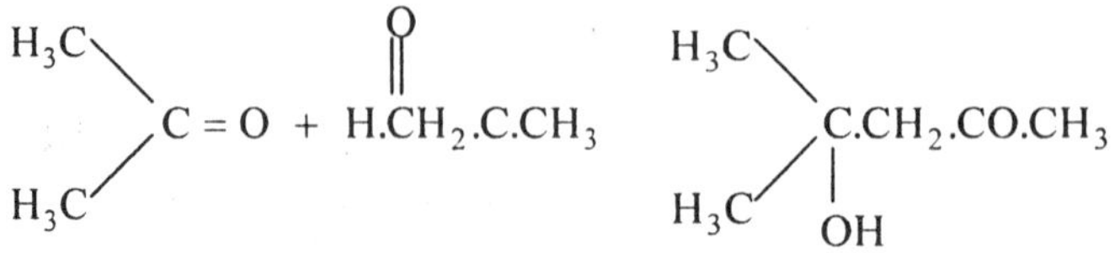

$$\underset{H_3C}{\overset{H_3C}{>}}C = O + H.CH_2.C.CH_3 \longrightarrow \underset{H_3C}{\overset{H_3C}{>}}\underset{OH}{\overset{|}{C}}.CH_2.CO.CH_3$$
Diacetone alcohol

On heating, these products eliminate water to form unsaturated compounds, e.g.:

$$CH_3.CH.CH_2.OH \quad \xrightarrow{\text{Heat}} \quad CH_3.CH = CH.CHO + H_2O$$
$$\underset{\displaystyle OH}{|}$$

Crotonaldehyde

$$(CH_3)_2.C.CH_2.CO.CH_3 \quad \xrightarrow{\text{Heat}} \quad (CH_3)_2.C = CH.COCH_3 + H_2O$$
$$\underset{\displaystyle OH}{|}$$

Mesityl oxide

Formaldehyde likewise has no α-hydrogen atoms and can be condensed with another aldehyde to yield formose in the presence of weak alkali (e.g. baryta).

$$H.CHO + H.CHO \quad \xrightarrow{Ba(OH)_2} \quad H - \underset{\displaystyle OH}{\overset{\displaystyle OH}{\underset{|}{|}}}CH.CHO \quad \xrightarrow[\text{H.CHO}]{Ba(OH)_2} \quad H.\underset{\displaystyle OH}{\overset{\displaystyle OH}{\underset{|}{|}}}CH.\underset{\displaystyle OH}{\overset{\displaystyle OH}{\underset{|}{|}}}CH.CHO$$

Glycollic aldehyde

$$\xrightarrow[3H.CHO]{Ba(OH)_2} \quad CH_2 - CH - CH - CH - CH - CH_2$$
$$\qquad\qquad\qquad\quad |\quad\ |\quad\ |\quad\ |\quad\ |\quad\ |$$
$$\qquad\qquad\qquad\quad OH\ \ OH\ OH\ OH\ OH\ OH$$

Formose

Aldol condensation is employed for the preparation of acrolein on commercial scale. In this process equimolecular quantities of acetaldehyde and formaldehyde are reacted.

$$H.CHO + H.CH_2.CHO \quad \xrightarrow[\text{Heat}]{\text{Cat.}} \quad [HO.CH_2.CH_2.CHO] \quad \xrightarrow{-H_2O} \quad H_2C = CH.CHO$$

Acrolein

Mechanism: In a base catalyst aldol condensation of aldehydes, the carbanion is formed first of all which then combines with a second molecule of acetaldehyde to form the anion of aldol.

$$H\bar{O} + H - CH_2.\overset{\displaystyle O}{\overset{\|}{CH}} \rightleftharpoons \left[\bar{C}H_2 - \overset{\displaystyle O}{\overset{\|}{C}} - H \longleftrightarrow CH_2 = \overset{\displaystyle \bar{O}}{\overset{|}{C}} - H \right] + H_2O$$

Carbanion

$$H_3C - \overset{\displaystyle O}{\overset{\|}{C}}H + \bar{C}H_2.CHO \rightleftharpoons \left[CH_3.\overset{\displaystyle \bar{O}}{\overset{|}{C}}H - CH_2.CHO \right] \rightleftharpoons CH_3.\overset{\displaystyle OH}{\overset{|}{C}}H.CH_2.CHO$$

Aldol anion

REACTIONS GIVEN BY ALDEHYDES ONLY

1. **Reaction with Schiff's reagent:** Schiff's reagent is rosaniline hydrochloride dye dissolved in water in which sulphur dioxide is passed until the magenta colour is discharged. Aldehydes restore the pink colour of magenta to the Schiff's reagent.

2. **Oxidation:**
   (i) **With potassium dichromate or potassium permanganate:** Aldehydes are easily oxidized and hence are powerful reducing agents. Oxidation with acidic dichromate and permanganate gives carboxylic acids containing the same number of carbon atoms as present in the aldehyde molecule.

$$R.CHO + (O) \xrightarrow[H^+]{KMnO_4} R.COOH$$

(ii) **With Fehling's solution:** Fehling's solution is an alkaline solution containing a complex of copper tartrate. When aldehydes are heated with it, a reddish brown precipitate of cuprous oxide is formed.

$$CuSO_4 + NaOH \longrightarrow Cu(OH)_2 + Na_2SO_4$$

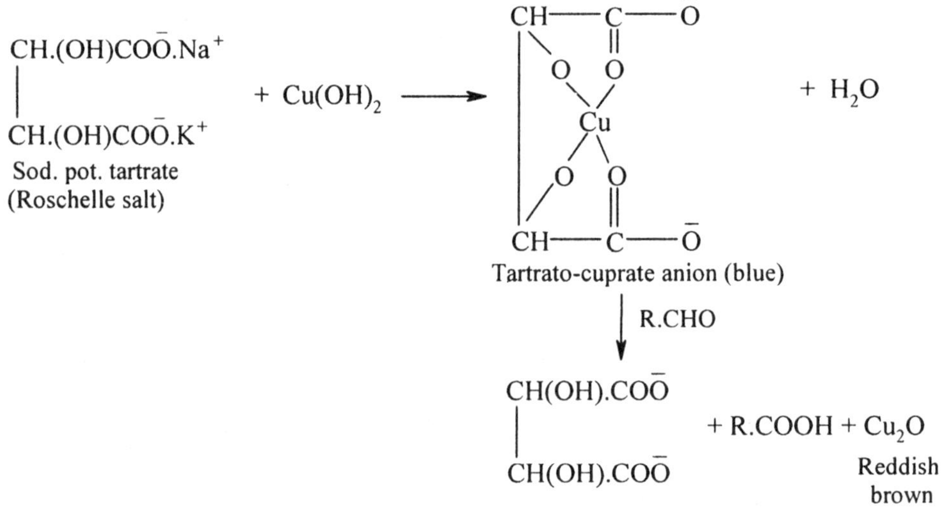

CH.(OH)COŌ.Na$^+$
|
CH.(OH)COŌ.K$^+$
Sod. pot. tartrate
(Roschelle salt)

$+ Cu(OH)_2 \longrightarrow$

Tartrato-cuprate anion (blue)

$\downarrow$ R.CHO

CH(OH).COŌ
| $+ R.COOH + Cu_2O$
CH(OH).COŌ   Reddish
                      brown

In short the reaction is represented as:

$$R.CHO + 2CuO \longrightarrow R.COOH + Cu_2O$$

(iii) **With Benedict's reagent:** Benedict's solution is the mixture of copper sulphate, sodium citrate and sodium bicarbonate. When an aldehyde is heated with it, reddish brown precipitate of cuprous oxide is formed.

$$2R.CHO + Na_2CO_3 + 4 \underset{\underset{CH_2.COONa}{|}}{\overset{\overset{CH_2.COONa}{|}}{HO.C.COO.Na}} \longrightarrow 4 \underset{\underset{CH_2.COONa}{|}}{\overset{\overset{CH_2.COONa}{|}}{C(OH).COO.Na}}$$

$$+ 2 R.COO.Na + H_2O + Cu_2O$$

(iv) **With Tollen's reagent:** Tollen's reagent is a solution of ammonical silver nitrate. With aldehydes it gives a precipitate of metallic silver which is deposited on the walls of the test tube forming a silver mirror (Silver mirror test).

$$R.CHO + 2Ag(NH_3)_2.NO_3 + H_2O \longrightarrow R.COO.NH_4 + NH_3 + 2NH_4NO_3 + Ag$$

3. **Addition of alcohols:** Aldehydes combine with alcohols in the presence of anhydrous acids (e.g., dry HCl) to form first the hemi-acetal and then acetal.

$$R.CHO + C_2H_5.OH \rightleftharpoons R.\overset{\overset{\displaystyle O.C_2H_5}{|}}{\underset{\underset{\displaystyle H}{|}}{C}} - OH \underset{-H_2O}{\overset{+C_2H_5.OH}{\rightleftharpoons}} R.\overset{\overset{\displaystyle O.C_2H_5}{|}}{\underset{\underset{\displaystyle H}{|}}{C}}.O.C_2H_5$$

Mechanism:

$$R-\overset{}{\underset{\underset{\displaystyle H}{|}}{C}}=O \overset{H^+}{\rightleftharpoons} R-\overset{+}{\underset{\underset{\displaystyle H}{|}}{C}}=OH \rightleftharpoons R-\overset{\oplus}{\underset{\underset{\displaystyle H}{|}}{C}}=OH \rightleftharpoons R-\overset{\overset{\displaystyle \overset{\oplus}{O}-C_2H_5}{|}}{\underset{\underset{\displaystyle H}{|}}{C}}=OH$$

$$\overset{-H^+}{\rightleftharpoons} R-\overset{\overset{\displaystyle O.C_2H_5}{|}}{\underset{\underset{\displaystyle H}{|}}{C}}=OH \overset{H^+}{\rightleftharpoons} R-\overset{\overset{\displaystyle O.C_2H_5}{|}}{\underset{\underset{\displaystyle H}{|}}{C}}\overset{+}{=}OH_2 \overset{\overset{\displaystyle 1.-H_2O}{2.C_2H_5.OH}}{\rightleftharpoons} R-\overset{\overset{\displaystyle O.C_2H_5}{|}}{\underset{\underset{\displaystyle H}{|}}{C}}=O.C_2H_5$$

Acetal

4. **Cannizzaro reaction:** The reaction, characteristic of aldehydes containing no α-hydrogens, undergoes self oxidation and reduction to yield a mixture of an alcohol and a salt of carboxylic acid in the presence of concentrated alkali. The reaction which bears the name of the Italian discoverer Stanislao Cannizzaro (1853), is generally brought about by allowing the aldehyde to stand at room temperature with aqueous or alcoholic sodium hydroxide.

$$2 \text{ H.CHO} \xrightarrow{50\% \text{ NaOH}} CH_3.OH + H.CO\overline{O}.Na^+$$

Formaldehyde   Methanol   Sodium formate

$$2 (CH_3)_2C.CHO \xrightarrow{\text{Conc. NaOH}} (CH_3)_3C.COO.Na + (CH_3)_3C.CH_2.OH$$

2,2-Dimethylpropanal   Sodium 2,2-dimethyl   2,2-Dimethylpropanol
                              propionate

A mixture of two aldehydes undergoes a Cannizzaro reaction to yield all possible product. However, if one of the aldehydes is H.CHO, reaction yields sodium formate (Crossed Cannizzaro's reaction).

$$C_6N_5.CHO + H.CHO \xrightarrow{\text{Conc. NaOH}} C_6H_5.CH_2.OH + H.CO\overline{O}.Na^+$$

Benzaldehyde   Benzyl alcohol

All other aldehydes when warmed with concentrated sodium hydroxide form resinous products via a series of condensation, e.g.:

$$2 CH_3.CHO \longrightarrow CH_3.CH(OH).CH_2 \xrightarrow{-H_2O} CH_3.CH=CH.CHO \xrightarrow{CH_3.CHO}$$

$$CH_3.CH=CH.CH(OH).CH_2.CHO \xrightarrow{-H_2O} CH_3.CH=CH.CH=CH.CHO \text{ etc.}$$

All aldehydes can be made to undergo the Cannizzaro's reaction by treatment with aluminium ethoxide. Under these conditions the acids and alcohol are combined as the ester and the reaction is known as Tischenko's reaction, e.g.:

$$2\ CH_3.CHO \xrightarrow{Al(O.C_2H_5)_3} [CH_3.COOH + C_2H_5.OH \longrightarrow CH_3.CO.OC_2H_5$$

Acetaldehyde   Ethyl acetate

5. **Reaction with ammonia:** Except formaldehyde, other aldehydes react with ammonia in ethanol solution to give a precipitate of aldehyde-ammonia, e.g.:

$$CH_3.CHO + NH_3 \longrightarrow CH_3.CH(OH).NH_2\ (50\%)$$

Formaldehyde reacts with ammonia to form hexamethylene tetramine or hexamine.

$$6\ H.CHO + 4NH_3 \longrightarrow (CH_2)_6N_4 + 6H_2O$$

Hexamamethylene tetramine

6. **Polymerization:** Polymerization is a process in which molecules of a compound are combined together without any elimination of water etc. so that the molecular weight of the product is a multiple of that of the original compound. In short polymerization is the process of joining together of many small molecules to make very large molecule.

(Polymer, Greek: Poly + Meros = Many parts). The simple compounds from which polymers are made are called monomers (mono = one).

The polymer may or may not show any close relationship in the properties to the monomer. Where only two or three monomers combine the process is usually termed as dimerization or trimerization.

Simple aliphatic aldehydes tend to polymerize under different reaction conditions to give different products. The usual mode of polymerization of aldehydes is linkage through oxygen. This can form ring compounds utilizing 3 or 4 aldehyde molecules by joining the ends of the chain. Higher polymers, on the other hand, are chain forms produced from a large number of aldehyde molecules such as:

$$X - CH - O.CH - O.CH - O.CH - O - Y$$
$$\qquad |\qquad\quad |\qquad\quad |\qquad\quad |$$
$$\qquad R\qquad R\qquad R\qquad R$$

Formaldehyde forms the following polymers:

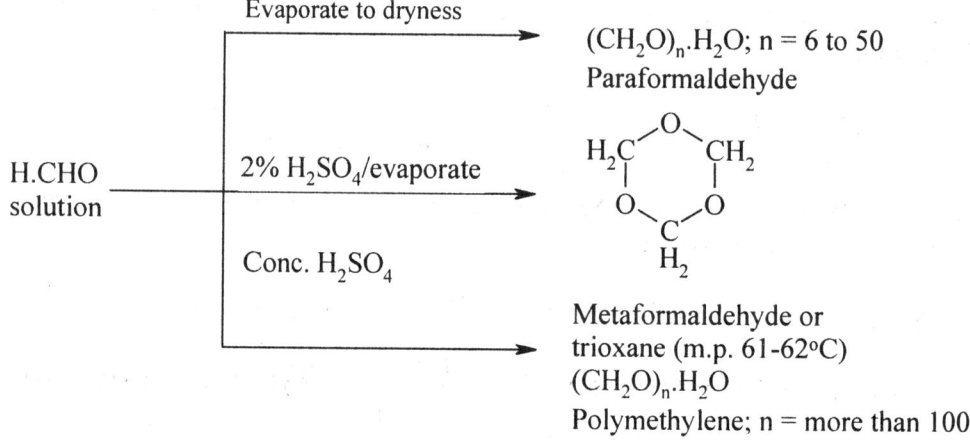

Evaporate to dryness → $(CH_2O)_n.H_2O$; n = 6 to 50
Paraformaldehyde

H.CHO solution

2% H_2SO_4/evaporate →

Metaformaldehyde or trioxane (m.p. 61-62°C)
$(CH_2O)_n.H_2O$

Conc. H_2SO_4 →

Polymethylene; n = more than 100

Acetaldehyde polymerizes to form sweet-smelling paraldehyde (b.p. 123°C) when treated with concentrated sulphuric acid and a white solid metaldehyde (m.p. 246°C) when treated with hydrogen chloride or sulphur dioxide.

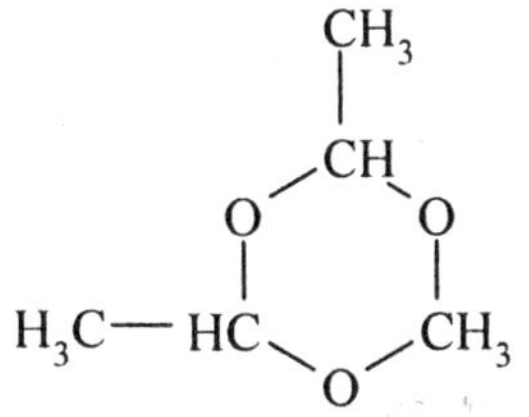

Paraldehyde

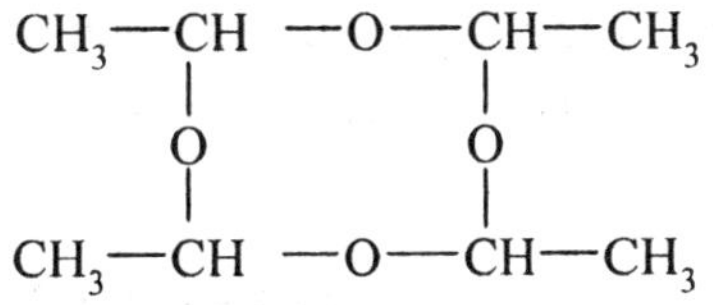

Metaldehyde

REACTIONS GIVEN BY KETONES ONLY

1. Ketones do not give Schiff's reaction. However, acetone gives pink colour very slowly.
2. Ketones do not reduce Fehling's solution, Benedict's and Tollen's reagents. However, with acidic potassium dichromate or permanganate they are oxidized to carboxylic acids on warming. The acids formed contain fewer carbon atoms than the starting ketone.

$$CH_3.CO.CH_3 \xrightarrow[KMnO_4]{[O]} \underset{\text{Acetic acid}}{CH_3.COOH} + \underset{\text{Formic acid}}{H.COOH}$$

3. Ketones react with ammonia to yield complex ketone amines, e.g.:

$$(H_3C)_2C=O + H.NH_2 + \underset{\text{Acetone}}{H.CH_2.CO.CH_3} \longrightarrow \underset{\text{Diacetone amine}}{(H_3C)_2C(NH_2)—CH_2.CO.CH_3} + H_2O$$

Similarly triacetone amine is formed.

4. Ketones do not react readily to form ketals when treated with alcohols in the presence of hydrogen chloride. Treatment of ketones, however, with triethyl orthoformate yields ketals.

$$R_2C=O + HC.(OC_2H_5)_3 \longrightarrow R_2C.(OC_2H_5)_2 + H.COOC_2H_5$$

5. When ketones are treated with nitrous acids, the half oxime of the α-dicarbonyl compound is formed.

$$CH_3.CO.CH_3 + HNO_2 \xrightarrow{C_2H_5.NO_2/HCl} CH_3CO.CN = N.OH + H_2O$$

6. Ketones condense with chloroform in the presence of potassium hydroxide to form chloro-hydroxy compounds.

$$CH_3.C.CH_3 + CHCl_3 \xrightarrow{KOH} (CH_3)_2 - C \underset{CCl_3}{\overset{OH}{\diagdown}}$$

Acetone   Chlorotone

7. Ketones form sodio-derivatives when treated with sodium or sodamide in ethereal solution.

$$CH_3.CO.CH_3 + NaNH_2 \xrightarrow[\text{Ether}]{} CH_3.CO.CH_2.Na + NH_3$$

Sodio-acetone

OFFICIAL COMPOUNDS
FORMALDEHYDE SOLUTION
(Syn. Formalin)

Formaldehyde solution is a solution of formaldehyde in water with methyl alcohol added to prevent polymerisation. It contains not less than 34.0 per cent w/w and not more than 38.0 per cent w/w of formaldehyde.

Description: It is a colourless liquid with characteristic pungent and irritating odour and burning taste. On long standing, especially in the cold, a white cloudy (amorphous) deposit of formaldehyde is formed which disappears on warming the solution.

It is miscible with water and alcohol and is tested for acidity and methanol. Its weight per ml at 20° is 1.079 to 1.094 g (App. III).

Assay: Weigh accurately about 3 g of formaldehyde and add it to a mixture of 50 ml solution of hydrogen peroxide and 60 ml of 1 N sodium hydroxide, warm on water bath till the effervescence ceases. Titrate the excess of alkali with 1 N sulphuric acid, using solution of phenolphthalein as an indicator. Repeat the experiment with the same quantities of the same reagents in the same manner omitting formaldehyde solution (i.e. blank titration). The difference between the titrations represents the sodium hydroxide required to neutralize the formic acid produced by the oxidation of formaldehyde.

$$H.CHO + H_2O_2 \longrightarrow H.COOH + H_2O$$
$$NaOH + H.COOH \longrightarrow H.COO.Na + H_2O$$

Each ml of 1 N sodium hydroxide is equivalent to 0.03003 g of CH_2O.

Formaldehyde solution is stored and preserved in a well closed container, preferably at a temperature not below 15°.

Uses: It is used as a disinfectant. It acts as a bactericidal and is used for disinfecting room etc. It is produced by heating paraformaldehyde and its required concentration in the air is 1–2 per cent.

N.B.: It is not now included as an independent monograph, but just as a solution.

PARALDEHYDE

Mol. Form.: $C_6H_{12}O_3$ Mol. Wt.: 132.16

Paraldehyde is a trimer of acetaldehyde. It contains upto 0.01 per cent w/v of a suitable antioxidant. It gets oxidized easily in atmosphere with the formation of peroxidized compounds and acetic acid. Hence it is stored in the dark in a small well-filled container in a cool place.

It is a colourless transparent liquid with a strong characteristic odour and disagreeable taste. At low temperature it solidifies to form a crystalline mass (the whole content of the container should be liquefied before use).

Solubility: It is soluble in water (8 parts), in boiling water (17 parts), miscible with alcohol (90%) chloroform, solvent ether and volatile oils.

Identity: It is identified by (a) heating with dilute sulphuric acid when acetaldehyde is produced; (b) by warming its saturated solution in water with solution of silver ammonia nitrate in a test tube, when silver is deposited as a mirror on the sides of the tube.

Tests for purity: It is tested for purity; for distillation range; melting point; wt. per ml; acetaldehyde; acidity; and peroxide compounds; chloride; sulphate; refractive index and non-volatile residues.

Uses: It is used as a central depressant and a basal anaesthetic.

Paraldehyde was introduced in the therapy in 1882 as a soporific (sleeping agent). Its usual dose being 3–5 ml (letahal dose 100–150 ml).

CHLORAL HYDRATE

Mol. Form.: $CCl_3.CH(OH)_2$ Mol. Wt.: 165.40

Chloral hydrate contains not less than 99.5 per cent and not more than 102.5% of $C_2H_3O_2Cl_3$. It is not now included as a monograph, but in I.P. appendices.

Chloral hydrate is manufactured by chlorinating ethanol, decomposing the resulting chloral half acetal with acid and treating chloral with water to get chloral hydrate as follows:

$$3CH_3.CH_2.OH \xrightarrow{Cl_2} CCl_3.CH(OH).O.C_2H_5 \xrightarrow{H_2SO_4} CCl_3.CHO \xrightarrow{H_2O} CCl_3.CH(OH)_2$$

Description: Chloral hydrate is a colourless or white transparent crystalline substance, having an aromatic, pungent odour and bitter taste. It volatilizes slowly on exposure to air. It is soluble in water (0.25 part), alcohol (1.3 parts) and solvent ether (1.5 parts).

It is identified by:

  (i) Taking 2 ml of a 10.0 per cent w/v solution and adding to it 1 ml of solution of sodium hydroxide when chloroform separates as a lower layer. The supernatant aqueous layer on acidifying with acetic acid followed by boiling with test solution of mercuric chloride gives a precipitate.

 (ii) Heating with a few drops each of aniline and solution of sodium hydroxide when phenyl isocyanate is produced.

(iii) Liquefying when it liquefies between 50 and 58.

Tests for identity: It is tested for purity for reaction; benzene; chloride; chloral alcoholate and sulphated ash (App. II).

Assay: In an earlier procedure a weighed quantity of the substance was left in contact with a measured volume of N/1 sodium hydroxide and the excess of alkali was then titrated with N/1 sulphuric acid and the calculations done on the basis of the equation given below:

$$NaOH + CCl_3.CH(OH)_3 \longrightarrow CH.Cl_3 + H.COO.Na + H_2O$$

The difficulty with this method was that even within a short time during which the decomposition of chloral hydrate by the alkali was done, a small quantity of the chloroform produced was also decomposed as per the reaction given below:

$$4NaOH + CHCl_3 \longrightarrow H.COO.Na + 3NaCl + H_2O$$

The process was, therefore, modified by inclusion of a correction for the small amount of alkali consumed in the reaction with chloroform as determined by titration with N/10 silver nitrate of the sodium chloride formed. Every 3 equivalents of silver nitrate used correspond to 4 equivalents of sodium hydroxide consumed (see equation above). Thus every 30 ml of N/10 silver nitrate are equivalent to 4 ml of N/10 alkali so that to the volume of N/10 sulphuric acid used in the blank titration there must be added 4/30 of the volume of N/10 silver nitrate.

Weigh accurately about 4 g of chloral hydrate, dissolve it in 10 ml of water and add 30 ml of 1 N NaOH solution to it. Allow the mixture to stand at room temperature for 2 minutes, and then titrate with 1 N H_2SO_4, using phenolphthalein solution as an indicator. Titrate the neutralized liquid with 0.1 N silver nitrate using solution of potassium chromate as indicator. Add two fifteenth of the amount of 0.1 N silver nitrate used to the amount of 1 N H_2SO_4 used in the first titration and deduct the figure so obtained from the amount of 1 N NaOH added.

Each ml of 1 N NaOH obtained as difference is equivalent to 0.1654 g of $C_2H_3O_2Cl_3$.

Storage: Chloral hydrate is stored and preserved in a tightly-closed glass container in a cool and dark place.

Uses: Chloral hydrate is used as a hypnotic and sedative. In the usual dose (500 mg) it causes sedation in just 10–15 minutes, while it induces sleep within an hour, which lasts upto 8 hours. The sleep is light and normal and the person can be easily aroused.

A dose of 6 g or over induces complete anaesthesia. But such doses cause respiratory depression and chloral hydrate cannot be safely used as an anaesthetic. Chloral hydrate causes local irritation, nausea, vomitting and diarrhoea, especially if taken with less amount of fluids.

Carboxylic Acids

An organic compound containing the carboxylic functional group (–COOH) is called carboxylic acid. The functional group is obtained by the combination of a **carbonyl** and a **hydroxyl** group. The carboxylic acids may be saturated or unsaturated. The saturated monocarboxylic acids are also known as the fatty acids, since higher members like palmatic acid and stearic acid occur in fats. They are classified as mono-, di-, tri- or polycarboxylic acids, according to the number of carboxylic groups present in the molecule. Their general formula is $C_nH_{2n}O_2$. But they are generally expressed as $C_nH_{2n+1}.COOH$ or R.COOH due to the presence of the functional group, –COOH. The monocarboxylic acids are monobasic acids since only the carboxyl group hydrogen is replaceable by a metal.

The structure of the carboxyl group is represented as:

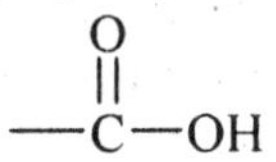

$$\overset{\displaystyle O}{\underset{\displaystyle \parallel}{}}$$
$$—C—OH \qquad or \qquad – COOH$$

The structure of carboxylic acid can be written by a resonance hybrid as shown below:

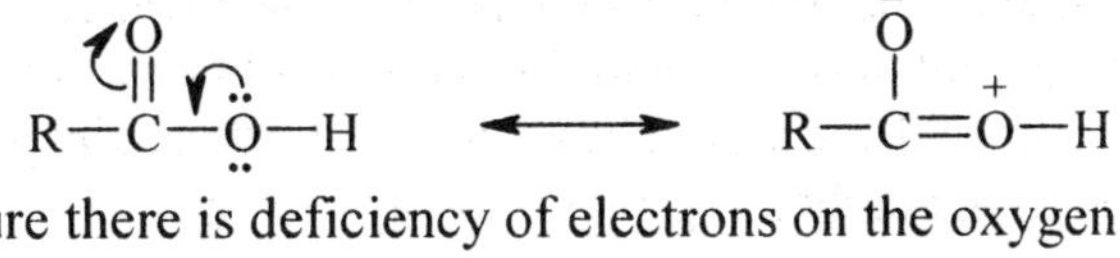

$$R—\overset{O}{\overset{\parallel}{C}}—\overset{..}{\underset{..}{O}}—H \qquad \longleftrightarrow \qquad R—\overset{\overset{\displaystyle \bar{O}}{\mid}}{C}=\overset{+}{O}—H$$

In the second structure there is deficiency of electrons on the oxygen atom of hydroxyl group. Proton is eliminated from this oxygen easily and carboxylate ion is formed. This ion is a resonance hybrid to which the equivalent contributing structures are represented as:

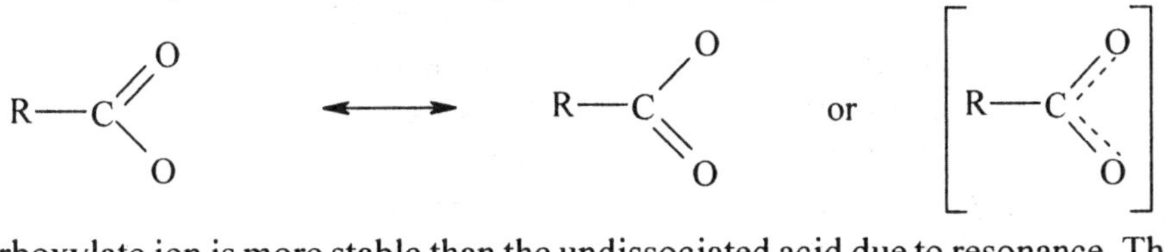

$$R—C\overset{\displaystyle O}{\underset{\displaystyle O}{}} \qquad \longleftrightarrow \qquad R—C\overset{\displaystyle O}{\underset{\displaystyle O}{}} \qquad or \qquad \left[R—C\overset{\displaystyle O}{\underset{\displaystyle O}{}} \right]$$

This carboxylate ion is more stable than the undissociated acid due to resonance. The resonance energy of the ion is much higher than that of the acid which dissociates into carboxylate ion and proton. Thus these compounds are acidic in nature.

Nomenclature: The following systems are used for naming the carboxylic acids.

(i) **Common names:** The carboxylic acids are usually known by the common names which have been derived from the source of the corresponding acid.

Formula	Source	Common name/ Trivial name
H.COOH	Formica (Red ant)	Formic acid
CH_3.COOH	Acetum (Vinegar)	Acetic acid
C_3H_7.COOH	Butyrum (Butter)	Butyric acid
C_3H_5.COOH	Croton oil	Crotonic acid
C_4H_9.COOH	Valerian plant root	Valeric acid
C_5H_{11}.COOH	Caper (goat) fat	Caproic acid
$C_{11}H_{23}$.COOH	Laurel oil	Lauric acid
$C_{17}H_{33}$.COOH	Olive oil	Oleic acid

The position of substituted acids is represented by Greek letters α, β, γ, δ etc., e.g.:

$$CH_3.CH_2.CH.COOH$$
$$|$$
$$NH_2$$
$$\alpha\text{-Aminobutyric acid}$$

$$CH_3.CH.CH.COOH$$
$$|\quad|$$
$$Cl\quad CH_3$$
$$\beta\text{-Chloro-}\alpha\text{-methylbutyric acid}$$

(ii) **Derived names:** In another system of naming the acids are considered as derivatives of acetic acid (except formic acid), e.g.:

Formula	Name
$CH_3.CH_2$.COOH	Methylacetic acid
$(CH_3)_2$.CH.COOH	Dimethylacetic acid
$(CH_3)_3$.C.COOH	Trimethylacetic acid
$(CH_3)_2$.CH.CH_2.COOH	Isopropylacetic acid

(iii) **IUPAC names:** According to this system the longest chain carrying the carboxyl group is considered the parent structure and the name is obtained by replacing the –e of the corresponding alkane with **oic acid**. The positions of side-chains are indicated by numbers, the number given to the carboxyl group is always 1. Thus:

Formula	IUPAC names
H.COOH	Methanoic acid
CH_3.COOH	Ethanoic acid
C_2H_5.COOH	Propanoic acid
C_3H_7.COOH	Butanoic acid
C_4H_9.COOH	Pentanoic acid
C_5H_{11}.COOH	Hexanoic acid
$\overset{5}{C}H_3.\overset{4}{C}H_2.\overset{3}{C}H.\overset{2}{C}H_2.\overset{1}{C}OOH$ $\quad$ $|$ $\quad$ CH_3	3-Metyl pentanoic acid

Besides these systems another method is also used for naming the carboxylic acids. The carboxyl group is considered as a substituent, and is denoted by the suffix carboxylic acid to the name of the corresponding hydrocarbon, e.g.:

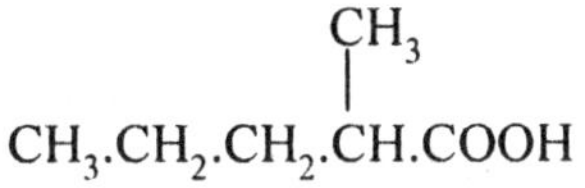

$$\overset{\displaystyle CH_3}{\underset{\displaystyle }{|}}$$

$$CH_3.CH_2.CH_2.CH.COOH$$

2-Methylbutane-1-carboxylic acid

ISOMERISM: Carboxylic acids show the following type of isomerism:

(i) Chain isomerism:

$$CH_3.CH_2.CH_2.CH_2.CH_2.COOH$$

Hexanoic acid

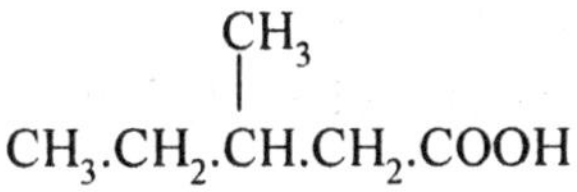

$$\overset{\displaystyle CH_3}{\underset{\displaystyle }{|}}$$

$$CH_3.CH_2.CH.CH_2.COOH$$

3-Methylpentanoic acid

(ii) Position isomerism:

$$CH_3.CH_2.CH_2.COOH$$

Butanoic acid

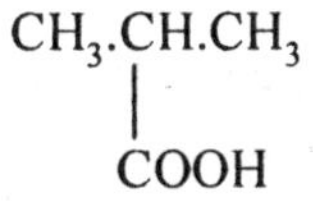

$$CH_3.CH.CH_3$$
$$|$$
$$COOH$$

Isobutanoic acid

(iii) Functional isomerism:

$$CH_3.CH_2.COOH$$

Propionic acid

$$CH_3.CO.OCH_3$$

Methyl acetate

$$H.CO.OC_2H_5$$

Ethyl formate

(iv) Optical isomerism:

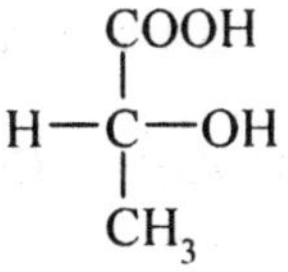

$$\begin{array}{c} COOH \\ | \\ H-C-OH \\ | \\ CH_3 \end{array}$$

d-Lactic acid

$$\begin{array}{c} COOH \\ | \\ HO-C-H \\ | \\ CH_3 \end{array}$$

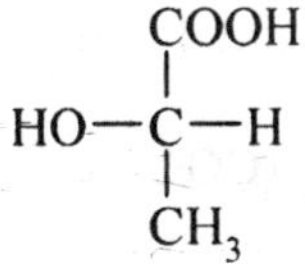

l-Lactic acid

(v) Geometrical isomerism:

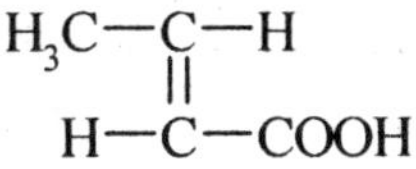

$$\begin{array}{c} H_3C-C-H \\ \| \\ H-C-COOH \end{array}$$

trans-Crotonic acid

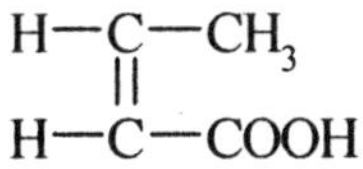

$$\begin{array}{c} H-C-CH_3 \\ \| \\ H-C-COOH \end{array}$$

cis-Isocrotonic acid

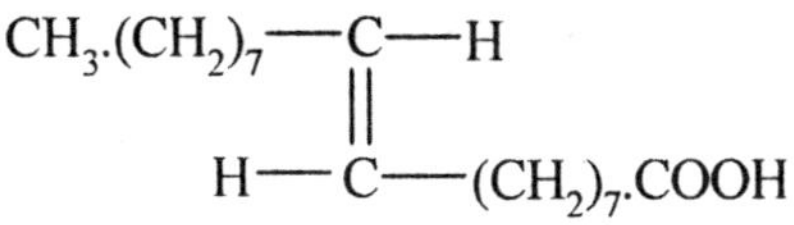

$$\begin{array}{c} CH_3.(CH_2)_7-C-H \\ \| \\ H-C-(CH_2)_7.COOH \end{array}$$

trans-Claidic acid

$$\begin{array}{c} CH_3.(CH_2)_7-C-H \\ \| \\ HOOC.(CH_2)_7-C-H \end{array}$$

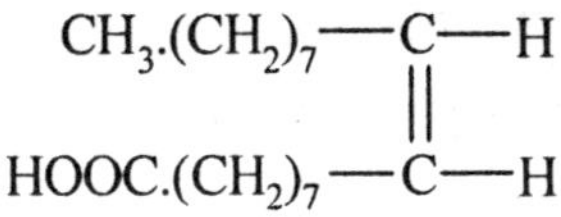

cis-Oleic acid

General Methods of Preparation

1. **Oxidation of alcohols and carbonyl compounds:** Oxidation of alcohols, aldehydes or ketones with acid dichromate affords carboxylic acids.

$$CH_3.CH_2OH \xrightarrow{[O]} CH_3.CHO \xrightarrow{[O]} CH_3.COOH$$

Ethanol   Acetaldehyde   Acetic acid

$$CH_3.CH.CH_3 \xrightarrow{[O]} CH_3.CO.CH_3 \xrightarrow{[O]} H.COOH + CH_3.COOH$$

|
OH

Isopropyl alcohol   Acetone   Formic acid   Acetic acid

2. **Hydrolysis of cyanides:** Hydrolysis of cyanides with acid or alkali gives fatty acids in very good yields.

$$R.C \equiv N + H_2O \longrightarrow \left[\begin{array}{c} OH \\ | \\ R.C = NH \end{array} \right] \longrightarrow R.C.NH_2 \xrightarrow{H_2O} R.COOH + NH_3$$

3. **From Grignard reagents:** In an alternate synthetic method, carboxylic acids are prepared by reacting Grignard reagents with either gaseous CO_2 in ether solution or crushed dry ice (solid CO_2). The reagent adds to the carbon-oxygen double bond to form an adduct which on hydrolysis with a mineral acid gives acid.

$$R.Mg.I + CO_2 \longrightarrow R.C.O.MgI \xrightarrow{H_2O} R.C.OH$$

Grignard's   Adduct   Acid
reagent

4. **From dicarboxylic acids:** When dicarboxylic acids, containing two carboxyl groups on the same carbon atom, are heated then monocarboxylic acids are obtained.

$$CH_2.(COOH)_2 \xrightarrow{Heat} CH_3.COOH + CO_2$$

Malonic acid   Acetic acid

5. **From sodium alkoxides:** Sodium salts of acids are obtained by the action of carbon monoxide on sodium alkoxides under pressure. These salts on hydrolysis yield fatty acids.

$$R.O.Na + CO \longrightarrow R.COO.Na \xrightarrow{HCl} R.COOH$$

Sodium alkoxide   Sodium salt   Fatty acid

6. **Hydrolysis of malonic and acetoacetic esters:** Acid hydrolysis of these esters gives carboxylic acids as shown below:

$$CH_3.CO.CH.R.CO.OC_2H_5 \xrightarrow{H^+} R.CH_2.COOH + CH_3.COOH + C_2H_5.OH$$

HO–H HO–H
| |

Besides these esters the hydrolysis of lower common esters yields acids. Higher members are produced by the hydrolysis of glycerides (e.g. oils and fats).

$$CH_3.CO.OC_2.H_5 + NaOH \longrightarrow CH_3.CO.ONa + C_2H_5.OH$$

Ethyl acetate (ester)   Sodium acetate

7. **Oxidation of higher hydrocarbons:** Higher fatty acids are obtained by the oxidation of long chain hydrocarbons at 120° in the presence of air and manganous stearate as a catalyst.

$$2R.CH_3 + 3O_2 \longrightarrow 2R.COOH + 2H_2O$$

Higher   Fatty acid
alkane

8. **Hydrolysis of trihaloalkanes:** Trihaloalkanes having three halogen atoms on the same carbon atom give fatty acids on hydrolysis in small yields.

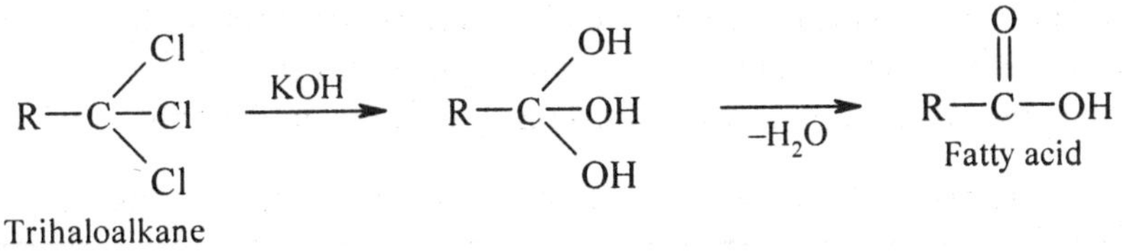

Trihaloalkane

9. **From olefins:** Monocarboxylic acids may be prepared by heating an alkene with carbon monoxide and steam under pressure at high temperature (300–$400^\circ C$) in the presence of phosphoric acid as a catalyst.

$$CH_2 = CH_2 + CO + H_2O \longrightarrow CH_3.CH_2.COOH$$

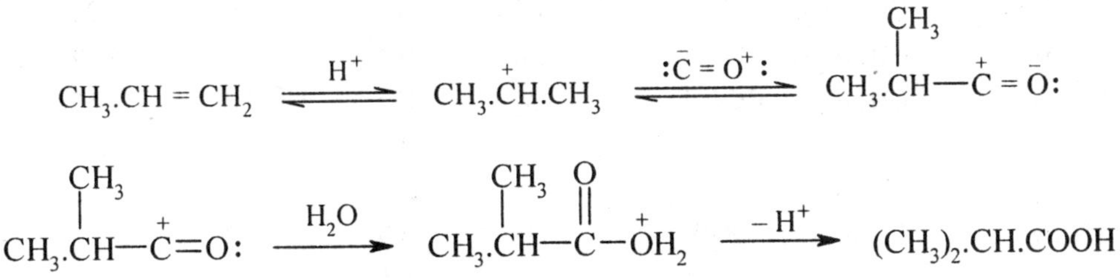

General Physical Properties

1. The first three acids are colourless and pungent - smelling liquids. The acids from butyric ($C_3H_7.COOH$) to nonanoic ($C_8H_{17}.COOH$) acids are oils having goat butter like smell. The acids higher than decanoic acid ($C_9H_{19}.COOH$) are odourless waxy solids.

2. Lower members upto C_4 are very soluble in water. Solubility decreases with increase in the molecular weight. Acids from C_{10} onwards are water insoluble. But they are soluble in less polar solvents like ether, alcohol, benzene, etc.

3. The lower members are far less volatile than is to be expected from their molecular weights. For example, propionic acid (b.p. 141°) boils more than twenty degree higher than the alcohol of comparable molecular weight, n-butyl alcohol (b.p. 118°). This can be explained on the basis of hydrogen bonding. Electron diffraction studies and X-ray crystallographic measurements

indicate that an eight-membered ring is present, i.e., the acids exist as cyclic dimers formulated as shown:

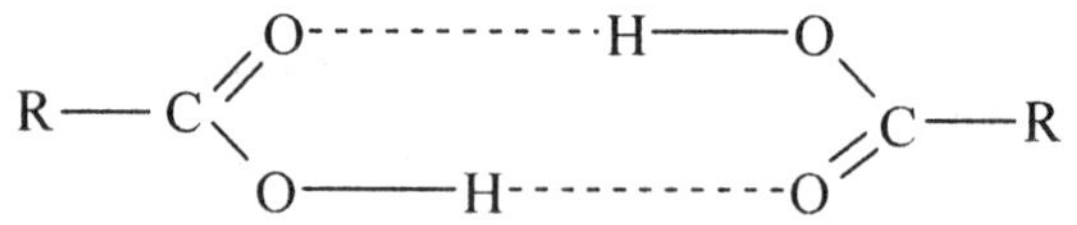

4. The melting points of the n-monocarboxylic acids show alternation from one member to the next. The melting point of an **even** acid being higher than that of the **odd** acid below and above it in the series. This is due to the close packing of the molecules in the solid state. The boiling point increases with increase in the molecular weight.

5. Only the first two members are heavier than water. The specific gravity of fatty acids decreases gradually (1.22 for formic acid and 0.85 for stearic acid).

6. Fatty acids are relatively weak acids. Formic acid is the strongest acid. Their acid character decreases with increase in the molecular weight. The acid strength is expressed either in a term of dissociation constant (K_a) or by the negative logarithm (pK_a) of dissociation constant. The physical constants of monocarboxylic acids are shown in the Table 15.1 given below:

Table 15.1. Physical constants of monocarboxylic acids

Name	Formula	M.P. ^oC	B.P. ^oC	Solub. g/100 g H_2O	K_a at 25^oC
Formic	H.COOH	8	100.5	∞	17.7×10^{-5}
Acetic	CH_3.COOH	16.6	118	∞	1.84
Propionic	$CH_3.CH_2$.COOH	-22	141	∞	1.22
Butyric	$CH_3.(CH_2)_2$.COOH	-6	164	∞	1.50
Valeric	$CH_3.(CH_2)_3$.COOH	-34	187	3.7	1.56
Caproic	$CH_3.(CH_2)_4$.COOH	-3	205	1.0	1.40
Caparylic	$CH_3.(CH_2)_6$.COOH	16	238	0.7	
Capric	$CH_3(CH_2)_8$.COOH	31	269	0.2	
Lauric	$CH_3.(CH_2)_{10}$.COOH	44	225	Insol.	
Myristic	$CH_3.(CH_2)_{12}$.COOH	54	251	Insol.	
Palmitic	$CH_3.(CH_2)_{14}$.COOH	63	269	Insol.	
Stearic	$CH_3.(CH_2)_{16}$.COOH	70	287	Insol.	
Oleic	$C_{17}H_{33}$.COOH	16	223	Insol.	
Linoleic	$C_{17}H_{31}$.COOH	-5	230	Insol.	
Linolenic	$C_{17}H_{29}$.COOH	-11	232	Insol.	
Cyclohexane	C_6H_{11}.COOH	31	233	0.20	

General Chemical Properties

The chemical properties of carboxylic acids are due to the presence of functional group Carboxyl, –COOH. One carbonyl group (C = O) and one hydroxyl group (–OH) are present in the carboxylic group. The –OH group loses one proton (H^+) in a chemical reaction. This proton may be replaced by another group. The carbonyl group has pronounced effect in releasing the proton.

The rest of the molecule undergoes reaction characteristic of its structure.

A. Reactions Due to Carboxyl Group

1. **Reaction involving proton replacement:** Carboxylic acids undergo ionization like inorganic acids to give proton and acid anion.

$$R.COOH \rightleftharpoons R.CO\bar{O} + H^+$$

Strongly electropositive metals or their salts react with acids with the liberation of hydrogen and formation of a salt:

$$R.COOH + Na \longrightarrow R.CO\bar{O}Na^+ + \frac{1}{2}H_2$$

$$R.COOH + KOH \longrightarrow R.CO\bar{O}K^+ + H_2O$$

$$2R.COOH + ZnO \longrightarrow (R.COO)_2Zn + H_2$$

$$2R.COOH + Na_2CO_3 \longrightarrow 2R.CO\bar{O}Na^+ + H_2O + CO_2$$

2. **Reactions involving hydroxyl group:**
    (i) **Formation of esters:** A carboxylic acid is converted directly into an ester when heated with an alcohol under the influence of an acid catalyst (HCl, H_2SO_4). The reaction is reversible and an equilibrium is obtained when there are appreciable quantities of both reactants and products.

$$\underset{\text{Acid}}{R.COOH} + \underset{\text{Alcohol}}{R'OH} \overset{H^+}{\rightleftharpoons} \underset{\text{Ester}}{R.CO.OR'} + H_2O$$

The hydrogen ion, catalyzes the forward reaction (esterification) as well as the reverse reaction (hydrolysis). The order of esterification for alcohol is $CH_3OH > 1^0 > 2^0 > 3^0$, and for acids is: $H.COOH > CH_3.COOH > R.CH_2.COOH > R_2.CH.COOH > R_3.C.COOH$.
Mechanism of the reaction:

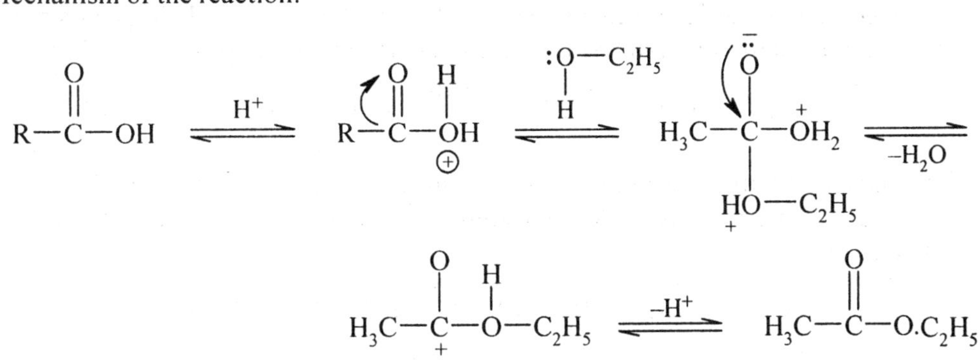

    (ii) **With phosphorus halides and thionyl chloride:** An acid halide is formed by replacing the –OH group of acids with a halogen. The reaction is carried out with the reagents like phosphorus pentahalides, phosphorus trihalides, and thionyl chloride.

$$3R.COOH + PCl_3 \longrightarrow 3R.CO.Cl + H_3PO_3$$

$$CH_3.COOH + PCl_5 \longrightarrow CH_3.CO.Cl + POCl_3 + HCl$$
Acetic acid   Acetyl chloride

$$C_2H_5.COOH + SOCl_2 \longrightarrow C_2H_5.CO.Cl + SO_2 + HCl$$
Propionic acid   Propionyl chloride

Thionyl chloride particularly is a convenient reagent, since the by-products formed are gases and thus easily separated from the acid chloride formed.

(iii) **With ammonia:** Carboxylic acids react with ammonia to form ammonium salts. These salts when heated produce amides as the final compounds.

$$R.COOH + NH_3 \longrightarrow R.CO\bar{O}NH_4^+ \xrightarrow{\text{Heat}} R.CO.NH_2 + H_2O$$
Acid

(iv) **Dehydration:** Acid anhydrides are obtained when fatty acids are dehydrated in the presence of phosphorus pentoxide. These anhydrides are also formed when sodium salts of acids are reacted with their chlorides.

$$CH_3.COOH + HOOC.CH_3 \xrightarrow{P_2O_5} (CH_3.CO)_2O + H_2O$$
Acetic acid (2 moles)   Acetic anhydride

$$CH_3.COO.Na + Cl.CO.CH_3 \longrightarrow (CH_3.CO)_2O + H_2O$$
Sodium acetate   Acetyl chloride

3. **Reduction of carbonyl group:** Due to resonance the carbon-oxygen double bond has some single bond character and thus the double bond character of C = O group is reduced to some extent. Therefore, the C = O group of an acid does not undergo addition reactions as in case of ketones i.e., they do not form oximes, phenylhydrazones, semicarbazones etc.

However, the carbonyl group of acids is reduced to methylene group ($-CH_2-$) either by hydrogen under pressure and in the presence of nickel catalyst or by lithium aluminium hydride, e.g.:

$$4R.COOH + 3LiAlH_4 \longrightarrow 4H_2 + 2LiAlO_2 + (R.CH_2O)_4AlLi \xrightarrow{H_2O} 4R.CH_2.OH$$
1° alcohol

Higher members are more easily reduced than the lower ones. Hydrogenation of these acids with copper chromium catalyst is used for the preparation of primary alcohols.

$$C_{11}H_{23}.COOH + 2H_2 \xrightarrow{CuCr_2O_4} C_{11}H_{23}.CH_2.OH + H_2O$$
Lauryl alcohol

Reduction of fatty acids with hydriodic acid red phosphorus mixture under pressure, or with hydrogen under pressure at elevated temperature in the presence of a nickel catalyst produces an alkane.

$$R.COOH + 3H_2 \xrightarrow{Ni} R.CH_3 + 2H_2O$$
Alkane

4. **Reaction involving carbonyl group as a whole:**

(i) **Formation of alkanes:** When the anhydrous sodium salt of a fatty acid is heated with soda-lime an alkane is formed along with other side products.

$$R.COO.Na + NaOH \xrightarrow{\text{Heat}} \underset{\text{Alkane}}{R.H} + Na_2CO_3$$

Mechanism of the reaction:

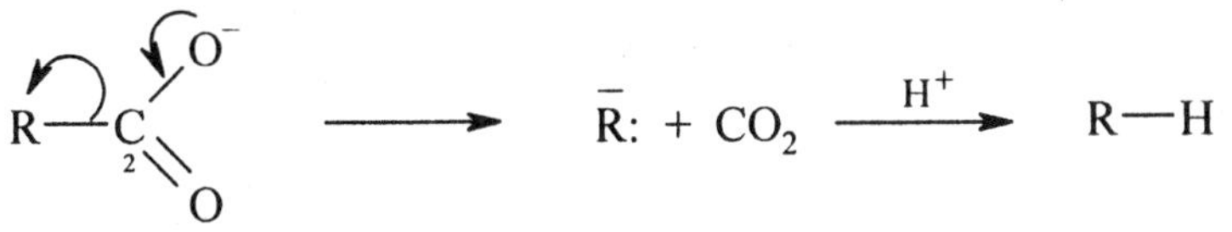

$$\xrightarrow{} \bar{R}: + CO_2 \xrightarrow{H^+} R-H$$

(ii) **Kolbe's reaction:** A higher alkane is formed when electrolysis of sodium or potassium salt of a fatty acid is carried out in concentrated aqueous solution.

$$R.COO.Na \underset{}{\overset{\text{Electrolysis}}{\rightleftharpoons}} R.CO\bar{O} + Na^+$$

At anode:

$$2R.CO\bar{O} \longrightarrow R.R + 2CO_2 + 2\bar{e}$$

At cathode:

$$2Na + 2\bar{e} \longrightarrow 2Na \xrightarrow{2H_2O} 2NaOH + H_2$$

(iii) **Formation of carbonyl compounds:** Calcium salts give ketones when heated strongly; while aldehydes are obtained when a mixture of calcium formate and a calcium salt of other fatty acid is heated.

$$\underset{\text{Calcium acetate}}{(CH_3.COO)_2Ca} \xrightarrow{\text{Heat}} \underset{\text{Acetone}}{(CH_3)_2CO} + CaCO_3$$

$$\underset{\text{Calcium formate}}{(CH_3.COO)_2Ca + (H.COO)_2Ca} \xrightarrow{\text{Heat}} \underset{\text{Acetaldehyde}}{2CH_3.CHO} + 2CaCO_3$$

$$\underset{\text{Calcium formate}}{(H.COO)_2Ca} \xrightarrow{\text{Heat}} \underset{\text{Formaldehyde}}{H.CHO} + CaCO_3$$

(iv) **Formation of alkyl halides:** Alkyl halides are formed when wilver salts of fatty acids are reacted with halogens, e.g.:

$$2 R.COO.Ag + 2 Br_2 \longrightarrow \underset{\text{Alkyl halide}}{2 R.Br} + 2 CO_2 + 2 AgBr$$

(v) **Formation of primary amines (Schmidt reaction):** Hydrazoic acid reacts with carboxylic acids to yield primary amines at 50–55°.

$$\underset{\text{Acid}}{R.COOH} + \underset{\substack{\text{Hydrazoic} \\ \text{acid}}}{HN_3} \xrightarrow[H_2SO_4]{50-55°C} \underset{\substack{\text{Primary} \\ \text{amine}}}{R.NH_2} + N_2 + CO_2$$

B. Reactions Due to Alkyl Group

1. **Halogenation:** Carboxylic acids react smoothly with chlorine or bromine in the presence of phosphorus to produce a compound in which α-hydrogen has been replaced by halogen.

$$CH_3.CH_2.COOH \xrightarrow[-HCl]{Cl_2/P} CH_3.CHCl.COOH \xrightarrow[-HCl]{Cl_2/P} CH_3.CCl_2.COOH$$

Propionic acid

$$\downarrow Cl_2/P$$

No further substitution

2. **Oxidation:** Carboxylic acids when heated with powerful oxidizing agents are oxidized to give carbon dioxide and water. However, with mild oxidizing agents like 3% H_2O_2 they are oxidized to β-hydroxy acids.

$$CH_3.CH_2.CH_2.COOH \xrightarrow[H_2O_2]{[O]} CH_3.CH.CH_2.COOH$$

Butyric acid

$$|$$
$$OH$$

β-Hydroxybutyric acid

Acetic Acid, $CH_3.COOH$

Acetic acid occurs in free form in a number of fermented juices of fruits. It is the main constituent of vinegar (Latin: acetone = vinegar). In the combined state it is found in biological fluids and plant extracts as salt and ester and as glyceride in croton oil.

Preparation: Acetic acid can be prepared by any general method described for the general preparations of monocarboxylic acids. However, it can be manufactured by the following general methods.

1. **From pyroligneous acid:** Pyroligneous acid is obtained during the preparation of methanol by destructive distillation of wood. It is a mixture of acetic acid (10%), methanol (2–4%), acetone (0.5%) and water. It is treated with lime-water and evaporated to get calcium acetate as a residue. This is purified by crystallization and then hydrolyzed with dilute sulphuric acid in 10–15% amount. The dilute solution is neutralized with sodium carbonate and the sodium acetate so obtained is crystallized. The crystals are dried by heating and then distilled with calculated amount of concentrated sulphuric acid to get pure glacial acetic acid.

2. **From vinegar:** Vinegar contains 7–8% acetic acid which is obtained when cane-juice or malt liquor is fermented. A dilute solution of alcohol (15%) is fermented by **Acetobacter aceti** in the presence of air and inorganic salts. The temperature is maintained between 30–35°C. Alcohol is oxidized to acetic acid.

$$C_2H_5.OH + O_2 \longrightarrow CH_3.COOH + H_2O$$

Vinegar is reacted with lime when calcium acetate is formed. This is crystallized from the solution and then distilled with concentrated sulphuric acid to get acetic acid in pure form.

3. **From acetylene:** Acetylene is passed into dilute sulphuric acid (42%) at 60° in the presence of mercuric sulphate (1%). Acetaldehyde is produced which is then oxidized to acetic acid in about 80% yield by passing its vapours along with air over manganese acetate at 70°.

$$HC \equiv CH + H_2O \xrightarrow[\text{HgSO}_4]{\text{H}_2\text{SO}_4} CH_3.CHO \xrightarrow{[O]} CH_3.COOH$$

4. **From methanol:** Methanol reacts with carbon monoxide under pressure in the presence of cobalt octacarbonyl at about 210°C.

$$CO + CH_3.OH \longrightarrow CH_3.COOH$$

Physical properties: Acetic acid is a colourless, pungent smelling, corrosive liquid, m.p. 16.6°C, b.p. 118°C with sharp vinegar smell and sour taste. It is miscible in all proportions with, water ethanol and ether. Its specific gravity is 1.08 at 0°C and occurs in dimer form due to association. It is commonly used as a solvent for sulphur, iodine and phosphorus, and in the preparation of acetates, acetone, acetic anhydride, etc. At low temperature, it solidifies to form icy and hygroscopic crystals, and therefore, it is named as glacial acetic acid.

Chemical properties: Acetic acid gives the usual properties of an organic acid as described earlier.

Uses: It is used:

   (i) As vinegar for table purpose.

  (ii) For manufacture of various dyestuffs, perfumes, rayon, rubber from latex, casein from milk, pickles, non-inflammable cinematographic films and organic chemicals such as acetone, acetic anhydride etc.

 (iii) Aluminium and chromium acetates are used as mordants.

 (iv) Alkali acetates as diuretics, basic lead acetate for fractures and burns and phenacetin for headache.

  (v) White lead and basic copper acetate as paint.

 (vi) Lead tetracetate as an oxidizing agent and aluminium acetate as water proofing of fabrics and as antiseptic and astringent.

Trichloroacetic Acid, $CCl_3.COOH$

Preparation:

1. Chlorination of acetic acid in the presence of a trace of iodine, red phosphorus or with exposure to sunlight leads to the formation of chloroacetic acid, di- and trichloroacetic acid.

$$CH_3.COOH \xrightarrow{\text{Cl}_2/\text{P}} CH_2.Cl.COOH \xrightarrow{\text{High temp.}} CHCl_2.COOH \xrightarrow{\text{High temp.}} CCl_3.COOH$$

The iodine acts as a catalyst as well as halogen carrier. Probably iodine trichloride is formed which chlorinates most effectively.

$$I_2 + 3Cl_2 \longrightarrow 3ICl_3$$
$$ICl_3 + 2CH_3.COOH \longrightarrow ICl + 2CH_2.Cl.COOH$$
$$ICl + Cl_2 \longrightarrow ICl_3$$

2. It is prepared most conveniently by oxidation of chloral hydrate with concentrated nitric acid.

$$CCl_3.CH(OH_2) + [O] \longrightarrow CCl_3.COOH + H_2O$$

Properties: It is a crystalline, colourless, deliquescent solid, m.p. 58°C with sharp pungent smell. It is strongly corrosive and is soluble in water, alcohol and ether. It is one of the strongest organic acids.

The presence of three chlorine atoms on a carbon atom attached to a carbonyl group causes the C–C bond to break very easily. Thus, when trichloroacetic acid is boiled with dilute alkali, or even with water, chloroform is achieved.

$$CCl_3.COOH \longrightarrow CHCl_3 + CO_2$$

Three chlorine atoms attract electrons towards themselves due to inductive effect. Thus, C–C bond is readily cleaved and a possible mechanism of the reaction is demonstrated below:

$$Cl_3C-COO^- \longrightarrow CO_2 + C\bar{C}l_3 \xrightarrow{H_2O} CHCl_3$$

Use: It is used:
   (i) as a reagent for detection of albumin;
   (ii) in medicine and as herbicide; and
   (iii) in organic synthesis.

Oleic Acid, cis-Octadec-9-enoic Acid
$CH_3.(CH_2)_7CH = CH.(CH_2)_7.COOH$

It occurs as glyceryl ester in oils and fats especially in olive oil (76–86%), the fruit fat of *Olea europaea*; almond-kernel oil (77%), the seed fat of *Prunus amygdalus*; linseed oil and cotton seed oil. It is also the major acid of depot fats of herbivorous animals; mutton and beef tallows (50%), and oil from ox hoof (80%).

Preparation: Oleic acid can be obtained by hydrolysis of olive oil with hot, dilute alkalis or superheated steam. The hydrolyzed product is a mixture of sodium salts of palmitic, stearic and oleic acids.

$$
\begin{array}{l}
CH_2.O.CO.C_{15}H_{31} \\
| \\
CH.O.CO.C_{17}H_{35} + 3NaOH \xrightarrow{Heat} \\
| \\
CH_2.O.CO.C_{17}H_{33}
\end{array}
\quad
\begin{array}{l}
CH_2.OH \\
| \\
CH.OH \\
| \\
CH_2.OH
\end{array}
+
\begin{array}{l}
C_{15}H_{31}.COO.Na \\
\text{Sodium palmitate} \\
+ \\
C_{17}H_{35}.COO.Na \\
\text{Sodium stearate} \\
+ \\
C_{17}H_{33}.COO.Na \\
\text{Sodium oleate}
\end{array}
$$

Oleopalmitostearin   Glycerol

These salts are treated with aqueous lead acetate when insoluble salts of fatty acids are formed. The dry lead salts are dissolved in ether. Only lead oleate is soluble in ether leaving behind the two insoluble salts. The ethereal solution is filtered, evaporated and the residue so obtained is heated with sulphuric acid (dilute). Oleic acid is liberated as oily layer which is separated, dehydrated with anhydrous calcium chloride and distilled in vacuum.

Physical properties: Pure oleic acid is a colourless oil (b.p. 286°, m.p. 16°). It is insoluble in water, but soluble in alcohol and ether. On exposure to air, it gradually becomes yellow due to slow oxidation and develops a rancid odour. It dissolves in alkalis with formation of soaps.

Chemical properties: Oleic acid is an unsaturated acid. Catalytic reduction converts it into stearic acid. It is easily oxidized with cold, dilute alkaline solution of potassium permanganate. It combines with bromine to form the dibromide, dihydroxy compound with either $KMnO_4$ or hydrogen peroxide which on oxidation with periodic acid or lead tetraacetate gives normal perlargonic aldehyde and azelaic aldehyde. These products are also obtained when oleic acid is ozonized. Formation of these products indicates that the position of double bond in oleic acid is 9.10.

1. $CH_3.(CH_2)_7.CH = CH.(CH_2)_7.COOH \xrightarrow[Ni]{H_2} CH_3.(CH_2)_{16}.COOH$

     Oleic acid   Stearic acid

2. $CH_3.(CH_2)_7.CH = CH.(CH_2)_7.COOH \xrightarrow{Br_2} CH_3.(CH_2).CH - CH.(CH_2)_7.COOH$

                                                            Br   Br

                                                9,10-dibromostearic acid

3. $CH_3.(CH_2)_7.CH = CH.(CH_2)_7.COOH + H_2O + O_2 \xrightarrow[\text{or } H_2O_2]{\text{Dil. alkaline } KMnO_4}$

$CH_3.(CH_2)_7.CH - CH.(CH_2)_7.COOH \xrightarrow[(CH_3.COO)_4 Pb]{HIO_4 \text{ or}} CH_3.(CH_2)_7.CHO + OHC.(CH_2)_7.COOH$

                                                         Perlargonic aldehyde   Azelaic half aldehyde

4. $CH_3.(CH_2)_7.CH{=}CH.(CH_2)_7.COOH \xrightarrow[\substack{Acidic \\ KMnO_4}]{[O]} CH_3.(CH_2)_7.COOH + HOOC.(CH_2)_7.COOH$

                                                     Nonanoic acid   Azelaic acid

5. $CH_3.(CH_2)_7.CH{=}CH.(CH_2)_7.COOH + O_3 \longrightarrow$

$$CH_3.(CH_2)_7.\underset{\displaystyle |}{CH}\overset{\displaystyle O}{\overbrace{}}\underset{\displaystyle |}{CH}.(CH_2)_7.COOH$$

                                          O——O

                                          Ozonide

                                           $\downarrow H_2O$

$$H_2O_2 + CH_3.(CH_2)_7.CHO + CHO.(CH_2)_7.COOH$$

                           Nonanoic   Azelaic half

                           aldehyde   aldehyde

Oleic acid is the cis form. The trans form is elaidic acid (m.p. 51°C), which is obtained when oleic acid is reacted with nitrous acid or by heating at 180–200° with a small amount of selenium.

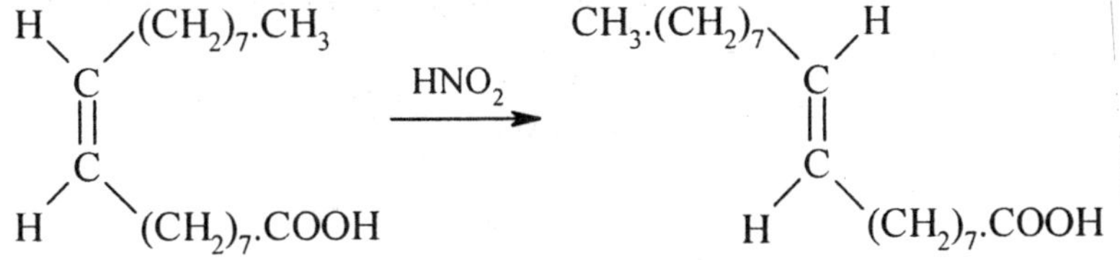

               Oleic acid   Elaidic acid

Uses: Oleic acid is used in the manufacture of soaps and for oiling wool before spinning.

Oxalic Acid, Ethanedioic Acid $(COOH)_2$

Oxalic acid occurs in rhubarb, in soyrel and other plants of **oxalis** group (hence the name). Its potassium and calcium salts are found in plants of rumex family. Rhubarb rhizome contains about 7 per cent of calcium oxalate. Calcium and ferrous oxalates also occur in minerals.

Preparation:

1. When carbon dioxide is passed over potassium or sodium at high temperature ($360°$) salt of oxalic acid is obtained. Hydrolysis of the salt gives oxalic acid.

$$2CO_2 + 2Na \longrightarrow \begin{matrix} COO.Na \\ | \\ COO.Na \end{matrix} \xrightarrow[-2NaCl]{2HCl} \begin{matrix} COOH \\ | \\ COOH \end{matrix}$$

2. Oxidation of the following compounds gives oxalic acid.

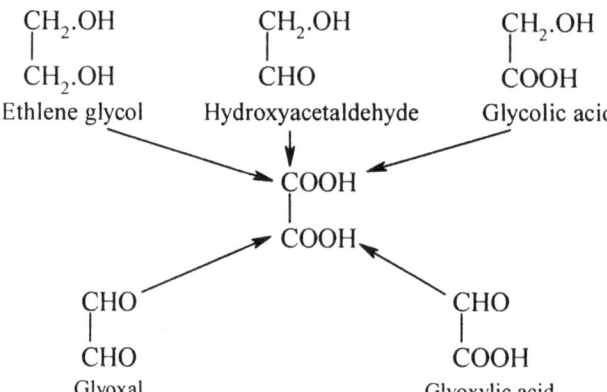

$$\begin{matrix} CH_2.OH \\ | \\ CH_2.OH \end{matrix} \qquad \begin{matrix} CH_2.OH \\ | \\ CHO \end{matrix} \qquad \begin{matrix} CH_2.OH \\ | \\ COOH \end{matrix}$$

Ethlene glycol   Hydroxyacetaldehyde   Glycolic acid

$$\begin{matrix} COOH \\ | \\ COOH \end{matrix}$$

$$\begin{matrix} CHO \\ | \\ CHO \end{matrix} \qquad\qquad \begin{matrix} CHO \\ | \\ COOH \end{matrix}$$

Glyoxal   Glyoxylic acid

3. In the laboratory, oxalic acid is prepared by the oxidation of sucrose with nitric acid. A mixture of sucrose (10 gm), concentrated nitric acid (75 ml) and vanadium pentaoxide catalyst (0.05 gm) is slightly heated in a flask on a steam bath. A vigorous reaction takes place and brown fumes of nitrogen dioxide are evolved. The flask is cooled if the reaction becomes extremely violent. When the reaction is completed, the mixture is left for several hours. Colourless crystals of oxalic acid separate out which are filtered on the pump and purified by recrystallization from water.

Cyanogen is converted into oxalic acid by hydrolysis as shown below:

$$\begin{matrix} CN \\ | \\ CN \end{matrix} + 4H_2O \longrightarrow \begin{matrix} COOH \\ | \\ COOH \end{matrix} + 2NH_3$$

4. Reaction of carbon monoxide on sodium hydroxide gives sodium formate which on heating yields sodium oxalate.

$$CO + NaOH \xrightarrow[8-10\ Atm.]{200°C} H.COO.Na$$
Sodium formate

$$2H.COO.Na \xrightarrow[-H_2]{360°C} \begin{matrix} COO.Na \\ | \\ COO.Na \end{matrix}$$
Sodium oxalate

Sodium oxalate is dissolved in water and reacted with lime water. Calcium oxalate is precipitated which is filtered, washed and treated with the calculated amount of dilute sulphuric acid. The insoluble calcium sulphate is filtered off and the filtrate is evaporated to give the concentrated solution. Oxalic acid is crystallized on cooling.

5. Cellulose on oxidation gives oxalic acid. Saw dust is the cheap raw material which is mixed with a mixture of caustic potash and caustic soda. The paste so prepared is spread in thin films on iron sheets and fused at 200–220°. Cellulose is oxidized to give sodium and potassium oxalates. After cooling, the residue is extracted with water and the alkali oxalates are reacted with lime water. The calcium oxalate is worked up for obtaining oxalic acid as described earlier.

Physical properties: Oxalic acid is a colourless, crystalline solid containing two molecules of water. The melting point of hydrate is 101.5°C and that of anhydrous acid is 190°C. It is soluble in water and alcohol but insoluble in ether. It is a poisonous compound.

Chemical properties: Oxalic acid shows all the usual reactions of dicarboxylic acids. It consists of two carboxyl groups only and does not contain the hydrocarbon chain. Its important chemical properties are given below:

1. **Action of heat:** The dihydrate loses water when heated at 100–150°C and when heated at about 200°C it partly sublimes and partly decomposes into carbon dioxide, carbon monoxide, formic acid and water. If sulphuric acid is used then the decomposition takes place at lower temperatures, and in this case the formic acid is transformed into carbon monoxide and water.

$$(COOH)_2.2H_2O \xrightarrow{100–105°C} (COOH)_2 + H_2O$$

Crystalline oxalic acid   Anhydrous oxalic acid

$$(COOH)_2 \xrightarrow{200°C} CO_2 + H.COOH \xrightarrow{Heat} 2CO_2 + H_2O$$

The anhydrous acid is conveniently prepared by heating the hydrate with carbon tetrachloride.

2. **With concentrated sulphuric acid:** When heated with concentrated sulphuric acid at 90°C oxalic acid is decomposed into a mixture of carbon monoxide, carbon dioxide and water.

$$(COOH)_2 \xrightarrow[90°C]{Conc. H_2SO_4} CO + CO_2 + H_2O$$

3. **Oxidation:** It differs from other members of the series in being that it is oxidized by hot acidic potassium permanganate to carbon dioxide in which rupture of a weakened linkage between two highly active carbon atoms takes place.

$$(COOH)_2 + [O] \xrightarrow{KMnO_4} 2CO_2 + H_2O$$

The reaction is used in volumetric analysis for standardization of $KMnO_4$ solution as the reaction is quantitative and oxalic acid dihydrate is an easily purified crystalline substance. Slow oxidation takes place with concentrated nitric acid. When it is fused with potassium hydroxide, hydrogen gas is evolved.

$$(COO.K)_2 + 2KOH \longrightarrow 2K_2CO_3 + H_2$$

4. **With ethylene glycol:** Oxalic acid forms cyclic compound, ethylene oxalate, when heated with ethylene glycol.

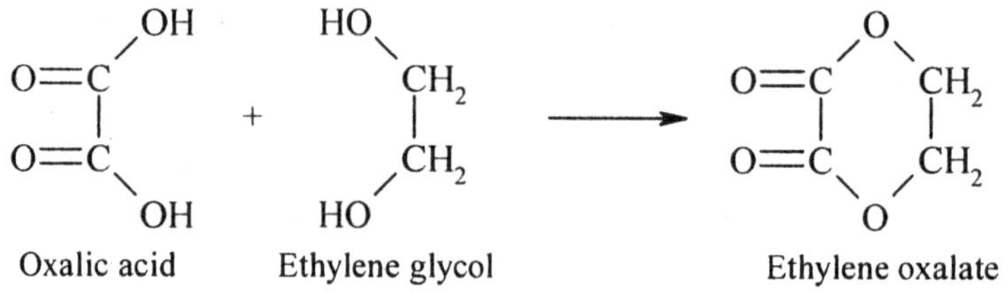

$$\text{Oxalic acid} + \text{Ethylene glycol} \longrightarrow \text{Ethylene oxalate}$$

5. **Reduction:** Oxalic acid is reduced to glycolic acid with zinc and dilute sulphuric acid whereas glyoxylic acid is obtained on electrolytic reduction using lead cathode.

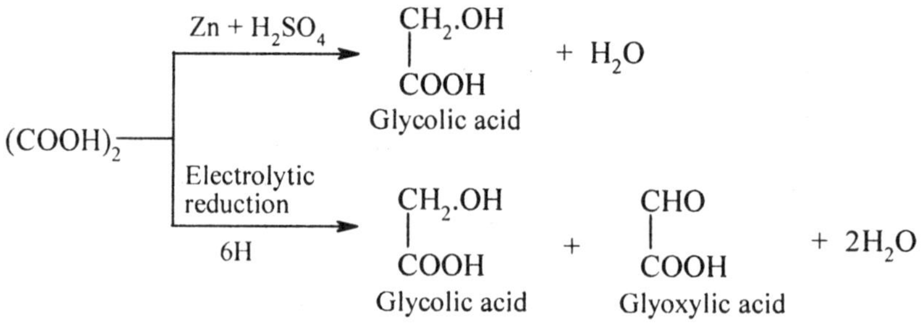

$$(COOH)_2 \xrightarrow{\quad Zn + H_2SO_4 \quad} \begin{matrix} CH_2.OH \\ | \\ COOH \end{matrix} + H_2O$$

Glycolic acid

$$(COOH)_2 \xrightarrow[\text{6H}]{\begin{matrix}\text{Electrolytic}\\\text{reduction}\end{matrix}} \begin{matrix} CH_2.OH \\ | \\ COOH \end{matrix} + \begin{matrix} CHO \\ | \\ COOH \end{matrix} + 2H_2O$$

Glycolic acid   Glyoxylic acid

6. **Reaction with glycerol:** Oxalic acid reacts with glycerol to give different products under different reaction conditions. When excess of oxalic acid is heated with glycerol at 110°C then glycerol monoxalate is formed which on decarboxylation forms glycerol monoformate. This on hydrolysis (with water of crystallization) yields formic acid and glycerol.

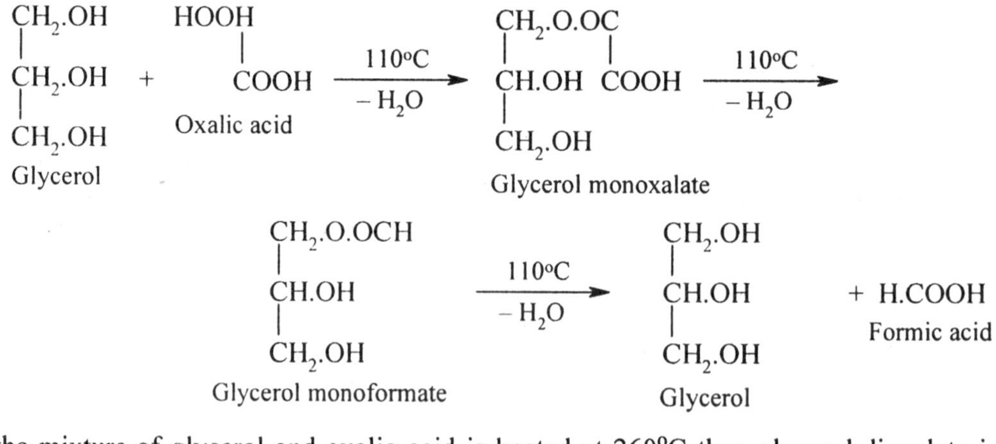

$$\begin{matrix} CH_2.OH \\ | \\ CH_2.OH \\ | \\ CH_2.OH \end{matrix} + \begin{matrix} HOOH \\ | \\ COOH \end{matrix} \xrightarrow[-H_2O]{110°C} \begin{matrix} CH_2.O.OC \\ | \quad\quad | \\ CH.OH \quad COOH \\ | \\ CH_2.OH \end{matrix} \xrightarrow[-H_2O]{110°C}$$

Glycerol   Oxalic acid   Glycerol monoxalate

$$\begin{matrix} CH_2.O.OCH \\ | \\ CH.OH \\ | \\ CH_2.OH \end{matrix} \xrightarrow[-H_2O]{110°C} \begin{matrix} CH_2.OH \\ | \\ CH.OH \\ | \\ CH_2.OH \end{matrix} + H.COOH$$

Glycerol monoformate   Glycerol   Formic acid

If the mixture of glycerol and oxalic acid is heated at 260°C then glycerol-dioxalate is obtained which on decomposition yields allyl alcohol.

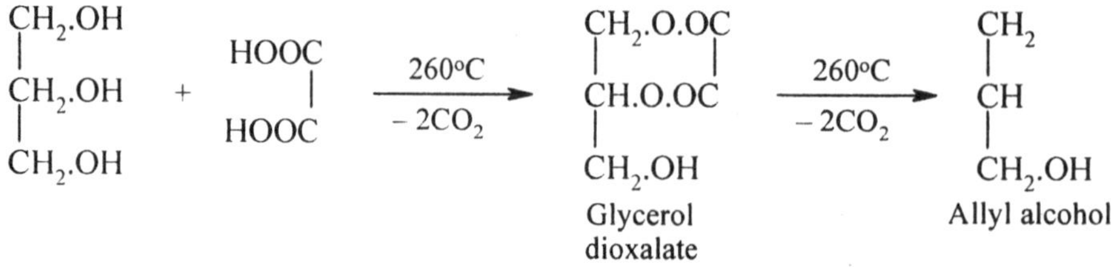

$$\begin{matrix} CH_2.OH \\ | \\ CH_2.OH \\ | \\ CH_2.OH \end{matrix} + \begin{matrix} HOOC \\ | \\ HOOC \end{matrix} \xrightarrow[-2CO_2]{260°C} \begin{matrix} CH_2.O.OC \\ | \quad\quad | \\ CH.O.OC \\ | \\ CH_2.OH \end{matrix} \xrightarrow[-2CO_2]{260°C} \begin{matrix} CH_2 \\ \| \\ CH \\ | \\ CH_2.OH \end{matrix}$$

Glycerol   Glycerol   Allyl alcohol
dioxalate

7. **Derivatives formation:** Due to the presence of two carbonyl groups oxalic acid forms series of salts, esters, amides, and other acid derivatives.

   (i) **Salt formation:** Potassium oxalate $K_2C_2O_4.H_2O$ is prepared by reacting solutions of oxalic acid and potassium carbonate in molecular proportion. The salt crystallized out is isolated. If oxalic acid and potassium carbonate are reacted in proportion of $2:1$ then potassium hydrogen oxalate, KHC_2O_4, is formed. Calcium oxalate, $CaC_2O_4.H_2O$, is insoluble in water and is prepared when calcium salt is added to a neutral solution of oxalate.

$$\underset{}{\begin{array}{c} COOH \\ | \\ COOH \end{array}} \xrightarrow{KOH} \underset{\substack{\text{Pot. hydrogen} \\ \text{oxalate}}}{\begin{array}{c} COO.K \\ | \\ COOH \end{array}} \xrightarrow{KOH} \underset{\substack{\text{Potassium} \\ \text{oxalate}}}{\begin{array}{c} COO.K \\ | \\ COO.K \end{array}}$$

   (ii) **Esterification:** When anhydrous oxalic acid is reacted with alcohol in the presence of a dehydrating agent, two series of esters – acid and normal esters are formed.

$$\underset{}{\begin{array}{c} COOH \\ | \\ COOH \end{array}} \xrightarrow{C_2H_2.OH} \underset{\substack{\text{Ethyl hydrogen} \\ \text{oxalate}}}{\begin{array}{c} COO.C_2H_5 \\ | \\ COOH \end{array}} \xrightarrow{C_2H_2.OH} \underset{\substack{\text{Ethyl oxalate}}}{\begin{array}{c} COO.C_2H_5 \\ | \\ COO.C_2H_5 \end{array}}$$

   Generally a di-ester is prepared by heating a mixture of oxalic acid, alcohol, toluene and concentrated sulphuric acid. The acid is used as a catalyst and the toluene removes the water by forming an azeotrope of alcohol, water and toluene.

   (iii) **Amide formation:** Ammonium salts of oxalic acid form half and normal amides on heating. Oxamic acid is prepared by the action of concentrated ammonium hydroxide solution on ethyl hydrogen oxalate or by heating ammonium hydrogen oxalate. Dehydration of oxamic acid forms oximide.

$$\underset{\substack{\text{Acid ammonium} \\ \text{oxalate}}}{\begin{array}{c} COO.NH_4 \\ | \\ COOH \end{array}} \xrightarrow[-H_2O]{Heat} \underset{\text{Oxamic acid}}{\begin{array}{c} CO.NH_2 \\ | \\ COOH \end{array}} \xrightarrow[-H_2O]{P_2O_5} \underset{\text{Oximide}}{\begin{array}{c} CO \\ | \quad \diagdown NH \\ CO \diagup \end{array}}$$

$$\underset{\text{Ammonium oxalate}}{\begin{array}{c} COO.NH_4 \\ | \\ COO.NH_4 \end{array}} \xrightarrow[-H_2O]{\text{Dry distillation}} \underset{\text{Oxamide}}{\begin{array}{c} CO.NH_2 \\ | \\ CO.NH_2 \end{array}}$$

   Oxamide may be prepared more conveniently by shaking ethyl oxalate with concentrated ammonium hydroxide solution or by passing cyanogen into cold concentrated hydrochloric acid.

$$\begin{array}{c} CO.OC_2H_5 \\ | \\ CO.OC_2H_5 \end{array} + 2NH_3 \longrightarrow NH_2.CO.CO.NH_2 + C_2H_5.OH$$

$$(CN)_2 + 2H_2O \xrightarrow{HCl} (CO.NH_2)_2$$

(iv) **Acid chloride formation:** When oxalic acid is treated with excess of phosphorus pentachloride, oxalyl chloride is formed.

$$
\begin{array}{c}
\text{COOH} \\
| \\
\text{COOH}
\end{array}
\;+\; 2PCl_5 \;\longrightarrow\;
\begin{array}{c}
\text{CO.Cl} \\
| \\
\text{CO.Cl}
\end{array}
\;+\; 2POCl_3 \;+\; 2HCl
$$

Oxalyl chloride

Uses: It is used:

1. As a mordant in calico printing and dyeing.
2. In the manufacture of carbon monoxide, formic acid, allyl alcohol, dyes and inks.
3. As a reagent and as a standard in volumetric analysis, ferrous potassium oxalate is used as developer in photography.
4. For bleaching wood, leather and straw.
5. For removing stains of ink and rust.

Succinic Acid, Butane 1,4-Dioic Acid
$HOOC.CH_2.CH_2.COOH$

Succinic acid occurs widely in nature. It was originally obtained by Agricola in 1550 by destructive distillation of amber (Latin: Succinum = amber) and can be obtained by fermentation of sugar and other substances.

Preparation:

1. By treating ethylene bromide with potassium cyanide and hydrolyzing the cyanide so obtained.

$$
\begin{array}{c}
\text{CH}_2.\text{Br} \\
| \\
\text{CH}_2.\text{Br}
\end{array}
\xrightarrow{\text{KCN}}
\begin{array}{c}
\text{CH}_2.\text{CN} \\
| \\
\text{CH}_2.\text{CN}
\end{array}
\xrightarrow{\text{H}_2\text{O}}
\begin{array}{c}
\text{CH}_2.\text{COOH} \\
| \\
\text{CH}_2.\text{COOH}
\end{array}
$$

Ethylene bromide   Ethylene cyanide   Succinic acid

2. By reducing malic acid or tartaric acid with hydriodic acid and red phosphorus in a sealed tube.

$$
\begin{array}{c}
\text{HO}-\text{CH.COOH} \\
\| \\
\text{CH}_2.\text{COOH}
\end{array}
\xrightarrow[-\text{H}_2\text{O}, -\text{I}_2]{\text{2HI, Red P}}
\begin{array}{c}
\text{CH}_2.\text{COOH} \\
| \\
\text{CH}_2.\text{COOH}
\end{array}
\xleftarrow[-2\text{H}_2\text{O}, -2\text{I}_2]{\text{4HI, Red P}}
\begin{array}{c}
\text{CH(OH).COOH} \\
| \\
\text{CH.(OH).COOH}
\end{array}
$$

Malic acid   Succinic acid   Tartaric acid

3. By catalytic or electrolytic reduction of maleic acid.

$$
\begin{array}{c}
\text{CH.COOH} \\
\| \\
\text{CH.COOH}
\end{array}
\;+\; \text{H}_2 \;\xrightarrow{\text{Ni}}\;
\begin{array}{c}
\text{CH}_2.\text{COOH} \\
| \\
\text{CH}_2.\text{COOH}
\end{array}
$$

Maleic acid

4. By the reaction between malonic ester (1 molecule) and ethyl chloroacetate or between malonic ester (2 molecules) and iodine.

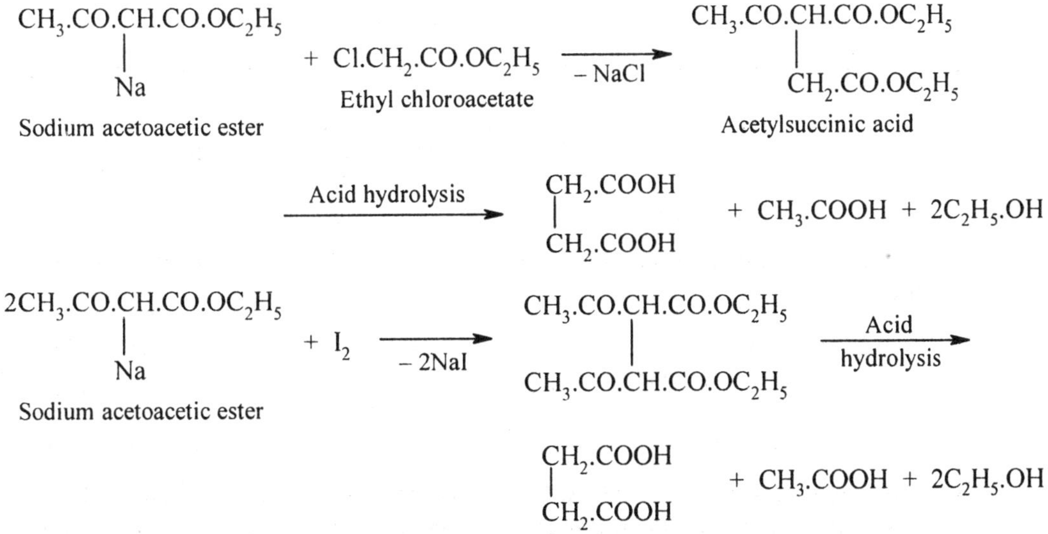

$$
\underset{\substack{| \\ Na \\ \text{Sodium acetoacetic ester}}}{CH_3.CO.CH.CO.OC_2H_5} + \underset{\text{Ethyl chloroacetate}}{Cl.CH_2.CO.OC_2H_5} \xrightarrow[-NaCl]{} \underset{\substack{| \\ CH_2.CO.OC_2H_5 \\ \text{Acetylsuccinic acid}}}{CH_3.CO.CH.CO.OC_2H_5}
$$

$$
\xrightarrow{\text{Acid hydrolysis}} \underset{\substack{| \\ CH_2.COOH}}{CH_2.COOH} + CH_3.COOH + 2C_2H_5.OH
$$

$$
\underset{\substack{| \\ Na \\ \text{Sodium acetoacetic ester}}}{2CH_3.CO.CH.CO.OC_2H_5} + I_2 \xrightarrow{-2NaI} \underset{\substack{| \\ CH_3.CO.CH.CO.OC_2H_5}}{CH_3.CO.CH.CO.OC_2H_5} \xrightarrow{\substack{\text{Acid} \\ \text{hydrolysis}}}
$$

$$
\underset{\substack{| \\ CH_2.COOH}}{CH_2.COOH} + CH_3.COOH + 2C_2H_5.OH
$$

5. By electrolysis of aqueous solution of potassium ethyl malonate (Crum-Brown and Walker's method).

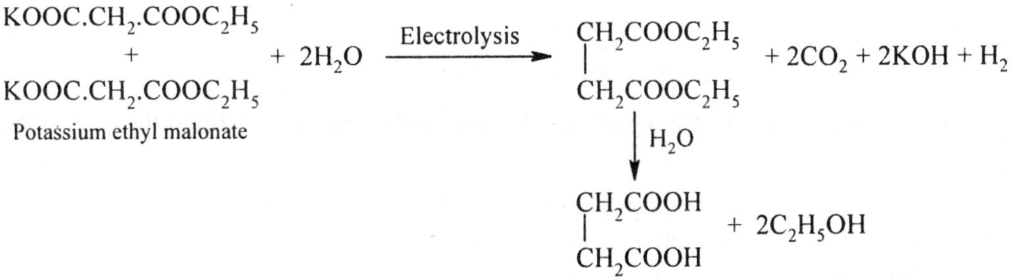

$$
\underset{\text{Potassium ethyl malonate}}{\substack{KOOC.CH_2.COOC_2H_5 \\ + \\ KOOC.CH_2.COOC_2H_5}} + 2H_2O \xrightarrow{\text{Electrolysis}} \underset{\substack{| \\ CH_2COOC_2H_5}}{CH_2COOC_2H_5} + 2CO_2 + 2KOH + H_2
$$

$$
\downarrow H_2O
$$

$$
\underset{\substack{| \\ CH_2COOH}}{CH_2COOH} + 2C_2H_5OH
$$

6. From Grignard's reagent of ethylene bromide.

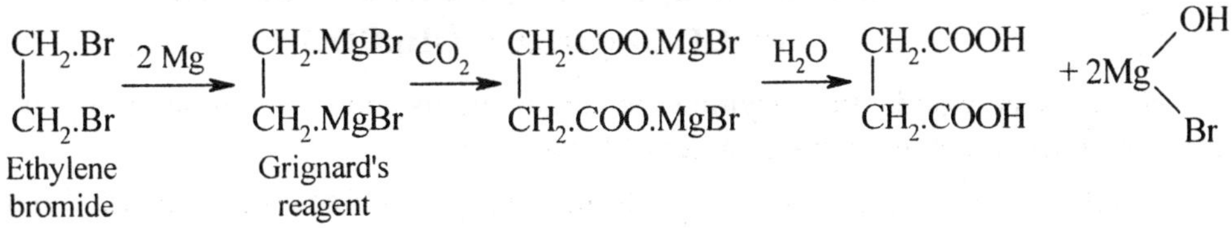

$$
\underset{\substack{\text{Ethylene} \\ \text{bromide}}}{\underset{|}{\overset{CH_2.Br}{CH_2.Br}}} \xrightarrow{2\ Mg} \underset{\substack{\text{Grignard's} \\ \text{reagent}}}{\underset{|}{\overset{CH_2.MgBr}{CH_2.MgBr}}} \xrightarrow{CO_2} \underset{|}{\overset{CH_2.COO.MgBr}{CH_2.COO.MgBr}} \xrightarrow{H_2O} \underset{|}{\overset{CH_2.COOH}{CH_2.COOH}} + 2Mg\overset{OH}{\underset{Br}{<}}
$$

Physical properties: Succinic acid is a colourless, crystalline solid (m.p. $185°$) and is sparingly soluble in water and alcohol.

Chemical properties: Like oxalic acid it is a dibasic acid and undergoes the following reactions in addition to the general reactions of carboxylic acids.

1. **Action of heat:** When heated above its melting point, a large amount of the compound sublimes and the rest is converted into the cyclic anhydride. Dehydration also takes place when succinic acid is refluxed with acetic anhydride or acetyl chloride.

$$\underset{\overset{|}{CH_2.COOH}}{\overset{CH_2.COOH}{|}} \xrightarrow[-H_2O]{Heat} \underset{\overset{|}{CH_2.CO}}{\overset{CH_2.CO}{|}} \!\!\!> O$$

Succinic anhydride

2. **Action of ammonia:** Ammonia reacts with succinic acid or its anhydride to form succinimide.

$$\underset{\overset{|}{CH_2.CO}}{\overset{CH_2.CO}{|}}\!\!\!> O + NH_3 \xrightarrow[-H_2O]{} \underset{\overset{|}{CH_2.CO}}{\overset{CH_2.CO}{|}}\!\!\!> NH$$

Succinic anhydride   Succinimide

Succinimide, obtained by reacting ethyl succinate with ammonia gives succinimide on heating.

$$\underset{\overset{|}{CH_2.CO.OC_2H_5}}{\overset{CH_2.CO.OC_2H_5}{|}} + 2NH_3 \xrightarrow{C_2H_5.OH} \underset{\overset{|}{CH_2.CO.NH_2}}{\overset{CH_2.CO.NH_2}{|}} \xrightarrow{Heat} \underset{\overset{|}{CH_2.CO}}{\overset{CH_2.CO}{|}}\!\!\!> NH$$

Ethyl succinate   Succinamide   Succinimide

Succinimide reacts with bromide at 0°C in the presence of sodium hydroxide to yield N-bromosuccinimide which is an important reagent for brominating olefinic compounds in the allyl position.

$$\underset{\overset{|}{CH_2.CO}}{\overset{CH_2.CO}{|}}\!\!\!> NH + Br_2 \xrightarrow[-HBr]{NaOH,\ 0°} \underset{\overset{|}{CH_2.CO}}{\overset{CH_2.CO}{|}}\!\!\!> N.Br \xrightarrow{-CH_2.CH=CH_2} \underset{Br}{\overset{-CH.OH=CH_2}{|}} + \underset{\overset{|}{CH_2.CO}}{\overset{CH_2.CO}{|}}\!\!\!> NH$$

N-Bromosuccinimide

It forms both types of salts, normal and acid salts, same as obtained in case of oxalic acid.

Uses: It is used:
1. In the manufacture of high polymer esters, dyes and perfumes.
2. As a laboratory reagent in volumetric analysis.
3. In medicine.

Tartaric Acid, α,α-Dihydroxysuccinic Acid
HOOC.CH(OH).CH(OH).COOH

Tartaric acid has two identical asymmetric carbon atoms and exists in the d-, l-, and dl- (racemic and meso-forms) (details in the Chapter of Isomerism).

Naturally occurring tartaric acid is in d-form and occurs in free state in tamarind and as potassium acid salt in juices of grapes, prunes, berries etc. During the fermentation of grapes the acid potassium salt is obtained as a reddish brown crystalline solid which is called as **argol**.

Preparation:
1. **From argol:** Crude argol is purified by crystallization from hot water. White mass known as cream of tartar (potassium hydrogen tartrate) is dissolved in hot water and treated with lime water to neutralize it. In this way half of the original tartrate separates as insoluble calcium tartrate and the rest remains in solution as normal potassium tartrate.

$$2 \begin{array}{c} CH(OH).COOH \\ | \\ CH(OH).COOK \end{array} + Ca(OH)_2 \xrightarrow{-2H_2O} \begin{array}{c} CH(OH).COO \\ | \\ CH(OH).COO \end{array}\Big\rangle Ca + \begin{array}{c} CH(OH).COO.K \\ | \\ CH(OH).COO.K \end{array}$$

Pot. hydrogen tartrate   Pot. tartrate

The insoluble calcium salt is filtered and the filtrate is treated with calcium chloride solution to get precipitated calcium tartrate from potassium tartrate.

$$K_2C_4H_4O_6 + CaCl_2 \longrightarrow Ca.C_4H_4O_6 + 2KCl$$
Pot. tartrate   Cal. tartrate

The whole of the calcium tartrate obtained in both the steps is then decomposed with calculated amount of dilute sulphuric acid. Calcium sulphate is removed by filtration and the filtrate is decolourized with animal charcoal. The clear solution is concentrated under reduced pressure go get d-tartaric acid.

$$\begin{array}{c} CH(OH).COO \\ | \\ CH(OH).COO \end{array}\Big\rangle Ca + H_2SO_4 \longrightarrow \begin{array}{c} CH(OH).COOH \\ | \\ CH(OH)COOH \end{array} + CaSO_4$$

Calcium tartrate   Tartaric acid

2. By treating fumaric acid with dilute alkaline potassium permanganate.

$$\begin{array}{c} H-C-COOH \\ | \\ HOOC-C-H \end{array} \xrightarrow[KMnO_4]{[O]} \begin{array}{c} CH(OH).COOH \\ | \\ CH(OH).COOH \end{array}$$

Fumaric acid   dl-Tartaric acid

Maleic acid under the same conditions forms meso-tartaric acid.

3. By hydrolysis of α,α′-dibromosuccinic acid with silver oxide in water.

$$\begin{array}{c} CHBr.COOH \\ | \\ CHBr.COOH \end{array} + 2AgOH \xrightarrow{Boil} \begin{array}{c} CH(OH).COOH \\ | \\ CH(OH).COOH \end{array} + 2AgBr$$

dl-Tartaric acid

4. By hydrolysis of glyoxal cyanohydrin.

$$\begin{array}{c} CHO \\ | \\ CHO \end{array} \xrightarrow{HCN} \begin{array}{c} CH(OH).CN \\ | \\ CH(OH).CN \end{array} \xrightarrow{H_2O} \begin{array}{c} CH(OH).COOH \\ | \\ CH(OH).COOH \end{array}$$

Glyoxal   Glyoxal   dl-Tartaric acid
                        cyanohydrin

Physical properties: Tartaric acid is a colourless, crystalline solid. It is readily soluble in water and in alcohol but is insoluble in ether. Some physical constants of various forms of tartaric acid are listed in Table 15.2.

Chemical properties: Tartaric acid shows the properties of a dicarboxylic acid and those of secondary alcohol. All the four forms behave in the same way chemically.

1. **Salt formation:** Two series of salts are formed with electropositive metals or their carbonates and hydroxides.

Table 15.2. Physical constants of tartaric acid

Tartaric acid	Dextro	Laevo	Meso	Racemic
m.p.	167–170°C	167–170°C	140°C	205–206°C
Sp. gr.	1.760	1.760	1.697	1.667
[α] D	+12	–12	0	0
Crystal form	Prism	Prism	Plates	Rhombic
Solubility at 20° g/100 in water	139	139	125	206
K_a at 25°C ($\times 10^{-3}$)	1.30	1.30	0.60	1.03

CH(OH).COOH
|
CH(OH).COO.K
Sodium hydrogen
tartrate

CH(OH).COO.Na
|
CH(OH).COO.K
Sodium Pot. tartrate
(Rochelle salt)

CH(OH).COO(SbO)
|
CH(OH).COO.K
Pot. antimonyl
tartrate

2. **Ester formation:** With alcohol, formation of both types of esters, acid and normal esters, takes place as usual.

CH(OH).COOH
|
CH(OH).CO.OC$_2$H$_5$
Ethyl hydrogen tartrate

CH(OH).COO.OC$_2$H$_5$
|
CH(OH).CO.OC$_2$H$_5$
Diethyl tartrate

3. **Action of ammonia:** With ammonia it forms ammonium tartrate which is converted into amide on heating.

CH(OH).COONH$_4$
|
CH(OH).COONH$_4$
$\xrightarrow{\text{Heat}}$
CH(OH).CO.NH$_2$
|
CH(OH).CO.NH$_2$

4. **Effect of heat:** Tartaric anhydride is formed on heating the acid at 150°. If the compound is heated strongly then it chars to form pyruvic acid.

CH(OH).COOH
|
CH(OH).COOH
$\xrightarrow{150°C}$
CH(OH).CO
| \textbackslash O
CH.(OH).CO /

CH(OH).COOH
|
CH(OH).COOH
$\xrightarrow{\text{Strong heating}}$
CH$_3$.CO.COOH + CO$_2$ + H$_2$O
Pyruvic acid

5. **Action of hydrogen bromide:** Dibromuccinic acid is formed when it is reacted with hydrogen bromide.

CH(OH).COOH
|
CH(OH).COOH
+ 2HBr $\longrightarrow$
CHBr.COOH
|
CHBr.COOH
+ 2H$_2$O

6. **Action of hydrogen iodide:** Tartaric acid is reduced with hydriodic acid in the presence of red phosphorus to yield malic acid and then succinic acid.

$$
\begin{array}{l}
CH(OH).COOH \\
| \\
CH(OH).COOH
\end{array}
\;+\; 2HI \;\xrightarrow[-H_2O, -I_2]{red\ P}\;
\begin{array}{l}
CH(OH).COOH \\
| \\
CH_2.COOH
\end{array}
\;\xrightarrow[-H_2O, -I_2]{+\,2HI,\ red\ P}\;
\begin{array}{l}
CH_2.COOH \\
| \\
CH_2.COOH
\end{array}
$$

Malic acid   Succinic acid

7. **Action of concentrated sulphuric acid:** Sulphuric acid decomposes it into carbon monoxide, carbon dioxide, sulphur dioxide, etc.

$$
\begin{array}{l}
CH(OH).COOH \\
| \\
CH(OH).COOH
\end{array}
\;+\; H_2SO_4 \;\longrightarrow\; CO_2 \;+\; 3CO \;+\; SO_2 \;+\; 5H_2O
$$

8. **Acetylation:** With acetic anhydride or acetyl chloride it gives monodiacetyl derivatives.

$$
\begin{array}{l}
CH(OH).COOH \\
| \\
CH(OH).COOH
\end{array}
\;\xrightarrow[-HCl]{CH_3.CO.Cl}\;
\begin{array}{l}
CH_3.CO.O.CH.COOH \\
| \\
HO.CH.COOH
\end{array}
\;\xrightarrow[-HCl]{CH_3.CO.Cl}\;
\begin{array}{l}
CH_3.CO.O.CH.COOH \\
| \\
CH_3.CO.O.CH.COOH
\end{array}
$$

Monoacetyl derivative   Diacetyl derivative

9. **Oxidation:** Mild oxidizing agents convert tartaric acid into tartronic acid while oxalic acid is formed with strong oxidizing agents (like conc. HNO_3).

$$
\begin{array}{l}
CH(OH).COOH \\
| \\
CH(OH).COOH
\end{array}
\;\xrightarrow{[O]}\;
\begin{array}{l}
CH(OH).COOH \\
| \\
COOH
\end{array}
\;\xrightarrow{[O]}\;
\begin{array}{l}
COOH \\
| \\
COOH
\end{array}
$$

Tartronic acid   Oxalic acid

However, Fenton's reagent (alk. H_2O_2 + $FeSO_4$) oxidizes it into dihydroxymaleic acid.

$$
\begin{array}{l}
CH(OH).COOH \\
| \\
CH(OH).COOH
\end{array}
\;+\; H_2O_2 \;\xrightarrow{FeSO_4}\;
\begin{array}{l}
CH(OH).COOH \\
|| \\
C(OH).COOH
\end{array}
\;+\; H_2O
$$

Dihydroxymaleic acid

It reduces Tollen's reagent (ammonical silver nitrate) to form silver mirror.

10. **Action of phosphorus pentachloride:** It reacts with PCl_5 to yield dichlorosuccinyl chloride.

$$
\begin{array}{l}
CH(OH).COOH \\
| \\
CH(OH).COOH
\end{array}
\;\xrightarrow{PCl_5}\;
\begin{array}{l}
CH(OH).COOH \\
| \\
C(OH).COOH
\end{array}
$$

Dichlorosuccinyl
chloride

11. **With Fehling's solution:** Fehling's solution is the mixture of copper sulphate, potassium sodium tartrate (Rochelle salt) and sodium hydroxide. The tartrate forms a complex with insoluble copper hydroxide and thus checks the precipitation as:

$$\begin{bmatrix} \bar{O}OC.CH-O \diagdown & \diagup O-CH.CO\bar{O} \\ & Cu^{-2} \\ \bar{O}OC.CH-O \diagup & \diagdown O-CH.CO\bar{O} \end{bmatrix} 6\overset{+}{N}a$$

Sodium cupritartrate (soluble)

1-Tartaric acid: It does not occur in nature. It may be obtained by the resolution of dl-tartaric acid.

dl-Tartaric acid: It is manufactured by the oxidation of fumaric acid with dilute alkaline permanganate. In the solid state dl-tartaric acid exists as the racemic compound; but in solution it is dissociated into d- and l-form.

meso-Tartaric acid: It may either be prepared by heating d-tartaric acid with alkali or by the oxidation of maleic acid with dilute alkaline solution of potassium permanganate.

Uses: d-Tartaric acid is used:

1. In the preparation of effervescent drinks.
2. As potassium sodium tartrate in the preparation of mirrors and in Fehling's solution.
3. As cream of tartar in making baking powder.
4. Potassium antimonyl tartrate as medicine for eliminating poisons from stomach by causing nausea and vomiting and also used in dyeing and calico printing.

Lactic acid, α-Hydroxypriopionic Acid
$CH_3.CH(OH).COOH$

It is found in sour milk (L. lactum = milk), gastric juice, opium and cucumber.

Preparation:

1. **By fermentation of cane-sugar:** It is manufactured by fermentation of sugary material, such as molasses, cane-sugar, and glucose by lactic acid bacteria.

   A mixture of dilute solution of sugar and a little of sour milk of decayed cheese is kept at 40–45° for about one week. The chalk is added which keeps the acidity of the medium below 1% which is suitable for the bacteria. In the end of fermentation the solution is neutralized with lime water when insoluble calcium lactate is precipitated. This is filtered off and decomposed by calculated amount of dilute sulphuric acid. Calcium sulphate is separated on the pump and the filtrate is evaporated under reduced pressure to obtain the crystals of lactic acid.

$$C_{12}H_{22}O_{11} \xrightarrow{H_2O} \underset{\text{Glucose}}{C_6H_{12}O_6} + \underset{\text{Fructose}}{C_6H_{12}O_6} \xrightarrow[\text{40–45°C}]{\text{B. acidi lactiti}} \underset{\text{Methyl glyoxal}}{2CH_3.CO.CHO} \xrightarrow{2H_2O}$$

$$\underset{\text{Lactic acid}}{2CH_3.CH(OH).COOH} \xrightarrow{CaCO_3} \underset{\text{Calcium lactate}}{CH_3.CH(OH).COO_2.Ca} \xrightarrow{H_2O} 2CH_3.CO(OH).COOH + CaSO_4$$

In another procedure sugar may be fermented by *Rhizopus oryzae.*

2. **From acetylene:** Hydration of acetylene with dilute sulphuric acid under the catalytic

influence of mercuric sulphate produces acetaldehyde which reacts with hydrogen cyanide to give cyanohydrin. Lactic acid is achieved when cyanohydrin is hydrolyzed.

$$2C + H_2 \xrightarrow{\text{Electric arc}} HC \equiv CH \xrightarrow[1\% H_2SO_4, 80^0]{\text{dil. } H_2SO_4} CH_3.CHO \xrightarrow{HCN}$$

Acetylene   Acetaldehyde

$$CH_3.CH(OH).CN \xrightarrow{\text{dil. HCl}} CH_3.CH(OH).COOH$$

Acetaldehyde   dl-Lactic acid
cyanohydrin

3. **From propane:** Addition of bromine to propene gives 1,2-dibromopropane which on hydrolysis with dilute alkali yields dihydroxypropane. Oxidation of the dihydroxy compounds leads to the formation of lactic acid.

$$CH_3.CH = CH_2 + Br_2 \rightarrow CH_3.CH - CH_2 \xrightarrow{\text{dil. NaOH}} CH_3.CH - CH_2 \xrightarrow{[O]} CH_3.CH(OH).COOH$$

Propene | | | | dl-Lactic acid
                        Br   Br   OH   OH

Isomers of lactic acid: Lactic acid contains one asymmetric carbon atom, hence it is optically active compound. It occurs in the following three isomeric forms:

(i) **d-Lactic acid:** It is found in meat and, therefore, called as sarcolactic acid (Greek: sarkos = flesh). During muscular activities glycogen is converted into sarcolactic acid which is changed back into glycogen during rest. Fatigue is due to the formation of this acid in muscles. It may either be extracted from the meat or by resolution of racemic mixture using **Penicillium glaucum** which utilizes the laevo form leaving behind the d-form.

(ii) *l*-**Lactic acid:** Fermentation of sucrose with **Bacillus acidi laevolactiti** yields l-lactic acid. It may also be obtained by resolution of racemic form (dl-) with strychnine.

(iii) *dl*-**(Racemic) Lactic acid:** This form occurs in sour milk. It may be obtained by any one procedure described above.

Physical properties: Racemic lactic acid is a colourless oily liquid m.p. 18°, b.p. 120° with decomposition, and has a sour taste. It is hygroscopic and soluble in water in all proportions.

Chemical properties: Lactic acid besides containing a carboxylic group also has a secondary alcoholic group. It shows the properties of both the groups. Its important chemical reactions are given below:

1. **Oxidation:** It is oxidised under controlled oxidation using Fenton's reagent (H_2O_2 + $FeSO_4$) to pyruvic acid.

$$CH_3.CH(OH).COOH \xrightarrow[\text{[O]}]{H_2O_2 / FeSO_4} CH_3.CO.COOH$$

Pyruvic acid

Permanganate oxidation, however, converts it into acetic acid and carbon dioxide.

$$CH_3.CH(OH).COOH \xrightarrow[\text{[O]}]{KMnO_4} CH_3.CHO + CO_2 + H_2O \xrightarrow{[O]} CH_3 - \overset{\displaystyle OH}{\underset{\displaystyle |}{CO}}$$

2. **Action of sulphuric acid:** Treatment of lactic acid with sulphuric acid results in the fission of the molecule to acetaldehyde and formic acid.

$$CH_3.CH(OH).COOH \xrightarrow{\text{Conc. } H_2SO_4} CH_3.CHO + H.COOH$$

With concentrated sulphuric acid the formic acid formed is decomposed into carbon monoxide and water.

$$H.COOH \xrightarrow{\text{Conc. } H_2SO_4} CO + H_2O$$

3. **Iodoform reaction:** Formation of iodoform takes place when lactic acid is allowed to react with iodine and caustic soda.

$$CH_3.CH(OH).COOH \xrightarrow{I_2} \underset{\text{Pyruvic acid}}{CH_3.CO.COOH} \xrightarrow{I_2} \underset{\text{Tri-iodopyruvic acid}}{CI_3.CO.COOH} \xrightarrow{NaOH} \underset{\text{Iodoform}}{CH.I_3} + \underset{\substack{\text{Sodium} \\ \text{oxalate}}}{(COO.Na)_2}$$

Uses: It is used:

1. In tanning and dyeing industries, in soft drinks for improving their flavours, in food of infants and in the preparation of useful lactates.
2. Ethyl lactate is used as a solvent for cellulose nitrate.
3. Calcium lactate is used for removing calcium deficiency, in baking powder and as blood coagulant.
4. Silver lactate is used as antiseptic and astringent.
5. Titanium lactate is used in tanning.
6. Antimony lactate is used in wool dyeing and in calico printing.

Citric Acid, 2-Hydroxypropane-1,2,3-tricarboxylic Acid
$HOOC.CH_2.C(OH).COOH.CH_2.COOH$

Citric acid occurs in the fruit juice of various species of **citrus** group (e.g., lemons, limes, bergamots, galgal etc.) and in unripe fruits. Lemon juice contains about 6–10 per cent of citric acid.

Preparation:

1. **From lemon juice:** In this old commercial process the juice is boiled to coagulate proteins and then filtered. The filtrate is neutralized with lime and boiled. The insoluble calcium citrate is separated from the hot solution on pump and decomposed with calculated amount of dilute sulphuric acid. The precipitated calcium sulphate is separated by filtration and the volume of the filtrate is reduced to get the compound in crystallized form.
2. **From sugars:** A dilute solution of glucose, sucrose or cane.

Physical properties: Citric acid forms large, colourless crystals containing one molecule of water of crystallization. Melting point of crystalline acid is $101°$, and of anhydrous acid is $153°$. It has a pleasant acid taste. It is readily soluble in water and alcohol and less soluble in ether.

Chemical properties: Citric acid behaves as an alcohol and a tribasic acid. Its specific reactions are given below:

1. **Salt formation:** Due to the presence of three carboxylic groups the acid forms three series of salts with alkalis, e.g.:

CH$_2$.COO.Na   CH$_2$.COO.Na   CH$_2$.COO.Na
|
CH(OH).COOH   C(OH).COOH   CH(OH).COO.Na
|
CH$_2$.COOH   CH$_2$.COO.Na   CH$_2$.COO.Na

Monosodium citrate   Disodium citrate   Trisodium citrate

2. **Esterification:** Three series of esters are obtained when the acid is treated with alcohol.

CH$_2$.CO.OC$_2$.H$_5$ CH$_2$.CO.OC$_2$H$_5$ CH$_2$.CO.OC$_2$H$_5$
|
C(OH).COOH   C(OH).COOH   C(OH).CO.OC$_2$H$_5$
|
CH$_2$.COOH   CH$_2$.CO.OC$_2$H$_5$ CH$_2$.CO.OC$_2$H$_5$

Monoethyl citrate   Diethyl citrate   Triethyl citrate

3. **Acetylation:** With acetic anhydride or acetyl chloride alcoholic group reacts to form monacetyl derivative.

CH$_2$.COOH   CH$_2$.COOH
|
C(OH).COOH + (CH$_3$.CO)$_2$O $\longrightarrow$ C(O.CO.CH$_3$).COOH
|
CH$_2$.COOH   CH$_2$.COOH

Acetyl citric acid

4. **Reduction:** Chemical reduction of citric acid with hydriodic acid and red phosphorus yields tricarballylic acid.

CH$_2$.COOH   CH$_2$.COOH
| Red P
2 C.(OH).COOH + 2Hi $\xrightarrow{\quad}$ CH.COOH + H$_2$O + I$_2$
| |
CH$_2$.COOH   CH$_2$.COOH

Tricarballylic acid

5. **Action of heat:** When heated alone citric acid is charred to some extent and irritating vapours are formed. At 150° it loses a molecule to water yielding an unsaturated acid called as aconitic acid. At higher temperature citric acid is pyrolyzed to give a number of products, such as aconitic acid, mesaconic acid, citraconic acid and its anhydride, itaconic acid and its anhydride and acetone. These products can be isolated under carefully regulated conditions. If anhydrous acid is rapidly distilled it yields citraconic acid and its anhydride as the main products.

$$2KOH + Br_2 \longrightarrow K.Br + K.OBr + H_2O$$

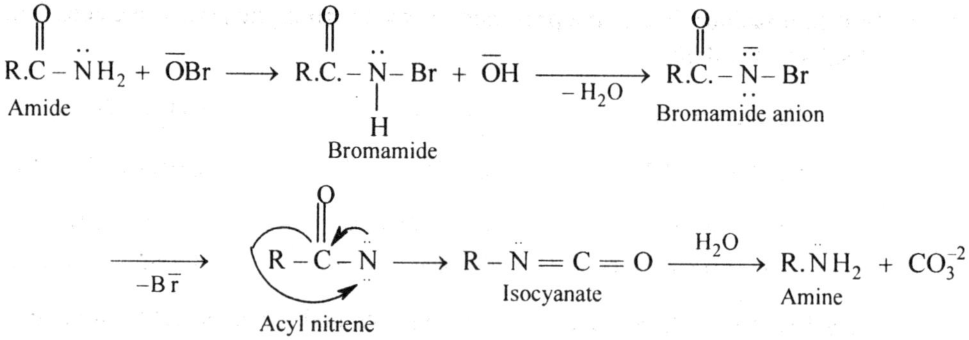

$$\text{R.C}-\overset{\overset{O}{\|}}{\underset{\cdot\cdot}{N}}H_2 + \bar{O}Br \longrightarrow \text{R.C.}-\underset{\overset{|}{H}}{\overset{\overset{O}{\|}}{N}}-Br + \bar{O}H \xrightarrow{-H_2O} \text{R.C.}-\underset{\cdot\cdot}{\overset{\overset{O}{\|}}{\overset{\cdot\cdot}{N}}}-Br$$

Amide   Bromamide   Bromamide anion

$$\xrightarrow[-B\bar{r}]{} \quad \overset{\overset{O}{\|}}{R-C-N} \longrightarrow R-N=C=O \xrightarrow{H_2O} R.NH_2 + CO_3^{-2}$$

Acyl nitrene   Isocyanate   Amine

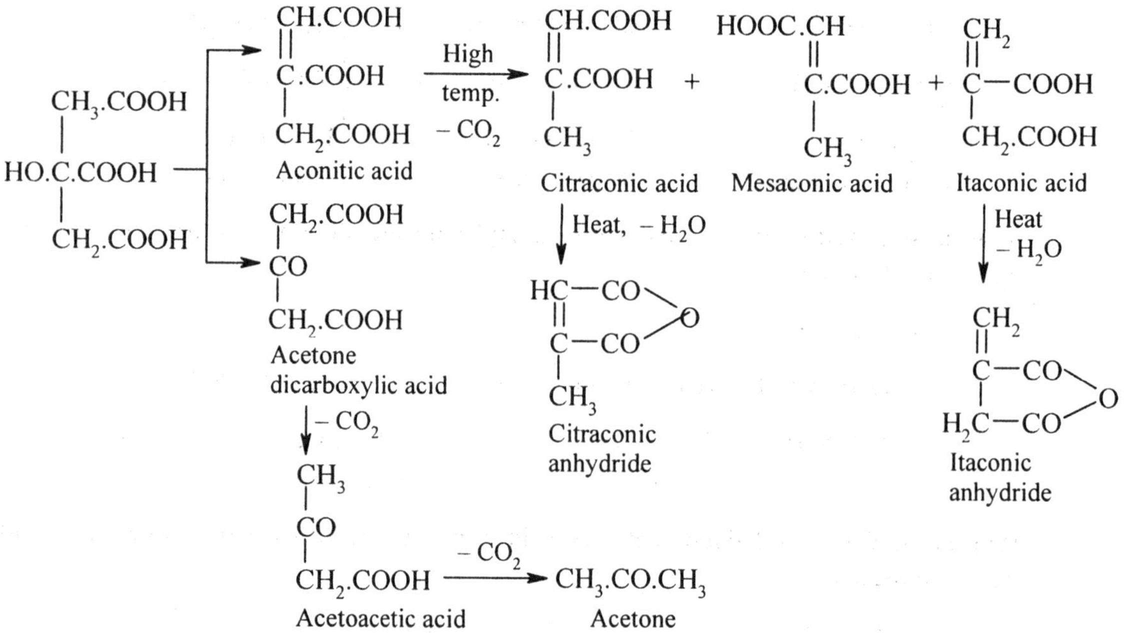

Reduction of aconitic acid produces tricarballytic acid.

6. **Action of sulphuric acid:** With concentrated sulphuric acid aconitic acid is obtained at low temperature but charring of the compounds takes place under reflux condition. With sulphuric acid, citric acid yields acetone dicarboxylic acid in high yield (85–90%).

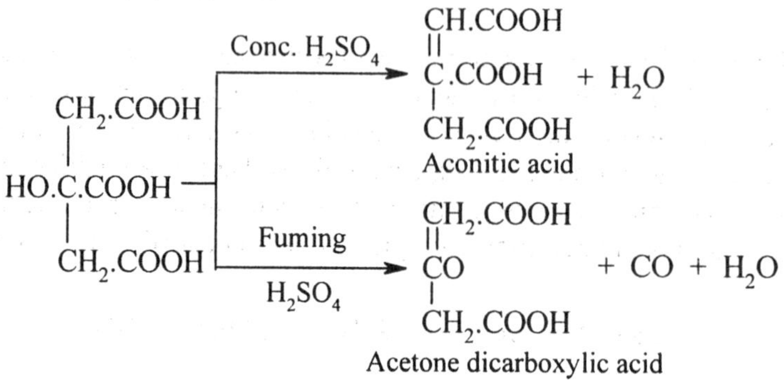

7. **Complex formation:** With certain metallic hydroxides it forms soluble complexes and thus prevents the precipitation as in case of tartaric acid.

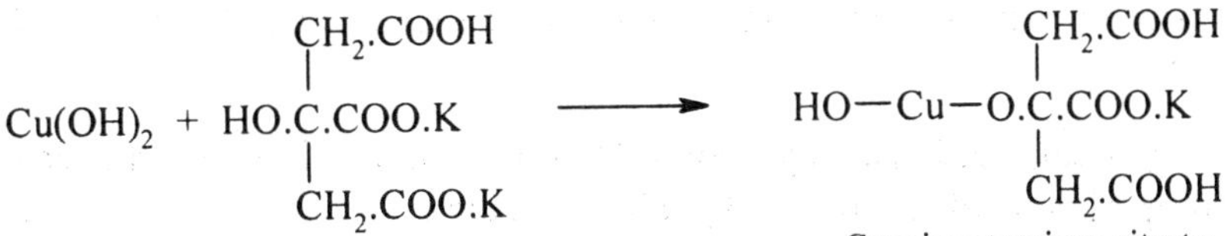

$$Cu(OH)_2 \;+\; \underset{\displaystyle \underset{CH_2.COO.K}{|}}{\overset{\displaystyle \overset{CH_2.COOH}{|}}{HO.C.COO.K}} \;\longrightarrow\; \underset{\displaystyle \underset{CH_2.COOH}{|}}{\overset{\displaystyle \overset{CH_2.COOH}{|}}{HO-Cu-O.C.COO.K}}$$

Cupriopotassium citrate
(soluble complex)

Benedict's reagent, used for the identification of aldehydes, is a soluble complex of $CuSO_4$, Na_2CO_3 and sodium citrate. The probable structure of the reagent is as:

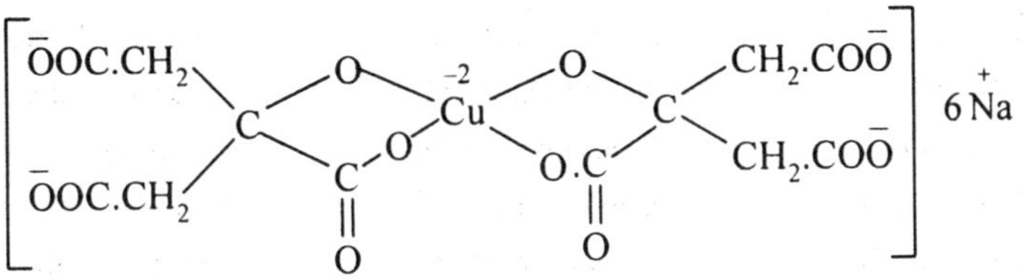

$$\left[\underset{\displaystyle \overline{O}OC.CH_2}{\overset{\displaystyle \overline{O}OC.CH_2}{}} C \underset{\displaystyle C}{\overset{\displaystyle O}{}} \underset{\displaystyle O}{\overset{\displaystyle Cu^{-2}}{}} \underset{\displaystyle O.C}{\overset{\displaystyle O}{}} C \underset{\displaystyle CH_2.CO\overline{O}}{\overset{\displaystyle CH_2.CO\overline{O}}{}} \right] \; 6\,\overset{+}{N}a$$

Uses: It is used as:

1. A mordant in dyeing and printing and for making synthetic fruit drinks.
2. Tributyl citrate as solvent in plastic industry.
3. Magnesium citrate as laxative.
4. Sodium citrate as infant food and in preparing the Benedict's reagent.
5. Ferric ammonium citrate in preparing blueprints and as medicine for iron deficiency.

CARBOXYLIC ACID DERIVATIVES

Acid derivatives are obtained when –H or –OH of carboxylic group is replaced by another atom or group like –Cl, $-NH_2$, –OCO.R or –R.

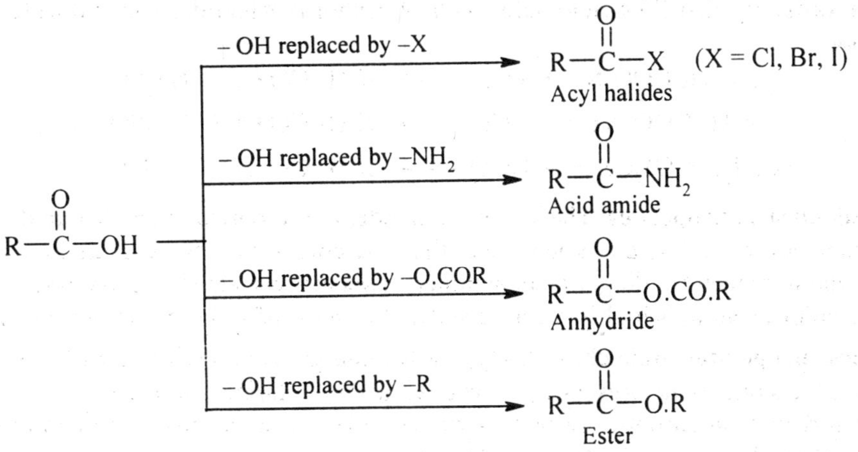

Acyl Halides

Acyl halides, also known as acid halides, have the general formula $R - \overset{\overset{\displaystyle O}{\|}}{C} - X$ in which the group $R - \overset{\overset{\displaystyle O}{\|}}{C} -$ is generally called as acyl group. They are reactive, low-boiling derivatives in which the hydroxyl group of an acid is replaced by a halogen atom.

Nomenclature: The common names of acyl halides are obtained by replacing the suffix '-ic acid' of the common names of the corresponding acid by 'yl halide'. To name them in the systematic system the ending 'e' of parent alkane is replaced by 'oyl halide'.

Formula	Common name	IUAPC name
H.CO.Cl	Formyl chloride	Methanoyl chloride
CH_3.CO.Cl	Acetyl chloride	Ethanoyl chloride
C_2H_5.CO.Cl	Propionyl chloride	Propanoyl chloride
C_3H_7.CO.Cl	Butyryl chloride	Butanoyl chloride
C_4H_9.CO.Cl	Valeryl chloride	Pentanoyl chloride

General Methods of Preparation

1. **From acids:** Treatment of acids with phosphorus trihalides or pentahalides or thionyl chlorides under reflux condition affords acid halides.

$$3.R.COOH + PCl_3 \longrightarrow \underset{\text{Acyl halide}}{3.R.CO.Cl} + \underset{\text{Phosphoric acid}}{H_3PO_3}$$

$$\underset{\text{Acetic acid}}{CH_3.COOH} + PCl_5 \longrightarrow \underset{\text{Acetyl chloride}}{CH_3.CO.Cl} + POCl_3 + HCl$$

$$\underset{\text{Propionic acid}}{CH_3.CH_2.COOH} + SOCl_2 \longrightarrow \underset{\text{Propionyl chloride}}{CH_3.CH_2.CO.Cl} + SO_2 + HCl$$

2. **From salts:** By distilling acid salts with phosphorus trihalides, oxychloride on sulphuryl chloride.

$$3CH_3.COO.Na + PCl_3 \longrightarrow 3CH_3.CO.Cl + Na_2PO_3$$

$$3CH_3.COO.Na + POCl_3 \longrightarrow 3CH_3.CO.Cl + Na_3PO_4$$

$$(CH_3.COO)_2Ca + SO_2Cl_2 \longrightarrow 2CH_3.CO.Cl + CaSO_4$$

General physical properties: The lower acyl halides are colourless, volatile liquids with irritating odours. Their boiling points are much lower than the corresponding acids due to the absence of intermolecular hydrogen bonding. Lower members fume in moist air. Higher members are colourless solids. The chlorine atom is highly reactive and so the acid chlorides are important reagents.

Chemical properties: Acid chlorides typically undergo nucleophilic substitution more rapidly than alkyl halides due to the presence of carbonyl group. Polarization of carbonyl group results in low electron density at carbonyl carbon. A nucleophile attacks at this carbon and the chlorine is removed as chloride ion or as hydrogen chloride.

1. **Acylation:** Acid chlorides react with compounds which have replaceable hydrogen atom such as water, alcohols, amines etc. In these reactions the hydrogen atom is replaced by acyl group (R.CO–) and, therefore, these reactions are referred as acylation reactions. Thus:

   Hydrolysis: The acid chlorides are very much sensitive to hydrolysis. They are readily hydrolyzed by water to form the parent acids.

   $$R\,CO\,Cl + H_2O \longrightarrow R.COOH + HCl$$

   Mechanism of the reaction:

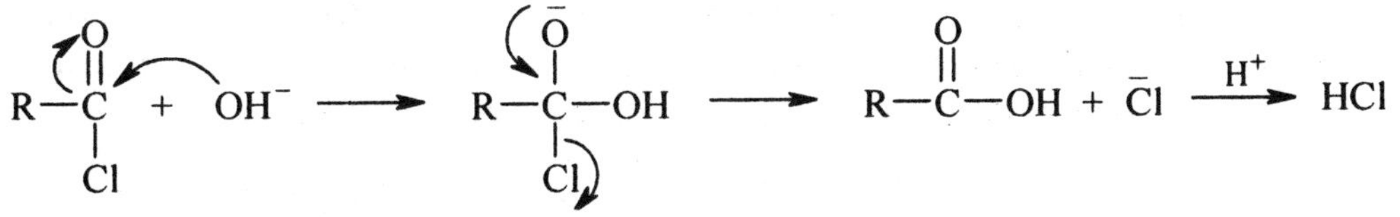

2. **Alcoholysis:** Acyl halides readily undergo alcoholysis with alcohols and yield the corresponding esters.

   $$R.CO.Cl + C_2H_5.OH \longrightarrow \underset{\text{Ester}}{R.CO.O.C_2H_5} + HCl$$

3. **Ammonolysis:** Ammonia reacts with acid chlorides to form amides, while the derivatives of ammonia such as primary and secondary amines give N-substituted amides.

   $$R.CO.Cl + NH_3 \longrightarrow \underset{\text{Amide}}{R.CO.NH_2} + NH_4Cl$$

   $$R.CO.Cl + \underset{\text{Primary}}{R.NH_2} \longrightarrow \underset{\substack{\text{N-substutited}\\\text{amide}}}{R.CO.NH.R} + HCl$$

   $$CH_3.CO.Cl + \underset{\text{Diethyl amine}}{NH(C_2H_5)_2} \longrightarrow \underset{\text{N,N-Diethyl acetamide}}{CH_3.CO.N(C_2H_5)_2} + HCl$$

   Hydrazides and hydroxamic acids are obtained when acid chlorides are allowed to react with hydrazine and hydroxylamine respectively.

   $$R.CO.Cl + \underset{\text{Hydrazine}}{H_2.N.NH_2} \longrightarrow \underset{\text{Hydrazide}}{R.CO.NH.NH_2} + HCl$$

   $$R.CO.Cl + \underset{\substack{\text{Hydroxy}\\\text{lamine}}}{H_2N.OH} \longrightarrow \underset{\text{Hydroxamic acid}}{R.CO.NH.OH} + HCl$$

4. **Reduction:** Catalytic reduction of acid chlorides in the presence of hydrogen and a catalyst such as palladium or platinum supported on barium sulphate leads to the formation of aldehydes.

   $$R.CO.Cl + H_2 \xrightarrow{Pd/BaSO_4} R.CHO + HCl$$

   However, primary alcohols are obtained when the reaction is carried out with lithium aluminium hydride by further reducing the initially formed aldehyde.

   $$CH_3.CO.Cl + 4[H] \xrightarrow{LiAlH_4} CH_3.CH_2.OH + HCl$$

5. **Reaction with Grignard reagents:** Grignard reagents readily react with acid chlorides, like an ester, to yield ketones and then tertiary alcohols according to the conditions of the reaction.

$$R.CO.Cl + CH_3.MgBr \longrightarrow \underset{\text{Ketone}}{R.CO.CH_3} + MgCl_2 \xrightarrow[\text{2. H}_2\text{O}]{\text{1. CH}_3\text{.MgBr}} \underset{\text{Tertiary alcohol}}{\overset{R}{\underset{H_3C}{\diagdown}}C - OH}$$

The initial step proceeds more rapidly than the corresponding reaction of an ester.

6. **Friedel-Crafts reaction:** Aromatic compounds react with acid chlorides in the presence of anhydrous aluminium trichloride to produce aromatic ketones.

$$\underset{\text{Benzene}}{CH_3.CO.Cl + C_6H_6} \xrightarrow{\text{AlCl}_3} \underset{\text{Acetophenone}}{C_6H_5.CO.CH_3} + HCl$$

7. **Halogenation:** Acid chlorides are easily halogenated in α-position. This is due to the presence of chlorine atom attached to the carbonyl carbon, the α-carbon atom becomes more active than that of acids.

$$\underset{\text{Propionyl chloride}}{CH_3.CO_2CO.Cl + Cl_2} \longrightarrow \underset{\underset{\text{α-Chloropropionyl chloride}}{|}}{CH_3.CH.CO.Cl} + HCl$$
$$\underset{\text{Cl}}{}$$

8. **Action of potassium cyanide:** They react with potassium cyanide to yield acyl cyanides. Hydrolysis of the cyanides results in the formation of keto acids.

$$CH_3.COCl + KCN \longrightarrow \underset{\text{Acetyl cyanide}}{CH_3.CO.CN} \xrightarrow{\text{H}_2\text{O}} \underset{\text{Pyruvic acid}}{CH_3.CO.COOH}$$

9. **Action of acid salts:** Acid chlorides give acid anhydrides when they are heated with salts of acids.

$$CH_3.CO.Cl + \underset{\text{Sodium acetate}}{NaO.CO.CH_3} \xrightarrow{\text{Heat}} \underset{\text{Acetic anhydride}}{(CH_3.CO)_2O} + NaCl$$

10. **Action of ethers:** In the presence of anhydrous zinc chloride, they react with ethers to form esters and alkyl halides.

$$CH_3.CO.Cl + C_2H_5.O.C_2H_5 \xrightarrow{\text{ZnCl}_2} \underset{\text{Ethyl acetate}}{CH_3.CO.O.C_2H_5} + C_2H_5.Cl$$

11. **Reaction with alkenes:** Acid chlorides are added to the double bond of an alkene to give chloro ketones in the presence of a catalyst like zinc chloride or aluminium chloride.

$$\underset{\text{Isobutylene}}{(CH_3)_2CH = CH_2} + CH_3CO.Cl \xrightarrow{\text{ZnCl}_2} \underset{\underset{\text{Cl}}{|}}{(CH_3)_2C - CH_2 - COCH_3}$$
$$\downarrow \text{Heat}$$
$$HCl + \underset{\text{Mesityl oxide}}{(CH_3)_2C = CH.CO.CH_3}$$

From glycerol: The following reactions are involved in the synthesis of citric acid from glycerol:

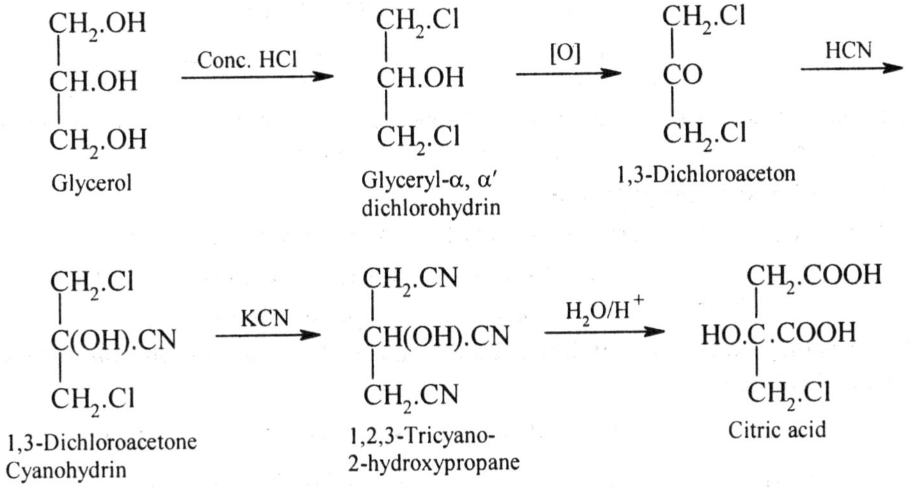

$$
\begin{array}{c}
\overset{|}{\underset{|}{CH_2.OH}} \\
CH.OH \\
CH_2.OH
\end{array}
\xrightarrow{\text{Conc. HCl}}
\begin{array}{c}
CH_2.Cl \\
CH.OH \\
CH_2.Cl
\end{array}
\xrightarrow{[O]}
\begin{array}{c}
CH_2.Cl \\
CO \\
CH_2.Cl
\end{array}
\xrightarrow{\text{HCN}}
$$

Glycerol ; Glyceryl-α, α' dichlorohydrin ; 1,3-Dichloroaceton

$$
\begin{array}{c}
CH_2.Cl \\
C(OH).CN \\
CH_2.Cl
\end{array}
\xrightarrow{\text{KCN}}
\begin{array}{c}
CH_2.CN \\
CH(OH).CN \\
CH_2.CN
\end{array}
\xrightarrow{H_2O/H^+}
\begin{array}{c}
CH_2.COOH \\
HO.C.COOH \\
CH_2.Cl
\end{array}
$$

1,3-Dichloroacetone Cyanohydrin ; 1,2,3-Tricyano-2-hydroxypropane ; Citric acid

of hydrogen chloride is eliminated and an unsaturated ketone is produced.

$$(CH_3)_2.CH = CH_2 + CH_3.CO.Cl \xrightarrow{ZnCl_2} (CH_3)_2.C.CH_2.CO.CH_3 \xrightarrow{\text{Heat}}$$

Isobutylene

$$(CH_3)_2.C = CH.CO.CH_3 + HCl$$

Mesityl oxide

Uses: Acetyl chloride is used as acetylating agent; for detection and estimation of hydroxy and amino groups, and in the preparation of organic compounds like acetic anhydride, acetamide and acetanilide.

Acid Anhydrides

The acid anhydrides may be considered as acyloxy derivatives which may be regarded theoretically as being derived from an acid by the elimination of one molecule of water from two molecules of the acid.

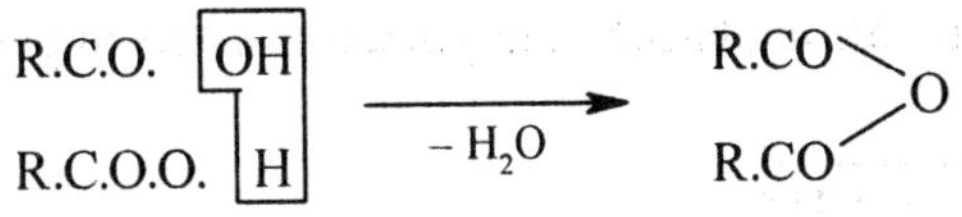

$$
\begin{array}{c}
R.C.O.\ \boxed{OH} \\
R.C.O.O.\ \boxed{H}
\end{array}
\xrightarrow{-H_2O}
\begin{array}{c}
R.CO \\
\diagdown \\
\diagup \quad O \\
R.CO
\end{array}
$$

2 mol. acids ; Acid anhydride

The acid anhydrides may be divided into two classes:

  (i) Simple anhydrides: When both acyl groups are similar, and
  (ii) Mixed anhydrides: When the acyl groups are different.

The anhydrides are named as the anhydride of the acid groups present from which they are obtained. For example:

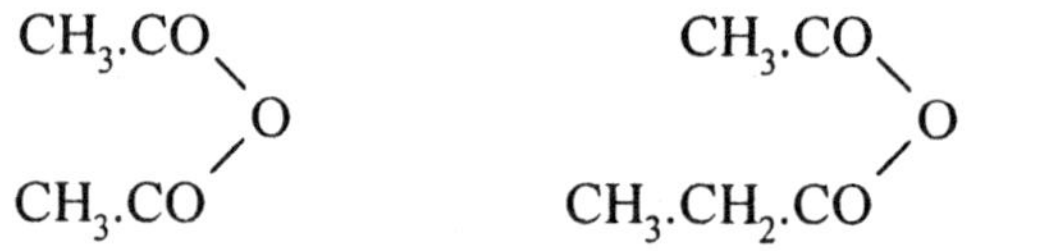

$$\begin{array}{ll} CH_3.CO \diagdown \\ \qquad\qquad O \\ CH_3.CO \diagup \end{array} \qquad \begin{array}{ll} CH_3.CO \diagdown \\ \qquad\qquad O \\ CH_3.CH_2.CO \diagup \end{array}$$

Acetic anhydride   Acetic propionic anhydride
(simple)   (mixed)

Formic anhydride is not known, but mixed anhydride like formic acetic anhydride, H.CO.O.CO. CH_3, exists. Formic acid yields carbon monoxide on dehydration.

General methods of preparation:

1. By heating an acid chloride with anhydrous sodium salt of the acid.

$$CH_3.CO.Cl + Na.O.CO.CH_3 \longrightarrow CH_3.CO.O.CO.CH_3 + NaCl$$

Acetyl chloride   Sodium acetate   Acetic anhydride

2. By treating excess of anhydrous sodium salt of the acid with phosphorus oxychloride or thionyl chloride.

$$3CH_3.COO.Na + POCl_3 \longrightarrow 3CH_3.CO.Cl + Na_3PO_4$$

$$CH_3.CO.Cl + Na.O.CO.CH_3 \longrightarrow (CH_3.CO)_2O + NaCl$$

$$2R.COO.Na + SOCl_2 \longrightarrow (R.CO)_2O + SO_2 + 2NaCl$$

Acid anhydride

3. By the dehydration of anhydrous acids in the presence of suitable dehydrating agents like P_2O_5,

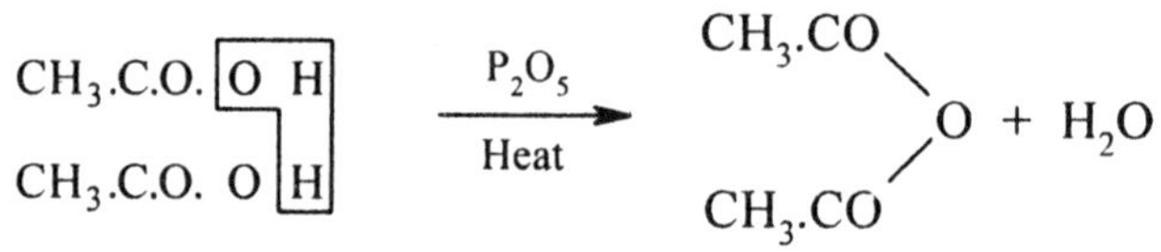

$$\begin{array}{ll} CH_3.C.O.\boxed{O\ H} \\ \qquad\qquad\qquad \xrightarrow[\text{Heat}]{P_2O_5} \\ CH_3.C.O.\ O\boxed{H} \end{array} \qquad \begin{array}{ll} CH_3.CO \diagdown \\ \qquad\qquad O + H_2O \\ CH_3.CO \diagup \end{array}$$

4. Anhydrides of higher acids are obtained when their salts are heated with acetic anhydride.

$$2R.COO.Na + (CH_3.CO)_2O \longrightarrow (R.CO)_2O + 2CH_3.COOH$$

5. Acetic anhydride is also prepared by passing acetylene into glacial acetic acid in the presence of mercuric sulphate catalyst and distilling the resulting diacetate derivative so obtained.

$$CH \equiv CH + 2CH_3COOH \xrightarrow{HgSO_4} CH_3.CH(OCO.CH_3)_2 \xrightarrow{\text{Distillation}} (CH_3.CO)_2O + CH_3.CHO$$

Another method of preparation of acetic anhydride consists in passing of ketene into glacial acetic acid.

$$\begin{array}{ll} \qquad\qquad\quad CH_3 \\ \qquad\qquad\quad | \\ H\!-\!CH_2 - C = O \xrightarrow[\text{Cracking}]{700\text{-}750^o} CH_2 = C = O + CH_4 \end{array}$$

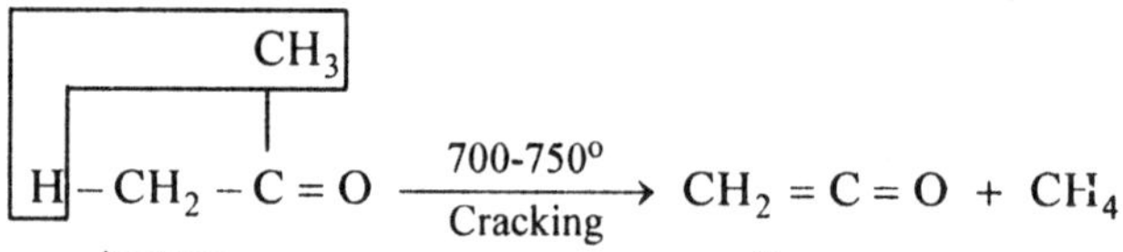

Acetone   Ketene

$$CH_2 = C = O + CH_3.COOH \longrightarrow (CH_3.CO)_2O$$

Industrially it is prepared (in USA) by passing chlorine into a mixture of sodium acetate and sulphur dichloride. The mixture is then distilled for obtaining the anhydride.

$$8CH_3.COO.Na \; + \; SCl_2 \; + \; 2Cl_2 \; \longrightarrow \; 4(CH_3.CO)_2O \; + \; 6NaCl \; + \; Na_2SO_4$$

Sulphur
dichloride

General physical properties: Acid anhydrides are colourless typical liquids or solids with irritating smell having higher boiling points than the acyl chlorides. They do not fume in air like acid chlorides. They resemble acid chlorides in their reactions, but are less reactive. This is due to the fact that electron deficiency at the carbonyl carbon in the anhydrides is compensated by donating electrons by oxygen. In acid chlorides the deficiency is increased due to strong inductive effect of carbon-chlorine bond. Chlorine atom attracts the electrons by its donor action.

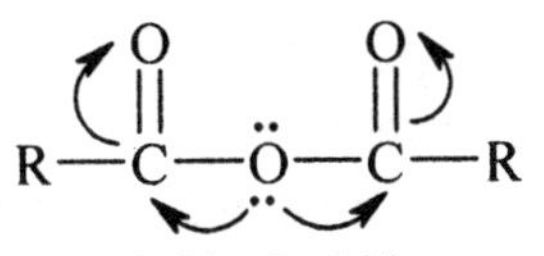

Acid anhydride

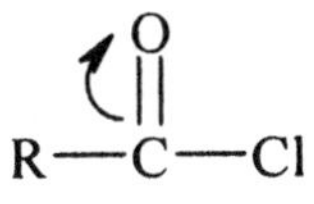

Acid chloride

They are generally insoluble in water but soluble in alcohol and ether.

General chemical properties: Like acyl halides anhydrides also undergo hydrolysis and ammonolysis and form acetyl derivatives. They are better acetylating agents because the reactions are less vigorous.

1. **Action with compounds containing 'active hydrogen':** Acid anhydrides like acetic anhydride react with compounds like water, alcohol, ammonia, amines etc. to form acetyl derivatives. One half of the molecule is used up in acetylation and the other half is converted into acid.

$$(R.CO)_2O \; + \; H_2O \; \longrightarrow \; 2R.COOH$$
Acid

$$(CH_3.CO)_2O \; + \; C_2H_5.OH \; \longrightarrow \; CH_3.CO.O.C_2H_5 \; + \; CH_3.COOH$$
Ethyl acetate

$$(CH_3.CO)_2O \; + \; NH_3 \; \longrightarrow \; CH_3.CO.NH_2 \; + \; CH_3.COOH$$
Acetamide

$$(CH_3.CO)_2O \; + \; H_2N.C_2H_5 \; \longrightarrow \; CH_3CONHC_2H_5 \; + \; CH_3.COOH$$
Ethylamine   N-Ethylacetamide

$$(CH_3.CO)_2O \; + \; HN(C_2H_5)_2 \; \longrightarrow \; CH_3.CO.N.(C_2H_5)_2 \; + \; CH_3.COOH$$
Diethylamine   N,N-Diethylacetamide

2. **Action with dry hydrogen chloride:** Acetic anhydride reacts with dry hydrogen chloride in the presence of a catalyst like pyridine, sodium acetate or conc. sulphuric acid to give acetyl chloride.

$$(CH_3.CO)_2O \; + \; HCl \; \longrightarrow \; CH_3.CO.Cl \; + \; CH_3.COOH$$

3. **Action of chlorine:** Chlorine reacts with acetic anhydride to yield acetyl chloride and monochloroacetic acid.

$$(CH_3.CO)_2O \; + \; Cl_2 \; \longrightarrow \; CH_3.CO.Cl \; + \; Cl.CH_2.COOH$$

4. **Action of aldehydes:** Acetic anhydride reacts with aldehydes to form alkylidene diacetate.

$$(CH_3.CO)_2O + CH_3.CHO \longrightarrow CH_3.CH.(O.CO.CH_3)_2$$
$$\text{Acetaldehyde} \qquad\qquad \text{Ethylene diacetate}$$

5. **Action of phosphorus pentachloride:** Formation of acetyl chloride takes place when it reacts with PCl_5.

$$(CH_3.CO)_2 + PCl_5 \longrightarrow 2CH_3.CO.Cl + POCl_3$$

6. **Friedel-Crafts' acylation:** Aromatic hydrocarbons react with acid anhydrides in the presence of anhydrous aluminium chloride to form aromatic ketones.

$$C_6H_6 + (CH_3.CO)_2O \xrightarrow{\ AlCl_3\ } C_6H_5.CO.CH_3 + CH_3.COOH$$
$$\text{Acetophenone}$$

Uses: Acetic anhydride is used as an acetylating agent; for detection and estimation of hydroxyl and amino groups; in the manufacture of dyes; drugs like aspirin, phenacetin; and polymers like acetate rayon from cellulose and amyl acetate which are utilized in the preparation of celluloid.

Acid Amides, $R.CO.NH_2$

Acid amides, which contain amide group $-CONH_2$, are the derivatives of acids which are obtained by replacing the hydroxyl or carboxyl group by the amino group, $-NH_2$.

$$R.COOH \xrightarrow[+NH_2]{-OH} R.CO.NH_2$$
$$\text{Acid} \qquad\qquad \text{Acid amide}$$

Alternately, they may be considered as acyl derivatives of ammonia obtained by substituting hydrogen atom of ammonia with acyl group.

$$NH_3 \xrightarrow[+RCO^-]{-H} R.CO.NH_2$$

Amides are divided into three classes: Primary amides, $R.CONH_2$; secondary amides, $(R.CO_2)$. NH; and tertiary amides, $(R.CO)_3.N$. Only the primary amides are the important compounds.

Nomenclature: They are usually named by replacing the suffix '-ic acid' by 'amide' of the corresponding acid. In IUPAC system the ending 'e' of the parent hydrocarbon is replaced by 'amide' to name them.

Formula	Parent acid	Common name	Parent alkane	IUPAC name
$H.CO.NH_2$	Formic acid	Formamide	Methane	Methanamide
$CH_3.CO.NH_2$	Acetic acid	Acetamide	Ethane	Ethanamide
$C_2H_5.CO.NH_2$	Propionic acid	Propionamide	Propane	Propanamide
$C_3H_7.CO.NH_2$	Butyric acid	Butyramide	Butane	Butanamide
$C_4H_9.CO.NH_2$	Valeric acid	Valeramide	Pentane	Pentanamide

General methods of preparation:

1. By ammonolysis of acid chlorides, acid anhydrides or esters.

$$R.CO.Cl + NH_3 \longrightarrow R.CO.NH_2 + HCl$$
$$\text{Acid chloride} \qquad\qquad \text{Amide}$$

$$(R.CO)_2O + NH_3 \longrightarrow R.CO.NH_2 + R.COOH$$
Acid anhydride

$$R.CO.OR' + NH_3 \longrightarrow R.CO.NH_2 + R.OH$$
Ester

2. By heating ammonium salts of carboxylic acids.

$$RCOOH + NH_3 \longrightarrow RCO\overline{O}NH_4^+ \xrightarrow{\text{Heat}} RCONH_2 + H_2O$$

3. By partial hydrolysis of alkyl cyanides with concentrated sulphuric acid or by shaking the alkyl cyanide with cold concentrated hydrochloric acid.

$$R.C \equiv N + H_2O \xrightarrow{\text{HCl}} R.CO.NH_2$$

General physical properties: Only formamide is a liquid. All other amides are colourless, crystalline neutral solids. Amides of low molecular weight are soluble in water. Their melting points are much higher than the corresponding acids due to the presence of intermolecular hydrogen bonding.

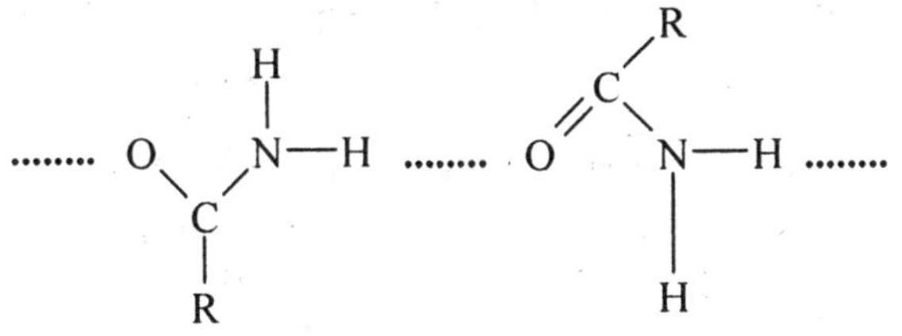

Intermolecular hydrogen bonding

Solubility of amides in water is due to the formation of intermolecular hydrogen bonding between the amide and water.

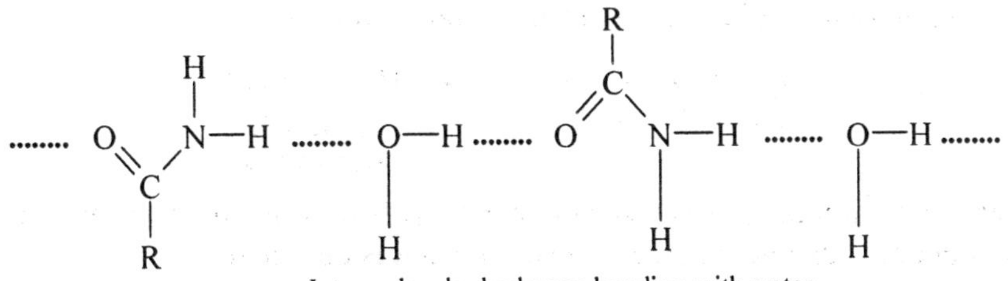

Intermolecular hydrogen bonding with water

General chemical properties: Amides have carbonyl and amino groups. The electron deficiency on the carbonyl carbon is compensated by the electron donor action of nitrogen atom. Therefore, the amides do not show the reactions of carbonyl group. They are not used as acylating agents as acid chlorides and acid anhydrides are utilized. The important reactions of amides are discussed below.

1. **Hydrolysis:** Unlike acid chlorides and acid anhydrides, the amides are not hydrolyzed by water easily. They are hydrolyzed slowly by water, readily by acids and more readily by alkalis.

$$R.CO.NH_2 + H_2O \longrightarrow R.COOH + NH_3$$

Mechanism of the reaction:

(i) Base hydrolysis:

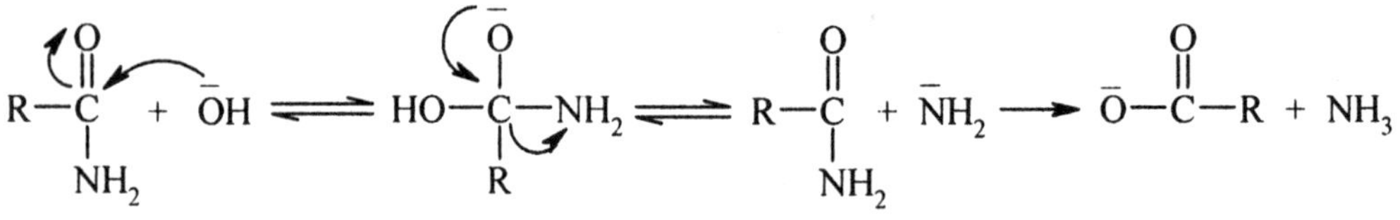

$$R-\underset{NH_2}{\overset{O}{\overset{||}{C}}} + \bar{O}H \rightleftharpoons HO-\underset{R}{\overset{\bar{O}}{\overset{|}{C}}}-NH_2 \rightleftharpoons R-\underset{NH_2}{\overset{O}{\overset{||}{C}}} + \bar{N}H_2 \longrightarrow \bar{O}-\overset{O}{\overset{||}{C}}-R + NH_3$$

(ii) Acid hydrolysis:

$$R-\underset{NH_2}{\overset{O}{\overset{||}{C}}} + \overset{+}{H} \rightleftharpoons R-\overset{O}{\overset{||}{C}}-\overset{+}{N}H_3 \overset{H_2O}{\rightleftharpoons} R-\underset{\overset{OH_2}{+}}{\overset{\bar{O}}{\overset{|}{C}}}-\overset{+}{N}H_3 \underset{+NH_3}{\overset{-NH_3}{\rightleftharpoons}} R-\underset{\overset{OH_2}{+}}{\overset{}{C}}=O$$

$$\underset{R-\overset{O}{\overset{||}{C}}-OH + \overset{+}{N}H_4}{\downarrow}$$

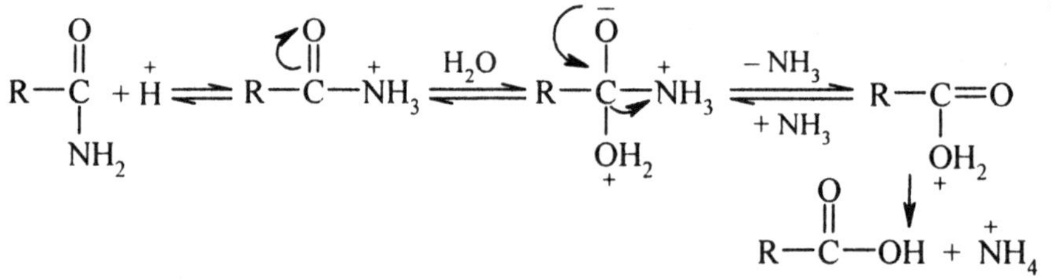

2. **Amphoteric character:** An amide can be represented by the following tautomeric form:

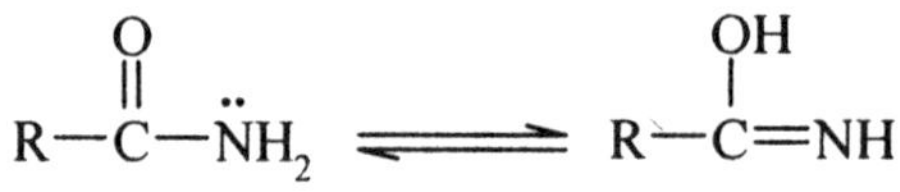

$$R-\overset{O}{\overset{||}{C}}-\overset{..}{N}H_2 \rightleftharpoons R-\overset{OH}{\overset{|}{C}}=NH$$

(Keto form)   (Enol form)
I   II

In the structure I the nitrogen atom has a lone pair of electrons indicating the basic character of amide whereas a proton can be removed from the hydroxyl group in the structure II. This indicates that amides also have acidic character. Therefore, amides form salts with acids and bases both.

With strong inorganic acids amides form unstable salts as:

$$CH_3.CO.NH_2 + HCl \longrightarrow CH_3.CO.\overset{+}{N}H_3\bar{Cl}$$

Acetamide   Acetamide
                                  hydrochloride

They react with inorganic bases like mercuric oxide to form covalent mercury compounds. With sodium or sodamide in ether the sodium salt is obtained.

$$2CH_3.CO.NH_2 + HgO \longrightarrow (CH_3.CO.NH)_2 Hg + H_2O$$

Mercuric acetamide

$$CH_3.\underset{}{\overset{OH}{\overset{|}{C}}} = NH + NaNH_2 \overset{Ether}{\longrightarrow} [CH_3.\overset{\bar{O}}{\overset{|}{C}} = NH]\ Na^+ + NH_3$$

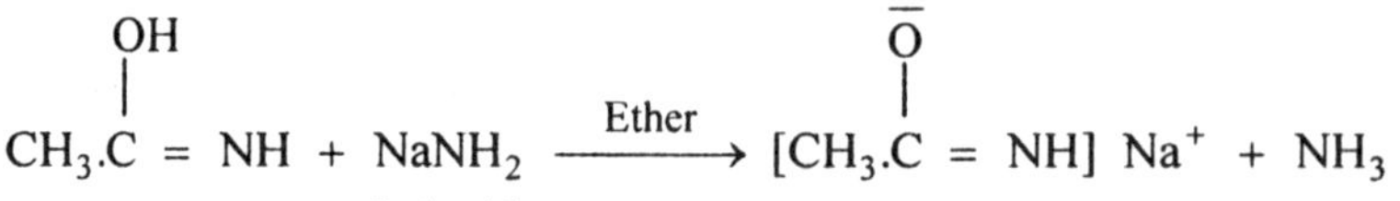

Sodamide

3. **Reduction:** Chemical reduction with sodium and ethanol or lithium aluminium hydride gives primary amines.

$$R.CO.NH_2 + 4[H] \xrightarrow[\text{or LiAlH}_4]{Na/C_2H_5.OH} R.CH_2.NH_2 + H_2O$$

4. **Action of phosphorus pentachloride:** Treatment of amides with phosphorus pentachloride under reflux affords alkyl cyanides.

$$CH_3.CO.NH_2 + PCl_5 \xrightarrow[-POCl_3]{} CH_3.CCl_2.NH_2 \xrightarrow{Heat} CH_3.CN + HCl$$
$$\text{Methyl}$$
$$\text{cyanide}$$

5. **Action of nitrous acid:** When amides are reacted with nitrous acid nitrogen is evolved and the acid is formed.

$$R.CO.NH_2 + HNO_2 \longrightarrow R.COOH + N_2 + H_2O$$

6. **Dehydration:** When heated with dehydrating agent like phosphorus pentoxide, amides eliminate a molecule of water forming cyanides.

$$CH_3.CO.NH_2 \xrightarrow{P_2O_5} CH_3.CN + H_2O$$
$$\text{Acetamide} \qquad\qquad \text{Methyl cyanide}$$

Alkyl cyanides are also obtained when the amides of the higher acids are heated at a high temperature.

$$2R.CO.NH_2 \longrightarrow R.CN + R.COOH + NH_3$$

7. **Hofmann degradation of amides:** When a mixture of amide, bromine and alkali is heated, then the amide is converted into a primary amine with one carbon atom less than the amide. The overall reaction is represented as shown hereunder:

$$R.CO.NH_2 + Br_2 + 4KOH \longrightarrow R.NH_2 + 2KBr + K_2CO_3 + 2H_2O$$

Mechanism of the reaction: The reaction is believed to proceed by the following reaction steps:

$$2KOH + Ba_2 \longrightarrow K.Br + K.OBr + H_2O$$

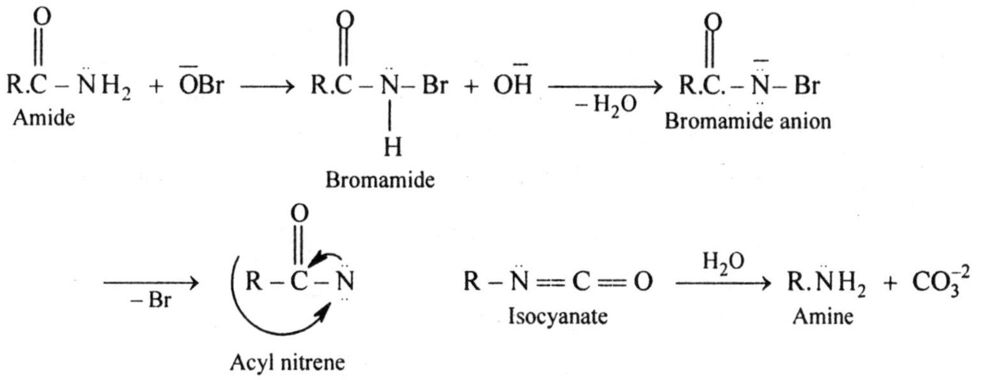

OFFICIAL COMPOUNDS

ACETIC ACID

Mol. Form.: $C_2H_4O_2$ Mol. Wt.: 60.1

Acetic acid contains not less than 32.5 per cent w/w and not more than 33.5 per cent w/w of $C_2H_4O_2$.

It is a clear, colourless liquid with pungent odour and sharp acidic taste. It is miscible with water, alcohol and glycerine.

It is identified (i) due to its being strongly acidic even when diluted freely and (ii) due to the characteristic reactions given by its neutralized solution for acetates (App. I, Inorganic Pharmaceutical Chemistry by the same author).

Tests for purity: It is tested for weight per ml; arsenic; heavy metals; chloride; sulphate; certain aldehydic substances; formic acid and oxidisable impurities and odorous impurities; readily oxidizable impurities and non-volatile matter.

Assay: It is assayed by simple titration with N/1 sodium hydroxide, using phenolphthalein as indicator. For the assay 5 g of acetic acid is weighed into a stoppered flask containing 50 ml of water and the solution titrated with N/1 sodium hydroxide.

$$NaOH + CH_3.COOH \longrightarrow CH_3.COO.Na + H_2O$$

Each ml of N/1 sodium hydroxide is equivalent to 0.06005 g of $C_2H_4O_2$.

Acetic acid is used as a pharmaceutical aid (see also page ....).

DILUTE ACETIC ACID

Dilute acetic acid is prepared by diluting the acid with purified water. The mixture contains 6.0 per cent w/w of $C_2H_4O_2$ (acetic acid 182 g is mixed with 818 g of purified water).

It is tested for purity in the same way as acetic acid.

It is assayed in the similar way as Acetic acid by using 20 g.

Dilute acetic acid is used as a pharmaceutical aid and is an ingredient of Ipecacuanha and Urginea Vinegar.

GLACIAL ACETIC ACID

Mol. Form.: $C_2H_4O_2$ Mol. Wt.: 60.1

Glacial acetic acid (mol. wt. 60.05) contains not less than 99.0 per cent w/w of $C_2H_4O_2$. It is assayed in the same way as acetic acid, using 1 g accurately weighed, and is used as a pharmaceutical aid. It is an ingredient of Strong Ammonium Acetate solution.

I.P. 2007 gives a complete monograph only on Glacial Acetic Acid (page 685).

TRICHLOROACETIC ACID

Trichloroacetic acid ($CCl_3.COOH$) is included in Appendix of I.P. page No. 536 and is used as caustic. See also its full account on previous page 265–66.

LACTIC ACID

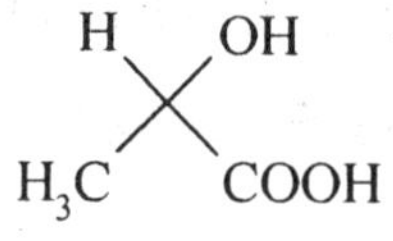

Mol. Form.: $CH_3.CH(OH).COOH$ Mol. Wt.: 90.08

Lactic acid is a mixture of lactic acid and lactic anhydride and contains the equivalent of not less than 87.5 per cent and not more than 90.0 per cent w/w of $C_3H_6O_3$. It is a colourless or slightly yellow syrupy hygroscopic liquid; odourless or with slight pleasant odour and sour taste. It is miscible with water, alcohol (95 per cent) and solvent ether. It is identified by warming (1 g) with potassium permanganate (0.1 g) when it yields acetaldehyde, recognisable by its odour.

Tests for purity: It is tested for weight per ml; arsenic; heavy metals; iron; chloride; sulphate; citric, oxalic, phosphoric and tartaric acids; readily carbonisable substances; reducing sugars; sulphated ash; either insoluble substances; volatile fatty acids and methanol and methyl esters (p. 1275),

Assay[1]: Weigh accurately about 3 g of lactic acid and dilute with 50 ml of water, add 50 ml of 1 N sodium hydroxide and boil gently for five minutes, titrate the excess of alkali with 1 N sulphuric acid using solution of phenolphthalein as indicator. Repeat the experiment with the same quantities of the same reagents in the same manner omitting the lactic acid. The difference between the two titrations represents the alkali required to convert the lactic acid and the lactic anhydride into sodium lactate.

$$CH_3.CH(OH).COOH + NaOH \longrightarrow CH_3.CH(OH).COO.Na + H_2O$$

Each ml of 1 N sodium hydroxide is equivalent to 0.9008 g of $C_3H_6O_3$.

Storage: Lactic acid should be stored in a well-closed container.

Uses: It is used as a pharmaceutical aid as metabolic neutralizer (see also p. 278–80).

In concentrated form it is caustic and hence it is seldom used. It is added to infant formulae to aid digestion. It is employed as a spermatocidal agent in contraceptives.

Preparation: Compounds Sodium Lactate Injection.

OLEIC ACID

Oleic acid consists chiefly of $C_{17}H_{33}.COOH$ and may be obtained by the hydrolysis of fats or fixed oils and separation of the liquid acids by expression or by other suitable methods.

Description: It is a yellowish to pale brown oily liquid with characteristic odour and taste. It is insoluble in water but soluble in alcohol, chloroform and solvent ether. (See also p. 263–65).

Tests for purity: It is tested for purity; for acid value; iodine value; mineral acids, neutral fats and mineral oils; stearic acid and congealing temperature; and sulphated ash.

Storage: Oleic acid is preserved in a well-closed container and is used as pharmaceutical aid.

UNDECYLENIC ACID
(Undecenoic acid)

Mol. Form.: $CH_2.CH.(CH_2)_8.COOH$ Mol. Wt.: 184.3

Undecylenic acid consists mainly of undec-10-enoic acid and contains not less than 9.0 per cent and not more than 1.0 per cent $C_{11}H_{20}O_2$. It is obtained from the products of pyrolysis of castor oil.

Description: It is a colourless to yellowish liquid which solidifies on cooling and has characteristic odour. It is almost insoluble in water, but is miscible with alcohol, chloroform, solvent ether and benzene.

---

1. I.P. 2007 has modified a little the assay method, but based on the same principle of titration. See also a full descriptive account on p. 288–90.

Tests for purity: It is tested for freezing point; iodine value; reflective index; neutral fats and minerals; water-soluble acids and sulphated ash.

Assay[1]: It is assayed by titration with N/10 potassium hydroxide in alcoholic solution, using phenolphthalein as an indicator. About 0.5 g of the acid is used in 20 ml alcohol.

$$C_{10}H_{19}.COOH + KOH \longrightarrow C_{10}H_{19}.COO.K + H_2O$$

Each ml of N/10 KOH is equivalent to 0.01843 g of $C_{11}H_{20}O_2$.

It is stored in tightly packed container, protected from light and air.

Uses: It is used as fungistatic agent, chiefly in ointments and dusting powders. Zinc Undecylenate ointment is official in I.P. 1965.

BEMEGRIDE

Mol. Form.: $C_8H_{13}O_2N$ Mol. Wt.: 155.2

Bemegride is β-ethyl-β-methylglutarimide and is a respiratory stimulant. It is a specific antagonist of barbiturate and is useful in barbiturate poisoning. It is a good material for terminating barbiturate anaesthesia. It has been official in I.P., B.P., U.S.P. etc. It has been excluded from I.P. 2007.

Bemegride is a white, crystalline powder with no odour but with a bitter taste. It melts at 126–128°.

It is tested for purity for melting point; acidity; and sulphated ash.

Assay: It is assayed by nitrogen determination.

Weigh accurately about 0.3 g of bemegride and transfer to a long-necked flask; add 10 ml of nitrogen-free sulphuric acid, 3 g of anhydrous sodium sulphate and 0.3 g of nitrogen-free mercuric oxide; heat the mixture until it is decolourized and boil gently for further two hours and cool. Transfer with the aid of water to an ammonia distillation apparatus and add water to give a volume of about 30 ml. Add a small piece of granulated zinc and 15 ml of solution containing 2 g of sodium thiosulphate and such quantity of sodium hydroxide that after addition the mixture is strongly alkaline. Distil the liberated ammonia in 25 ml of 0.1 N hydrochloric acid. Titrate the excess of hydrochloric acid with 0.1 N sodium hydroxide using solution of methyl red as indicator. Repeat the experiment with the same quantity of the same reagents in the same manner omitting Bemegride. The difference between the two titrations represents the acid required to neutralize the ammonia. Each ml of 0.1 N hydrochloric acid is equivalent to 0.01552 g of $C_8H_{13}O_2N$.

Bemegride injection has also been official in I.P.

1. I.P. 2007 has modified assay method. It uses 0.5 M sodium hydroxide in place of N/10 potassium hydroxide (p. 1845).

CITRIC ACID

Mol. Form.: $C_6H_8O_7$ Mol. Wt.: 192.1

According to I.P., citric acid contains not less than 99.0 per cent and not more than the equivalent of 101.0 per cent of $C_6H_8O_7.H_2O$, calculated on anhydrous basis.

Description: Citric acid occurs as a colourless translucent crystals or as white crystalline powder. In moist air it is hygroscopic but is slightly efflorescent in warm dry air. It is odourless with strongly acid taste. It is soluble in water (1 : 0.5), alcohol (1 : 2) and ether (1 : 3) and is insoluble in organic solvents.

Identity: It is identified from its neutralized solution which yields reactions characteristic of citrates.

Tests for purity: It is tested for arsenic; copper and iron; lead; sulphate; oxalic acid; readily carbonisable substances; and sulphated ash (I.P. 942).

Assay: It is assayed by dissolving 3 g in 100 ml of water and titrating the solution with 1 N sodium hydroxide using solution of thymol blue as indicator. The end point indicates the completion of formation of the trisodium salt as shown in the reaction below:

$$C_6H_8O_7 + 3NaOH \longrightarrow Na_3C_6H_5O_7 + 3H_2O$$

Each ml of 1 N sodium hydroxide is equivalent to 0.07005 g of $C_6H_8O_7.H_2O$.

I.P. 2007 uses a somewhat modified assay, by titrating with 1 M sodium hydroxide, using phenolphthalein solution as an indicator.

Citric acid is stored in well-closed container. It is used as a pharmaceutical aid.

N.B.: See also p. 280–83 for full account on citric acid.

CITRIC ACID MONOHYDRATE

Mol. Form.: $C_6H_8O_7.H_2O$ Mol. Wt.: 210.1

I.P. 2007 also includes citric acid monohydrate as an official monograph. It is 2-hydroxypropane-1,2,3-tricarboxylic acid monohydrate, and contains not less than 99.0% and not more than 101.0% of $C_6H_8O_7$, calculated on anhydrous basis.

The compound meets all the requirements i.e. tests for identity, tests for purity, assay method etc. as are stipulated for Citric Acid.

Anhydrous citric acid has been used in pharmaceutical industry for preparing Soluble Aspirin Tablets and also for Soluble Compound Tablets.

Esters

Esters are compounds which are formed by the interaction of an alcohol with an acid, the acid may be organic or inorganic. Depending on the acid from which they are obtained the esters are divided into two classes: (i) inorganic esters e.g., ethyl nitrate and (ii) organic esters, e.g., ethyl acetate. The organic esters are most important and have the general formula $C_nH_{2n}O_2$ which is the same as that of the carboxylic acids. Volatile esters are liquids possessing fruity odours. They are responsible for the flavour and fragrance of many fruits and flowers. The artificial flavouring substances are synthetic esters.

The process of formation of an ester is termed as esterification. It is a slow and reversible process. The reaction is speeded up by the presence of small amounts of inorganic acids as catalysts especially with a dehydrating agent. In the formation of esters the –OH of the carboxylic group reacts with hydrogen of the hydroxyl group of the alcohol, but in case of inorganic acids, reverse is the case.

$$CH_3.COOH + HO.C_2H_5 \rightleftharpoons CH_3.CO.O.C_2H_5 + H_2O$$

$$C_2H_5.OH + HCl \rightleftharpoons C_2H_5.Cl + H_2O$$

Organic esters may be regarded as alkyl derivatives of organic acids. They occur in plants, fruits, flowers etc. Oils and fats, called as glycerides in chemical language, are esters of higher fatty acids like stearic acid, palmitic acid and oleic acid. Esters of higher fatty acids (e.g., palmitic and cerotic acids) with higher monohydric alcohols such as myricyl, cetyl, stearyl alcohols are called waxes.

Nomenclature: The common name of esters is alkyl carboxylate. In IUPAC system alkyl group is named first followed by the name of the acid and changing the 'ic acid' by 'ate'. For example:

Formula	Common name	IUPAC name
$H.CO.O.CH_3$	Methyl formate	Methyl methanoate
$CH_3.CO.O.C_2H_5$	Ethyl acetate	Ethyl ethanoate
$C_2H_5.CO.O.CH_3$	Methyl propionate	Methyl propanoate

Isomerism: Esters show the following types of isomerism:

(i) **Chain isomerism:**

$C_5H_{10}O_2$:

$CH_3.CH_2.CH_2.CO.O.CH_3$ $CH_3CH.CO.O.CH_3$

        Methyl butyrate |

                                                CH_3

                                Methyl isobutyrate

(ii) **Functional isomerism:**

$C_3H_6O_2$: $H.CO.OC_2H_5$ $C_2H_5.COOH$ $CH_3.CO.O.CH_3$

                     Ethyl formate   Propanoic acid   Methyl acetate

(iii) **Metamerism:**

$C_3H_6O_2$: $H.CO.O.C_2H_5$ $CH_3.CO.O.CH_3$

                     Ethyl formate   Methyl acetate

General methods of preparation:

1. **Esterification:** The method of esterification was introduced by E. Fischer in which a carboxylic acid is converted directly into an ester by refluxing an alcohol in the presence of a little mineral acid catalyst, usually concentrated sulphuric acid or dry hydrogen chloride. The reaction is reversible, and generally reaches equilibrium when there are appreciable quantities of both reactants and products.

$$R.COOH + R'.OH \underset{}{\overset{H^+}{\rightleftharpoons}} R.CO.O.R' + H_2O$$

   Acid   Alcohol   Ester

Esterification may also be carried out by passing vapours of alcohol and acid over metallic catalyst, e.g. thoria at 300°C.

Mechanism of the reaction:

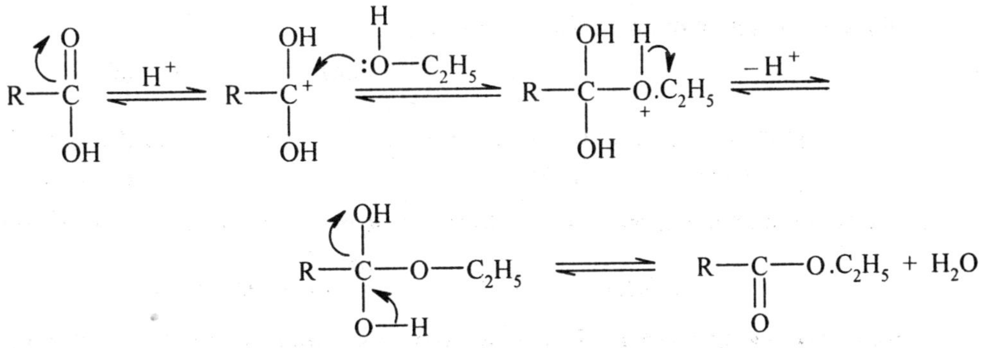

The presence of bulky groups near the site of reaction slows down the esterification. The ease of esterification is:

Alcohol : $CH_3.OH > 1° > 2° > 3°$.

Acids : $H.COOH > CH_3.COOH > R.CH_2.COOH > R_2.CH.COOH > R_3.C.COOH.$

2. **By the action of alcohol on acid anhydrides or chlorides:**

$$(CH_3.CO)_2O + C_2H_5.OH \longrightarrow CH_3.CO.O.C_2H_5 + CH_3.COOH$$

    Acetic anhydride   Ethyl acetate

$$CH_3.CO.Cl + C_2H_5.OH \longrightarrow CH_3.CO.O.C_2H_5 + HCl$$

    Acetyl chloride

Tertiary alcohols react with acid anhydrides and their chlorides slowly yielding side products.

3. **By refluxing the silver salts of acids with alkyl halides in alcoholic solution:**

$$R.COO.Ag + I.C_2H_5 \longrightarrow R.CO.O.C_2H_5 + AgI$$

    Silver salt

4. By the action of ethereal solution of diazomethane on carboxylic acids (methyl esters are easily prepared by this method).

$$CH_3.COOH + CH_2.N_2 \longrightarrow CH_3.CO.O.CH_3 + N_2$$

                Diazomethane   Methyl acetate

5. By condensing aldehydes in the presence of aluminium ethoxide (Tischenko's reaction):

$$CH_3.\overset{O}{\overset{\|}{C}} - H + O == \overset{H}{\overset{|}{C}} - CH_3 \xrightarrow{Al(O.C_2H_5)_3} CH_3.CO.O.C_2H_5$$

    Acetaldehyde (2 moles)   Ethyl acetate

6. By the combination of an ether with carbon monoxide at 125–180°C, under 500 atm. pressure in the presence of boron trifluoride and water.

$$R - O - R + CO \xrightarrow[150-180°C]{BF_3-H_2O} R.CO.O.R.$$

                                                Ester

7. By the interaction of an alcohol with ketene:

$$H_2C = C = O + HO.R \longrightarrow [CH_3 - \overset{OH}{\overset{|}{C}} - OR] \longrightarrow CH_3\overset{O}{\overset{\|}{C}} - O.R$$

    Ketene   Alcohol   Ester

8. By the addition of a carboxylic acid to an alkene in the presence of boron trifluoride catalyst:

$$R.COOH + CH_2 = CH_2 \xrightarrow{BF_3} R.CO.O.C_2H_5$$

General physical properties: Esters are colourless liquids or solids with pleasant smell like that of fruits and flowers. Lower esters are fairly soluble in water and the solubility decreases with increase in the molecular weights. All esters are soluble in most organic solvents. The boiling points of the straight-chain isomers are higher than those of the branched chain compounds. Since there is no association due to hydrogen bonding, they have low melting and boiling points than the corresponding acids. Their boiling and melting points are tabulated as follows:

Physical constants of esters of carboxylic acids

Name	M.P. °C	B.P. °C	Name	M.P. °C	B.P. °C
Methyl acetate	– 98	57.5	Ethyl formate	– 80	54
Ethyl acetate	– 84	77	Ethyl propionate	– 74	99
n-Propyl acetate	– 92	102	Ethyl n-butyrate	– 93	121
n-Butyl acetate	– 77	126	Ethyl n-valerate	– 91	146
n-Pentyl acetate	–	148	Ethyl stearate	– 34	215
Isopentyl acetate	– 78	142	Methyl propionate	–	80
n-Octyl acetate	–	210	Methyl n-valerate	–	102
Isoamyl isovalerate	–	194	Methyl isovalerate	–	127
Isoamyl n-valerate	–	178	Ethyl n-heptylate	–	187

General chemical properties: Like acid amide esters can be represented by the following resonating structures:

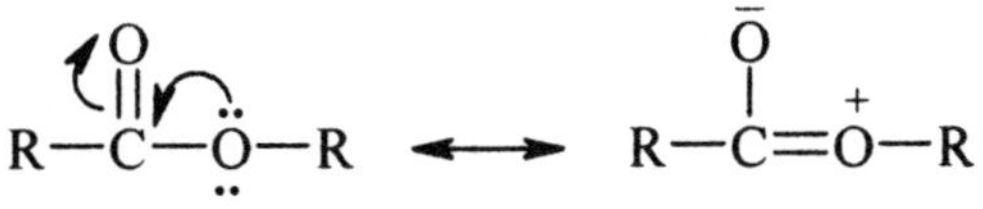

$$R-\overset{O}{\overset{||}{C}}-\overset{..}{\underset{..}{O}}-R \longleftrightarrow R-\overset{\bar{O}}{\overset{|}{C}}=\overset{+}{O}-R$$

The electron deficiency created at the carbonyl carbon has been compensated by the lone pair of electrons present on adjacent oxygen atom. Hence, the esters do not respond the reaction of carbonyl group $\left[\underset{/}{\overset{\backslash}{C}}=O \right]$.

Esters undergo the nucleophilic substitution reaction as in case of other acid derivatives. Attack occurs at the electron deficient carbonyl carbon. The alkoxy group, –OR, is replaced by the nucleophilic group such as $-\bar{O}H$, $-\bar{O}R''$, $-\bar{N}H_2$ etc. For example:

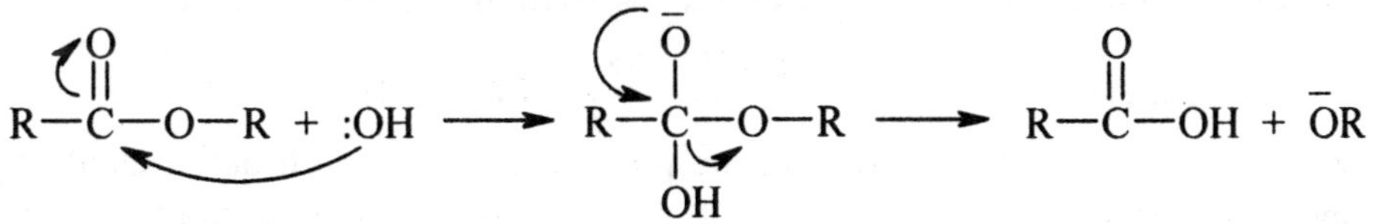

$$R-\overset{O}{\overset{||}{C}}-O-R + :OH \longrightarrow R-\overset{\bar{O}}{\underset{\underset{OH}{|}}{C}}-O-R \longrightarrow R-\overset{O}{\overset{||}{C}}-OH + \bar{O}R$$

The carboxyl carbon in esters is less electron deficient than in case of other acid derivatives. Hence with nucleophilic reagents esters undergo slower reactions than in case of acid chlorides and acid anhydrides.

1. **Hydrolysis:** An ester is hydrolyzed to a carboxylic acid and an alcohol when heated with an aqueous acid or an aqueous base. Under alkaline conditions the salt of the carboxylic acid is formed from which the acid can be liberated by the addition of a mineral acid.

$$R.COO.R' + H_2O \underset{}{\overset{HCl}{\rightleftharpoons}} R.COOH + R'.OH$$

$$CH_3.CO.O.C_2H_5 + NaOH \rightleftharpoons CH_3.COO.Na + C_2H_5.OH$$

Salts of higher fatty acids (stearic, palmitic and oleic acids) are called soaps. When esters of these acids with glycerol (glycerides) are hydrolyzed with a base then soaps are obtained. This process is called saponification which is more rapid than hydrolysis.

Mechanism of the hydrolysis:

(i) **Acid hydrolysis:**

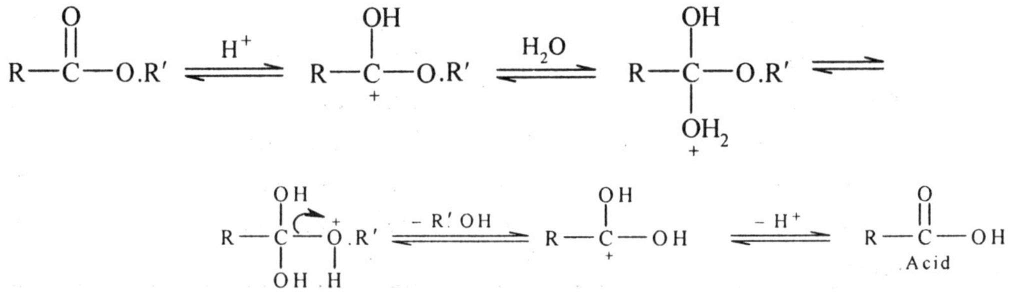

(ii) **Alkaline hydrolysis:**

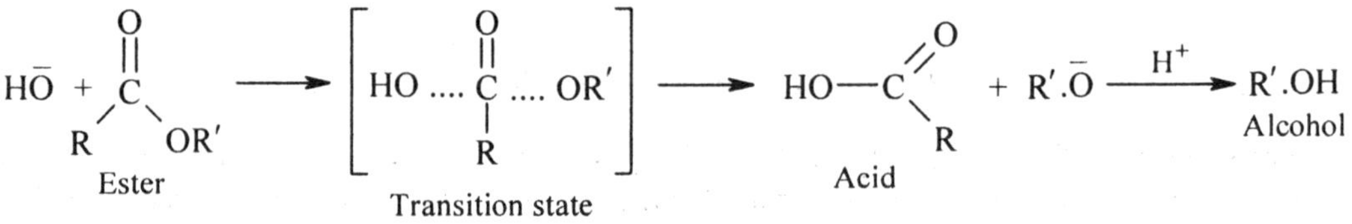

2. **Ammonolysis:** Esters are converted by interaction with ammonia or its alkyl derivatives (e.g. amines) into amides and alcohols.

$$CH_3.CO.O.C_2H_5 + NH_3 \longrightarrow CH_3.CO.NH_2 + C_2H_5.OH$$

Ethyl acetate   Acetamide

3. **Reduction:** Chemical reduction of esters using sodium and absolute alcohol yields alcohols.

$$R.CO.O.R' + 4H \xrightarrow{C_2H_5.OH + Na} R.CH_2.OH + R'.OH$$

However, catalytic hydrogenation in the presence of copper chromite catalyst at higher temperature and pressure or with metallic hydrides like lithium aluminium hydride forms primary alcohols.

$$R.CO.O.R' + 2H_2 \xrightarrow[\substack{100-300 \text{ atm.} \\ 200-300^\circ C}]{CuCr_2O_4-CuO} R.CH_2.OH + R'.OH$$

$$R.CO.O.R' + LiAlH_4 \longrightarrow (R.CH_2.O)_2 (OR)_2 LiAl \xrightarrow{H_2O} 2R.CH_2.OH + 2R'.OH$$

4. **Alcoholysis (splitting by alcohol):** Partial exchange of alcohol residue takes place when an ester is refluxed with excess of alcohol in the presence of a base or acid catalyst. The process is usually effective in replacing a higher alcohol by a lower one, e.g.:

$$\underset{}{CH_3.CO.O.C_5H_{11} + C_2H_5.OH} \underset{}{\overset{C_2H_5.O.Na}{\rightleftharpoons}} \underset{\text{Ethyl acetate} \quad \text{Pentanol}}{CH_3.CO.O.C_2H_5 + C_5H_{11}.OH}$$

This alcoholysis (cleavage by an alcohol) of an ester is called **transesterification**.

5. **Acidolysis (splitting by acid):** In this process the acid residue is displaced from its lower ester by another acid residue.

$$\underset{\text{Ethyl acetate} \qquad \text{Valeric acid}}{CH_3.CO.O.C_2H_5 + C_4H_9.COOH} \rightleftharpoons \underset{\text{Ethyl valerate}}{CH_3.COO + C_4H_9.CO.OC_2H_5}$$

6. **Reaction with hydrazine:** Acid hydrazides are obtained when esters are allowed to react with hydrazine.

$$R.CO.O.R' + \underset{\text{Hydrazine}}{NH_2NH_2} \longrightarrow \underset{\text{Hydrazide}}{R.CO.NH.NH_2} + R'.OH$$

7. **Action of phosphorus pentachloride:** Esters react with phosphorus pentachloride to yield acyl chloride.

$$Cl - PCl_3 - Cl$$
$$CH_3.CO - O - C_2H_5 \longrightarrow \underset{\text{Acetyl chloride}}{CH_3.CO.Cl} + POCl_3 + C_2H_5.Cl$$

Acid chlorides are also formed when phosphorus pentachloride is replaced by thionyl chloride in this reaction.

8. **Halogenation:** Esters readily react with halogens in the presence of red phosphorus to produce α-halogenated esters.

$$CH_3.CO.O.C_2H_5 + Br_2 \xrightarrow{\text{Red P}} \underset{\alpha\text{-Bromoethyl acetate}}{CH_2Br.CO.O.C_2H_5} + HBr$$

9. **Claisen condensation:** In the presence of a base catalyst one molecule of an ester combines with other molecule of ester, an aldehyde or a ketone. Such type of condensation is known as Claisen condensation.

$$\underset{CH_3.\overset{\overset{O}{\|}}{C}.O.C_2H_5}{} \xrightarrow{C_2H_5.O.Na} \underset{CH_3 - \overset{\overset{O.Na}{|}}{\underset{\underset{OC_2H_5}{|}}{C}} - O.C_2H_5}{} \xrightarrow[-2C_2H_5.OH]{CH_3.CO.O.C_2H_5}$$

$$\underset{CH_3.\overset{\overset{O.Na}{|}}{C} = CH.CO.O.C_2H_5}{} \xrightarrow{H^+} \underset{\text{Enol form}}{CH_3.\overset{\overset{OH}{|}}{C} = CH.CO.O.C_2H_5} \quad \underset{\underset{\text{(Keto form)}}{\text{Acetoacetic ester}}}{CH_3.\overset{\overset{O}{\|}}{C}.CH_2.COOC_2H_5}$$

10. **Pyrolysis:** When esters are heated alone at high temperature, alkenes are formed.

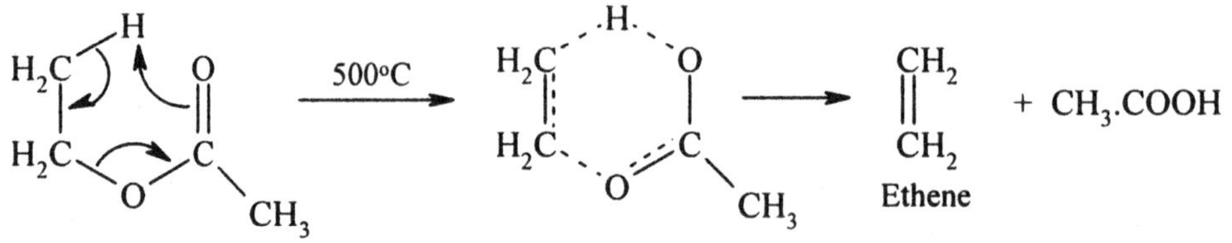

11. **Action of sodamide:** Esters containing α-hydrogen atoms react with sodamide in liquid ammonia solution to yield the acid amide and the condensation product involving two molecules of ester, e.g.

$$\underset{\text{Ethyl acetate}}{CH_3.CO.O.C_2H_5} + \underset{\text{Sodamide}}{NaNH_2} \longrightarrow \underset{\text{Acetamide}}{CH_3.CO.NH_2} + C_2H_5.O.Na$$

$$CH_3.CO.O.C_2H_5 + NaNH_2 \longrightarrow NH_3 + [CH_2.CO.O.C_2H_5]^- Na^+$$

$$\xrightarrow[CH_3.CO.O.C_2H_5]{} \underset{\text{Acetoacetic ester}}{CH_3.CO.CH_2.CO.O.C_2H_5} + C_2H_5.OH$$

12. **Action of Grignard reagents:** Esters react with Grignard reagents to produce tertiary alcohols.

$$R-\overset{\overset{O}{\|}}{C}-O.R \xrightarrow{R''.MgX} [R-\underset{\underset{.R.O.MgX}{|}}{\overset{\overset{O}{\|}}{C}}-R'] \xrightarrow{R''.MgX} R-\underset{\underset{O.MgX}{|}}{\overset{\overset{R''}{|}}{C}}-R \xrightarrow{H_2O} \underset{\text{3° alcohol}}{R''-\underset{\underset{OH}{|}}{\overset{\overset{R''}{|}}{C}}-R''}$$

Use: Esters are used:

1. As solvent for cellulose, oils, gums, resins etc.
2. As plasticiser.
3. For making artificial flavours and essences, e.g. isoamyl isovalerate (apple), methyl butyrate (pineapple), etc.

Ethyl acetoacetate or Acetoacetic ester

$$CH_3-\overset{\overset{O}{\|}}{C}-CH_2-\overset{\overset{O}{\|}}{C}-OC_2H_5$$

It is a β-ketonic ester. It is extensively used in organic synthesis. It is a liquid made by acting upon ethyl acetate with sodium and decomposing the initial product (a sodium salt) with dil. acid. It is an example of Claisen condensation.

$$\underset{\text{Ethyl acetate (2 molar)}}{CH_3.COO.C_2H_5 + CH_3.COO.C_2H_5} \longrightarrow CH_3.CO.CH_2.COO.C_2H_5 + C_2H_5OH$$

It exists in keto and enol tautomeric forms.

$$\underset{\text{Keto form}}{CH_3-\overset{\overset{O}{\|}}{C}-CH_2COOC_2H_5} \rightleftharpoons \underset{\text{Enol form}}{CH_3-\overset{\overset{OH}{|}}{C}=CH-COOC_2H_5}$$

Ordinary ethyl acetoacetate is a mixture of 93% keto and 7% enol forms. They have been separated at low temperature.

Reaction of ethyl acetoacetate

Ketonic hydrolysis and acid hydrolysis: This ester undergoes hydrolytic fission on one side or other side of α-carbon atom giving rise to ketones or acids (acid hydrolysis).

Ketonic hydrolysis:

$$CH_3 - CO - CH_2 - COOC_2H_5 \xrightarrow{\text{2KOH}} CH_3COCH_3 + K_2CO_3 + C_2H_5OH$$

Acid hydrolysis:

$$CH_3 - CO - CH_2COOC_2H_5 \xrightarrow{\text{2KOH}} CH_3COOK + CH_3COOK + C_2H_5OH$$

Malonic ester (or Ethyl malonate)

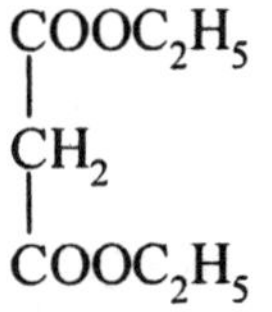

$$\begin{array}{c} COOC_2H_5 \\ | \\ CH_2 \\ | \\ COOC_2H_5 \end{array}$$

Synthetic uses of malonic ester are many.

Example: Most of barbiturates are made by condensing urea with an appropriately substituted malonic ester.

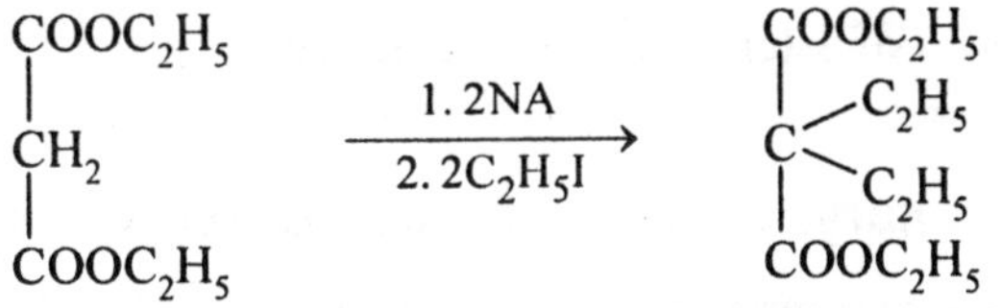

Ethyl diethyl malonate

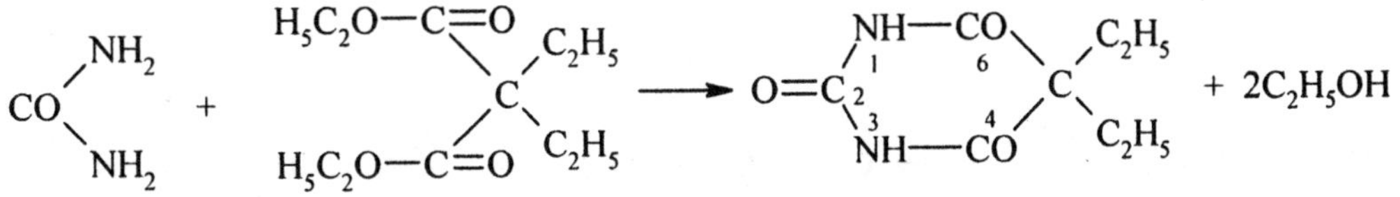

Urea   Ethyl diethyl malonate   Barbitone
(5,5-diethyl barbituric acid)

Similarly other homologues of barbitone are:

1. **Butobarbitone:**

(5-butyl-5-ethyl barbituric acid) =

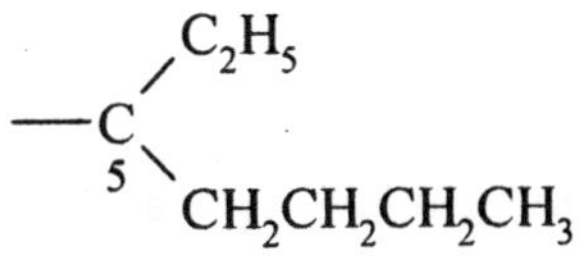

2. **Amylobarbitone:**

(5-ethyl-5-isopentyl barbituric acid) = $-\underset{5}{C}\Big\langle\substack{C_2H_5 \\ CH_2CH_2-CH\langle\substack{CH_3 \\ CH_3}}$

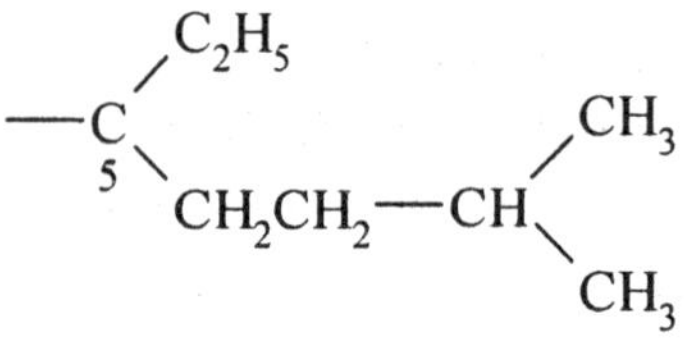

3. **Pentobarbitone:**

(5-ethyl-5 (1-methyl butyl barbituric acid) = $-\underset{5}{C}\Big\langle\substack{C_2H_5 \\ CH-CH_2CH_2CH_3 \\ | \\ CH_3}$

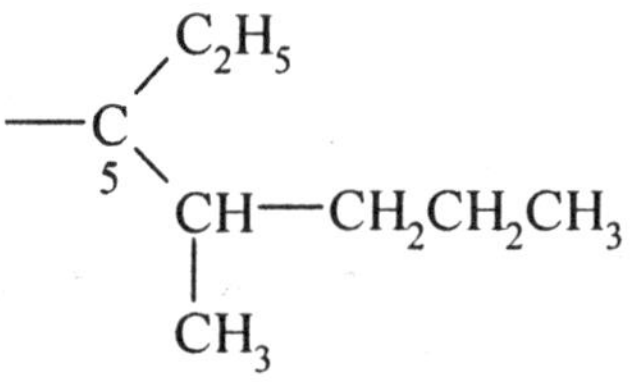

Likewise malonic ester is extensively used in the organic synthesis of various compounds.

Ethyl Acetate ($CH_3.CO.O.C_2H_5$)

Ethyl acetate is an organic ester. It is obtained by the interaction of ethanol with acetic acid or acetyl chloride or acetic anhydride as discussed earlier.

It is a colourless, mobile liquid having a pleasant fruity odour. It boils at 77°, has sp. gr. 0.9. It is slightly soluble in water but miscible with alcohol, ether and chloroform in all proportions.

It shows all general reactions of ester as mentioned above.

Ethyl Lauryl Sulphate ($C_{12}H_{25}.O.SO_2.O.Na$)

This is the sodium salt of inorganic ester and is obtained by treating lauryl alcohol (dodecyl alcohol, $C_{12}H_{25}.OH$) with sulphuric acid and then with sodium.

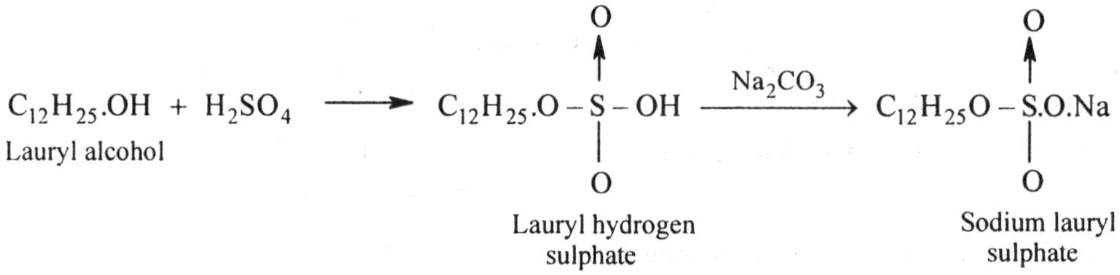

$$C_{12}H_{25}.OH + H_2SO_4 \longrightarrow C_{12}H_{25}.O-\overset{\overset{O}{\uparrow}}{\underset{O}{S}}-OH \xrightarrow{Na_2CO_3} C_{12}H_{25}O-\overset{\overset{O}{\uparrow}}{\underset{O}{S}}.O.Na$$

Lauryl alcohol   Lauryl hydrogen   Sodium lauryl
                           sulphate   sulphate

The product is hydrolyzed easily by refluxing it with dilute hydrochloric acid.

$$C_{12}H_{25}.O.SO_2.O.Na + H_2O \xrightarrow{Heat} C_{12}H_{25}.OH + NaHSO_4$$

It is used as an ingredient for emulsifying wax and for lowering the surface tension.

OFFICIAL COMPOUNDS

Ethyl Oleate

Mol. Form.: $C_{20}H_{38}O_2$ Mol Wt.: 310.5

Ethyl oleate contains not less than 98.0 per cent w/w of esters calculated as $C_{20}H_{38}O_2$. It is obtained by esterifying oleic acid with ethyl alcohol.

It is a pale yellow oil which possesses strong and disagreeable odour and taste. It is practically insoluble in water, but is miscible with fixed oils.

It is tested for purity for acid value; iodine value; weight per ml and peroxide.

Assay: It is carried out by using the method for determination of esters.

It is used as a pharmaceutical aid in making certain preparations for intramuscular injections, like injections of progesterone, oestradiol benzoate, testosterone propionate, testosterone phenylpropionate, deoxycortone acetate. These injections are less viscous and hence they flow through the needle more readily than those prepared by using arachis or other oils.

Sodium Lauryl Sulphate

Sodium lauryl sulphate is a mixture of sodium and normal primary alkyl sulphates, consisting chiefly of sodium dodecyl sulphate, $CH_3.(CH_2)_{10}.CH_2O.SO_3.Na$. It contains equivalent of not less than 58.0 per cent w/w of total alcohols.

It is prepared by converting commercial lauryl alcohol into the hydrogen sulphate and converting this into the sodium salt.

It is a white or light yellow powder or crystals with slight but characteristic odour. It is soluble in water (1 : 10) and partly in alcohol.

It is identified through the reactions characteristic of sodium and sulphate from its solution.

It is tested for alkalinity; sodium chloride; sodium sulphate and unsulphated alcohols.

Assay: It is assayed by hydrolyzing the sodium alkyl sulphate by boiling under reflux with dilute hydrochloric acid. The reaction is as follows:

$$C_{12}H_{25}.O.SO_2.O.Na + H_2O \longrightarrow C_{12}H_{25}.OH + NaHSO_4$$

The alcohols are extracted with ether. Ether is evaporated and the residue is dried and weighed.

Uses: Sodium lauryl sulphate is used as a detergent and emulsifier. It is an ingredient of emulsifying wax and in emulsions it is used to lower the surface tension. It is a good base for soapless shampoos and an ideal tablet lubricant. It is widely used in textile industry.

Busulphan

Mol. Form: $C_6H_{14}O_6S_2$ Mol. Wt.: 246.3

Busulphan is 1,4-di(methanesulphonyloxy)butane and contains not less than 98.0 per cent of $C_6H_{14}O_6S_2$ calculated with reference to the substance dried to constant weight in vacuum at 60°.

It occurs as a white crystalline powder which is practically insoluble in water but is slightly soluble in alcohol.

It is tested for melting point; loss on drying and sulphated ash.

Assay: It is assayed by hydrolyzing about 0.8 g with boiling water under reflux, and titrating the resulting methanesulphonic acid with N/10 sodium hydroxide using phenylhydrazine as an indicator.

$$CH_3.SO_3.H + NaOH \longrightarrow CH_3.SO_3.Na + H_2O$$

Each ml of N/10 NaOH is equivalent to 0.006158 of $C_6H_{14}O_6S_2$.

It is used as neoplastic suppressant. It is highly poisonous. Busulphan tablets are official in I.P.

Doses: 2 to 4 mg daily.

Amines

Alkyl amines are derivatives of ammonia in which one or more hydrogen atoms of NH_3 molecule have been replaced by alkyl groups. They are classified as primary, secondary and tertiary amines according to the number of groups attached to the nitrogen atom, e.g.:

$$
\begin{array}{cccc}
\overset{\displaystyle H}{\underset{\displaystyle |}{}} & \overset{\displaystyle H}{\underset{\displaystyle |}{}} & \overset{\displaystyle H}{\underset{\displaystyle |}{}} & \overset{\displaystyle R}{\underset{\displaystyle |}{}} \\
H\!-\!N\!-\!H & R\!-\!N\!-\!H & R\!-\!N\!-\!R & R\!-\!N\!-\!R \\
\text{Ammonia} & \text{Primary amine} & \text{Secondary amine} & \text{Tertiary amine}
\end{array}
$$

Each amine is characterized by the presence of the amino group $-NH_2$, the imino group $\diagdown NH$, and the tertiary nitrogen atom $-\overset{|}{N}-$ respectively.

The alkyl groups attached to the nitrogen may be the same or different. Thus they may be simple or mixed amines according to the presence of the same or different groups.

Besides these amines tetra-alkyl derivatives of ammonium salts are also known and they are called as quaternary ammonium salts, e.g. $[(CH_3)_4 N]^+ I^-$ Tetramethyl ammonium iodide.

Nomenclature: Amines are named by naming the alkyl groups attached to nitrogen, and following these by the word 'amine'. According to the IUPAC system of nomenclature the names for primary, secondary and tertiary amines are aminoalkanes, alkyl aminoalkanes, and dialkyl aminoalkanes respectively (Table 17.1).

Salts of amines are generally named by replacing 'amine' by 'ammonium' and adding the name of the anion such as chloride, nitrate, sulphate etc. For example:

$$(CH_3.NH_3)_2^{++} SO_4^{--} \qquad (C_2H_5)_3 N^+ HNO_3^-$$

Methylammonium sulphate   Triethylammonium nitrate

Table 17.1.

Formula	Common name	IUPAC
$CH_3.NH_2$	Methyl amine	Aminomethane
$(CH_3)_2NH$	Dimethylamine	Methylaminomethane
$C_2H_5.NH_2$	Ethyl amine	Aminoethane
$(C_2H_5)_2NH$	Diethyl amine	N-Ethylaminoethane
$CH_3.NH.C_2H_5$	Methylethyl amine	N-Methylaminoethane
$(CH_3)_3N$	Trimethyl amine	N-N-Dimethylaminomethane
$\begin{array}{c} H_3C \\ C_2H_5 \!-\! N \\ C_3H_7 \end{array}$	Methyethylpropyl amine	N-Methyl-N-ethylaminopropane

The method of naming a quaternary ammonium salt is illustrated by the following examples:

$$(CH_3)_4N^+OH^- \qquad\qquad [(CH_3)_3N^+.C_2H_5]\overline{Cl}$$

Tetramethyl ammonium hydroxide   Ethyl trimethyl ammonium chloride

Isomerism: Amines show the following types of isomerism.

1. Position isomerism:

C_3H_9N : $CH_3.CH_2.CH_2.NH_2$ $CH_3.CH.CH_3$

1-Aminopropane
(n-Propylamine)

NH_2

2-Aminopropane
(Isopropylamine)

2. Chain isomerism:

$C_4H_{11}N$: $CH_3.CH_2.CH_2.CH_2.NH_2$ $CH_3.CH.CH_2.NH_2$

n-Butylamine

CH_3

Isobutylamine

3. Metamerism:

$C_4H_{11}N$: $C_2H_5.NHC_2H_5$ $CH_3.NH.C_3H_7$

Diethylamine   Methylpropylamine

4. Functional isomerism:

C_3H_9N : $CH_3CH_2.CH_2NH_2$ $CH_3.NH.C_2H_5$ $(CH_3)_3N$

Propylamine
(Primary)

Methylethylamine
(Secondary)

Trimethylamine
(Tertiary)

General methods of preparation: All types of amines including quaternary ammonium salts can be prepared only by few methods while others yield only primary, secondary or tertiary amine. These methods are discussed in the following pages.

(A) Methods for all Types of Amines

1. **From alkyl halides (Hofmann's method, 1849):** Ammonolysis of alkyl halides with aqueous or alcoholic solution of ammonia in a sealed tube at $100°C$ produces a mixture of all types of amines along with quaternary ammonium salts.

$$C_2H_5.I + NH_3 \longrightarrow C_2H_5NH_2HI \xrightarrow[-HI]{C_2H_5.I} (C_2H_5)_2NH.HI \xrightarrow[-HI]{C_2H_5.I}$$

Ethylamine   Diethylamine
hydroiodide   hydroiodide

$$(C_2H_5)_3NHI \xrightarrow[-HI]{C_2H_5.I} [(C_2H_5)_4N]^+I^-$$

Triethylamine   Tetraethylammonium
hydroiodide   iodide

The order of reactivity of halides is $RI > RBr > RCl$. If excess of ammonia is reacted the main product formed is primary amine. However, tertiary amine is formed in excess if excess of alkyl halide is used.

2. **From alcohols:** A mixture of three types of amines is obtained by the ammonolysis of alcohols. In this process, vapours of an alcohol and ammonia are passed over a heated catalyst like alumina, copper chromite, thoria, or silica gel at $360°$.

$$C_2H_5.OH + NH_3 \xrightarrow[-H_2O]{} C_2H_5.NH_2 \xrightarrow[-H_2O]{C_2H_5.OH} (C_2H_5)_2NH \xrightarrow[-H_2O]{C_2H_5.OH} (C_2H_5)_2N$$

3. **By methylation of ammonia:** All types of amines are also achieved when acidic solution of ammonia is heated with formaldehyde solution.

$$2NH_3 + 3HCHO \xrightarrow{HCl} 2CH_3.NH_2 + CO_2 + H_2O$$

$$2CH_3.NH_2 + 3HCHO \xrightarrow{HCl} 2(CH_3)_2NH + CO_2 + H_2O$$

$$2(CH_3)_2.NH + 3HCHO \xrightarrow{HCl} 2(CH_3)_3N + CO_2 + H_2O$$

Secondary and tertiary amines may be obtained by methylating primaryamines with dimethyl sulphate.

$$CH_3.NH_2 + (CH_3)_2SO_4 \longrightarrow (CH_3)_2NH + CH_3.HSO_4$$

$$(CH_3)_2.NH + (CH_3)_2SO_4 \longrightarrow (CH_3)_3N + CH_3.HSO_4$$

(B) Methods of Yielding Primary Amines

1. **By reduction of nitroalkanes:** The nitro compounds can be reduced by catalytic hydrogenation using molecular hydrogen or by chemical reduction using a metal and acid or lithium aluminium hydride.

$$R.NO_2 + 6H \longrightarrow R.NH_2 + 2H_2O$$

2. **By reduction of alkyl cyanides:** The reduction of nitriles may be carried out using molecular hydrogen and a catalyst or by sodium and alcohol or with lithium aluminium hydride. The reaction involves addition of two pairs of hydrogen atoms to the triple bond ($-C \equiv N$).

Primary amines are obtained that have one more carbon than the alkyl halides from which the nitriles are formed.

$$R.CH_2.Br + NaCl \xrightarrow[NaBr]{} R.CH_2.C \equiv N \xrightarrow[140°C]{H_2, Ni} R.CH_2.CH_2.NH_2$$

3. **By reduction of acid amides:** Chemical reduction of amides with lithium aluminium hydride or sodium and ethanol leads to the formation of primary amines.

$$R.CO.NH_2 + 4H \xrightarrow{LiAlH_4} R.CH_2.NH_2 + H_2O$$

4. **By reduction of oxides and hydrazones:** Oximes and hydrazones, obtained by condensation of hydroxylamine and hydrazines with carbonyl compounds, are also reducible to primary amines by addition of hydrogen to the double bond and replacement of hydroxyl group by hydrogen.

$$R.CH = N.OH + 4H \longrightarrow R.CH_2.NH_2 + H_2O$$
Aldoxime

$$R_2C = N.OH + 4H \longrightarrow R_2.CH.NH_2 + H_2O$$
Ketoxime

$$R.CH = N.NH_2 + 4H \longrightarrow R.CH_2.NH_2 + NH_3$$
Hydrazone

5. **By Hoffmann's bromamide method (1881):** Acid amides containing upto six carbon atoms on treatment with bromine and caustic potash produce primary amines in excellent yields, with one carbon less than that of the parent amide.

$$R.CO.NH_2 + Br_2 + 4KOH \longrightarrow R.NH_2 + 2KBr + K_2CO_3 + 2H_2O$$

The mechanism of this remarkable reaction has been discussed earlier.

6. **By Gabriel's phthalimide reaction (1887):** This method was developed by Gabriel in which the acidic hydrogen of phthalimide is removed by an active metal in alcohol. The salt so secured is heated with an alkyl halide to form N-alkyl phthalimide. On hydrolysis with 20 per cent hydrochloric acid under pressure this gives pure primary amine and phthalic acid. This method has many applications in the synthesis of amino acids.

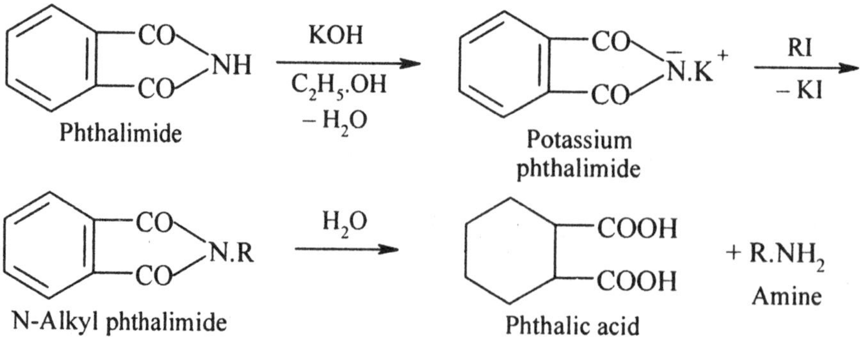

Phthalimide → Potassium phthalimide → N-Alkyl phthalimide → Phthalic acid + R.NH₂ (Amine)

7. **By the action of carbonyl compounds with ammonium formate or with formamide (Leuckart reaction):** In this reaction formyl derivatives of primary amines are formed which on hydrolysis yield primary amines.

$$R.CHO + 2H.COO.NH_4 \longrightarrow R.CH_2.NH.CHO + 2H_2O + CO_2 + NH_3$$

  Aldehyde   Ammonium formate   N-Formyl deriv.

$$R_2.C = O + 2H.CO.NH_2 \longrightarrow R_2.CH.NH.CHO + CO_2 + NH_3$$

  Ketone   Formamide

$$R.CH_2.NH.CHO \xrightarrow{H_2O} R.CH_2.NH_2 + H.COOH$$

$$R.CH_2.NH.CHO \xrightarrow{H_2O} R.CH_2.NH_2 + H.COOH$$

8. **By reductive amination:** By passing a mixture of aldehyde or ketone with excess of ammonia and hydrogen under pressure over nickel catalyst at 40–150°C.

$$R_2.C = O + NH_3 \xrightarrow[-H_2O]{H_2/Ni} [R_2.C = NH] \xrightarrow{H_2/Ni} R_2.CHNH_2$$

  Ketone   Imine

9. **By the action of chloramine on Grignard reagents:**

$$R.MgX + Cl.NH_2 \longrightarrow R.NH_2 + Mg(Cl)X$$

10. **By decarboxylation of amino acids:**

$$H_2N.CH_2.COOH \xrightarrow[Heat]{Ba(OH)_2} CH_3.NH_2 + CO_2$$

  Glycine   Methylamine

11. **By hydrolysis of isocyanide or isocyanate (Wurtz's reaction):**

$$R.NC + KOH + H_2O \longrightarrow R.NH_2 + H.COO.K$$

  Alkyl isocyanide

$$R.N = C = O + 2KOH \longrightarrow R.NH_2 + K_2CO_3$$

  Alkyl isocyanate

12. **Curtius reaction (1894):** Primary amines are also prepared by utilizing the Curtius reaction, but the method is less widely used than the method of Hofmann. In this procedure esters are reacted with hydrazine to form hydrazides which are converted to acid azides. The azides when boiled with benzene or chloroform form isocyanates which on hydrolysis with alkali afford primary amines.

$$RCOOH + C_2H_5.OH \xrightarrow{H_2SO_4} R.CO.O.C_2H_5 \xrightarrow{NH_2.NH_2} R.CO.NH.NH_2$$

$$\xrightarrow[-2H_2O]{HNO_2} R.CON_3 \xrightarrow[Boil]{Benzene} R.N. = C = O \xrightarrow{KOH} R.NH_2$$

     Acid azide   Isocyanate   Amine

13. **Schmidt reaction:** Carboxylic acids react with hydrazoic acid to yield primary amine.

$$R.COOH + HN_3 \xrightarrow{H_2SO_4} R.NH_2 + CO_2 + N_2$$

  Hydrazoic acid

(C) Methods Yielding Secondary Amines

1. By reduction of alkyl isocyanide with sodium and alcohol.

$$R.NC + 4H \xrightarrow{\text{Na/C}_2\text{H}_5.\text{OH}} R.NH.CH_3$$

2. By heating an alcoholic solution of a primary amine with a calculated amount of alkyl halide.

$$R.NH_2 + R'X \longrightarrow R.R'.NH.HX$$

3. By hydrolysis of p-nitrosodialkylaniline, obtained from aniline, by boiling with strong alkali.

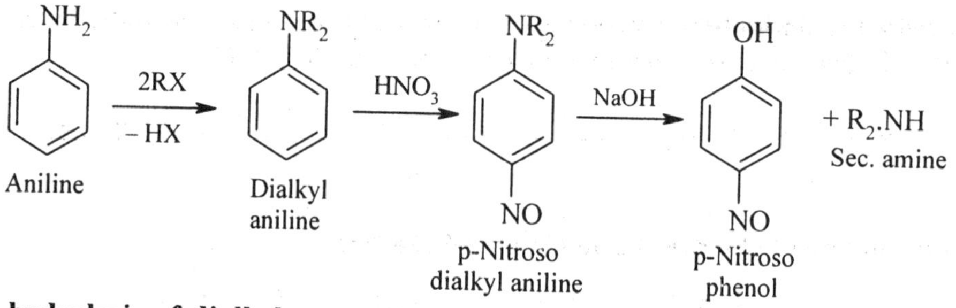

4. **By hydrolysis of dialkyl cyanamides:** Dialkyl cyanamides are obtained from sodium cyanamide which on hydrolysis yield N,N-dialkyl carbamic acids. These acids undergo decarboxylation on heating when secondary amines are produced.

$$Na_2.N-C\equiv N + 2RX \xrightarrow[-2NaX]{} R_2N.C\equiv N \xrightarrow[-NH_3]{2H_2O} R_2N.COOH \xrightarrow[-CO_2]{Heat} R_2NH$$

Sodium cyanamide   Dialkyl cyanamide   Dialkyl carbamic acid   Sec. amine

(D) Methods Giving Tertiary Amines Only

1. By heating an alcoholic solution of ammonia with excess of alkyl halide.

$$3RX + NH_3 \longrightarrow R_3N + 3HI$$

2. By reduction of aldehyde or ketone with hydrogen in the presence of primary or secondary amine.

$$R'.CHO + R''_2.NH + H_2 \xrightarrow{Ni} R'.CH_2.N.R''_2 + H_2O$$

Tert. amine

3. By the hydrolysis of a quaternary ammonium salt with moist silver oxide and then heating tertiary alkyl ammonium hydroxide so obtained.

$$(C_2H_5)_4N^+I^- + AgOH \xrightarrow[-AgI]{} (C_2H_5)_4N^+\overline{O}H \xrightarrow{Heat} (C_2H_5)_3N + C_2H_4 + H_2O$$

Tert. ethyl ammonium iodide   Triethyl amine

When tetramethyl ammonium hydroxide is strongly heated then the following decomposed products are obtained.

$$(CH_3)_4\overset{+}{N}\overline{O}H \xrightarrow{Heat} (CH_3)_3N + CH_3.OH$$

General Physical Properties

The lower members are gases at ordinary temperature, the members from C_3 to C_{11} are volatile liquids and higher members are solids. The lower members are volatile, highly soluble in water, have a powerful fishy smell and are combustible. Their solubility in water decreases with increase in molecular weights but boiling points increase with increase in molecular weight. The aqueous solutions are alkaline to litmus and conduct electricity.

Like ammonia, primary and secondary amines are polar compounds and form intermolecular hydrogen bonds. But these bonds are not so strong as in case of alcohols and carboxylic acids. Due to this they have lower boiling points than the corresponding alcohols or acids. The boiling points are, however, higher than the corresponding nonpolar hydrocarbons.

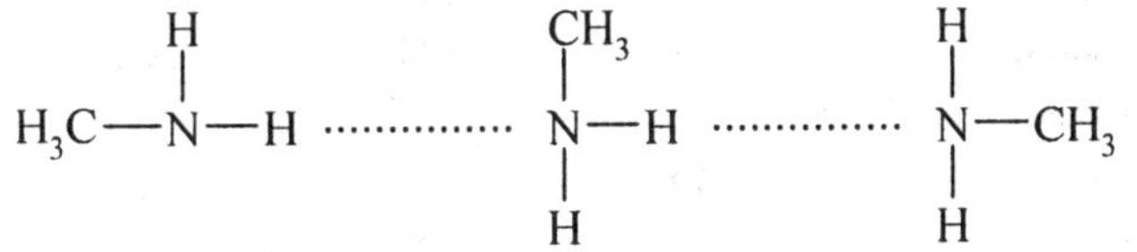

Intermolecular hydrogen bonding in methylamine

All amines form hydrogen bondings with water. Amines are soluble in less polar solvents like ether, benzene, etc. Their physical constants are given in Table 17.2.

General Chemical Properties

Like ammonia, all types of amines contain nitrogen that bear an unshared pair of electrons. Due to the presence of these electrons most of chemical behaviour of amines resembles very closely to the chemical behaviour of ammonia.

Amines are more basic than ammonia due to the presence of unshared electron pair on nitrogen atom. Alkyl groups have positive inductive effect (+I) due to which electron density at nitrogen atom increases and makes the unshared electron pair more available for protonation. Thus basicity of amines should be in the order: tertiary > secondary > primary, but the order is found to be as secondary > primary > tertiary. The reason for this order is not known. It has been suggested that a steric factor operates. Addition of the proton increases crowding and thus a strain is set up. This is greatest in the tertiary amines and so the stability of these molecules is decreased.

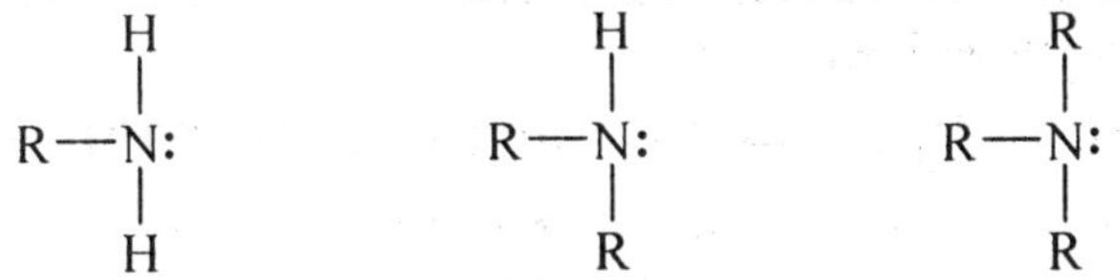

Primary, secondary and tertiary amines have different properties in many respects which are discussed separately for the sake of convenience.

Table 17.2. Physical constants of amines

Name	M.P. °C	B.P. °C	Solubility g/100 g of H_2O	K_b
Methylamine	– 92	7.5	1156	4.4×10^{-4}
Dimethylamine	– 96	7.5	v. sol.	5.1
Trimethylamine	– 117	3.5	91	0.662
Ethylamine	– 80	17	α	4.7
Diethylamine	– 39	55	v. sol	9.5
Triethylamine	– 115	89	14	5.5
n-Propylamine	– 83	49	α	3.8
Di-n-propylamine	– 63	110	s. sol.	8.1
Tri-n-propylamine	– 93	157	s. vol.	4.0
Isopropylamine	– 101	34	α	–
n-Butylamine	– 50	78	v. sol.	4.1
Isobutylamine	– 85	68	α	–
sec-Butylamine	– 104	63	α	–
tert-Butylamine	– 67	46	α	–
Allylamine	–	53.2	–	0.761
Cyclohexylamine	–	134	s. sol.	–
Ethylenediamine	8	117	α	–
Tetramethylenediamine	27	158	v. sol.	–
Hexamethylenediamine	39	196	v. sol.	–
Trimethylenediamine	–	135.5	–	0.884
Pentamethylenediamine	9	178	–	0.855
n-Amylamine	– 55	104	–	0.766
n-Iexylamine	– 19	130 (742 mm)	–	–
Laurylamine	28	135 (15 mm)	–	–
Ethanolamine	–	171	–	1.022
Diethanolamine	28	270	–	1.097
Triethanolamine	21	279 (0.5 mm)	–	1.124

A. Reactions Given by Primary, Secondary and Tertiary Amines

1. **Reaction with water:** Alkyl ammonium hydroxides are formed when amines combine with water like the reaction with ammonia.

$$CH_3NH_2 + H_2O \longrightarrow CH_3.NH_3.OH \rightleftharpoons CH_3 \overset{+}{N}H_3O\overline{H}$$

Methylamine   Methyl ammonium
                              hydroxide

$$(CH_3)_3N + H_2O \longrightarrow (CH_3)_3NH_3.OH \rightleftharpoons (CH_3)_3 \overset{+}{N}H_3 + \overline{O}H$$

Trimethyl   Trimethyl ammonium
amine   hydroxide

2. **Salt formation:** Formation of salts takes place when amines are reacted with mineral acids.

$$C_2H_5.NH_2 + HCl \longrightarrow C_2H_5 \overset{+}{N}H_3\overset{-}{Cl}$$

Ethylamine   Ethylamine hydrochloride

$$2(C_2H_5)_2NH + H_2SO_4 \longrightarrow [(C_2H_5)_2NH]_2.H_2SO_4$$

Diethylamine   Diethyl ammonium sulphate

$$(C_2H_5)_3N + HBr \longrightarrow (C_2H_5)_3N.HBr$$

Triethylamine   Triethylamine hydrogen bromide

3. **Reaction with alkyl halides:** All amines combine with alkyl halides to form quaternary ammonium salts as the final products.

$$C_2H_5NH_2 \xrightarrow[-HI]{C_2H_5.I} (C_2H_5)_2NH \xrightarrow[-HI]{C_2H_5.I} (C_2H_5)_3N \xrightarrow{C_2H_5.I} (C_2H_5)_4\overset{+}{N}.\overset{-}{I}$$

Ethylamine   Diethylamine   Triethylamine   Tetraethyl

(primary)   (sec.)   (tert.)   ammonium

                                                           iodide

4. **Reaction with nitrous acid:** All types of amines react with nitrous acid in different ways. Primary amines on treatment with nitrous acid yield unstable diazonium salts which break down to yield a mixture of alcohols and alkenes.

$$C_4H_9.NH_2 + HNO_2 \xrightarrow[HCl]{NaNO_2} [C_4H_9.\overset{+}{N_2}]\overset{-}{Cl} \xrightarrow{H_2O} C_4H_9.OH + C_4H_8 + N_2 + CH_3.\underset{\underset{OH}{|}}{CH}.CH_2.CH_3$$

n-Butylamine   n-Butyl   Butene

                                   alcohol   Isobutyl alcohol

However, methylamine forms methyl nitrite and dimethyl ether when it reacts with nitrous acid.

$$CH_3.NH_2 + 2HNO_2 \longrightarrow CH_3.ONO + N_2 + 2H_2O$$

Methyl nitrite

$$2CH_3.NH_2 + 2HNO_2 \longrightarrow CH_3.O.CH_3 + 2N_2 + 3H_2O$$

Dimethyl ether

Secondary amines react with nitrous acid to yield N-nitrosoamines which are generally yellow and neutral compounds and are insoluble in dilute aqueous mineral acids.

$$(CH_3)_2.NH + HNO_2 \longrightarrow (CH_3)_2.N - N = O + H_2O$$

Dimethylamine   N-Nitrosodimethylamine

Tertiary amines react with nitrous acid to yield N-nitroso derivatives of secondary amine. Although this reaction is not really understood, it seems that unstable nitrite is formed by the attack of $\overset{+}{N}O$ on nitrogen.

$$R_3.N + HNO_2 \, [R_3.\overset{+}{N}H]\overset{-}{NO_2} \xrightarrow{Heat} R_2N - NO + R.OH$$

                        Nitrite   Nitrosoamine

5. **Reaction with gold and platinum chlorides:** Double salts formation takes place when amines are allowed to react with auric and platinic chlorides.

$$CH_3.NH_2 + HCl + AuCl_3 \longrightarrow [CH_2.NH_3].AuCl_4$$

Methyl ammonium
chloroaurate

$$2(CH_3)_2.NH + 2HCl + PtCl_4 \longrightarrow [(CH_3)_2.NH_2]_2.PtCl_6$$

Diethyl ammonium
chloroplatinate

$$(CH_3)_3.N + HCl + AuCl_3 \longrightarrow [(CH_3)_3.NH].AuCl_4$$

Trimethyl ammonium
chloroaurate

Pure metal is obtained when these crystalline salts are decomposed by heating. In this way molecular weights of amines may be determined.

6. **Oxidation:** Different oxidizing products are obtained when amines are oxidized with different oxidizing agents. Generally powerful oxidizing agents such as Caro's acid (H_2SO_5) and potassium permanganate are required for the oxidation of amines.

(a) **Oxidation with Caro's acid:**

(i) **Primary amines:**

$$R.CH_2.NH_2 \xrightarrow{[O]} R.C = N.OH + R.CH = N.OH + R.CH_2.NH.OH$$

|
OH

Primary amine with primary alkyl group — Hydroxamic acid — Aldoxime acid — N-Alkylhydroxyl amine

$$R_2.CH.NH_2 \xrightarrow{[O]} R_2.C = N.OH$$

Pri. amine with sec. alkyl group — Ketoxime

$$R_3.CH - NH_2 \xrightarrow{[O]} R_3.C - NO$$

Pri. amine with tert. alkyl group — Nitrosoalkane

(ii) **Secondary amine:**

$$R_2.NH \xrightarrow{[O]} R_2.N.OH$$

Sec. amine — Dialkylhydroxyl amine

(iii) **Tertiary amine:**

$$R_3.N \xrightarrow{[O]} R_3.N \rightarrow O$$

Amine oxide

(b) **Oxidation with potassium permanganate:**

(i) **Primary amine**

$$R.CH_2.NH_2 \xrightarrow{[O]} R.CH = NH \xrightarrow{H_2O} R.CHO + NH_3$$

Aldimine — Aldehyde

$$R_2.CH.NH_2 \xrightarrow{[O]} \underset{\text{Ketimine}}{R_2.C = NH} \xrightarrow{H_2O} \underset{\text{Ketone}}{R_2.C = O + NH_3}$$

$$R_3.C.NH_2 \xrightarrow{[O]} \underset{\text{Nitroalkane}}{R_3.C.NO_2}$$

(ii) Secondary amine

$$2R_2.NH \xrightarrow{[O]} \underset{\substack{\text{Tetraalkyl} \\ \text{hydrazine}}}{R_2.N - N.R_2} + H_2O$$

C. Reactions Given by Primary Amines Only

1. **Carbylamine reaction:** Primary amines form isocyanides when they are heated with chloroform and alcoholic caustic potash. Isocyanides have extremely unpleasant odour. Hence, this reaction is used to characterize primary amines.

$$C_2H_5.NH_2 + CHCl_3 + 3KOH \longrightarrow \underset{\text{Ethyl isocyanide}}{C_2H_5.N \equiv C} + 3KCl + 2H_2O$$

2. **Hofmann's mustard oil reaction:** When primary amines are warmed with carbon disulphide, dithiocarbamic acid is obtained which is decomposed to alkyl isothiocyanate by the addition of mercuric chloride.

$$R.NH_2 + CS_2 \longrightarrow S = C \underset{\substack{\text{Monoalkyl dithio-} \\ \text{carbamic acid}}}{\overset{\nearrow \text{NH.R}}{\underset{\searrow \text{SH}}{}}} \xrightarrow{HgCl_2} \underset{\substack{\text{Alkyl iso-} \\ \text{thiocyanate}}}{R.NCS} + HgS + 2HCl$$

This reaction is also used for the identification of primary amines.

3. **Reaction with aldehydes:** Imines are obtained when primary amines are allowed to combine with aldehydes.

$$\underset{\text{Benzaldehyde}}{C_6H_5.CHO} + R.NH_2 \longrightarrow \underset{\text{Imine}}{C_6H_5.CH = N.R} + H_2O$$

D. Reactions Given by Primary and Secondary Amines Only

1. **Reaction with acid chloride and acid anhydrides:** Primary and secondary amines combine with acid chlorides and acid anhydrides to yield acyl derivatives.

$$C_2H_5.NH_2 + \underset{\text{Acetyl chloride}}{Cl.CO.CH_3} \longrightarrow \underset{\text{Acetyl ethyl amine}}{C_2H_5.NH.CO.CH_3} + HCl$$

$$(CH_3)_2NH + \underset{\text{Acetic anhydride}}{(CH_3.CO)_2O} \longrightarrow \underset{\text{Acetyl dimethylamine}}{(CH_3)_2.N.CO.CH_3} + CH_3.COOH$$

2. **Reaction with sodium:** Sodium derivatives are formed when primary and secondary amines are heated with sodium.

$$2C_2H_5.NH_2 + 2Na \longrightarrow 2C_2H_5.NH.Na + H_2$$

$$2(C_2H_5)_2.NH + 2Na \longrightarrow 2(C_2H_5)_2.N.Na + H_2$$

3. **Reaction with phenyl lithium:** Proton of primary and secondary amines is replaced by lithium when they are reacted with phenyl lithium.

$$(CH_3)_2.NH + C_6H_5.Li \longrightarrow (CH_3)_2.\overline{N}.Li^+ + C_6H_6$$

Dimethyl amine   Phenyl lithium

4. **Reaction with Grignard's reagents:** Primary and secondary amines react with Grignard's reagents to produce hydrocarbons.

$$C_2H_5.NH_2 + CH_3.MgI \longrightarrow C_2H_5NHMgI + CH_4$$

Ethylamine   Methane

$$(C_2H_5)_2.NH + CH_3.MgI \longrightarrow (C_2H_5)_2NH.MgI + CH_4$$

5. **Reaction with nitroso chloride:** Alkyl halides are obtained when primary amines react with nitroso chloride whereas secondary amines form nitrosoamines.

$$R.NH_2 + NOCl \longrightarrow R.Cl + N_2 + H_2O$$

Primary
amine

$$R_2.NH + NOCl \longrightarrow R_2.N - NO + HCl$$

Secondary   Nitrosoamine
amine

6. **Reaction with halogens:** Protons of amino group are replaced by halogens when the reaction is carried out in the presence of an alkali.

$$R.NH_2 \xrightarrow[-HCl]{Cl_2/NaOH} R.NH.Cl \xrightarrow[-HCl]{Cl_2/NaOH} R.N.Cl_2$$

N-Chloroalkyl   N,N-Dichloro-
amine   alkyl amine

$$(C_2H_5)_2 NH \xrightarrow{Cl_2/NaOH} (C_2H_5)_2.N.Cl + HCl$$

N-Chlorodiethyl
amine

7. **Reaction with phenylisocyanate:** Phenylisocyanate forms well-defined crystals with amines as indicated below:

$$R.NH_2 + C_6H_5.NCO \longrightarrow R.NH.CO.NHC_6H_5$$

$$R_2.NH + C_6H_5.NCO \longrightarrow R_2.N.CO.NH.C_6H_5$$

D. Reactions Given by Secondary Amines Only

1. **Reaction with carbon disulphide:** Secondary amines form dithiocarbamic acids when heated with carbon disulphide, which are not decomposed by mercuric chloride to alkyl isothiocyanates as in case of primary amines.

$$S=C=S + R_2.NH \longrightarrow S=C\begin{smallmatrix} \diagup NR_2 \\ \diagdown SH \end{smallmatrix}$$

Dithiocarbamic acid

2. Secondary amines form enamines with aldehydes containing no hydrogen.

$$\begin{smallmatrix} R \\ \diagdown \\ \diagup \\ R' \end{smallmatrix} CH-C=O + HN.R_2'' \longrightarrow \begin{smallmatrix} R \\ \diagdown \\ \diagup \\ R' \end{smallmatrix} C=C-N.R_2''$$

Aldehyde   Enamine

E. Reactions Given by Tertiary Amines Only

1. **Reaction with cyanogen bromide:** Tertiary amines react with cyanogen to yield dialkylcyanamides which are hydrolyzed to secondary amines.

$$R_3.N + BrCN \longrightarrow [R_3.N.CN]^+ B\bar{r} \longrightarrow R.Br + R_2.N.CN \xrightarrow{H_2O} R_2.NH$$

2. **Oxidation:** Tertiary amines are oxidized at the α-hydrogen atoms by potassium permanganate, manganese dioxide or mercuric acetate to form enamines which are hydrolyzed to give aldehydes and secondary amines.

$$R'.CH_2CH_2N\begin{smallmatrix} \diagup R \\ \diagdown R \end{smallmatrix} + [O] \xrightarrow{Hg(O.CO.CH_3)_2} R.CH=CH.N\begin{smallmatrix} \diagup R \\ \diagdown R \end{smallmatrix} \longrightarrow R.CH_2.CHO + \begin{smallmatrix} R \\ \diagdown \\ \diagup \\ R' \end{smallmatrix} NH$$

Aldehyde

QUATERNARY AMMONIUM SALTS

Quaternary ammonium salts may be regarded as tetra-alkyl derivatives of ammonium salts. They are the products of the final stage of alkylation of nitrogen. For example, if all the hydrogen atoms of ammonium chloride are replaced by methyl groups then tetramethyl ammonium chloride is obtained. Generally they are represented by the formula $R_4N^+\bar{X}$ where four organic groups are covalently bonded to nitrogen, and the positive charge of this ion is balanced by some nitrogen ion. The alkyl groups attached to the nitrogen atom may be same or different when the salt of an amine is reacted with hydroxide ion, nitrogen gives up a hydrogen ion and free amine is obtained. However, the quaternary ammonium ion, which does not have a proton for elimination, is not affected by hydroxide ion.

$$\begin{bmatrix} R \\ R:\ddot{N}:R \\ R \end{bmatrix}^+ \bar{X} \xrightarrow{Ag_2O} \begin{bmatrix} R \\ R:\ddot{N}:R \\ R \end{bmatrix}^+ \bar{OH} + AgX$$

Insoluble

Quaternary   Quaternary
ammonium salt   ammonium hydroxide

Quaternary ammonium salts are prepared by the alkylation of amines. Treatment of an amine with an alkyl halide gives the product of an amine of the next higher class. The alkyl halide undergoes nucleophilic substitution. Due to the presence of lone pair of electrons on nitrogen an amine becomes basic and serves as the nucleophilic reagent. As the hydrogen attached to nitrogen has been replaced by an alkyl group, therefore, the reaction is referred to as alkylation of amines. The amine can be primary, secondary, tertiary, aliphatic or aromatic.

The quaternary ammonium salts are white crystalline solids. They are soluble in water and completely ionized in the solution. Formation of tertiary amines takes place when such salts are heated in vacuum.

$$[R_4N]^+ \overline{X} \xrightarrow{\text{Heat}} R_3N + R.X$$

Like the quaternary ammonium salts, their hydroxides are white, deliquescent, crystalline solids. They are represented by the structure $R_4\overset{+}{N}OH^-$ and are as strongly basic as sodium and potassium hydroxides. Their solutions eliminate ammonia from their salts and absorb carbon dioxide. The salts containing a long-chain alkyl group are used for the manufacture of detergents. It is due to the surface activity of the positive ion and not to negative ion as in alkyl hydrogen sulphate detergents.

When a quaternary ammonium hydroxide is heated at high temperature it yields a tertiary amine, an alkene and water on decomposition via the E_2 mechanism. For example, thermal decomposition of trimethyl n-propyl ammonium hydroxide gives trimethylamine and propylene:

$$\begin{array}{c}\overset{\displaystyle CH_3}{|}\\ CH_3 - \overset{+}{N} - CH_2.CH_2.CH_2.\overline{O}H \\ |\\ CH_3 \end{array} \xrightarrow{125-150^\circ C} \begin{array}{c}\overset{\displaystyle CH_3}{|}\\ CH_3 - N \\ |\\ CH_3 \end{array} + CH_2 = CH.CH_3 + H_2O$$

Propylene

Trimethylamine

This reaction is called as the Hofmann elimination which is identical to the dehydrohalogenation of an alkyl halide. Hydroxide ion abstracts a hydrogen ion from β-carbon. A molecule of tertiary amine is expelled from the adjacent carbon atom, and the double bond is formed.

$$\begin{array}{c} \overset{+}{R_3.N} \\ | \\ -\underset{1}{C} - \underset{3}{C} - \\ | \quad | \\ \quad H \\ \quad :\overline{O}H \end{array} \longrightarrow H_2C=CH.CH_3 + R_3.N + H_2O$$

The formation of quaternary ammonium salts followed by Hofmann elimination is used to prepare alkenes and in the determination of structures of nitrogen-containing compounds. Any type of amine may be converted into quaternary ammonium hydroxide by reacting it with excess of methyl iodide and silver oxide. Primary amine will combine with three molecules of methyl iodide, a secondary amine will react with two and a tertiary amine will take up only one. This process is known as **Hofmann exhaustive methylation of amines**.

Alternately, quaternary ammonium hydroxides decompose on heating to produce alkenes via **Cope reaction**. In this process amine oxides are prepared by treating tertiary amines with hydrogen peroxide. The oxides so secured yield alkenes on heating.

$$RCH_2.CH_2.\overset{\overset{\displaystyle CH_3}{|}}{N} - CH_2.CH_2.R' \xrightarrow{\ H_2O_2\ } R.CH_2.CH_2.\overset{\overset{\displaystyle CH_3}{|}}{\underset{\underset{\displaystyle O}{\downarrow}}{N}}.CH_2.CH_2.R' \xrightarrow{\ 140^\circ C\ }$$

A 3° amine

$$R.CH = CH_2 \ + \ CH_3.\overset{}{\underset{\underset{\displaystyle OH}{|}}{N}}.CH_2.CH_2.R'$$

Alkene

N,N–Dialkylhydroxyl amine

$$CH_3.\overset{\overset{\displaystyle CH_3}{|}}{\underset{\underset{\displaystyle O}{\downarrow}}{N}}.CH_2.CH_2.R' \xrightarrow[\ 140^\circ C\ ]{\ CH_3.I, Ag_2O\ } CH_3.\overset{\overset{\displaystyle CH_3}{|}}{\underset{\underset{\displaystyle OH}{|}}{N}} + CH_2 = CH.R'$$

If dimethylsulphoxide or tetrahydrofuran is used as a solvent then the reaction may be carried out at room temperature.

OFFICIAL COMPOUNDS

Ethylenediamine Hydrate

Mol. Form.: $C_2H_8N_2.H_2O$ Mol. Wt.: 78.12

Ethylenediamine hydrate contains not less than 97.5 per cent and not more than the equivalent of 101.5 per cent of $C_2H_8N_2.H_2O$ and is prepared from ethylene dichloride and ammonia. It is $H_2N.CH_2CH_2NH_2.H_2O$, ethane-1,2-diamine monohydrate.

Description: It is a colourless to light yellow liquid with ammonical odour and with alkaline, corrosive but characteristic taste. It is miscible with water and alcohol and is soluble in chloroform and alcohol. It is very irritating to skin and mucous membrane.

Tests for purity: It is tested for wt. per ml; boiling range; ammonia and other basic compounds; heavy metals; iron and non-volatile matter.

The test for ammonia and other bases is performed by converting it into its dihydrochloride which is dried and weighed.

$$C_2H_4(NH_2)_2, H_2O \longrightarrow C_2H_4(NH_2)_2, 2HCl$$

Thus 78.12 g of diamine should give 133.03 g of dihydrochloride. In case ammonia and other bases of lower or higher equivalent are present this weight ratio will be altered.

Assay: Weigh accurately about 1.5 g and dissolve in 75 ml of water and titrate with 1 M hydrochloric acid using solution of bromophenol blue as indicator until yellow colour is produced. Each ml of 1 M hydrochloric acid is equivalent to 0.03906 g of $C_2H_8N_2.H_2O$.

Storage: It is stored in tightly closed container away from light.

Uses: It is used as a pharmaceutical aid and is an ingredient of Aminophylline injection and tablets (I.P.).

Disodium Ethylenediamine Tetraacetate, $C_{10}H_{14}O_8N_2Na_2.H_2O$ is a white crystalline material and was included in Appendices of I.P. earlier.

Meprobamate

$$H_2N-\overset{\overset{O}{\|}}{C}-O.CH_2-\overset{\overset{CH_3}{|}}{\underset{\underset{CH_2-CH_2-CH_3}{|}}{C}}-CH_2.O-\overset{\overset{O}{\|}}{C}-NH_2$$

Mol. Form: $C_9H_{18}O_4N$ Mol. Wt.: 218.3

Meprobamate* is 2-methyl-2-propyl-1,3-propanediol dicarbamate and contains not less than 97.0 per cent of $C_9H_{18}O_4N_2$ when dried in vacuum at $60°$ for three hours.

Description: It is a white crystalline powder with characteristic odour and slight bitter taste. It is slightly soluble in water, freely in alcohol and sparingly in solvent ether. Its m.p. is $103-107°$.

It is tested for melting point, loss on drying, and sulphated ash.

Assay: The I.P. follows a different assay procedure as compared to the simple assay method used in B.P., which consists in hydrolyzing meprobamate with sulphuric acid and liberating the ammonia by addition of excess of sodium hydroxide solution and titrating the liberated ammonia with N/10 sulphuric acid. A blank titration is also done. The I.P. method is given in I.P. '66, on page 439.

Uses: Meprobamate is used as a tranquiliser. It was prepared for the first time in 1950 and was examined pharmaceutically for its muscle relaxing action. It has definite resemblance in its action with Methylpentinol, a tertiary alcohol, which is used to induce sleep. Meprobamate produces skeletal muscle relaxation and this action is 8 to 10 times more than that produced by mephenesin. Its main use is in the treatment of increased central nervous stimulation like insomnia. It is also used in attacks by epilepsy and in the treatment of alcoholism. Meprobamate is given in doses of 0.2 to 0.4 g orally (0.4–1.2 g daily). The action starts within half an hour and lasts upto 5 hours. 90% of it is excreted in the form of glucoronic acid while 10 per cent gets excreted unchanged. It is less toxic but there is danger for its addiction.

Meprobamate tablets are official in I.P. Usual strength of tablet is 0.4 g and dose of Meprobamate is 0.4–1.2 g daily in divided doses.

Urea

$$\overset{\overset{O}{\|}}{\underset{H_2N \quad\quad NH_2}{C}}$$

Mol. Form.: $NH_2.CO.NH_2$ Mol. Wt.: 60.06

Urea, also known as carbamide, is the diamide of carbonic acid. It contains not less than 99.0 per cent and not more than 101.0 per cent of CH_4ON_2.

---

* It was official in earlier I.P.s. It continues to be official in other pharmacopoeias, and being important is still retained here.

It is a colourless to white prismatic crystals or white crystalline powder. It is odourless, but on long standing develops odour of ammonia. It has cooling and saline taste. It is soluble in water (1 : 15) or in alcohol (1 : 10) and its aqueous solution is neutral to litmus. Its m.p. is 132 to 134°. It is slightly hygroscopic.

It is tested for melting point; alcohol insoluble matters, and sulphated ash, loss on drying and biuret.

Assay: It can be assayed by a Kjeldahl nitrogen determination method. For full details of assay method now see I.P. 2007.

Urea is diuretic. It is a normal excretion product of human beings (5–6 g per day). It is used locally to treat infected wounds as it is said to possess antiseptic activity.

Urea Stibamine and Urea Stibamine Injection were also official in I.P. '66. Urea cream is now official in I.P.

Urethane

Mol. Form.: $NH_2.CO.O.C_2H_5$ Mol. Wt.: 89.10

Urethane is ethyl carbamate and contains not less than 98.0 per cent of $C_3H_7O_2N$.

It can be prepared by the action of ammonia on ethyl chloroformate, as per the reaction below.

$$2NH_3 + Cl.CO.O.C_2H_5 \longrightarrow NH_2.CO.O.C_2H_5 + NH_4Cl$$

It occurs as colourless, odourless, prismatic crystals and has a saline, slightly bitter taste. It melts at 50°C. It is easily hydrolysed by alkalis and acids to ammonia (or ammonium salt), carbon dioxide (or a carbonate) and ethyl alcohol; these reactions help to identify it.

The esters of carbamic acid are usually designated by the term urethane.

It is used as neoplastic suppressant.

Appendices

Melting Point /Melting Range

The melting point determination is one of the foremost and fundamental of a number of physical properties of a substance which has been at the service of scientists in characterizing and identifying the substance.

The melting point of a substance is the temperature at which the material changes from a solid to a liquid state. Pure crystalline substances have a clear sharp melting point and hence should melt at a precisely defined temperature. During the melting process all of the energy added to a substance is consumed as heat of fusion and the temperature remains constant. In other simpler words it can be expressed as "The melting point of a substance is the temperature at which the solid phase converts to the liquid phase under one atmosphere of pressure. A pure substance normally should have a melting point range no larger than $1–1.5^{\circ}C$.

Melting range or temperature is now the usually used modern expression, and rightly so, by the Indian Pharmacopoeia. This expression has full justification because of the fact that although there should be a single temperature at which a pure solid and a liquid are in equilibrium, almost all the samples melt over a small temperature range, as stated above. This is because of the fact that with capillary or block melting points, the temperature of the bath or block rises a little during the time it takes for the sample to melt. The presence of impurities in the sample can also cause the sample to melt over a range of temperatures. Thus, a sharp melting point (actually, a melting range of less than about $1^{\circ}C$) is often taken as evidence that the sample is fairly pure, and a wide melting range is evidence that it is not pure.

Identification and characterization by use of melting points: When two samples have different melting points, their molecules must differ either in structure or in configuration. They must be either structural isomers or diastereomers. If the melting points of two samples are the same, the structures of their molecules must be the same, although they might have enantiomeric configurations.

These statements apply only to pure substances, and do not take into account the fact that some substances can exist in different crystalline forms that have different melting points.

Mixture/Mixed Melting Points

Mixtures of different substances generally melt over a range of temperatures, and melting is usually complete at a temperature that is below the melting point of at least one of the components. Thus, the nonidentity of two substances of the same melting point can often be established by determining that the melting point of a mixture of the two is *depressed.* If each individual sample melts "sharply" (and at the same temperature, of course), and if an intimate mixture of the two, made by rubbing approximately equal amounts together, melts over a wide range, the two substances are not the same.

According to I.P. 2007, melting range or temperature of a substance is defined as those points of temperature within which, or the point at which, the substance begins to coalesce and is completely melted as defined otherwise for certain substances.

The I.P. describes four procedures for determining the melting points suitable for substances included in it. However, Method I is the one which is used for most of the substances. Other methods, if required to be used, are also specified in the individual monograph.

Melting point apparatuses: A few melting point apparatuses are also available in different laboratories engaged in determining the melting points. An apparatus is a scientific instrument used to determine the melting point of a substance. Four types of melting point apparatuses are the Thiele tube, Fisher-John's apparatus, Gallenkamp (electronic) melting point apparatus and the automatic melting point apparatus. Some specific models of these include the Büchi B-540, the MEL-TEMP 3.0, and the Fisher-John's apparatus.

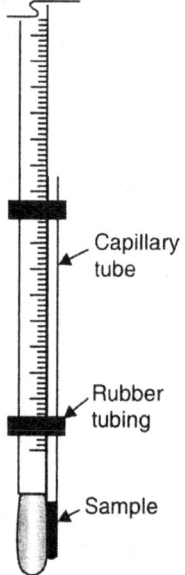

Fig. A-1. Arrangement of sample and thermometer for use in melting point determination.

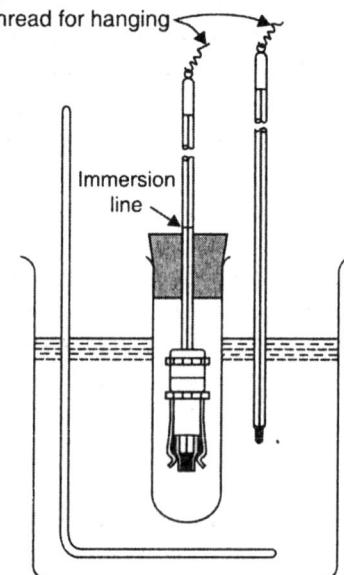

Fig. A-2. Apparatus for determination of melting range or temperature for use in I.P. method IV (p. 137).

They have different designs. However, generally a sample is loaded into a sealed capillary (*melting point capillary*). It is placed in the machine and the sample may be heated electrically, either via a heating block, or an oil bath. A control panel allows the starting and final temperatures, as well as the temperature gradient (in °C per minute) to be programmed.

I.P. Method I, as described in I.P. 2.4.21, p. 135, is outlined hereunder:

Apparatus

(a) A glass heating vessel of suitable construction and capacity containing one of the following or any other suitable bath liquid, to a height of not less than 14 cm:

    (1) Water for temperatures upto 150.

    (2) Glycerin for temperatures upto 150.

    (3) Liquid paraffin of sufficiently high boiling range for temperatures upto 250.

    (4) Sesame oil or a suitable grade of silicone oil for temperatures upto 300.

(b) A suitable stirring device capable of rapidly mixing the liquids.

(c) An accurately standardized thermometer suitable for the substance under examination. The thermometer should be positioned in the bath liquid to its specified immersion depth and yet leave the bulb about 2 cm above the bottom of the bath.

(d) Thin-walled capillary glass tubes of hard glass, closed at one end, about 12 cm long with a thickness of 0.2 to 0.3 mm and an internal diameter of 0.8 to 0.11 mm. The tubes should preferably be kept sealed at both ends and cut as required. A suitable magnifying glass may be used for observation of melting in the capillary tube.

(e) A source of heat (open flame or electric heater).

Procedure: Reduce the substance to a very fine powder and unless otherwise directed, dry it at a temperature considerably below its melting temperature or at a pressure of 1.5 to 2.5 kPa over *self-indicating silica gel* for 24 hrs. Introduce into a capillary glass tube a sufficient quantity of the dry powder to form a compact column of 4 to 6 mm high. Heat the bath until the temperature is about 10 degrees below the expected melting temperature. Remove the thermometer and quickly attach the capillary tube to the thermometer by wetting both with a drop of the liquid of the bath or otherwise and adjust its height so that the closed end of the capillary is near the middle of the thermometer bulb. Replace the thermometer and continue the heating, with constant stirring, sufficiently to cause the temperature to rise at a rate of about 10 degrees per minute. Continue the heating and note the temperature at which the column of the sample collapses definitely at the side of the tube at any point, when melting may have been considered to begun and note also the temperature at which the sample becomes liquid throughout as seen by the formation of a definite meniscus. The two temperatures fall within the limits of the melting range.

APPENDIX II

Determination of Ash Values

The total ash, acid-insoluble ash, water-soluble ash and sulphated ash contents of drugs of Indian materia medica, drugs and pharmaceuticals have been widely used as one of the indices to illustrate the quality as well as purity of herbal drugs and other forms of medicines. Such an approach has also been adopted by many official organizations in writing monographs for pharmacopoeia worldwide. Indian Pharmacopoeia is no exception; rather it is, with Chinese, world's leading country which includes Ash Values as the important tests for thousands of crude drugs used in the various indigenous systems of medicines, including Ayurveda and Unani. Almost all the drugs included in the number of volumes of Ayuvedic Pharmacopoeia include Ash Values determinations as tests for evaluation of Ayurvedic drugs and their products. Fortunately the pharmacists are already familiar with the Ash Values determinations, as they have been already exposed to these procedures in different subjects, including, of course, pharmacognosy. I.P. 2007 mentions these determinations in its appendix 2.3.18/19.

The ash values determination procedures are very simple in both involving the apparatuses and/ or the chemicals and the nature of practical work. There is a little difference in the procedure for crude vegetable drugs and for all other substances. Further for calculating the acid-insoluble ash and water-insoluble ash first the total ash has to be made (calculated, if required).

Total ash: The methods for crude vegetable drugs and for all other materials are mentioned here as Method A and Method B respectively, like they are given in I.P. 2.3.19.

In Method A 2 to 3 g of the air-dried material is weighed in a tared platinum or silica dish and incinerated at a temperature not exceeding 450°C until free from carbon. The material is cooled and weighed. The percentage of ash on the dried drug basis is calculated (I.P. 2.3.19).

In Method B a platinum or silica crucible is heated to red heat for 30 minutes, cooled in a desiccator and weighed. About 1 g of the substance, accurately weighed, is evenly distributed in the crucible, dried at 100 to 105°C for 1 hour and ignited to constant weight in a muffle furnace at 600± 25°C. The crucible is cooled in the desiccator after each ignition. If need be the crucible is further ignited to constant weight. The percentage of ash on dry basis is calculated (I.P. 2.3.19).

Acid-insoluble ash: The ash obtained from Method A or B is boiled with 25 ml of 2 M hydrochloric acid for 5 mins and the insoluble matter is collected in a Gooch crucible or on an ashless filter paper, washed with hot water and ignited. After cooling the desiccator the weight is taken and the percentage of the acid insoluble ash on the dried drug basis is calculated (I.P. 2.3.19).

Water-soluble ash: The ash obtained in Method A or B is boiled with 25 ml of water and the insoluble matter is collected in a Gooch crucible or on ashless filter paper and washed with hot water. The crucible is ignited for 15 minutes at a temperature not exceeding 450°C. The weight of the insoluble matter is subtracted from the weight of ash and the difference in weight represents the water-soluble ash. The percentage of the water soluble ash on the dried basis is calculated (I.P. 2.3.19).

Sulphated ash: A silica or platinum crucible is heated to redness for 10 minutes and allowed to cool in a desiccator and weighed. To the crucible 1 g of the substance under examination is transferred and the crucible is weighed with the contents accurately. The crucible is ignited gently until the substance is thoroughly charred. After cooling the residue is moistened with 1 ml of sulphuric acid and the heating continued gently until the white fumes are no longer evolved. The ignition is continued at $800 \pm 25^{\circ}C$ until all black particles have disappeared. After cooling the crucible a few drops of sulphuric acid are added and heat continued till the material is ignited as before. The crucible is cooled and weighed. The operation is repeated until two successive weighings do not differ by more than 0.5 mg (I.P. 2.3.18).

APPENDIX III

Weight Per Millilitre and Relative Density
Specific Gravity (Weight per ml)

I.P. defines wt. per ml as the weight per millilitre of a liquid is the weight, in g of 1 ml of a liquid when weighed in air at 25°C, unless otherwise specified.

On this subject matter the following remarks/definitions are worth additional mention:

Density and specific gravity have very similar, but not quite identical definitions.

Density is the amount of something per unit volume. Most typically, one expresses the mass per unit volume for a solid or liquid. For example, 5.2 g/cm^3. For gases or dusts we might express this as g/m^3.

Specific gravity is a ratio of the mass of a material to the mass of an equal volume of water at 4°C. Because specific gravity is a ratio, it is a unit less quantity. For example, the specific gravity of water at 4°C is 1.0 while its density is 1.0 g/cm^3.

Relative density is essentially the same as specific gravity; however, the temperature used for the water (or even another material) is not necessarily 4°C. For this reason, a relative density measurement will include the temperatures used for both materials. For example, "relative density 15/0: 0.87" indicates that the density of the material was determined at 15°C and it is being divided by the density of water at 0°C. The temperatures may also be indicated as a superscript (material) and subscript (water) after the numeric value.

Specific gravities can be determined in many ways including pycnometry (weighing a known volume).

The specific gravity of a liquid can be determined with a hydrometer, a hollow, sealed, calibrated glass tube. The depth to which the hydrometer sinks is inversely proportional to the specific gravity of the liquid.

The I.P. method for determining weight per ml is given below.

Select a thoroughly clean and dry pycnometer. Calibrate the pycnometer by filling it with recently boiled and cooled water at 25° and weighing the contents. Assuming that the weight of 1 ml of water at 25° when weighed in air of density 0.0012 g per ml is 0.99602 g, calculate the capacity of the pycnometer (ordinary deviations in the density of air from the value given do not affect the result of a determination significantly). Adjust the temperature of the substance under examination to about 20° and fill the pycnometer with it. Adjust the temperature of the filled pycnometer to about 25°, remove any excess of the substance and weigh. Subtract the tare weight of the pycnometer with the filled weight of the pycnometer. Determine the weight per millilitre by dividing the weight in air, in g of the quantity of the liquid which fills the pycnometer at the specified temperature, by the capacity expressed in ml, of the pycnometer at the same temperature.

Relative density: The relative density of a substance is the ratio of the mass of a given volume of the substance to the mass of an equal volume of water, both weighed at 25°, unless otherwise specified.

Method: Proceed as described under Weight per millilitre. Divide the weight of the substance in the pycnometer by the weight of the water contained, both determined at 25°, unless otherwise directed in the individual monograph.

APPENDIX IV

Determination of Congealing Point
Congealing Range or Temperature

The congealing point of a liquid or of a melted solid is the highest temperature at which it solidifies. The congealing point of the liquid is the same as the melting temperature of the solid, but since the liquid may be cooled to a temperature below its congealing point without assuming the solid form, the method described below is used to determine the congealing point of a liquid or of a melted solid.

Apparatus: A suitable apparatus consists of a test-tube of about 2 cm internal diameter and about 10 cm in length, suspended by means of a bored cork inside a larger tube, about 3 cm in diameter and 12 cm in length, a vessel with water or suitable freezing mixture, and an accurately standardized thermometer. The I.P. 2007 gives the figure of the apparatus used for the determination of congealing range or temperature.

Procedure: Unless otherwise specified in the monograph, place in the inner test-tube about 10 ml of the liquid, or 10 g of the melted solid, to be tested and cool together the inner and the outer tubes in water or in a suitable freezing mixture to a temperature about 5°C below the expected congealing point of the liquid; with the thermometer gently stir the liquid until it begins to solidify. At first there is a gradual fall in temperature. Then, as the solid phase forms, the temperature remains constant for some time or rises before becoming constant. The highest temperature observed is regarded as the congealing point. If the liquid does not start to congeal within 2°C of the expected temperature, congelation may be induced by adding a small crystal of the substance to the liquid or by rubbing the inner walls of the test-tube with the thermometer. The I.P. gives its general method on page 117.

APPENDIX V

Dynamic Viscosity

Viscosity is a measure of the resistance of a fluid which is being deformed by either shear stress or tensile stress. Generally when we talk about fluids, viscosity refers to their "thickness". Thus, water is "thin", having a lower viscosity, while honey is "thick", having a higher viscosity. Viscosity describes a fluid's internal resistance to flow and may be thought of as a measure of fluid friction. In simple words, if something i.e. some materiel is less viscous, it will make its movement (fluidity) with greater ease. All real fluids have some resistance to experience and express stress. Hence a fluid which has no resistance to shear stress is known as an ideal fluid or inviscid fluid. The study of viscosity is also known as rheology.

In general, in any flow, layers move at different velocities and the fluid's viscosity arises from the shear stress between the layers that ultimately oppose any applied force.

Isaac Newton postulated that, for straight, parallel and uniform flow, the shear stress, τ, between layers is proportional to the velocity gradient, $\partial u / \partial y$, in the direction perpendicular to the layers.

Viscosity determination: The determination of viscosity of Newtonian liquids is carried out by means of a capacity viscometer, unless otherwise specified; Methods A and B described in I.P. are recommended. For non-Newtonian liquids Method C using the rotating viscometer can be used.

For measurement of viscosity, the temperature of the substance being measured must be accurately controlled, since small temperature changes may lead to marked changes in viscosity. For usual pharmaceutical purposes, the temperature should be maintained to within $\pm 0.1^{\circ}C$. These methods using viscometers with figures of Oswald-Type Viscometer, Suspended-Level Viscometer and Rotating Viscometer with dimensions are given on pages 163 to 165 in detail, and do not deserve space here for a few compounds included here.

APPENDIX VI

Determination of Boiling Range of Temperature and Distillation Range

Distillation is the process of heating a liquid until it boils. The principles of distillation have been in use for thousands of years. Distillation was probably first used by ancient Arab chemists to isolate perfumes. Vessels with a trough on the rim to collect the distillate, called *diqarus*, date back to 3500 BC.

In the modern organic chemistry laboratory, distillation is a powerful tool, both for the identification and the purification of organic compounds. The boiling point of a compound, determined by distillation, is well-defined and thus is one of the physical properties of a compound by which it is identified. Distillation is also used to purify a compound by separating it from a non-volatile or less-volatile material. If different compounds in a mixture have different boiling points, it is possible to separate them into individual components provided the mixture is carefully distilled. The boiling points are usually measured by recording the boiling point (or range) on a thermometer during the process of distillation.

The boiling or distilling range of a liquid is the temperature interval, corrected for a pressure of 101.3 kPa within which the liquid, or a special fraction of the liquid, distils under the conditions specified in the test. The lower limit of the range is the temperature indicated by the thermometer when the first drop of the condensate leaves the tip of the condenser, and from the lowest point in the distillation task; it may also be the temperature observed when the proportion specified in the individual monograph has been collected.

The method for determining the boiling range is given at I.P. pp. 114 & 115. It gives details of the apparatuses used; consisting of distillation flask, condenser, receiver and thermometer. However, the method of I. P. is outlined below in full to help understand the process and apply the variation of correction factor with temperature.

Method: If the liquid under examination distils under 80°C, cool it to between 10 and 15°C before measuring the sample for distillation.

Assemble the apparatus and place in the flask 100 ml of the liquid being examined, taking care not to allow any of the liquid to enter the side-arm. Insert the thermometer and shield the entire heating and flask assembly from external air currents. Add a few pieces of porous material and heat rapidly to boiling using a Bunsen burner (or an electric heater or mantle with arrangement of adjustment of the applied heat) and an asbestos plate pierced by a hole 33 mm in diameter. Record the temperature at which the first drop of distillate falls into the receiver and adjust the rate of heating to obtain a regular distillation rate of 4 to 5 ml per minute. Record the temperature when the first drop of liquid evaporates from the lowest point in the distillation flask or when the specified percentage has distilled over. Correct the observed temperature readings for any variation in the barometric pressure from the normal (101.3 kPa) using the following expression.

$$T_1 = T_2 + K(a - b),$$

where,

$T_1 =$ the corrected temperature

$T_2 =$ the observed temperature

$a =$ 101.3, when the barometric pressure is measured in kilopascals (kPa), or 760 when measured in torr

$b =$ barometric pressure at the time of determination

$K =$ the correction factor indicated in Table A-1.

Table A-1. Variation of correction factor with temperature

Boiling range $^o C$	K (KPa)	K (torr)
Less than 100	0.30	0.040
100 to 140	0.34	0.045
141 to 190	0.38	0.050
191 to 240	0.41	0.055
More than 240	0.45	0.060

Determination of Benzene and Related Substances

The Determination of Benzene and Related Substances is done by using the gas chromatographic technique. The I.P. describes in its Appendix 2.4.13 the complete process of gas chromatography, also known as gas liquid chromatography. However, it gives under each monograph of the official compound and/or its preparation, to be tested for purity, preliminary treatment before it is subjected to the test via the use of chromatography. These instructions are to be followed before using the gas chromatographic process to arrive at the purity result.

Under this Appendix VII here, there is no need to describe the whole process of gas chromatography, and hence the readers are advised to look for the complete gas chromatographic technique (as also other branches of chromatography) in Chapter on chromatographic techniques.

Determination of Refractive Index

Refractive Index (RI) can be defined as a measure of the bending or refraction of a beam of light on entering a denser medium (the ratio between the sine of the angle of incidence of the ray of light and the sine of the angle of refraction). It is constant for pure substances under standard conditions. RI is used as a measure of sugar or total solids in solution, purity of oils, etc.

For Refractive Index (RI) measurements in refractometry only a small volume of samples is required. For routine applications one can now a days choose from different flow-through cells to suit one's analysis and get RI results in seconds.

Refractometry theory: The speed of light in vacuum is always the same, but when light moves through any other medium it travels more slowly since it is constantly being absorbed and reemitted by the atoms in the material. The ratio of the speed of light in vacuum to the speed of light in another substance is defined as the index of refraction also known as refractive index or n for the substance.

$$\text{Refractive index of substance } (n) = \frac{\text{Speed of light in vacuum}}{\text{Speed of light in substance}}$$

According to I.P. the refractive index (n) of a substance with reference to air is the ratio of the sine of the angle of incidence to the sine of the angle of refraction of a beam of light passing from air into the substance. It varies with the wavelength of the light used in its measurement. Generally (unless otherwise specified in individual monograph) the refractive index is measured at $20^{\circ}C \pm 0.5$ with reference to the wavelength of the D line of sodium ($\lambda = 589.3$ nm). The temperature should be carefully adjusted and maintained since the refractive index varies significantly with temperature.

The Abbe's refractometer (a refractometer is a laboratory or field device for the measurement of index of refraction) is convenient for most measurements of refractive index but other refractometers of equal or greater accuracy may be used. Commercial refractometers are normally constructed for use with white light but are calibrated to give the refractive index in terms of the D line of sodium. The apparatus is provided with a water jacket to control the temperature of measurements. The manufacturer's instructions relating to a suitable light source should be followed subject to the directions given in the Pharmacopoeia. To achieve accuracy, the apparatus should be calibrated against distilled water which has refractive index of 1.3325 at $25^{\circ}C$ or against the reference liquids given in the following Table A-2.

Table A-2.

Reference liquid		Temperature coefficient $\Delta n/\Delta t$
Carbon tetrachloride	1.4603	-0.00057
Toluene	1.4969	-0.00056
α-Methylnaphthalene	1.6176	-0.00048

APPENDIX IX

Determination of Water

Methods for moisture and water content determinations are prescribed due to the fact that the moisture content influences the physical properties of a substance such as weight, density, viscosity, refractive index, electrical conductivity etc. Chemical, thermo-gravimetric or loss on drying techniques are used to determine this undesirable content.

Most natural products contain moisture. The water content per se is seldom of interest. Rather, its presence questions whether a product intended for use as such or in production has standard properties such as storability, agglomeration in the case of powders, microbiological stability, flow properties, viscosity, concentration or purity, compliance with quality agreements, nutritional value of the product and legal conformity (statutory regulations governing medicines and pharmaceutical products).

The I.P. 2007 prescribes three methods for the determination of water content, as:

Method 1. Titrimetric Method

Method 2. Azeotropic Distillation Method

Method 3. Coulometric Titration Method

The Titrimetric Method is the oldest well known Karl Fischer Method, which utilizes the Karl Fischer Reagent. I.P. always follows this method A, unless otherwise directed in its monograph. The method further comprises of two Methods: Method A and Method B.

The Determination of Water Content by Karl Fischer Titration Method

Since its introduction in 1935, the Karl Fischer (KF) titration has become one of the most widely used techniques for the determination of water content in a variety of substances including food products, industry chemicals, pharmaceutical products and compounds and preparations included in I.P. monographs. This technique is based on one specific water-consuming reaction, which involves two steps and is commonly written as shown below:

$$ROH + SO_2 + RN \longrightarrow (RNH)SO_3R$$

$$(RNH)SO_3R + 2RN + I_2 + H_2O \longrightarrow (RNH)SO_4R + 2(RNH)I$$

ROH: Alcohol, typically methanol; RN: base

Basically, the alcohol works as the solvent and involves in the reaction as well. It reacts with sulfur dioxide and forms an alkyl sulphite. The oxidation of the alkyl sulphite to alkyl sulphate by iodine consumes water and water reacts with iodine at a 1:1 stoichiometrical ratio. Once all the water available is consumed, excess iodine appears and signals the end point of the titration. Here, the base, classically pyridine but nowadays replaced by other bases, behaves as a buffer and keeps an optimum pH range of 5–8.

340

Over the years, KF titration method has been studied extensively. A variety of improvements and modifications have been introduced on reagent composition, end-point determination, titration type, instrument design/automation and other aspects. Currently, KF titration can be carried out in two different ways: volumetric titration and coulometric titration. The main difference between these two is the way of the iodine addition. In volumetric titration, the iodine solution is added automatically to the sample with a burette. Conversely, the iodine is generated electrochemically by the anodic oxidation of iodide during coulometric titration. The volumetric titration measures water level in a range of 100 ppm to 100%, while the coulometric titration is primarily used for the determination of water at trace levels of 1 ppm to 5%. For the in process control samples, the water content is relatively a small amount. Therefore, the coulometric titration technique is more popular for in-process control. In the pharmaceutical industry, in-process control for drug substance synthesis mainly involves reaction monitoring and final product testing. Water determination is performed at all the stages during the scale-up process because water content is a very important factor which influences the chemical and physical properties of the pharmaceutical products, such as stability, solubility, and reactivity. As a safe, rapid, accurate and reliable technique, KF titration is chosen as a major method for water determination in most in-process control labs.

The I.P. outlines all the methods in its appendix 2.3.43 and hence after the above useful discussion, it is not considered advisable to repeat the methods here.

APPENDIX X

Determination of pH

pH is a short form of potential for hydrogen ion concentration. It is a measure of the acidity or basicity of a solution. It approximates but is not equal to p[H], the negative logarithm (base 10) of the molar concentration of dissolved hydrogen ions (H^+).

It is defined as the negative common logarithm of the concentration of hydrogen ions [H^+] in moles/litre: $pH = -\log_{10} [H^+]$.

Pure water is said to be neutral, with a pH close to 7.0 at 25°C. Solutions with a pH less than 7 (at 25°C) are said to be acidic and solutions with a pH greater than 7 (at 25°C) are said to be basic or alkaline. Thus:

- when the pH is above 7 the solution is basic (alkaline)
- when the pH is below 7 the solution is acidic

pH measurements are important in medicine, biology, chemistry, food science, environmental science, and many other applications. It forms one of the tests for purity in I.P. monographs.

The I.P. gives values in its monographs, which conveniently represent the acidity and alkalinity of an aqueous solution. In the pharmacopoeia, standards and limits of pH have been provided for those pharmacopoeial substances in which pH as a measure of hydrogen ion activity is important from the standpoint of stability or physiological suitability. The determination is carried out at a temperature of 25°C ± 2°C, unless otherwise specified in the individual monograph.

Apparatus: The pH value of a solution is determined potentiometrically by means of a glass electrode, a reference electrode and a pH meter either of the digital or analogue type.

The pH meter is operated according to the manufacturer's instructions. The apparatus is calibrated using *buffer solution D* as the primary standard, adjusting the meter to read the appropriate pH value given in the table, corresponding to the temperature of the solution. To set the scale, use a second reference buffer solution, either *buffer solution A, buffer solution E or buffer solution G* and carry out a check with a third buffer solution of intermediate pH. The pH reading of the intermediate solution must not differ by more than 0.05 from the corresponding value indicated in the table.

The I.P. gives a list of nine Reference Buffer Solutions with their composition and their pH at various temperature in a table.

Method: Immerse the electrodes in the solution under examination and measure the pH at the same temperature as for the standard solutions. At the end of a set of measurements, record the pH of the solution used to standardize the meter and the electrodes. If the difference between this reading and the original value is greater than 0.05, the set of measurements must be repeated.

When measuring pH values above 10.0, ensure that the glass electrode is suitable for use under alkaline conditions and apply any correction that is necessary.

All solutions and suspensions of substances under examinations must be prepared using *carbon dioxide-free water*.

Index